T0334518

This is the first comprehensive volume to look at the importance of short-chain fatty acids in digestion, the function of the large intestine and their role in human health. Short-chain fatty acids are the major product of bacterial fermentation of dietary carbohydrates in the human and animal large intestine. Through their absorption from the caecum and colon they provide a means whereby energy can be salvaged from carbohydrates not digested in the upper gut. It is now increasingly recognized that they may have a significant role in protecting against large-bowel diseases and in metabolism in other tissues. This volume has been prepared by an international team of contributors who are at the forefront of this area of research. The volume will be an essential source of reference for gastroenterologists, nutritionists and others active in this area.

PHYSIOLOGICAL AND CLINICAL ASPECTS OF SHORT-CHAIN FATTY ACIDS

PHYSIOLOGICAL AND CLINICAL ASPECTS OF SHORT-CHAIN FATTY ACIDS

Edited by

JOHN H. CUMMINGS
Scientific Staff, Medical Research Council Dunn Clinical Nutrition Centre, and Honorary Consultant Physician, Addenbrooke's Hospital, Cambridge

JOHN L. ROMBEAU
Professor of Surgery, Department of Surgery, Hospital of University of Pennsylvania

and

TAKASHI SAKATA
Associate Professor in Biology, Department of Basic Sciences, Ishinomaki Senshu University, Japan

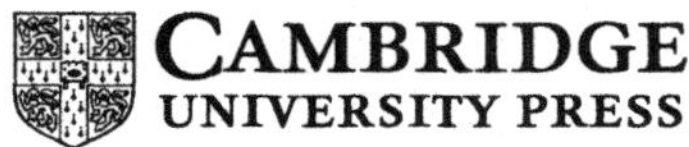
CAMBRIDGE
UNIVERSITY PRESS

PUBLISHED BY THE PRESS SYNDICATE OF THE UNIVERSITY OF CAMBRIDGE
The Pitt Building, Trumpington Street, Cambridge, United Kingdom

CAMBRIDGE UNIVERSITY PRESS
The Edinburgh Building, Cambridge CB2 2RU, UK
40 West 20th Street, New York NY 10011–4211, USA
477 Williamstown Road, Port Melbourne, VIC 3207, Australia
Ruiz de Alarcón 13, 28014 Madrid, Spain
Dock House, The Waterfront, Cape Town 8001, South Africa

http://www.cambridge.org

First published 1995
First paperback edition 2004

A catalogue record for this book is available from the British Library

Library of Congress cataloguing in publication data
Physiological and clinical aspects of short-chain fatty acids / edited
by John H. Cummings, John L. Rombeau, and Takashi Sakata.
p. cm.
ISBN 0 521 44048 3 (hardback)
1. Fatty acids – Metabolism. 2. Fatty acids – Physiological effect.
3. Intestines. I. Cummings, John H. II. Rombeau, John L.
III. Sakata, Takashi.
[DNLM: 1. Fatty Acids, Volatile – physiology. QU 90 P578 1995]
QP752.F35P48 1995
612.3′97 – dc20 94-7853 CIP
DNLM/DLC
for Library of Congress

ISBN 0 521 44048 3 hardback
ISBN 0 521 61613 1 paperback

Contents

List of contributors *page* xi
Preface xix

1 Definitions and history
O. M. Wrong 1
2 Chemistry of short-chain fatty acids
M. Fukushima 15
3 Measurement of acetate by enzymatic methods
M. Elia and G. Jennings 35
4 Biochemistry and microbiology in the rumen
R. J. Wallace 57
5 Short-chain fatty acids in the hindgut
G. Breves and K. Stück 73
6 Microbiological aspects of the production of short-chain fatty acids in the large bowel
G. T. Macfarlane and G. R. Gibson 87
7 Reductive acetogenesis in animal and human gut
M. Durand and A. Bernalier 107
8 Flow dynamics of digesta and colonic fermentation
I. D. Hume 119
9 Transport of short-chain fatty acids in the ruminant forestomach
G. Gäbel 133
10 Absorption of short-chain fatty acids from the large intestine
W. v. Engelhardt 149
11 Metabolism of short-chain fatty acids in the liver
C. Rémésy, C. Demigné and C. Morand 171

12 Effects of short-chain fatty acids on gastrointestinal motility
C. Cherbut 191

13 Sensory mechanisms for short-chain fatty acids in the colon
T. Yajima 209

14 Effects of short-chain fatty acids on exocrine and endocrine pancreatic secretion
K. Katoh 223

15 Effect of short-chain fatty acids on salivary flow in ruminants
P. Nørgaard 233

16 Utilization of short-chain fatty acids in ruminants
E. R. Ørskov 243

17 Short-chain fatty acids, pancreatic hormones and appetite control
A. de Jong 257

18 Effects of butyrate on cell proliferation and gene expression
J. Kruh, N. Defer and L. Tichonicky 275

19 Effects of short-chain fatty acids on the proliferation of gut epithelial cells *in vivo*
T. Sakata 289

20 Short-chain fatty acids and colon tumorigenesis: animal models
J. R. Lupton 307

21 Butyrate and the human cancer cell
G. P. Young and P. R. Gibson 319

22 The place of short-chain fatty acids in colonocyte metabolism in health and ulcerative colitis: the impaired colonocyte barrier
W. E. W. Roediger 337

23 Management of diversion colitis, pouchitis and distal ulcerative colitis
W. Scheppach, P. Bartram and F. Richter 353

24 The effects of short-chain fatty acids on phagocytic cell function
G. F. Brisseau and O. D. Rotstein 361

25 Short-chain fatty acids, antibiotic-associated diarrhoea, colonic adenomas and cancer
P. B. Mortensen and M. R. Clausen 373

26 *In vivo* and *in vitro* effects of short-chain fatty acids on intestinal blood circulation
F. V. Mortensen and H. Nielsen 391

27 Short-chain fatty acids and intestinal surgery: rationale and clinical implications
J. L. Rombeau, K. J. Reilly and R. H. Rolandelli 401

28 Short-chain fatty acids as an energy source in the colon: metabolism and clinical implications
G. Livesey and M. Elia 427

29 Short-chain fatty acids and carbohydrate metabolism
T. M. S. Wolever 483

30 Short-chain fatty acids and hepatic lipid metabolism: experimental studies
D. L. Topping and I. Pant 495

31 Short-chain fatty acids and lipid metabolism: human studies
J. W. Anderson 509

32 Colonic short-chain fatty acids in infants and children
C. H. Lifschitz 525

33 Short-chain triglycerides in clinical nutrition
S. J. DeMichele and M. D. Karlstad 537

Index 561

Contributors

Prof. J. W. Anderson
VA Medical Center
Lexington
KY 40502
USA

P. Bartram
Department of Medicine
University of Würzburg
Josef-Schneider-Strasse 2
D-8700 Würzburg
Germany

Dr A. Bernalier
Laboratoire de Nutrition et Sécurité Alimentaire
INRA
Centre de Recherche de Jouy-en-Josas
Domaine de Vilvert
78352 Jouy-en-Josas Cédex
France

Prof. G. Breves
Justus-Liebig-Universität Giessen
Fachbereich Veterinarmedizin
Institut für Veterinär-Physiologie
Frankfurterstrasse 100
D-6300 Giessen
Germany

G. F. Brisseau
Department of Surgery
Toronto General Hospital
200 Elizabeth Street
Eaton North 9-236
Toronto, Ontario M5G 2C4
Canada

Dr C. Cherbut
INRA Nantes
BP 527-Rue de la Geraudiere
F-44026 Nantes Cédex 03
France

Dr M. R. Clausen
Department of Medicine A
Rigshospitalet
University of Copenhagen
Denmark

Dr J. H. Cummings
Dunn Clinical Nutrition Centre
Hills Road
Cambridge CB2 2DH
UK

Dr N. Defer
ICGM Biochimie
Faculté De Médecine Cochin Port-Royal
24 rue du Faubourg-St-Jacques
75014 Paris Cédex 14
France

Dr A. de Jong
Institute of Animal Nutrition
Veterinary Division
Bayer
51368 Leverkusen
Germany

Dr S. J. DeMichele
Medical Nutrition Research and Development
Ross Laboratories (A Division of Abbott Laboratories USA)
625 Cleveland Avenue
Columbus
Ohio 43215
USA

Dr C. Demigné
Laboratoire des Maladies Métaboliques
INRA CRNH de Clermont-Ferrand/Theix
63122 St Genès-Champanelle
France

Dr M. Durand
Laboratoire de Nutrition et Sécurité Alimentaire
INRA
Centre de Recherche de Jouy-en-Josas
Domaine de Vilvert
78352 Jouy-en-Josas Cédex
France

Dr M. Elia
Dunn Clinical Nutrition Centre
Hills Road
Cambridge, CB2 2DH
UK

Prof. Dr W. v. Engelhardt
Department of Physiology
School of Veterinary Medicine
Bischofsholer Damm 15
D-3000 Hanover 1
Germany

Dr M. Fukushima
Department of Basic Science
Ishinomaki Senshu University
Minamisakai Shinmito 1
Ishinomaki 986
Japan

Dr G. Gäbel
Veterinär-Physiologisches Institut
Veterinärmedizinische Fakultät
Universität Leipzig
Semmelweisstrasse 2
D-04103 Leipzig
Germany

Dr G. R. Gibson
Dunn Clinical Nutrition Centre
Hills Road
Cambridge, CB2 2DH
UK

Dr P. R. Gibson
University Department of Medicine
Royal Melbourne Hospital
Melbourne
VIC 3050
Australia

Prof. I. D. Hume
School of Biological Sciences A08
University of Sydney
NSW 2006
Australia

Dr G. Jennings
Dunn Clinical Nutrition Centre
Hills Road
Cambridge, CB2 2DH
UK

Dr M. D. Karlstad
Department of Anesthesiology
University of Tennessee Medical Center
1924 Alcoa Highway
Knoxville
TN 37920
USA

Dr K. Katoh
Department of Animal Physiology
Faculty of Agriculture
Tohoku University
Sendai
Aoba-ku 981
Japan

Prof. J. Kruh
ICGM Biochimie
Faculté de Médecine Cochin Port-Royal
24 rue du Faubourg-St-Jacques
75014 Paris Cedex 14
France

Prof. C. H. Lifschitz
Department of Pediatrics
Baylor College of Medicine
1100 Bates
Houston
TX 77030
USA

Dr G. Livesey
AFRC Institute of Food Research
Norwich Research Park
Colney
Norwich, NR4 7UA
UK

Dr J. R. Lupton
Graduate Faculty of Nutrition
Texas A & M University
College Station
Texas 77843
USA

Dr G. T. Macfarlane
Dunn Clinical Nutrition Centre
Hills Road
Cambridge, CB2 2DH
UK

Dr C. Morand
Laboratoire des Maladies Métaboliques
INRA CRNH de Clermond-Ferrand/Theix
63122 St Genès-Champanelle
France

Prof. F. V. Mortensen
Department of Gastrointestinal Surgery
Amtssygehuset
Aarhus University Hospital
8000 Aarhus C
Denmark

Dr P. B. Mortensen
Department of Medicine A
Rigshospitalet
University Hospital
Blegdamsvej 9
DK-2100 Copenhagen
Denmark

Dr H. Nielsen
Department of Pharmacology and
Danish Biomembrane Research Center
University of Aarhus
8000 Aarhus C
Denmark

Dr P. Nørgaard
The Royal Veterinary and Agricultural University
Division of Animal Nutrition
Bulowsvej 13
DK-2000 Frederiksberg
Copenhagen
Denmark

Dr E. R. Ørskov
Rowett Research Institute
Greenburn Road
Bucksburn
Aberdeen. AB2 9SB
UK

Dr I. Pant
CSIRO
Division of Human Nutrition
Glenthorne Laboratory
Majors Road
O'Halloran Hill
SA 5158
Australia

Dr K. J. Reilly
Hospital of University of Pennsylvania
Department of Surgery
3400 Spruce Street
Philadelphia, Pennsylvania 19104
USA

Dr C. Rémésy
Director of Research
Laboratoire des Maladies Métaboliques
INRA CRNH de Clermond-Ferrand/Theix
63122 St Genès-Champanelle
France

Dr F. Richter
Department of Medicine
University of Würzburg
Josef-Schneider-Strasse 2
D-8700 Würzburg
Germany

Prof. W. E. W. Roediger
Department of Surgery
Queen Elizabeth Hospital
Woodville, SA 5011
Australia

Dr R. H. Rolandelli
Medical College of Pennsylvania/Hahnemann University
Department of Surgery
Broad and Vine
Philadelphia, Pennsylvania 19102
USA

Dr J. L. Rombeau
Hospital of University of Pennsylvania
Department of Surgery
3400 Spruce Street
Philadelphia, Pennsylvania 19104
USA

Mr O. D. Rotstein
Toronto General Hospital
200 Elizabeth Street
Eaton, North 9-236
Toronto, Ontario M5G 2C4
Canada

Dr T. Sakata
Ishinomaki Senshu University
Minamisakai Shinmito 1
Ishinomaki, Miyagi 986
Japan

Dr W. M. Scheppach
Department of Medicine
University of Würzburg
Josef-Schneider-Strasse 2
D-8700 Würzburg
Germany

Dr K. Stück
Justus-Liebig-Universität Giessen
Fachbereich Veterinarmedizin
Institut für Veterinar-Physiologie
Frankfurter Strasse 100
D-6300 Giessen
Germany

Dr L. Tichonicky
ICGM Biochimie
Faculté De Médecine Cochin Port-Royal
24 rue du Faubourg-St-Jacques
75014 Paris Cédex 14
France

Dr D. L. Topping
CSIRO
Division of Human Nutrition
Glenthorne Laboratory
Majors Road
O'Halloran Hill
SA 5158
Australia

Dr R. J. Wallace
Rowett Research Institute
Greenburn Road
Bucksburn
Aberdeen, AB2 9SB
UK

Prof. T. M. S. Wolever
Department of Nutritional Sciences
University of Toronto
Toronto
Ontario M5S 1A8
Canada

Prof. O. M. Wrong
Division of Nephrology
Institute of Urology and Nephrology
Middlesex Hospital
Mortimer Street
London, W1N 8AA
UK

Dr T. Yajima
Central Research Institute
Meiji Milk Products Co. Ltd
1-21-3 Sakae-Cho
Higashimurayama-Shi
Tokyo, J-189
Japan

Prof. G. P. Young
University Department of Medicine
Royal Melbourne Hospital
Melbourne, VIC 3050
Australia

Preface

In both the forestomach of ruminants and the hindgut of many animals, including man, short-chain fatty acids are produced from the breakdown of dietary carbohydrates. Thus, many species are able to obtain energy through symbiosis with anaerobic bacteria. The principal substrates that contribute to the production of short-chain fatty acids are the polysaccharides of the plant cell wall, starch, oligosaccharides, some sugars and mucus. Short-chain fatty acids may also be produced from amino acids arising from the degradation of proteins of dietary or endogenous sources. The process of breakdown of these substrates is collectively known as fermentation and the products, apart from short-chain fatty acids, include branched-chain fatty acids from amino acids, lactate, ethanol, hydrogen, methane, carbon dioxide and stimulation of the increase in bacterial biomass.

It has been known for more than 100 years that short-chain fatty acids exist in the gut. In animal nutrition they have been frequently studied, since they are the major energy source, especially for ruminants. Consequently, there is a substantial literature on this subject. Their role in human health, however, is only just emerging. It was not until the 1960s that short-chain fatty acids first became a focus for study in man. The literature on short-chain fatty acids covers many species and we therefore now have considerable knowledge of the bacterial metabolism necessary for the production of short-chain fatty acids, their epithelial transport, cellular metabolism, effects on cell growth and differentiation, and subsequent uptake by liver and muscle. Already, clinical uses for short-chain fatty acids have been suggested and their effects on lipid metabolism, glucose and insulin, the control of cellular proliferation and health of the colonic and other epithelial tissues have been observed. There are likely to be other effects both within and distant from the gut. These findings are of relevance to the cause of large-bowel cancer and management of ulcerative colitis and diversion colitis. It is also evident that fermentation may provide a route for salvaging energy from undigested carbohydrates in man which could be of vital importance for the nutrition of developing countries.

The term 'short-chain fatty acid', as used throughout the book, and as defined by Oliver Wrong and Michiko Fukushima in the opening chapters, refers to saturated unbranched alkyl monocarboxylic acids of 2–4 carbon atoms. Many of the contributing authors also refer to other organic acids produced during fermentation, including C5 (valerate) and C6 (caproate) in addition to formate, lactate and succinate. Moreover, fatty acid isomers of C4–6 are also recognized products of bacterial fermentation from the branched-chain amino acids, valine, leucine and isoleucine. However, the convention that most authors have adopted in the book is to use the term 'short-chain fatty acid' for acetic, propionic and butyric acids.

Thus, the study of short-chain fatty acids is an emerging field of great importance to human health. The literature is very scattered and research is currently being carried forward by investigators in many disciplines, including veterinary and animal scientists, human physiologists, biochemists, cell biologists and clinicians. It is our intention, therefore, in this book, to draw together into a scholarly, comprehensive and authoritative reference source the literature and current thinking on this subject. We hope that, from it, readers will be able to integrate observational and mechanistic studies, and ultimately develop a fuller understanding of the role of short-chain fatty acids in human and animal health.

John H. Cummings, Cambridge, UK
John L. Rombeau, Philadelphia, USA
Takashi Sakata, Ishinomaki, Japan

1

Definitions and history

O. M. WRONG

Definitions

This book is primarily concerned with the acetic, propionic and *n*-butyric acids that are generated by microbial fermentation within the digestive tract. They are substances which present a slight problem in terminology. Originally they were described as 'volatile fatty acids' (VFA), the word 'volatile' being used because they were measured by steam-distillation, after acidification, of intestinal contents. Now that steam-distillation has been superseded by gas–liquid chromatography, this terminology has been largely abandoned, and they are usually called 'short-chain fatty acids' (SCFA). The term 'fatty acid' is misleading in several ways. It is in general use by organic chemists, because the longer members of the series, particularly stearic and palmitic acids, are present in the triglycerides of natural fats. But SCFA are biochemically more closely related to carbohydrates than to fats, some of them are not constituents of natural fats, and they are not 'fatty', as the layman envisages the term, as they are completely miscible with water. If we wished to be absolutely precise, we would describe the SCFA that interest us as 'saturated unbranched alkyl monocarboxylic acids of 2–4 carbon atoms'. Certainly 'SCFA' is a more convenient term, despite its faults.

The digestive tract contains other carboxylic acids of small molecular size, usually in much smaller amounts. By general agreement, those with further substitutions – dicarboxylic acids (e.g. succinic), carbonyl acids (e.g. pyruvic) or hydroxy-acids (e.g. lactic) – are not described as 'SCFA', nor are they sufficiently volatile to be measured in the same gas–liquid chromatographic systems as the cardinal three SCFA. There is less agreement on what length the molecule of an unsubstituted acid should be to qualify as 'SCFA' – are acids with five, six or seven carbon atoms too long, and is formic acid with its single carbon atom too short to be included? These questions tend to disappear in practice, for these unsubstituted acids (formic, valeric, hexanoic, heptanoic and the branched-chain isomers of butyric and the last two acids), although easily measured in the chromatographic systems that record the main three SCFA, are present in digesta in such small amounts that most workers either disregard them as 'SCFA', or specify them separately. In practice, therefore, the term 'SCFA' is usually applied in a restricted sense to acetic, propionic and *n*-butyric acids, the three organic acids that are most abundant in the digestive tract.

In physiological terms these three SCFA are moderately strong acids, with p*K* values of about 4.8. Intestinal contents are more alkaline than this, so within the intestine SCFA are predominantly present as negatively charged *anions*, and not as free *acids*. But by convention many workers in the field refer to SCFA as *acids* even when describing their physiological properties as *anions*. SCFA are not volatile when ionized (hence the need to acidify samples to liberate free acids when they are measured by steam-distillation or gas–liquid chromatography), as can be realized by comparing the smell of a solution of sodium acetate with one of the acetic acid.

Ruminant studies

Most of the work on SCFA is performed by comparative zoologists and veterinary physiologists, and not (with a few notable exceptions) by human physiologists or clinical gastroenterologists. Emphasis on animals rather than humans, and particularly on herbivorous animals, has been a feature of work on the physiology of SCFA since it began in the nineteenth century, when the importance of microbial fermentation within the rumen to the nutrition of cattle and sheep was first realized and provided a strong commercial inducement to veterinarians to work in this field. In contrast, clinicians and alimentary physiologists working mainly with humans have tended to regard intestinal bacteria as unfortunate contaminants, of little metabolic significance for their hosts. Despite a recent awakening of interest among physicians, the subject is relatively neglected even today, as shown by meetings of the American Gastroenterological Association and the British Society of Gastroenterology: out of a grand total of 3738 research abstracts submitted to the two societies at their 1992 annual meetings, only 40 were in any way concerned with SCFA, an unimpressive 1.1%. Ignorance of veterinary (particularly ruminal) discoveries is still widespread among research gastroenterologists, and has led to some wasteful reduplication of effort, by myself among others.

The 1962 and 1966 monographs by Blaxter and Hungate, respectively, are useful starting points for those interested in the function of the rumen. In his introduction on the history of his subject, Hungate pointed out that some basic facts were known as long as 160 years ago; in 1831 Tiedemann & Gmelin found evidence of acetic and butyric acids in rumen contents, and a year later Sprengel, in his two-volume textbook, *Chemistry for Landowners, Foresters and Accountants* (my translation), pointed out that plant materials decomposed in the rumen to yield volatile breakdown products (Sprengel, 1832). In 1888 Tappeiner found that cellulose incubated with rumen contents was fermented to acetic and butyric acids. Protozoa, chiefly highly motile ciliates, were found to be abundant in the rumen as early as 1843 (Gruby & Delafond), and were subsequently shown to be involved in the fermentation of several forms of fibre, including cellulose, though they also feed by ingesting ruminal bacteria. These ciliates are of particular interest to zoologists, as most varieties have no close similarity to existing free-living protozoa, which suggests that they have evolved over millions of years in close association with the evolution of their hosts. However, the main agents of fibre fermentation are the abundant anaerobic bacteria in the rumen. Hungate explained the energy yield of microbial fibre digestion, in a form comprehensible to non-biochemists, by pointing out that the carbon in carbohydrates (—CHOH— groups), is at an intermediate stage of oxidation, and the anaerobic rearrangement, by which some carbon atoms become more oxidized (CO_2 and —COOH) and others more reduced (CH_4 and —CH_2—), produces energy that is available to micro-organisms for the synthesis of high-energy molecules such as ATP. The main end-products of these reactions are methane, carbon dioxide, and the three cardinal SCFA already defined, the actual proportions of these metabolites depending on the type of fibre digested and the organisms responsible. The three SCFA derived from plant fibre are all metabolized by the ruminant host, and calculations of the proportion of the original polysaccharide energy available to the host SCFA have produced estimates of 65–75% (Marston, 1948; Blaxter, 1962; Hungate, 1966). In addition to SCFA, some other organic acids, including lactic, succinic and formic acids, are produced in much smaller amounts, along with ethyl alcohol and hydrogen. Plant fibre is the predominant but not the only ruminal source of SCFA, which are also derived from microbial metabolism of proteins. The branched-chain amino acids from this metabolism give rise to the isobutyrate and isovalerate found in the rumen. Fats do not figure greatly in ruminal fermentation, but glycerol is partially converted to propionic acid, and unsaturated fatty acids are largely hydrogenated to their saturated analogues.

Non-ruminant studies

The importance of microbial fermentation of plant fibre to non-ruminant mammals has only slowly been realized. In 1885 Louis Pasteur suggested that the presence of bacteria in the alimentary tract was essential for the life of rabbits and guinea-pigs, and although this suggestion was subsequently disproved by the successful rearing of germ-free specimens of these animals, their shortened survival supported the principle that the intestinal flora was important for normal nutrition. The anatomical studies of Flower (1872) and Mitchell (1905) led to the appreciation that all predominantly herbivorous animals have, at some site in their digestive tract, an expanded fermention chamber that is often sacculated or subdivided by septa (McBee, 1977; Wrong, Edmonds & Chadwick, 1981; Clemens & Maloiy, 1982; Argenzio & Stevens, 1984). A particularly useful source is the 1988 monograph by Stevens on comparative aspects of the vertebrate digestive tract, which points out that of the 20 mammalian natural orders that exist at the present day there are 11 containing species that subsist largely on the fibrous parts of plants. Similar adaptations to such a dietary regime have sometimes developed in species that are only distantly related genetically; conversely, animals that are closely related may have very different alimentary adaptations for fibre fermentations. The most fundamental distinction is between herbivores with a fermentation chamber in the foregut, and those in which it is in the hindgut. Ruminants are the most obvious examples of the former, but the stomach is modified into the form of a fermentation chamber in many herbivores that do not ruminate, such as the camel, llama, hippopotamus, many marsupials and some foliage-eating monkeys and sloths. The herbivores with a hindgut fermentation chamber, in the form of an enormously capacious caecum or colon, include the perissodactyla (the horse, tapir and rhinoceros), lagomorphs (rabbits and hares), elephants, most rodents, and many primates. Some of these hindgut fermenters practise coprophagy, which ensures that bacterial metabolites arising in the large intestine have a further opportunity to be absorbed by the host. Many herbivores, particularly some species of pig, have well-developed fermentation chambers in both foregut and hindgut. The hyrax (probably, in Chapter 11 of the book of Leviticus, the coney that Jehovah forbade the children of Israel to eat) is unique in possessing fermentation chambers at both sites and a further chamber in the midgut. Omnivorous animals such as humans and the rat have a moderately well-developed fermentation chamber in the large intestine, without a fermentation chamber in the foregut, whereas purely carnivous animals such as the dog and ferret have no obvious fermentation chamber at any level, though their large intestine contains bacteria that have the ability to ferment plant fibre. Whales are of particular interest, for both toothed and baleen species, although not herbivorous, ingest large amounts of insoluble polysaccharide in the chitin skeletons of their cephalopod and crustacean prey, and have voluminous and compartmentalized stomachs that are well adapted to bacterial fermentation of this material.

Further evidence of the role of SCFA in the digestion of plant fibre by herbivores was provided by the Cambridge school of animal physiology (Elsden *et al.*, 1946), which showed high levels of SCFA in the rumen of cattle, sheep and deer; these ruminants showed a second SCFA peak in the large intestine, corresponding to the peak shown by hindgut fermenters such as the horse, rabbit, rat and pig (Fig. 1.1). The carnivorous dog, despite its relatively poorly developed large intestine, also showed a peak of SCFA in that organ (Phillipson, 1947), presumably derived from microbial breakdown of protein; our own later observation of SCFA in the lumen of the cleansed and defunctioned human colon (Rubinstein, Howard & Wrong, 1969) suggests that endogenous mucoprotein is a contributor to this SCFA. Of interest was the finding that SCFA concentrations in the large intestine were similar in the various mammals studied, regardless of feeding habits or the existence of a foregut fermentation chamber, suggesting that the capacity of the large intestine, and sequestration of contents in the viscus, are more important than the composition of contents in determining the amount of SCFA produced.

The human gut

In humans, early studies on intestinal SCFA were confined to observations on faecal composition, initially by Brieger (1878) in Berne, later by several other European workers (Hecht, 1910; Schmidt & Strasburger, 1910; Bahrdt & McLean, 1914; Roux & Goiffon, 1921; Cecchini, 1923), who separated the individual components of SCFA after steam-distillation by differential precipitation of their metallic salts. Their recorded concentrations of total SCFA agreed well with more recent estimates, except for occasional improbably high values in infants' stools, possibly the result of continuing fermentation after the stool was passed. These early contributors recognized that SCFA arose from microbial fermentation, but speculated little on the nature of the substrate involved, or on any further role of SCFA in nutrition or intestinal function, other than to suggest that it might be important in fermentative diarrhoea. The 1929 articles from the St Louis group were a landmark; these investigators reviewed earlier work, improved the old methods, and studied the factors influencing faecal SCFA in normal humans (Olmsted *et al.*, 1929; Grove, Olmsted & Koenig, 1929). Three normal subjects had mean SCFA concentrations in their stools of 93–219 ml 0.1N acid/100 g of whole stool. In separate articles they later described the 'disappearance' (i.e. fermentation) of various fibre fractions during alimentary transit; in three subjects taking several forms of fibre supplement, disappearance of cellulose was 0–72%, and of 'hemicellulose' was 32–89% (Williams & Olmsted, 1935, 1936). Their methods of establishing faecal recovery of these forms of fibre were imperfect by modern standards, but these workers were the first to study the digestibility of these fibre fractions in humans, and to suggest that they were a major source of faecal SCFA.

My personal involvement with SCFA in the human large intestine was originally accidental, and arose in the sixties from my dissatisfaction, as a physician interested in the salt and water composition of body fluids, that very little was known about the ionic composition of human faeces, although on average 75% of their weight is water. Human stool had long been submitted to analysis after incineration or various forms of digestion by strong acids, but the information obtained gave no information about organic constituents, or indicated which faecal constituents are precipitated in an insoluble form or exist in solution in faecal water. Microscopic examination of stool showed that this faecal water must exist in two main forms: (1) a discontinuous intracellular phase sequestered in the numerous inclusion bodies (chiefly bacteria, but also pips and seeds, protozoal bodies and desquamated epithelial cells) that are present in faeces, and (2) a continuous extracellular phase, in which these inclusion bodies are suspended and which itself is in contact with the intestinal mucosa until faeces are expelled from the body. An analogy with the intracellular and extracellular compartments of total body water is obvious. However, it seems that gastroenterologists have not conceived of faecal water as composed of these compartments, for the few other attempts that have been made to analyse the water of healthy human faeces have treated it as a single compartment (Tarlow & Thom, 1974; Bjork, Soergel & Wood, 1976).

A further difficult problem in the analysis of faecal water arises from the fact that within the large intestine the material is alive, containing many millions of bacteria, most of which are obligatory anaerobes. The metabolism of these bacteria continues after a stool has been passed, but many die and autolyse when they are exposed to the hostile aerobic environment outside the body. An indication of the continuing effect of bacterial activity on the composition of stool outside the body was provided by the early demonstration that the material continues to evolve ammonia (Gamble, 1915). Exploring this phenomenon, we found that ammonia was generated under all conditions of faecal incubation, but increased more when conditions were unfavourable to bacterial survival (Vince *et al.*, 1976); its generation could not be prevented even by complete sterilization of faeces with gamma-irradiation, and in this

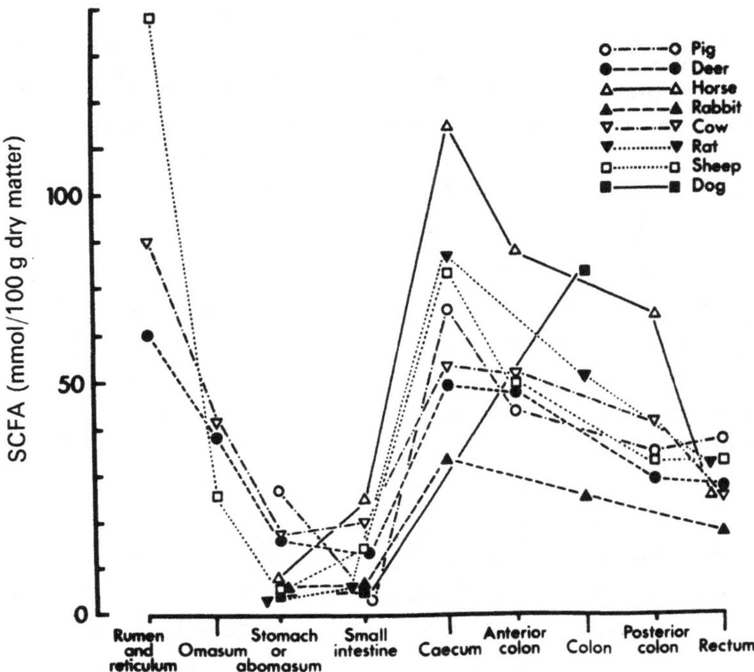

Fig. 1.1. SCFA concentrations at various levels in the digestive tract of different mammals. Redrawn from Elsden *et al.* (1946) and Phillipson (1947). From Wrong *et al.* (1981) with permission of the publishers.

circumstance we concluded that it was the result of deamination of bacterial proteins caused by residual bacterial enzymes. This study also showed that faeces incubated outside the body generated SCFA, whether or not conditions were favourable to bacterial survival. This practical problem of faecal generation of SCFA outside the body, despite efforts being made to bring these chemical processes to a stop, had previously been noted by Olmsted *et al.* (1929); history repeats itself, for it has recently been rediscovered, by a distinguished gastroenterology research unit, that generation of SCFA and osmoles by human stool continues even when specimens are kept on ice (Hammer *et al.*, 1989).

A less important problem has been the unit of measurement of intestinal concentrations. In the early literature these were variously expressed as per weight of water content (g/100 g), per weight of total contents, or per weight of solids (as in Fig. 1.1). The first of these is the most useful for readers, as it allows calculation of molal concentrations per litre of water; the other two units require assumptions regarding the proportion of intestinal solids, and simple adoption of a mean value of 25% (the average for human faeces)

Table 1.1. *Concentrations (mean values ± 1 SD) in stool water of human subjects, obtained by faecal dialysis* in vivo (*Wrong* et al., *1965; Rubinstein* et al., *1969*), *high-speed centrifugation* (*Tarlow & Thom, 1974*) *and ultrafiltration* (*Bjork* et al., *1976*)

	Dialysis *in vivo*	High-speed centrifugation	Ultrafiltration
mosmol/kg	376 ± 27	475 ± 66	410 ± 83
pH	7.0 ± 0.5	6.1 ± 0.7	—
Na (mmol/l)	32 ± 28	32 ± 19	24 ± 21
K (mmol/l)	75 ± 25	70 ± 33	83 ± 24
NH_4 (mmol/l)	14 ± 8	33	42 ± 11
Cl (mmol/l)	16 ± 8	23 ± 8	11 ± 4
Total CO_2 (mmol/l)	40 ± 15	7.3	18 ± 7
Organic anion (mmol/l)	172 ± 39	203 ± 27	196 ± 54

would produce errors with fluids of greatly different solid content. SCFA concentrations have usually been expressed as acetic-acid equivalents, or as millilitres of 0.1N mineral acid, from which it is easy to calculate SI units.

In vivo faecal dialysis

It was to get round these various problems that I and my colleagues introduced the technique of *in vivo* faecal dialysis, in which the contents of the large intestine were dialysed through small semipermeable cellulose capsules containing colloid, which were swallowed and later passed in the faeces. The contents of these dialysis capsules were removed for analysis as soon as a stool was passed, without further handling of stool samples (Wrong, Morrison & Hurst, 1961; Wrong *et al.*, 1965). Since the method was introduced, 32 years ago, we have recovered 5742 of these dialysis capsules from the faeces of 109 subjects, without clinical harm resulting, so the method is fairly safe, though we have deliberately avoided using it in infants or any subject whose past history suggests the possibility of an intestinal stricture. The fluid obtained by this technique can have equilibrated only with the extracellular component of faecal water, so it was to be expected that it should show some differences in composition from samples of total stool water obtained after faeces had been homogenized and either ultracentrifuged or ultrafiltered under aerobic conditions outside the body. However, the higher concentrations of organic anion and ammonia and higher osmolality (especially the last two), and the lower pH and concentration of bicarbonate of these samples of stool water, shown in Table 1.1, probably resulted mainly

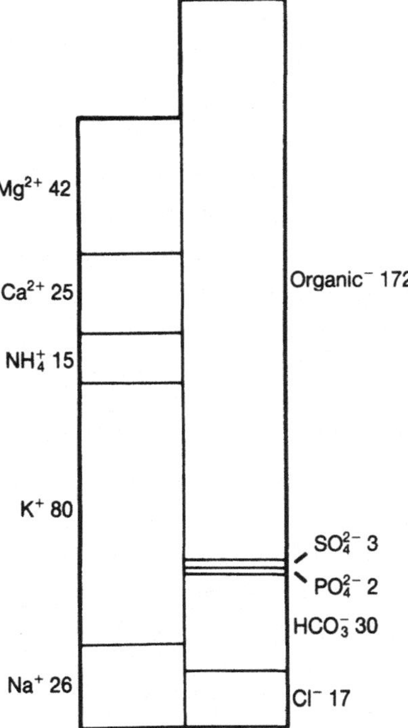

Fig. 1.2. Ionogram from faecal dialysate *in vivo* in humans. Mean values are shown, expressed in mequiv./l. From Wrong *et al.* (1981) with permission of the publishers.

from continued bacterial metabolism and autolysis outside the body, for the inorganic ion concentrations were very similar to those of the *in vivo* faecal dialysate, which would not be expected if they were samples of different compartments of faecal water.

The fluid produced by *in vivo* dialysis was usually clear, of a variable brown colour, with pH 7.0 ± 0.5 and osmolality 376 ± 27 mosmol/kg. This slight hypertonicity appeared to be the result of bacterial activity, for specimens became isotonic when intestinal bacterial activity was suppressed by oral use of insoluble broad-spectrum antibiotics (Wilson *et al.*, 1968). Ionic composition was very variable, mean values being shown as a Gamble ionogram (mequiv./l) in Fig. 1.2. To us the most surprising feature of the fluid was the vast gap between inorganic cations (potassium, sodium, ammonium, calcium and magnesium) and anions (chloride, bicarbonate, phosphate and sulphate), averaging 136 mequiv./l of missing anion. By exclusion, this gap could only be occupied by organic anion, and titration using a technique adapted from an old method for urine confirmed that it was indeed organic anion, with a mean p*K* value of just under 5. (This method tended to overestimate organic anion, and this overestimation, and the error caused by averaging small numbers of determination, were probably the main factors giving rise to the apparent higher mean anion than cation concentration in Fig. 1.2, a difference that cannot exist, as it implies that human faeces carry a negative charge of some millions of volts!) Glancing at an alphabetical table of p*K* values of organic acids, we were impressed that acetic acid appeared near the top of the table with a p*K* of 4.8. Subsequent gas chromatography showed that acetate was indeed the main organic anion in this fluid, followed by propionate and *n*-butyrate, in average proportions of 59:22:19 (Rubinstein *et al.*, 1969), ratios which are similar to those seen in the rumen. We also observed that faecal dialysate pH and total organic anion concentration were strongly negatively correlated, suggesting that faecal pH was largely determined by intestinal generation of SCFA.

This was probably the first time that the contribution of SCFA to the ionic and osmolar composition of faecal water was determined in humans. Its contribution was much greater than we had ever suspected, largely because we were ignorant of earlier work measuring SCFA in human faeces, which by 1965 was largely forgotten, or the observations on other mammals. Some colleagues in my own salt-and-water field expressed doubts whether our high SCFA values were correct; my suspicion is that they had become so used to the concept that the ionic and osmolar structure of body fluids is predominantly inorganic (the salt of 'salt and water'), that they found it hard to accept that here was one body fluid of which the major ionic and osmolar component was organic. The veterinary physiologists I met were not at all surprised; why, they reasoned, should humans be different from other mammals? (see Fig. 1.1).

SCFA as an energy source in humans

Standard texts on food composition, such as *McCance and Widdowson's The Composition of Foods* (Paul & Southgate, 1978), make the assumptions that in humans starch and glycogen are completely digested, but that no other dietary polysaccharides have any value as energy sources. These two assumptions may seem reasonable in texts used for the design of diets, but are oversimplifications in view of recent work both on the indigestibility of a variable portion of dietary starch (Cummings & Englyst, 1991), and on the extent of fibre breakdown in the large intestine. Because of the variability of starch and fibre intake in human diets, it is unlikely that the two errors (which in energy terms have opposite effects) will often cancel themselves out.

A study has indicated that in the human large intestine bacterial breakdown of pectin is complete (Cummings *et al.*, 1979), and our own studies of a faecal incubation system (Vince *et al.*, 1990) showed also that the normal faecal flora can completely ferment a hemicellulose, arabinogalactan. Most other forms of plant fibre appear to be incompletely broken down in the human gut, or are not fermented at all. In our faecal incubation studies, the yield of SCFA averaged 1.05 mol for each mole of hexose equivalent of fermentable substrate added. The metabolism of this SCFA in the body, if completely absorbed, would yield 45% of the energy originally present in the parent polysaccharide. A crude guess might estimate the average fermentation of dietary fibre in the human gut as 15 g/day; complete fermentation of this amount of fibre would, provided the resultant SCFA were completely absorbed and metabolized, contribute only 28 kcal (1 kcal ≈ 4.18 kJ), or about 1% of the daily energy needs of the body, an unimportant error when calculating diets. On the other hand, fermentation of 15 g of fibre, plus that of a similar amount of starch that had escaped digestion in the small intestine, would produce 200 mmol of SCFA, which might have a profound local effect on the large-bowel mucosa.

Absorption of SCFA through the intestinal mucosa is discussed later in this book. A possibility that has long intrigued me, because it is a passive mechanism involving other solutes and membranes elsewhere in the body, is that absorption might in part be dependent on coupled non-ionic diffusion (Wrong *et al.*, 1981). This process requires the presence of an anion/cation pair, of which both members can diffuse in non-ionic form. Coupled non-ionic diffusion of the bicarbonate/ammonium ion pair has been demonstrated in erythrocytes, sea-urchin eggs, and the urinary bladder, and more recently in both small and large intestines (Cohen, Stephens & Feldman, 1988). An ion pair of greater interest in the alimentary tract is the SCFA/ammonium combination, for both members of this pair arise from bacterial action (ammonium largely from deamination of protein); both are present in high concentration in rumen and large intestine, and both are of nutritional value to the host. Evidence suggesting that coupled non-ionic adsorption of this ion pair may operate in the rumen has been found by Hogan (1961), but so far the process has not been specifically sought in the large intestine.

References

Argenzio, R. A. & Stevens, C. E. (1984). The large bowel – supplementary rumen? *Proceedings of the Nutrition Society*, **43**, 12–23.

Bahrdt, H. & McLean, S. (1914). Untersuchungen über die Pathogenese der Verdauungsstörungen im Säuglingsalter. VIII. Ueber die flüchtingen Fettsäuren im Darm gesunder und magendarmkranker Säuglinde und ihre Beziehungen zu den Stoffwechselstörungen. *Zeitschrift für Kinderheilkunde*, **11**, 143–78.

Bjork, J. T., Soergel, K. H. & Wood, C. M. (1976). The composition of 'free' stool water. *Gastroenterology*, **70**, 864.

Blaxter, K. L. (1962). *The Energy Metabolism of Ruminants*. London: Hutchinson.

Brieger, L. (1878). Ueber die flüchtigen Bestandthiele der menschlichen Excremente. *Journal für praktische Chemie*, **17**, 124–38.

Cecchini, A. (1923). Sugli acidi grassi volatili nelle feci (ricerche chimico-cliniche). *Archivio di Patologia e Clinica Medica* (*Bologna*), **2**, 361–92.

Clemens, E. T. & Maloiy, G. M. O. (1982). The digestive physiology of three East African herbivores: the elephant, rhinoceros and hippopotamus. *Journal of Zoology* (*London*), **198**, 141–56.

Cohen, R. M., Stephens, R. L. & Feldman, G. M. (1988). Bicarbonate secretion modulates ammonium absorption in rat distal colon *in-vivo*. *American Journal of Physiology*, **254**, F657–76.

Cummings, J. H. & Englyst, H. N. (1991). Measurement of starch fermentation in the human large intestine. *Canadian Journal of Physiology and Pharmacology*, **69**, 121–9.

Cummings, J. H., Southgate, D. A. T., Branch, W. J., Wiggins, H. S., Houston, H., Jenkins, D. J. A., Jivraj, T. & Hill, M. J. (1979). The digestion of pectin in the human gut and its effect on calcium absorption and large bowel function. *British Journal of Nutrition*, **71**, 477–85.

Elsden, S. R., Hitchcock, M. W. S., Marshall, R. A. & Phillipson, A. T. (1946). Volatile acid in the digesta of ruminants and other animals. *Journal of Experimental Biology*, **22**, 191–202.

Flower, W. H. (1872). Lectures on the comparative anatomy of the organs of digestion of mammalia. *Medical Times and Gazette*, 12 lectures, Vol. 1, p. 215–Vol. 2, p. 647.

Gamble, J. L. (1915). The ammonia and urea content of infants' stool. *American Journal of Diseases of Children*, **9**, 519–22.

Grove, E. W., Olmsted, W. H. & Koenig, K. (1929). The effect of diet and catharsis on the lower volatile fatty acids in the stools of normal men. *Journal of Biological Chemistry*, **85**, 127–36.

Gruby, D. & Delafond, O. (1843). Recherches sur des animalcules se développant en grand nombre dans l'estomac et dans les intestins pendant la digestion des animaux herbivores et carnivores. *Comptes Rendus Hebdomadaires des Séances de L'Académie des Sciences*, **17**, 1304–8.

Hammer, H. F., Santa Ana, C. A., Schiller, L. R. & Fordtran, J. S. (1989). Studies of osmotic diarrhea induced in normal subjects by ingestion of polyethylene glycol and lactulose. *Journal of Clinical Investigation*, **84**, 1056–62.

Hecht, A. F. (1910). Das Verhalten der Fettsäurebildung im Darminhalt des Säuglings. *Munchener Medizinische Wochenschrift*, **57**, 62–7.

Hogan, J. P. (1961). The absorption of ammonia through the rumen of the sheep. *Australian Journal of Biological Sciences*, **14**, 448–60.

Hungate, R. E. (1966). *The Rumen and its Microbes*, pp. 245–6, 328. New York: Academic Press.

Marston, H. R. (1948). The fermentation of cellulose *in-vitro* by organisms from the rumen of sheep. *Biochemical Journal*, **42**, 564–74.

McBee, R. H. (1977). Fermentation in the hindgut. In *Microbial Ecology of the Gut*, ed. R. T. J. Clarke & T. Bauchop. London: Academic Press.

Mitchell, P. C. (1905). On the intestinal tract of mammals. *Transactions of the Zoological Society of London*, **17**, 437–536.

Olmsted, W. H., Duden, C. W., Whitaker, W. M. & Parker, F. F. (1929). A method for the rapid distillation of the lower fatty acids from the stools. *Journal of Biological Chemistry*, **85**, 115–26.

Pasteur, L. (1885). Discussion of paper by E. Duclaux. *Comptes Rendus Hebdomadaires des Séances de L'Académie des Sciences*, **100**, 68.

Paul, A. A. & Southgate, D. A. T. (1978). *McCance and Widdowson's The Composition of Foods*, 4th edn. London: HMSO/Amsterdam: Elsevier.

Phillipson, A. T. (1947). The production of fatty acids in the alimentary tract of the dog. *Journal of Experimental Biology*, **23**, 346–9.

Roux, J. C. & Goiffon, R. (1921). Les acides gras volatils et l'ammoniaque des selles d'adultes. *Archives des Maladies de l'Appareil Digestif et des Maladies de la Nutrition (Paris)*, **11**, 25–46.

Rubinstein, R., Howard, A. V. & Wrong, O. M. (1969). *In vivo* dialysis of faeces as a method of stool analysis. IV. The organic anion component. *Clinical Science*, **37**, 549–64.

Schmidt, A. & Strasburger, J. (1910). *Die Fäzes des Menschen im normalen und krankhaften Zustande mit besonderer Berücksichtigung der klinischen Untersuchungsmethoden*, 3rd edn. Berlin: Verlag von August Hirschwald.

Sprengel, K. (1832). *Chemie für Landwirthe, Forstmänner und Kameralisten.* Göttingen: Vandenhouk and Ruprecht.

Stevens, C. E. (1988). *Comparative Physiology of the Vertebrate Digestive System. Cambridge: Cambridge University Press.*

Tappeiner, H. (1888). Nachträge zu den Untersuchungen über die Gärung der Cellulose. *Zeitschrift für Biologie*, **24**, 105–19.

Tarlow, M. J. & Thom, H. (1974). A comparison of stool fluid and stool dialysate obtained *in vivo*. *Gut*, **15**, 608–13.

Tiedemann, F. & Gmelin, L. (1831). *Die Verdauung nach Versuchen*, 2nd edn. Heidelberg: Groos.

Vince, A., Down, P. F., Murison, J., Twigg, F. J. & Wrong, O. M. (1976). Generation of ammonia from non-urea sources in a faecal incubation system. *Clinical Science and Molecular Medicine*, **51**, 313–22.

Vince, A. J., McNeil, N. I., Wager, J. D. & Wrong, O. M. (1990). The effect of lactulose, pectin, arabinogalactan and cellulose on the production of organic acids and metabolism of ammonia in a faecal incubation system. *British Journal of Nutrition*, **63**, 17–26.

Williams, R. D. & Olmsted, W. H. (1935). A biochemical method for determining indigestible residue (crude fiber) in feces: lignin, cellulose, and non-water-soluble hemicelluloses. *Journal of Biological Chemistry*, **108**, 653–66.

Williams, R. D. & Olmsted, W. H. (1936). The effect of cellulose, hemicellulose and lignin on the weight of the stool: a contribution to the study of laxation in man. *Journal of Nutrition*, **11**, 433–49.

Wilson, D. R., Ing, T. S., Metcalfe-Gibson, A. & Wrong, O. M. (1968). *In-vivo* dialysis of faeces as a method of stool analysis. III. The effect of intestinal antibiotics. *Clinical Science*, **34**, 211–21.

Wrong, O., Metcalfe-Gibson, A., Morrison, R. B. I., Ng, S. T. & Howard, A. V. (1965). *In vivo* dialysis of faeces as method of stool analysis. I. Technique and results in normal subjects. *Clinical Science*, **28**, 357–75.

Wrong, O., Morrison, R. B. I. & Hurst, P. E. (1961). A method of obtaining faecal fluid by *in-vivo* dialysis. *Lancet*, **1**, 1208–9.

Wrong, O. M., Edmonds, C. J. & Chadwick, V. S. (1981). *The Large Intestine. Its Role in Mammalian Nutrition and Homeostasis.* Lancaster: MTP Press.

2

Chemistry of short-chain fatty acids

M. FUKUSHIMA

Introduction

Carboxylic acids (R—COOH) are defined as compounds that have carboxyl radicals (—COOH). Carboxylic acids that have alkyl or alkenyl groups as R— are called fatty acids. Chemically, there is little difference between the characteristics of carboxylic acids and those of fatty acids. Carboxylic acids having an alkenyl group are rarely found in the animal gut, although they do occur as intermediates in both bacterial and mammalian cellular metabolism.

Carboxylic acids have two different names: a name according to the IUPAC (International Union of Pure and Applied Chemistry) nomenclature and a common name (Table 2.1). The former is simpler and more systematic, though the latter is widely used outside chemical societies.

The physicochemical nature of short-chain fatty acids (SCFA) defines the behaviour of these acids in living organisms. This chapter briefly introduces the chemical characteristics of carboxylic acids that also apply to SCFA. Special attention is paid to factors that affect the acidity of these acids.

Isomers

Some fatty acids form geometrical and/or optical isomers according to their molecular forms. Although monocarboxylic acids with straight carbon chains do not form such isomers, information about isomers may help to understand the nature of branched-chain fatty acids and other SCFA derivatives.

Geometrical isomers

Examples of geometrical isomers are illustrated by fumaric acid (*trans*-1,2-ethylenedicarboxylic acid) and maleic acid (*cis*-1,2-ethylenedicarboxylic acid), both of which can be expressed as a common rational formula $(CHCOOH)_2$.

Table 2.1. *IUPAC and common names (with 'acid' omitted) and physicochemical constants of short-chain fatty acids*

Carbon number	Formula	IUPAC name	Common name	Molecular weight	pK_a	Boiling point (°C)
1	$HCOOH$	Methanoic	Formic	46.03	3.55	100.8
2	CH_3COOH	Ethanoic	Acetic	60.05	4.56	117.8
3	C_2H_5COOH	Propanoic	Propionic	74.08	4.67	140.8
4	C_3H_7COOH	Butanoic	*n*-Butyric	88.11	4.63	164
4	$(CH_3)_2CHCOOH$	2-Methylpropanoic	iso-Butyric	88.11	4.63	154.5
5	C_4H_9COOH	Pentanoic	*n*-Valeric	102.13	4.64	184
5	$(CH_3)_2CHCH_2COOH$	3-Methylbutanoic	iso-Valeric	102.13	4.58	176.5
6	$C_5H_{11}COOH$	Hexanoic	*n*-Caproic	116.16	4.63	205.8

pK_a at 25 °C, ionic strength 0.1 mol/l.
Data from Chemical Society of Japan (1984) and Japanese Society for Analytical Chemistry (1991).

Carboxylic acids that have asymmetric shapes due to a double bond between carbon atoms can be in two distinct forms (geometrical isomers) having two different names. A compound that has two substituents of interest on the same side of a double bond is called the *cis*-isomer, and if they are on different sides it is called the *trans*-isomer.

Optical isomers

The carbon atom is tetravalent. Thus, four atoms or atomic groups can make four single bonds with a carbon atom. When all the four substituents around a carbon atom are different from each other, as in lactic acid, the carbon atom is called asymmetric, and is sometimes shown with an asterisk to emphasize this (Fig. 2.1). Such a compound forms two isomers. The pair of isomers (e.g. (2) and (3) in Fig. 2.1) are mirror-images of each other. Such optical isomers are called enantiomers or antipodes. For monocarboxylic acids, only iso-carboxylic acids with a branched chain on the α-carbon can have enantiomers.

Enantiomers are detected with polarized light. If a polarized beam passes through an asymmetric material, the plane of polarization will be rotated. When the plane of polarization is rotated clockwise, the compound is called *dextro*-rotatory, and either '*d*' or (+) will be added in front of its name. When the optical rotation is anticlockwise, the compound is called *laevo*-

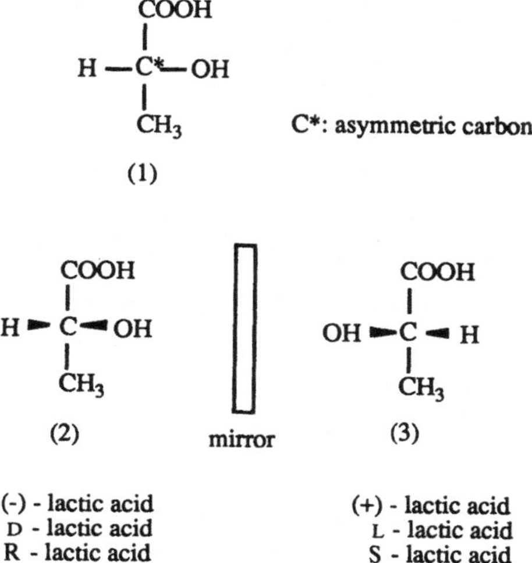

Fig. 2.1. Enantiomers of lactic acid. (−)- and (+)-lactic acid are the same as *l*- and *d*-lactic acid, respectively.

rotatory, and either '*l*' or (−) will be added (Fig. 2.1). A mixture of *d*- and *l*-isomers (50:50) is called racemate, and has no optical rotation.

Notation systems of optical isomers

Notation systems of optical isomers are complicated. The rules have changed several times, and different rules are used by different scientific societies. Apart from the (+)/(−) or *d*/*l* system, there are two other notation systems, and all three systems are independent of each other.

One system is the D/L system, which is familiar to biochemical societies. D or L is designated for compounds derived from (+)- or (−)-glyceraldehyde, respectively. As D/L reflects a metabolic pathway, it is a convenient indication of biological metabolism. However, it is important to note that the D/L system does not correspond to the stereochemical structure of compounds.

Another system, the S/R system, indicates the absolute configuration of compounds, regardless of their metabolic pathways, based on several stereochemical rules, which are beyond the scope of this book (Hendrickson, Cram & Hammond, 1970; Solomons, 1983; Carey, 1987).

Acidity

Carboxylic acids are strong acids in comparison with other organic compounds (Table 2.2). Acidity can be indicated by the acid dissociation constant, or pK_a for short. A model monoatomic acid, HA, where H represents the hydronium ion and A represents the carboxylate anion, will dissociate to some extent in an aqueous solution as follows:

$$HA + H_2O \rightleftharpoons H_3O^+ + A^- \tag{2.1}$$

where H_3O^+ is an aggregate of the hydronium ion with water. For convenience, the hydronium ion is written as H^+. Thus, eq. 2.1 can be written as follows:

$$HA \rightleftharpoons H^+ + A^- \tag{2.1'}$$

When this dissociation reaction attains equilibrium, the constant for acid dissociation, K_a, is defined as follows:

$$K_a = [H^+][A^-]/[HA] \tag{2.2}$$

It is more usual to use pK_a ($-\log K_a$) than K_a, just as pH ($-\log [H^+]$) is used instead of $[H^+]$.

Table 2.2. pK_a *values of several organic and inorganic compounds*

Compound	Formula	pK_a
Organic compound		
Formic acid	$HCOOH$	3.55
Acetic acid	CH_3COOH	4.56
Glycine	NH_2CH_2COOH	2.36 (pK_1) 9.57 (pK_2)
Ethylenediamine	$H_2NCH_2CH_2NH_2$	7.08
Phenol	C_6H_5OH	9.82
Acetylacetone	$CH_3COCH_2COCH_3$	8.80
Inorganic compound		
Carbonic acid	H_2CO_3	6.35
Hydrochloric acid	HCl	−8 (estimate)
Hydrogen cyanide	HCN	9.22
Phosphoric acid	H_3PO_4	2.15

pK_a at 25 °C, ionic strength 0.1 mol/l.
Data from Chemical Society of Japan (1984).

$$pK_a = -\log([H^+][A^-]/[HA]) = pH + \log([HA]/[A^-]) \qquad (2.3)$$

The pK_a of a compound means the pH of the solution at which half of the compound dissociates. At the same time, the pK_a of a compound represents the strength of the compound as an acid.

The pK_a values for dicarboxylic and tricarboxylic acids are defined in the same manner as for monocarboxylic acids, except that they dissociate stepwise. Thus, di- or tricarboxylic acids have two or three pK_a values, which represent each step of the dissociation. The first, second and third dissociation constants are expressed as pK_1, pK_2 and pK_3, respectively (Table 2.3).

When we refer to the pK_a of a compound, it must be kept in mind that the pK_a varies with the ionic strength and temperature of the aqueous solution. The pK_a decreases by 0.2 units when ionic strength increases from 0.0 to 0.1 in most carboxylic acids (Table 2.4). Ionic strength (μ) of a solution is defined as follows:

$$\mu = 1/2 \times \Sigma(C_i \times Z_i^2) \qquad (2.4)$$

where C_i (equivalents/l) denotes a concentration of an ionic species i, and Z_i denotes the charge of that ion. Ionic strength of 0.0 occurs when the solution is infinitely diluted. Ionic strength in the bulk phase of the gut lumen may not vary much. However, ionic strength of the microclimate at the luminal

Table 2.3. pK_a *of di- and tricarboxylic acids at 25 °C and ionic strength 0.1*

Carboxylic acid	Rational formula	pK_1	pK_2	pK_3
Dicarboxylic acid				
Oxalic acid	$(COOH)_2$	1.04	3.83	
Malonic acid	$CH_2(COOH)_2$	2.65	5.28	
Succinic acid	$(CH_2COOH)_2$	4.00	5.24	
Maleic acid	$(HCCOOH)_2$	1.75	5.83	
Fumaric acid	$(HCCOOH)_2$	2.85	4.10	
Tricarboxylic acid				
Citric acid	$C(CH_2COOH)_2OHCOOH$	2.87	4.35	5.69

Data from Chemical Society of Japan (1984).

surface of the epithelial cell can dramatically increase when secretion of cations or anions occurs.

The pK_a values of monocarboxylic acids, except for formic acid, vary little (Table 2.4). The pK_a values for chloroacetic acids are in the order of mono- > di- > tri-. This tendency is also seen for chlorinated derivatives of other carboxylic acids.

The pK_a values of monosubstituted butyric acid are in the order of γ- > β- > α-. This applies to other monosubstituted fatty acids (see below).

Acid dissociation of organic compounds in organic solvents (including organic solvent–water mixtures) is limited (Tables 2.5 and 2.6). Such behaviour of carboxylic acids may be seen in the hydrophobic climate of cell membranes. The dielectric constant of the solvent (Tables 2.5 and 2.6) is a measure of the force with which two opposite charges are separated; water has the greatest dielectric constant ($\varepsilon = 80$). Although the relationship between pK_a and the dielectric constant of organic solvents is unknown, we can see from Table 2.5 that the pK_a of a carboxylic acid becomes greater (i.e. it gets weaker as an acid) as the dielectric constant gets smaller. In other words, the acidity of a carboxylic acid becomes less in more hydrophobic conditions. Charged particles, such as dissociated protons or carboxylate anions, are unstable in a solvent of low dielectic constant. In such solvents the acid dissociation reaction is inhibited.

Factors affecting acidity

There are two major factors which influence the acidity of a compound. One is the ease with which the hydronium ion dissociates. The other is the stability of the anion produced by the dissociation of the hydronium ion.

Table 2.4. *pK_a values of several carboxylic acids at 25 °C*

Carboxylic acid (IUPAC name)	Rational formula	pK_a	Ionic strength (mol/l)
Monocarboxylic acids			
Formic (methanoic)	$HCOOH$	3.75	0.0
		3.55	0.1
Acetic (ethanoic)	CH_3COOH	4.76	0.0
		4.56	0.1
Propionic (propanoic)	C_2H_5COOH	4.87	0.0
		4.67	0.1
n-Butyric (butanoic)	C_3H_7COOH	4.63	0.1
iso-Butyric		4.63	0.1
n-Valeric (pentanoic)	C_4H_9COOH	4.64	0.1
iso-Valeric		4.58	0.1
t-Valeric		5.1[a]	(no description)
n-Caproic (hexanoic)	$C_5H_{11}COOH$	4.63	0.1
t-Butylacetic acid	$(CH_3)_3CCH_2COOH$	5.30[a]	(no description)
n-Enantic (heptanoic)	$C_6H_{13}COOH$	4.66	0.1
n-Caprylic (octanoic)	$C_7H_{15}COOH$	4.89	0.1
Substituted carboxylic acids			
Fluoroacetic acid	CH_2FCOOH	2.59	0.1
Chloroacetic acid	$CH_2ClCOOH$	2.68	0.1
Bromoacetic acid	$CH_2BrCOOH$	2.72	0.1
Iodoacetic acid	CH_2ICOOH	2.98	0.1
Dichloroacetic acid	$CHCl_2COOH$	1.30	0.0
Trichloroacetic acid	CCl_3COOH	0.66	0.1
α-Chlorobutyric acid	$CH_3CH_2CHClCOOH$	2.86	0.0
β-Chlorobutyric acid	$CH_3CHClCH_2COOH$	4.05	0.0
γ-Chlorobutyric acid	$CH_2ClCH_2CH_2COOH$	4.52	0.0

[a] Data from Carey (1987).
Data from Chemical Society of Japan (1984).

Resonance effect

Let us take acetic and ethyl alcohol as examples. These two compounds dissociate as follows:

$$CH_3COOH \rightleftharpoons CH_3COO^- + H^+$$

$$C_2H_5OH \rightleftharpoons C_2H_5O^- + H^+$$

The pK_a values (25 °C, ionic strength = 0.1 mol/dm^3) are 4.56 for acetic acid (Chemical Society of Japan, 1984) and 17 for ethyl alcohol (Hendrickson *et al.*, 1970) indicating that acetic acid is $10^{12.4}$ times $(17 - 4.56 = 12.44)$

Table 2.5. pK_a *of several carboxylic acids at 25 °C in various organic solvents (dielectric constants in parentheses; data from Chemical Society of Japan, 1984)*

	Dimethyl sulphoxide (46.7)	*N*,*N*-Dimethyl formamide (36.7)	Acetonitrile (36.2)	Methanol (32.63)	Ethanol (24.3)	Pyridine (12.3)	Acetic acid (6.2)
CH_3COOH	12.6	11.1	22.3	9.7	10.2	<12	
$CH_2ClCOOH$		9.0		7.8	8.5		
$CHCl_2COOH$		7.2		6.3	6.9		
CCl_3COOH							11.5
Benzoic acid	11.1	11.7	20.7	9.4	10.2	<11	

Table 2.6. pK_a *of acetic acid, benzoic acid and glycine in various mixtures*

	Dielectric constant	Acetic acid	Benzoic acid	Glycine (pK_1)	Glycine (pK_2)
Methonol (wt% in water)					
10	75.8	4.91	4.39		
20	71.0	5.07	4.72		
34.5			4.94		
40	61.2	5.45			
54.2			5.49		
60	46.5	5.90			
80	36.8	6.63			
90	32.4	7.31			
93.7			7.38		
95			7.99		
Ethanol (wt% in water)					
20	74.6	5.12	4.76		
35	58.7	5.43	5.24		
50	50.4	5.84	5.76		
65	40.6	6.29	6.19		
80	33.9	6.87	6.7		
100	24.3	10.32	10.25		
1,4-Dioxane (wt% in water)					
20	62.4	5.29	4.87	2.63	9.91
30	59.2		5.28		
40	56.3		5.79		
45	55.0	6.31		3.10	
50	53.4		6.38		10.24
70	48.2	8.28		3.97	
82		10.51			11.28

stronger an acid than is ethyl alcohol. These two compounds have approximately the same molecular weight, and approximately the same radical structure. What causes this big difference in acidity?

The reasonance effect explains why acetic acid is a strong acid. In general, the stability of a compound varies according to the number of canonical structures it has. Acetic acid has two canonical structures ((1) and (2) in Fig. 2.2), whilst ethyl alcohol does not have any.

In addition to this, the hydrogen atom (this will dissociate as a hydronium ion) in structure (2) in Fig. 2.2 has a positive charge, thereby making the electron density of its O—H bond lower than the O—H bond in ethyl alcohol. Thus, the hydrogen ion of acetic acid dissociates more easily than does that of ethyl alcohol.

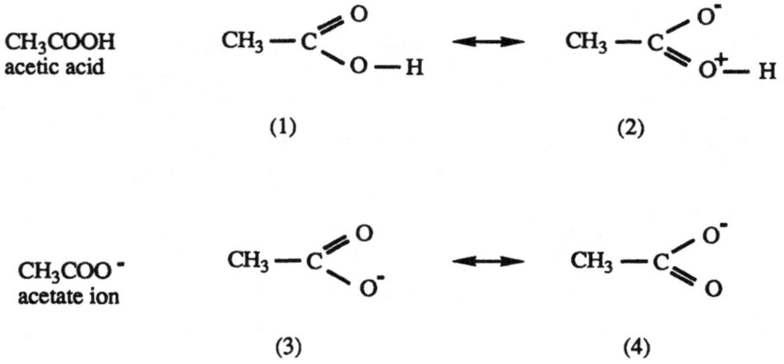

CH_3COOH acetic acid — $CH_3-C(=O)-O-H$ (1) ⟷ $CH_3-C(-O^-)=O^+-H$ (2)

CH_3COO^- acetate ion — $CH_3-C(=O)-O^-$ (3) ⟷ $CH_3-C(-O^-)=O$ (4)

Fig. 2.2. Resonance for acetic acid and acetate ion.

Furthermore, the acetate ion has two canonical structures ((3) and (4) in Fig. 2.2), and these two structures are symmetrical. In other words, dissociated carboxylate anion can take two different forms by exchanging oxygen atoms having either a double bond or a single bond, both of which are geometrically arranged on the same plane. This makes the resonance energy of acetic acid even greater; the degree of stabilization is indicated as resonance energy, which is the difference between the energy of the resonance hybrid and that of the non-resonant molecule.

These characteristics of acetic acid explain how acetate ion is stabilized by the resonance effect, and why the pK_a of acetic acid is lower than that of ethyl alcohol. This generally applies to other carboxylic acids; resonance effects make carboxylic acids strong acids, though the strength varies among acids.

Inductive and electrostatic effects

Every atom has electronegativity. When a pair of atoms with different electronegativity form a bond between them, a dipole moment will be generated between these atoms. The dipole moment has a direction from the relatively positive atom to the relatively negative atom. Electrons are attracted toward the negative dipole, as represented by the arrow in Fig. 2.3. The electron densities of atoms in a compound (such as H and O in Fig. 2.3) and those of free atoms are different according to the attraction force for electrons.

We can classify atoms and functional groups into those that have strong electron-withdrawing inductive effects, such as NO_2, CN, COOH, COOR, C=O, F, Cl, Br, I, NO, NR_3^+ and ONO, and those with electron-donating inductive effects, such as alkyl groups.

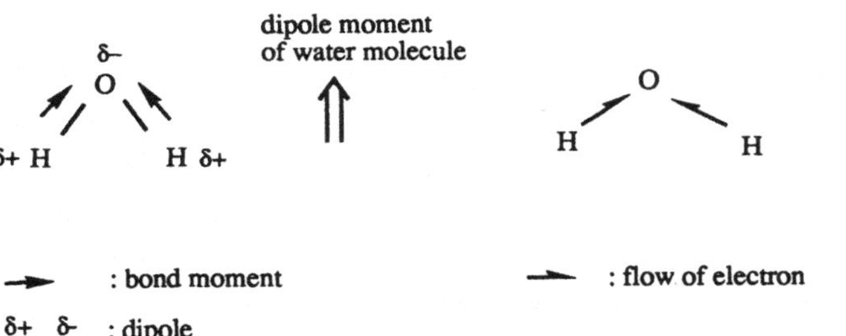

Fig. 2.3. Dipole and dipole moment of H_2O and flow of electrons.

Electron-withdrawing inductive effects and acidity

Substitution of a hydrogen atom on acetic acid with a chlorine atom produces a stronger acid than acetic acid (Table 2.4). The substituted halogen, being an electronegative atom, attracts electrons in the carboxyl group ((1) in Fig. 2.4). Such attraction of electrons lowers the electron density in the O—H

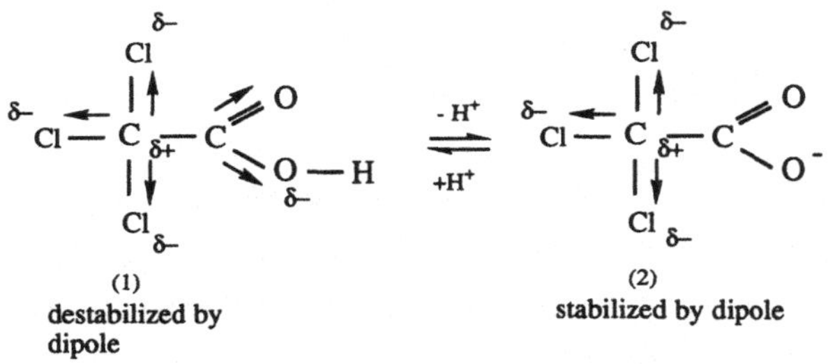

(1)
destabilized by dipole

- H^+ / + H^+

(2)
stabilized by dipole

Fig. 2.4. Dipole moment of acetic acid and acetate ion.

bond, thereby making it easier to dissociate. The strength of the halogen-substitution effect is in the order of F- > Cl- > Br- > I- and tri- > di- > monosubstitution (Fig. 2.5).

Such an effect of electron attraction is called the electron-withdrawing inductive effect. Accordingly, substitution of a carboxylic acid with electron-withdrawing functional groups produces a stronger acid than the original carboxylic acid.

Electron-donating inductive effect

In contrast, alkyl groups serve as electron donors. The electron density of the O—H bond of the carboxyl group of acetic acid is increased by the donation of electrons from the methyl group as shown in (2) of Fig. 2.4. Acetic

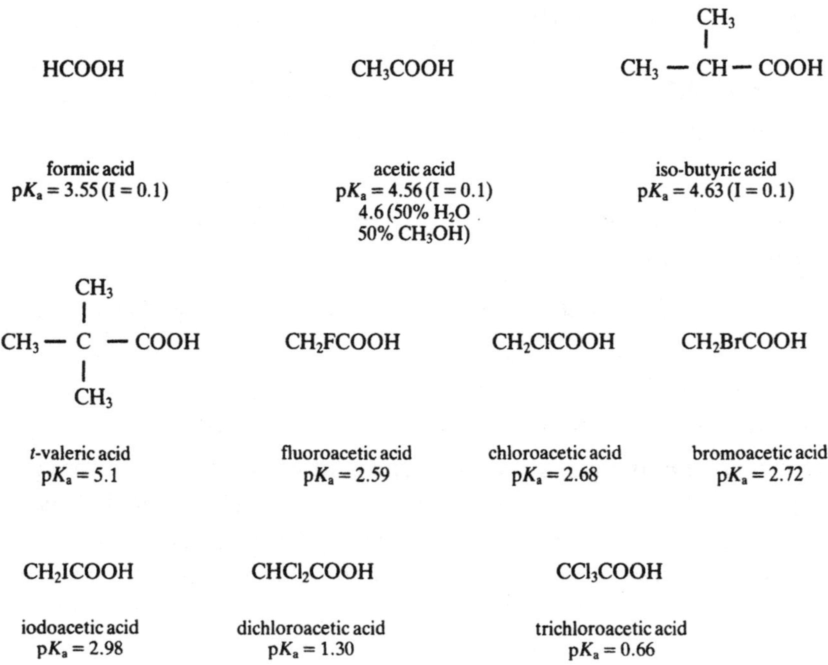

Fig. 2.5. pK_a values of several carboxylic acids.

acid is a weaker acid than formic acid, due to this effect, which is called the electron-donating inductive effect. This effect is almost independent of the number of carbon atoms of normal alkyl groups, as is shown in Table 2.4; the pK_a values of normal monocarboxylic acids are almost the same. The *t*-monocarboxylic acids are weaker acids than the corresponding normal acids (Table 2.4), although the precise conditions are not described. This means that the *t*-alkyl groups have a more electron-donating inductive effect than do normal alkyl groups.

Hydrogen bonding

Molecules of compounds containing O—H bonds are attracted to each other by an intermolecular force (dipole–dipole interaction) caused by the difference in the electronegativity of oxygen and hydrogen atoms. The water molecule has two O—H bonds and two bond-moments.The dipole moment of a molecule having only two atoms, such as HCl, is the same as the bond moment. Therefore, the dipole moment of a molecule having more than three atoms, such as H_2O or acetic acid, is a vector synthesized from each bond moment.

Hydrogen bonding is formed between H—O, H—F, H—Cl and H—N. Hydrogen bonding affects the dimerization, acidity and solubility of carboxylic acids. Thus, hydrogen bonding is the key factor determining the characteristics of SCFA in aqueous solutions.

Hydrogen bonding and acidity

There are two types of hydrogen bonding, intramolecular and intermolecular. When we discuss the effect of hydrogen bonding on boiling point, solubility and some other characteristics of chemical compounds, the discussion is about intermolecular hydrogen bonding in many cases. However, for acidity of some chemical compounds, such as maleic acid and salicylic acid, intramolecular hydrogen bonding has a considerable effect.

Maleic acid and fumaric acid are geometrical isomers of each other. The difference in their pK_1 and pK_2 values (Table 2.3) can be explained by the intramolecular hydrogen bonding. Maleic acid and the anion derived from it make intramolecular hydrogen bonds, but fumaric acid does not. Maleic acid and its first anion, caused by the first acid dissociation ((1) and (2) in Fig. 2.6, respectively) have intramolecular hydrogen bonding. Moreover, as

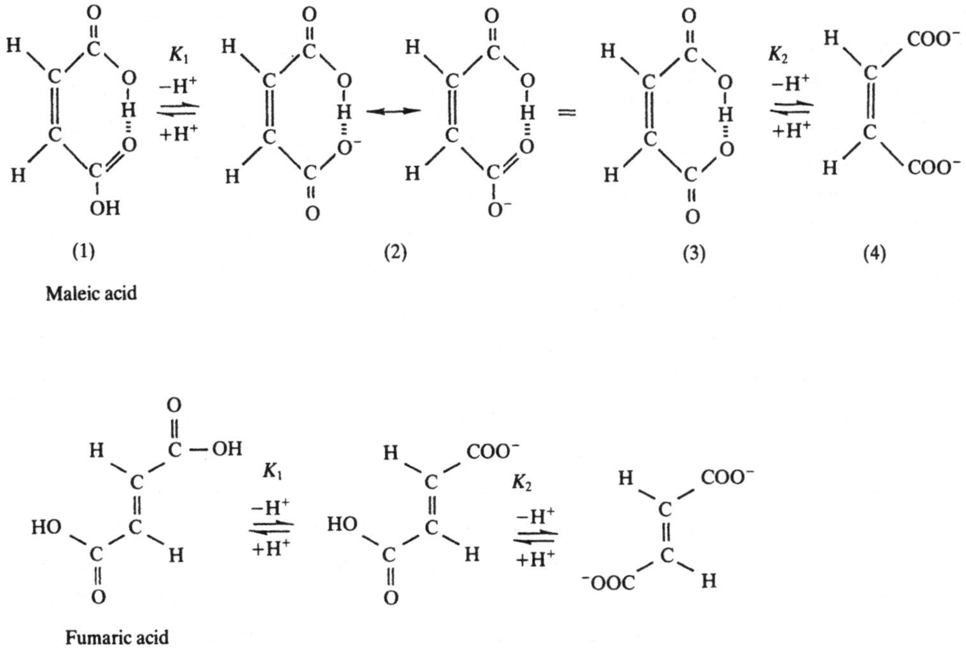

K_1 $-H^+$ $+H^+$ K_2 $-H^+$ $+H^+$

(1) (2) (3) (4)

Maleic acid

K_1 $-H^+$ $+H^+$ K_2 $-H^+$ $+H^+$

Fumaric acid

Fig. 2.6. The effect of hydrogen bonding on pK_a values.

the first anion has two canonical structures (Fig. 2.6 (3)), it may be thought that the anion (2) is very stable. However, the second anion (4) will be destabilized, because the second anion (4) cannot have intramolecular hydrogen bonding, and because of the repulsion between two negative charges on carboxyl anions. On the other hand, fumaric acid and its first and second anions have no canonical structures, no internal hydrogen bonding, and no repulsion. Thus the pK_1 of maleic acid is smaller than that of fumaric acid, but the pK_2 of maleic acid is greater than that of fumaric acid (Table 2.3).

Hydrogen bonding and solubility in water

Hydrocarbon groups of organic compounds are hydrophobic, but radicals that have dipole moments, such as —OH or —COOH, are hydrophilic. Accordingly, it is easy to understand why alcohols and carboxylic acids with low carbon numbers are water-soluble. This is due to hydrogen bonding between water and hydrophilic radicals.

Dimerization

Boiling point

Carboxylic acids form dimers in solid, liquid and gaseous states. It is also possible to couple two different carboxylic acids by the same mechanism. The boiling point reflects the formation of a dimer. Generally, the boiling point becomes higher as the molecular weight becomes larger and the intermolecular forces become stronger. Carboxylic acids have higher boiling points than those of alkanes of similar molecular weight, having neither intramolecular nor intermolecular hydrogen bonding (Table 2.7). For example, the boiling point of formic acid (M_r 46) is lower than that of propane (M_r 44) by 142.7 °C, but is similar to that of heptane (M_r 100). The boiling point of acetic acid (M_r 60) is similar to that of octane (M_r 114). This can be explained, if formic acid and acetic acid behave as quasi dimers with apparent molecular weight of 92 (46×2) and 120 (60×2), respectively.

Dimerization constant

The dimerization of carboxylic acids has been studied using solvent extraction, because almost the same level of polarity is required for extraction. Fatty acids are extracted as dimers with solvents of low dielectric constant, such as benzene, cyclohexane and carbon tetrachloride. Dimerization is necessary for fatty acids of low carbon number to be extracted into

Table 2.7. *Molecular weight and boiling point of some organic compounds*

	Molecular weight	Boiling point (°C)
Carboxylic acid		
HCOOH	46	100.7
CH_3COOH	60	118.1
C_2H_5COOH (*n*-)	74	141.1
C_3H_7COOH (*n*-)	88.1	163.5
$(CH_3)_2CHCOOH$	88.1	154.5
C_4H_9COOH (*n*-)	102.1	184
$(CH_3)_2CHCH_2COOH$	102.1	176.5
$C_5H_{11}COOH$ (*n*-)	116.2	205.8
$(CH_3CH_2)_2CHCOOH$	116.2	194
$(CH_3)_3CCH_2COOH$	116.2	190
Alkane		
C_3H_8	44	−42.1
C_4H_{10}	58	−0.5
C_5H_{12}	72	36.8
C_6H_{14}	86	68.7
C_7H_{16}	100	98.4
C_8H_{18}	114	125.7
C_9H_{20}	128	150.8
$C_{10}H_{22}$	142	174.1

Data from Japanese Society of Analytical Chemistry (1991).

organic solvents of low dielectric constant; fatty-acid monomers are too polar to be extracted by such solvents. Fatty-acid dimers are seldom observed when electron-donating solvents, such as alcohols or ketones, are used as organic solvents, because fatty acids and these solvents have different levels of polarity. Dipole moments of fatty acids compensate for each other when a pair of fatty acids form a dimer by hydrogen bonding. This compensation makes the polarity of the resultant dimer zero. This is the reason that non-polar dimers can be extracted with solvents of low dielectric constant.

In other words, fatty acids can form dimers according to the dielectric constant of the solvents. Thus, the physicochemical characteristics of fatty-acid monomers may not always apply to their actual behaviour *in vivo*. Further, we cannot simply adopt the physicochemical data of fatty acids in solvents of low dielectric constant such as hexane when we consider the behaviour of fatty acids in or across cell membranes that contain phospholipids more polar (higher dielectric constant) than hexane.

A pair of different fatty acids, e.g. acetic acid and propionic acid, can form a dimer. Interestingly, heterodimers are more easily formed than homodimers (Sekine *et al.*, 1967). This suggests that the behaviour of fatty acids may depend on whether they exist as the sole carboxylic acid or as different kinds of carboxylic acids.

To understand the formation of dimers, let us take the simplest system as an example: extraction of a monocarboxylic acid with a non-polar solvent. The monocarboxylic acid HA will dissociate into H^+ (hydronium ion) and A^- (carboxylate anion). HA, H^+ and A^- reach an equilibrium in an aqueous solution of HA. When this aqueous solution of HA is shaken with a non-polar organic solvent, three reactions occur:

(1) H^+ and A^- associate to become HA;
(2) HA is extracted with organic solvent; and
(3) HA monomers form dimers $(HA)_2$ in the organic solvent (Fig. 2.7).

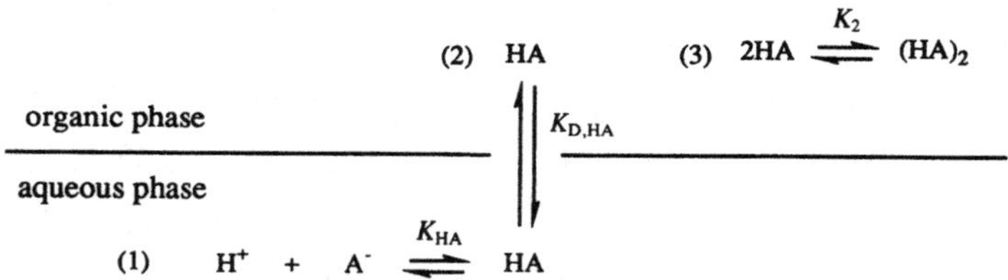

Fig. 2.7. Extraction scheme of monocarboxylic acid. HA, monocarbonic acid; K_{HA}, formation constant (the reciprocal of acid dissociation); $K_{D,HA}$, distribution coefficient of HA; K_2, dimerization constant.

Equilibrium constants K_{HA}, $K_{D,HA}$ and K_2 are defined as follows, where $[\ ]_O$ represents the concentration of the monomer or dimer in the organic solution:

$$K_{HA} = [HA]/[H^+][A^-] \tag{2.5}$$

$$K_{D,HA} = [HA]_O/[HA] \tag{2.6}$$

$$K_2 = [(HA)_2]_O/[HA]_2 \tag{2.7}$$

The distribution ratio (D) is a ratio of the total concentrations of chemical species in organic and aqueous phases.

$$D = \frac{[HA]_O + 2[(HA)_2]_O}{[HA] + [A^-]} \tag{2.8}$$

The distribution coefficient (K_D) is a ratio of concentrations of specific species in organic and aqueous phases. If $[HA]_O$, $[(HA)_2]_O$ and $[A^-]$

are substituted with K_{HA}, $K_{D,HA}$ and K_2 using eqs 2.5, 2.6 and 2.7, then we can obtain eq. 2.9:

$$D = \frac{K_{D,HA}(1 + 2K_2K_{D,HA}[HA])}{1 + ([H^+]K_{HA})^{-1}} \tag{2.9}$$

The initial concentration of HA (C_{HA}) is expressed as the sum of several concentrations of chemical species:

$$C_{HA} = [HA] + [A^-] + [HA]_O + 2[(HA)_2]_O \tag{2.10}$$

Fatty acids of low carbon number are polar, thus $K_{D,HA}$ is small enough to assume, from eq. 2.10, that

$$[HA] = C_{HA} \tag{2.11}$$

By using eq. 2.11, we can obtain eq. 2.9′ from 2.9:

$$D = \frac{K_{D,HA}(1 + 2K_2K_{D,HA}C_{HA})}{1 + ([H^+]K_{HA})^{-1}} \tag{2.9′}$$

These constants, obtained experimentally, are listed in Tables 2.8 and 2.9. In general, fatty acids become more extractable (larger $\log K_{D,HA}$ values) by organic solvents as their carbon number becomes larger (see $\log K_D$ in Table 2.8). Though these constants are useful when we estimate the behaviour of fatty acids in biological systems, we must maintain some reservations. The constants were obtained from experiments under precisely controlled conditions, e.g. constant temperature and salt concentration. However, the actual system *in vivo* is complicated by salts at high varying concentrations.

Several kinds of coexistent salts have two effects on solvent extraction: one is called the salting-out effect, and another is salting-in. When extractability becomes higher in the presence of a coexistent salt, it is said that the coexistent salt has a salting-out effect. For the salting-in effect, the extractability is reduced by the coexistence of a salting-in agent. For example, the extractability of the Co(II)-8-hydroxyquinoline complex to chloroform is reduced in the presence of NaBr, NaI and $CaCl_2$, and the order is NaBr > NaI > $CaCl_2$ (Bagreev & Zolotov, 1965). Data about salting effects are available (Zolotov & Lambrev, 1965; Zolotov, 1972).

There is a simple rule about solvent extraction: 'like dissolves like'. This means that polar compounds tend to dissolve in polar solvents. In the two phases (liquid–liquid or liquid–solid), compounds tend to be extracted into the solvent that has more affinity with the compound to be extracted. Thus, we may assume that the solubilities of the dimers of undissociated SCFA in

Table 2.8. *Distribution coefficient and dimerization constant of linear fatty acids at 25 °C*

	Benzene		1,2-Dichloroethane		Nitrobenzene		Isopropyl ether	
	$\log K_D$	$\log K_2$	$\log K_D$	$\log K_2$	$\log K_D$	$\log K_2$	$\log K_D$	$\log K_2$
CH_3COOH	−2.07	2.16	−1.60	1.47	−1.44	0.85	−0.76	−0.23
C_2H_5COOH	−1.36	2.21	−0.99	1.53	−0.86	0.97	−0.09	−0.30
C_3H_7COOH	−0.79	2.28	−0.39	1.45	−0.34	0.95	0.48	−0.37
C_4H_9COOH	−0.16	2.36	0.23	1.35	0.23	1.01	1.05	−0.20
$C_5H_{11}COOH$	0.31	2.45	0.82	1.19	0.77	0.96	1.48	−0.19

Data from Kojima, Yoshida & Tanaka, 1970.

Table 2.9. *Distribution coefficient and dimerization constant of propionic acid in various solvents*

	log K_D	log K_2
2-Ethyl hexyl alcohol	0.30	
Chloroform	−0.96	1.94
Carbon tetrachloride	−1.90	3.14
Cyclohexane	−2.54	3.71
n-Hexane	−2.56	3.94
Cyclohexanone	0.52	
Isopropylbenzene	−1.64	2.48
Chlorobenzene	−1.53	2.49
Toluene	−1.47	2.39

Data from Kojima *et al.* (1970).

neutral lipid are greater than those undissociated SCFA monomers. Accordingly, it is likely that SCFA form dimers when they exist in neutral lipid. Phospholipids constituting biological membranes are more polar than are neutral lipids, and therefore, the solubility of SCFA monomers in phospholipids will be greater than that in neutral lipids, making it possible for undissociated SCFA monomers to penetrate phospholipid phases more readily than do SCFA dimers.

Studies comparing the extraction behaviour of SCFA in non-polar solvents and polar solvents such as alkylphosphoric acids should provide us with more realistic ideas on the chemical behaviour of SCFA in biological systems. Solvent extraction experiments are a promising approach to understanding the transfer of polar materials such as SCFA in biological systems, especially across cell membranes.

Acknowledgements

I would like to express my gratitude to Mrs Kieko Suda, Hiromi and Tasuku Tominaga and their family for their support during the preparation of this chapter. I also thank Dr Takashi Sakata for his valuable suggestions and discussions during the preparation of this chapter.

References

Bagreev, V. V. & Zolotov, Y. A. (1965). Solvent extraction of chelate compounds in the presence of salts. Communication 3. Cobalt (II) and Uranium (VI) acetylacetonates. *Zhurnal Analyticheskoi Khimii*, **20**, 867–9.

Carey, F. A. (1987). *Organic Chemistry*, pp. 262–5. New York: McGraw-Hill.

Chemical Society of Japan (1984). *Kagakubinran*, 3rd edn. Tokyo: Maruzen Shuppan.

Hendrickson, J. B., Cram, D. J. & Hammond, G. S. (1970). *Organic Chemistry*, 3rd edn, pp. 175–230. Tokyo: McGraw-Hill.

Japanese Society for Analytical Chemistry (1991). *Bunsekikagakubinran*, 4th edn.

Kojima, I., Yoshida, M. & Tanaka, M. (1970). Distribution of carboxylic acids between organic solvents and aqueous perchloric acid solution. *Journal of Inorganic and Nuclear Chemistry*, **32**, 987–95.

Sekine, T., Isayama, M. Yamaguchi. S. & Moriya, H. (1967). Studies of liquid–liquid partition systems. V. The formation of mixed dimers with two carboxylic acids in carbon tetrachloride. *Bulletin of the Chemical Society of Japan*, **40**, 27–32.

Solomons, T. W. G. (1983). *Organic Chemistry*, 3rd edn, pp. 308–11. Toronto: John Wiley & Sons.

Zolotov, Y. A. (1972). *Chelate – kagoubutsu no Chuushutsu* (Extraction of chelate complexes), pp. 55–66. Tokyo: Baifuukann.

Zolotov, Y. A. & Lambrev, V. G. (1965). Solvent extraction of chelate compounds with 1-phenyl-3-methyl-4-benzoylpyrazolone-5. Extraction of calcium. *Zhurnal Analiticheskoi Khimii*, **20**, 659–64.

3

Measurement of acetate by enzymatic methods

M. ELIA AND G. JENNINGS

Despite the central role of acetate and its activated derivative, acetyl coenzyme A (acetyl-CoA), in mammalian metabolism, their accurate enzymatic measurement has proved difficult, especially in biological samples with low concentrations of these metabolites. The difficulties depend both on the type of sample (e.g. plasma, whole blood, tissue, wines, foodstuffs, bacterial products, etc.) and on the type of method used. To understand the advantages and disadvantages of the various enzymatic methods and how they compare with other non-enzymatic methods, it is necessary to consider the underlying principles of the techniques.

Since acetate has to be activated before it is metabolized, all enzymatic methods have involved an initial activation step, either to acetyl-CoA, as in mammals, or to acetyl phosphate, as in some bacterial species. Three types of enzymatic methods exist: those that measure acetyl-CoA (referred to as type-1 methods in this chapter), those that measure acetyl phosphate without subsequent formation of acetyl-CoA (referred to as type-2 methods) and those that measure a product of the activation process (i.e. measurement of ADP, which is formed during the phosphorylation of acetate to acetyl phosphate; referred to as type-3 methods). Figure 3.1 illustrates the major pathways involved in various enzymatic methods, but further details may be found in the appropriate sections.

Type-1 methods (1a–d) – measurement of acetate using acetyl-CoA as intermediate

Formation of acetyl-CoA (methods 1a–c)

Three methods are described for activating acetate to acetyl-CoA, giving rise to three type-1 methods for measuring acetate (1a–c).

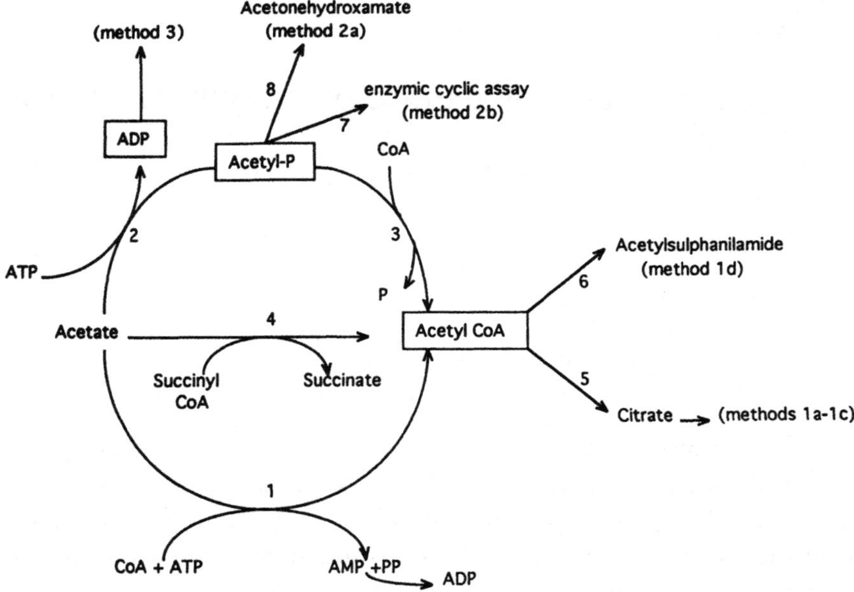

Fig. 3.1. Metabolic pathways involved in some enzymatic assays for acetate. Type-1 methods refer to measurements of acetyl-CoA, type-2 methods to measurement of acetyl-phosphate (Acetyl-P), and type-3 methods to measurement of ADP, formed during the activation of acetate to acetyl-phosphate (for details, see text). The enzymes involved are: 1, acetyl-CoA synthetase (ACS, EC 6.2.1.1); 2, acetate kinase (AK, EC 2.7.2.1); 3, phosphotransacetylase (PTA, EC 2.3.1.8); 4, acetate-CoA-transferase (EC 2.8.3.8); 5, citrate synthase (CS, EC 4.1.3.7); 6, arylamine-*N*-acetyl transferase (EC 2.3.1.5); 7, see text; 8, non-enzymatic. For further details of individual methods and enzymes, see text.

Method 1a

In method 1a, acetyl-CoA is formed from acetate with the use of the enzymes acetate kinase (AK, EC 2.7.2.1) and phosphotransacetylase (PTA, EC 2.3.1.8) (Bergmeyer & Möllering, 1966, 1974; Guynn & Veech, 1974; Seufert *et al.*, 1974; Jorfeldt & Juhlin-Dannfelt, 1978).

Method 1b

In method 1b, acetyl-CoA is formed directly from acetate with the use of the enzyme acetyl-CoA synthetase (ACS, EC 6.2.1.1) (Stegink, 1967; Seufert, Mewes & Soeling, 1984; Bartelt & Kattermann, 1985) (commercial kit from Boehringer Mannheim, kit no. 148261).

Method 1c

In method 1c, acetyl-CoA is formed directly from acetate with the use of the enzyme acetate CoA transferase (EC 2.8.3.8) from *Propionibacterium shermanii* (Schulmann & Wood, 1971).

The first two methods (1a and 1b) have been used much more widely than the third method (1c).

Measurement of acetyl-CoA using the malate dehydrogenase reaction as the preceding indicator reaction (methods 1a, b, c)

Acetyl-CoA, formed from actate, has been measured either by the use of a preceding indicator reaction (see below, methods 1a–c), which is described first, because it is by far the most common method, or by its reaction with sulphanilamide (method 1d).

In methods 1a–c, acetyl-CoA formed from acetate reacts with oxaloacetate to form citrate, under the catalytic activity of the enzyme citrate synthetase (CS, EC 4.1.3.7). The amount of oxaloacetate removed (and therefore the amount of acetate in the original sample) is measured by assessing the displacement of the malate–oxaloacetate equilibrium reaction. This reaction, which is catalysed by malate dehydrogenase (MDH, EC 1.1.1.37), acts as the indicator reaction. Removal of oxaloacetate is associated with the formation of NADH, which is measured by the change in absorbance (typically at 340 nm). The quantitative relationship between the substrate (acetate) and NADH formed is not a simple equimolar relationship, as it is for many other NAD/NADH-linked enzymatic assays, because the change in absorbance is due to removal of oxaloacetate (OA) from a near-equilibrium reaction. Therefore, 1 mol acetate is associated with the removal of 1 mol OA and the formation of less than 1 mol NADH.

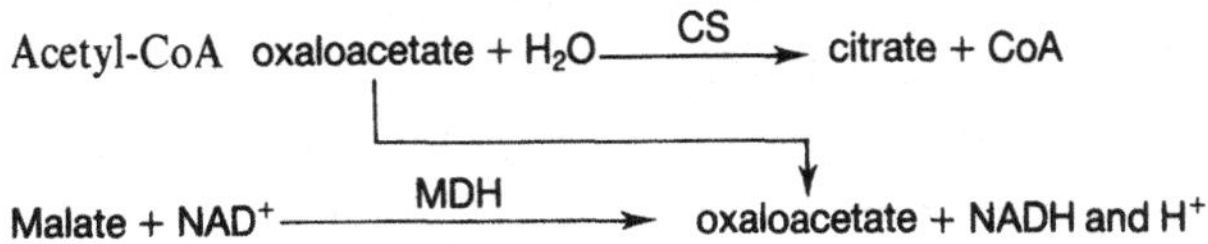

The extent of this inequality is also affected by the pH at which the reaction is performed, since hydrogen ions affect the equilibrium position (see equation above, and Bergmeyer & Möllering, 1974).

The principles of enzyme reactions coupled to a preceding enzyme indicator were first described in 1947 (Bücher, 1947), and 15–20 years later they were applied to the measurement of acetate in pure solutions (Pearson, 1965; Buckel & Eggerer, 1965) and in biological material (Bergmeyer & Möllering, 1966). One of the important requirements of such assays is that the equilibrium position of the indicator reaction favours the side of the starting material (in this case, malate – the equilibrium constant of the reaction, i.e. [OA][NADH][H]/[malate][NAD], is between 9×10^{-2} and 10×10^{-12} M at pH 7.4–8.0), and the overall reaction favours the other side (in this case, OA and NADH). Therefore, as oxaloacetate is removed to form citrate, a substantial amount of NADH (a little less than equimolar amounts) is formed. Two important implications follow. The first is that side reactions affecting the concentrations of the metabolites involved in the MDH reaction have important effects on the results. Removal of NADH (e.g. by contamination with the enzyme NADH oxidase) gives erroneously low results, whilst removal of oxaloacetate (e.g. to pyruvate by enzymatic contamination with OA decarboxylase) gives erroneously high results. The second is that when a low concentration of oxaloacetate, which is determined by the equilibrium constant of the MDH present in the reaction mixture, is associated with a low concentration of acetyl-CoA (e.g. due to low concentration of acetate in the sample), the reaction proceeds slowly and therefore large quantities of enzyme are required.

Since methods 1a–c require the enzymes that form acetyl-CoA from acetate (one or two enzymes – see Fig. 3.1) as well as enzymes for measuring acetyl-CoA (malate dehydrogenase and citrate synthase), up to four or sometimes five enzymes (see below for addition of lactate dehydrogenase in method 1a) are used in the assay. The last of the enzymes to be added to the mixture is the enzyme that activates acetate (i.e. acetate kinase in method 1a and 1c, and acetyl-CoA synthetase in method 1b – see above). The reaction is usually carried out in a buffer, such as triethanolamine pH 7.5–8.0 in the presence of ATP, CoA, NAD, NADH and magnesium chloride. Three absorbances are measured: the first after sample and buffer are mixed (A_0); the second after addition of malate dehydrogenase and citrate synthase (A_1); and the third after addition of the starter enzyme (A_2). In each case the plateau absorbance is used in the calculation (see Fig. 3.2). The general formula used to calculate the change in absorbance due to acetic acid (ΔA acetate) is not straightforward (for derivation see Bergmeyer & Möllering, 1974).

$$\Delta A \text{ acetate} = \left[(A_2 - A_0)\text{ sample } - \frac{(A_1 - A_0)^2 \text{ sample}}{(A_2 - A_0)\text{ sample}}\right] - \left[(A_2 - A_0)\text{ blank} - \frac{(A_1 - A_0)^2 \text{ blank}}{(A_2 - A_0)\text{ blank}}\right]$$

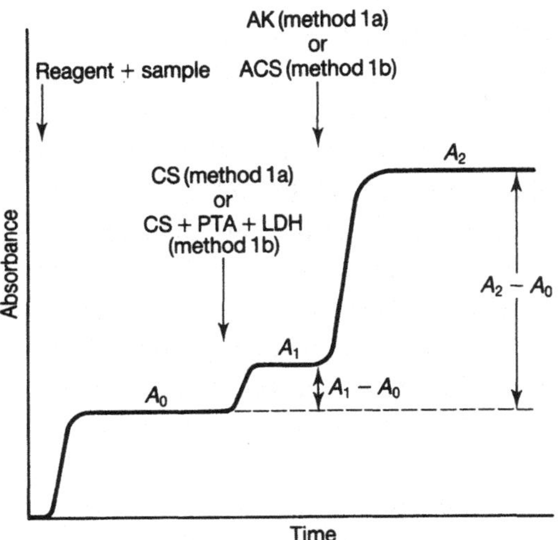

Fig. 3.2. Change in absorbance during the enzymatic determination of acetate using acetate kinase (AK) and phosphotransacetylase (PTA) (method 1a) or acetyl-CoA synthetase (ACS) (method 1b). The reagent containing CoA, ATP, NAD, malate dehydrogenase and citrate synthetase (CS) is added to the sample to produce absorbance A_0. The change in absorbance $(A_1 - A_0)$ is due to the presence in the sample of acetyl-CoA (method 1b) or acetyl-CoA + acetyl-phosphate (method 1a) as well as to the added enzymes. The further increase in absorbance following addition of the final 'start' enzymes is due to acetate. PTA, phosphotransacetylase; LDH, lactate dehydrogenase.

Purity of reagents

Because multiple enzymes are used in the assay, it is important to ensure that the enzymes are sufficiently pure to prevent side reactions from occurring. For example, malate dehydrogenase must be virtually free of all the other enzymes ($<0.05\%$). Citrate synthase should not contain acetate kinase ($<0.02\%$). None of the enzymes should be contaminated with enzymes that affect products of the malate hydrogenase reaction, e.g. NADH oxidase, aminotransferases and oxaloacetate decarboxylase ($<0.001\%$), or lactate dehydrogenase (unless this enzyme is added early on, to remove pyruvate – see below). It makes little difference if the final starter enzymes (acetate kinase in method 1a or acetyl-CoA synthetase in method 1b) contain the major enzymes already present in the incubation medium (e.g. MDH or CS).

Precision and recovery

This varies with the sample being tested and the concentration of acetate. For example, method 1a has been reported to measure acetate in wine

($\approx$5 mmol/l) with a coefficient of variation (CV) of 1.7% (Bergmeyer & Möllering, 1974). A microfluorimetric adaptation of the same method has been reported to measure plasma acetate ($\approx$0.85 mmol/l, after alcohol ingestion) with a CV of 4.4% and a recovery of 93–103% (Jorfeldt & Juhlin-Dannfelt, 1978). In another study, in which method 1b was automated on a centrifugal analyser in order to measure low plasma acetate concentrations (0.1 mmol/l), the CV was found to be $\approx$3% (G. Jennings & M. Elia, unpublished data). The use of method 1a to measure acetate in samples of rat tissue has been reported to be associated with a CV as low as $\approx$1%, and a recovery of 95–98% (Guynn & Veech, 1974).

Specificity

The assay is specific for acetate. In method 1a, acetate kinase reacts with propionic acid at about 2% of the rate as with acetate. This is of little significance for measurements in human peripheral blood, which contains little propionate.

Interference with the assay

Errors may also arise from the presence of samples of metabolites involved in the MDH equilibrium. However, in plasma the concentrations of malate, oxaloacetate, NAD and NADH are too low for such interference, although in tissue extracts the concentrations of NAD/NADH may be sufficiently high to cause some interference. The concentration of acetyl-CoA and acetyl phosphate in the sample should be relatively low in comparison to that of acetate. It is possible to separate acetate from the above interfering compounds as well as amino acids plus ketoglutarate, by prior distillation or freeze-transfer. NAD and NADH can also be absorbed on charcoal.

Incorrect results are obtained when the enzymes employed are contaminated with other enzymes that affect reactants or products of the MDH reaction: NADH oxidase removes NAD; oxaloacetate decarboxylase removes oxaloacetate; transaminases in the presence of amino acids and ketoglutarate remove oxaloacetate; lactate dehydrogenase (LDH, EC 1.1.1.27) forms NADH in the presence of pyruvate. Since the pyruvate/lactate equilibrium is very much in favour of lactate (the equilibrium constant is similar to that of the MDH reaction) extra LDH may be added to rapidly remove pyruvate, and prevent a subsequent reaction drift. However, such an addition is only necessary when LDH is likely to be a contaminant. In general, the presence of lactate (as opposed to pyruvate) in plasma and tissue samples has little effect on the results, because the equilibrium between lactate and pyruvate is strongly in favour of lactate. Interference due to insufficient purity of the various enzymes is suggested by a slow 'drift' in absorbance at the end of the reaction. If there is a constant drift in absorbance at the end of the reaction, this can be taken into account by extrapolating to the time of addition of the final starter enzyme. A change in absorbance (independent of drift) of more than about 0.1 absorbance units is desirable.

Measurement of acetyl-CoA using sulphanilamide (method 1d)

Another method for measuring acetyl-CoA, formed from acetate, employs sulphanilamide (method 1d). The enzymatic method (Soodak, 1948, 1957; Lundquist, Fugmann & Rasmussen, 1961; Lindeneg *et al.*, 1964; Murthy & Steiner, 1972; Lundquist *et al.*, 1973; Lundquist, 1974; Juhlin-Dannfelt, 1977), which has been used to measure acetate in tissue homogenates and blood, is included for completeness. It is not commonly used today, partly because the procedure is tedious and may be subject to interference from other compounds, and partly because of the lack of commercially available arylamine acetyltransferase (AAT) (acetyl-CoA: arylamine *N*-acetyltransferase – EC 2.3.1.5), which is used in the method.

The method, which employs a crude enzymatic preparation from pigeon liver (Lundquist, 1974), involves measurement of sulphanilamide (Bratton & Marshall, 1939), before and after it has reacted with the acetyl-CoA that is formed from acetate.

$$\text{Acetate} + \text{ATP} + \text{CoA} \xrightarrow{\text{ACS}} \text{acetyl-CoA} + \text{AMP} + \text{PP}$$

$$\text{Acetyl-CoA} + \text{sulphanilamide} \xrightarrow{\text{Non-enzymic}} \text{acetylsulphanilamide} + \text{CoA}$$

The recovery of acetyl sulphanilamide is variable and may be less than 85%. Therefore, appropriate standard curves are necessary. The acetylation of sulphanilamide (Lundquist *et al.*, 1961) is inhibited by alkali metal ions such as calcium ($\approx$50% inhibition by $CaCl_2$ at 100 mM, and to a much smaller extent by KCl and NaCl). Such interference may again be avoided by distillation or diffusion of acetate, although the error from this source is not likely to be significant in many biological samples. Plasma acetate has been reported to be measured with a precision of 5 μmol/l (Lundquist, 1974).

Other short-chain fatty acids produce little interference with this method. The colour changes with propionate, butyrate and valerate are 0.3–1.4% of that produced with an equivalent amount of acetate (Soodak, 1957; Lundquist *et al.*, 1961). Formate and pyruvate do not interfere (Soodak, 1957). However, the assay for sulphanilamide is not specific, since colour development occurs with therapeutic drugs such as paracetamol, metoclopramide and other sulphanamides. Furthermore, acetoacetate, which is normally found in plasma and tissues, especially during ketosis, produces almost the same colour change as equivalent amounts of acetate (Lundquist *et al.*, 1961). In order to remove this source of interference, and at the same time to improve the sensitivity of the method (e.g. when low tissue- or blood-acetate concentrations are measured), the acetate is separated and concentrated by distillation or diffusion. In the diffusion method, Conway dishes are used with potassium hydroxide (used to trap acetate) in the central well, and the sample in the outer well (Conway & Downey, 1950).

Type 2 methods (2a and 2b) – determination of acetate using acetyl phosphate (and not acetyl-CoA) as intermediate

Acetyl phosphate, formed from acetate under the catalytic activity of acetate kinase, can be used to assess the concentration of acetate in a sample by two separate methods (2a and 2b), neither of which involve acetyl-CoA. One of these methods (method 2a) is a colorimetric assay involving hydroxyamine, and is an order of magnitude less sensitive than other enzymatic assays, and the other (method 2b) is a cyclic enzymatic assay, which is up to an order of magnitude more sensitive than other enzymatic assays.

Determination with acetate kinase and hydroxylamine (method 2a)

This method (Rose, 1955; Holtz & Bergmeyer, 1974) is suitable for samples containing large amounts of acetate. It is not sensitive enough for assaying acetate in normal peripheral human blood.

The method depends on the principle that acyl phosphate (in this case acetyl phosphate formed from acetate in the presence of acetate kinase) forms

$$\text{Acetate} + \text{ATP} \xrightarrow{\text{AK}} \text{acetyl-P} + \text{ADP}$$

acetyl-P → (H_2NOH, non-enzymic; → P) → acetone hydroxamate ($CH_3CONHOH$)

hydroxamic acid, at a pH close to neutrality, and subsequently, a red- to red–violet-coloured ferric-hydroxamate complex (optimum absorbance 490 nm) in acid solution. The colour intensity is proportional to the amount of acetate.

Precision

The CV for measurement of acetate in wine (5–6 mmol/l) is reported to be 4–6% (Holtz & Bergmeyer, 1974).

Interference

Fatty acids, esters of fatty acids, lactones and acid amines may produce high blanks. The ATP used should be free of ADP, and acetate kinase should not be contaminated with ATPase.

Specificity

Acetate kinase reacts with acetate and to a slight extent with propionate ($\approx$2% of the rate observed with acetate). No reactions occur with acids such as formate, butyrate, valerate or long-chain fatty acids. Fluoroacetate also does not react. Hydroxylamine reacts with acetyl phosphate, other acyl phosphates, acid amines, acid anhydrides, aldehydes and esters (Pilz, 1958; Holz & Bergmeyer, 1974). A correction for the absorbance of these other substances can be made by treating an aliquot of the sample in exactly the same way as the test sample, with the exception that no acetate kinase is added.

Measurement of acetate by monitoring the rate of acetate–acetyl phosphate cycling, using acetate kinase and acetyl phosphate–hexose phosphotransferase (method 2b)

In this method (Buckley & Williamson, 1977) acetyl phosphate is formed from acetate in the presence of acetate kinase. The phosphate from acetyl phosphate is then transferred to glucose to form glucose-6-phosphate under the catalytic activity of acyl hexose phosphotransferase (EC 2.7.1.61). The glucose-6-phosphate is then oxidized using glucose-6-phosphate dehydrogenase (EC 1.1.1.49), and the resultant NADPH is measured spectrophotometrically (Fig. 3.3). Since acetate is utilized and produced simultaneously, its concentration remains constant, but for every revolution of the cycle, one equivalent of NADPH is formed. Because of the high K_m of acetate kinase for acetate ($\approx$0.3 M) and the low K_m of acyl phosphate–hexose phosphotransferase for acetyl phosphate ($\approx$0.5 mM) and glucose-6-

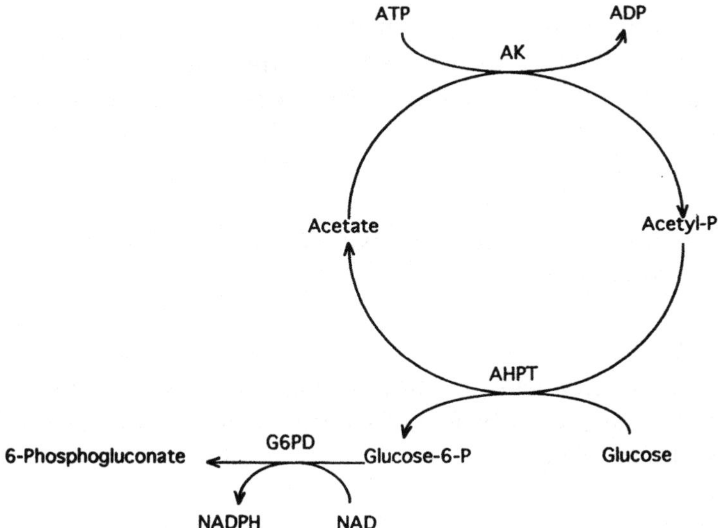

Fig. 3.3. Cyclic assay for measuring acetate. The enzymes are acetate kinase (AK, EC 2.7.2.1), acyl hexose phosphotransferase (AHPT, EC 2.7.1.61) and glucose-6-phosphate dehydrogenase (G6PD, EC 1.1.1.49).

phosphate dehydrogenase for glucose-6-phosphate ($\approx$20 μM), the rate of the cycle is linearly related to the acetate concentration in blood and tissues. Linear rates of reaction are reported for up to 60 min (Buckley & Williamson, 1977). The assay is a kinetic assay and is temperature-dependent.

Cyclic assays amplify the response by forming more end product or indicator (in this case NADPH). The assay is therefore more sensitive than the other enzymatic assays for acetate. The assay can be monitored continuously and assessed for linearity – unlike other cycling assays, which are end-point assays – and the use of NADPH, which is a more specific indicator than NADH, means that interference from contaminating enzymes and various tissue metabolites is less likely. In view of this, it has been argued (Buckley & Williamson, 1977) that there is less need for sample purification in this method compared with other enzymatic assays (Lundquist, 1963, 1974; Bergmeyer & Möllering, 1974). However, the presence of glucose in biological samples and as an enzyme contaminant in commercial preparations of acetate kinase that phosphorylate glucose is potentially an important problem (see below and method 3). The enzyme phosphohexose phosphotransferase, which is also used in the assay, is not generally available and therefore experience with this method is limited.

Interference

Negative interference Like other kinetic assays, this can be affected by substances that alter the activity of the rate-limiting enzyme. For example, tissue or plasma samples are normally deproteinized with perchloric acid and then neutralized with KOH, which largely removes the perchlorate, as potassium perchlorate is a precipitate. Residual perchlorate can have a substantial inhibitory effect on the cycling rate (Buckley & Williamson, 1977). The blanks and standards should therefore be prepared in the same way as the samples. Some tissues, such as liver obtained from the rat, also contain an inhibitory substance, but use of small sample volumes can overcome this effect, as assessed by recovery of added acetate (Buckley & Williamson, 1977). The recovery of 5 nmol of acetate added to blood samples, which are subsequently deproteinized and neutralized (0.05–1.0 ml/cuvette), is usually greater than 95%

Positive interference The assay cannot distinguish between the presence of acetate and acetyl phosphate in the samples. Acetyl phosphate is not considered to be an important intermediate in mammalian metabolism, but it may be in bacterial metabolism. Any glucose-6-phosphate present in the original sample reacts with glucose initially, but is not recycled. Similarly, other acyl phosphates may be involved with the phosphotransferase reaction, but they are not regenerated, due to the specificity of acetyl kinase. Therefore, the reaction mixture is allowed to stabilize for a few minutes before linearity measurements are made. However, some commercial batches of acetyl kinase contain a substantial amount of hexokinase, and therefore, a continuous independent supply of glucose-6-phosphate may produce erroneously high results for acetic acid. The batch-to-batch variation in hexokinase contamination may be substantial and the potential errors large. Absence of an absorbance change with a pure glucose solution indicates absence of such contamination. If enzymatic contamination is present, it may be necessary to remove glucose prior to the assay (see also method 3).

Type-3 method – measurement of ADP formed during activation of acetate

In this method it is not acetate carbon that is measured, but the ADP formed during the phosphorylation of acetate to acetyl phosphate (Ballard, Filsell & Jarrett, 1972; Knowles *et al.*, 1974; Skutches *et al.*, 1979; Trivin *et al.*, 1982; Akanji, Ng & Humphreys, 1988; Coppack *et al.*, 1990; Frayn *et al.*, 1990) (see

Fig. 3.1). Theoretically, there is also the opportunity of measuring ADP or AMP or PP, which are formed either directly or indirectly during the activation of acetate to acetyl-CoA (see Fig. 3.1). In the method described here, ADP formed during the activation of acetate to acetyl phosphate is linked to an NADH reaction. The change in absorbance due to the NADH is related to the amount of acetate in the sample.

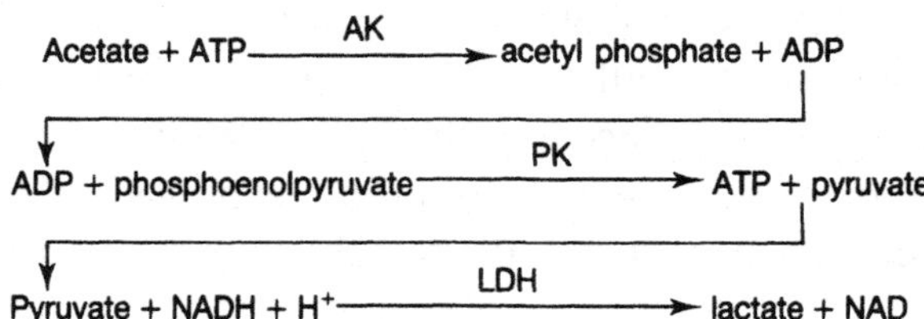

The reagent mixture containing ATP, NADH and the enzymes pyruvate kinase (PK) and lactate dehydrogenase is incubated with the sample to ensure removal of any pyruvate present in the sample, and to attempt to ensure that non-specific side reactions are complete, as indicated by steady absorbance readings relative to the control sample. The starter enzyme (acetate kinase) is then added and the absorbance monitored. The concentration of acetate is calculated either according to kinetic analysis (slope of the initial change in absorbance with time) or by the end-point method, which takes longer. Some workers have preferred to use the kinetic method, because of suspected time-dependent spontaneous hydrolysis of acetyl phosphate (Ballard *et al.*, 1972; Knowles *et al.*, 1974), although this has not been considered to be a problem by others (Akanji, 1987).

Precision

The between-batch variation for measurement of plasma acetate using this method has been reported to be 7–8% at a concentration of about 0.12 mmol/l, and 4.4% at a concentration of 0.55 mmol/l (Smith, Humphries & Hockaday, 1986). The same authors reported that the mean recovery of addition to plasma of 0.25, 0.5 and 1.0 mmol/l acetate was 108 ± 2%. In other studies the coefficient of variation ranged from 3.5 to 7.5% for acetate concentrations between 3.0 mmol/l and 0.3 mmol/l, respectively, and the analytical recovery by adding acetate to plasma (to increase the concentration by 0.5 to 4.0 mmol) ranged from 91 to 113% (Trivin *et al.*, 1982).

Possible interfering substances

Acetylcarnitine, which is found in plasma, has no detectable effect on the assay. Organic acetate, such as ethyl acetate, also has a negligible effect. Acetoacetate (0.25 M), pyruvate (0.25 mM), glycerol (0.25 mM), hydroxybutyrate (0.5 mM), lactate (1 M) and non-esterified fatty acids (1 mM), also have negligible effects on the assay, either alone or in combination (Akanji, 1987). Acetate kinase has been reported to react with propionate (Lipmann & Tuttle, 1945) but only to a small extent. The large change in blank absorbance, which may be two to three times greater than that due to the acetate (Smith, Humphries & Hockaday, 1986), is of some concern, and presumably results from degradation of NADH in non-specific side reactions that are activated by impurities in the added enzymes.

Another major problem encountered with some preparations of acetate kinase is their reported contamination with variable amounts of hexokinase (HK) (Smith *et al.*, 1986) to an extent that could more than double the apparent plasma acetate concentration.

$$\text{Glucose} + \text{ATP} \rightarrow \text{glucose-6-P} + \text{ADP}$$

This is because the method essentially measures ADP, and the formation of ADP during phosphorylation of glucose is an obvious source of interference. Each batch of acetate kinase should be routinely checked for this contamination (e.g. by running glucose standards), because there seems to be substantial batch-to-batch variation in the contamination of some commercial preparations (Smith *et al.*, 1986). If contamination is confirmed the glucose in the samples should be removed prior to analysis (e.g. by incubating the sample with glucose oxidase). Some workers have chosen to remove glucose routinely from the sample (Smith *et al.*, 1986), although this had not been practised previously by those using this method (Ballard *et al.*, 1972; Knowles *et al.*, 1974; Trovin *et al.*, 1982).

Sample preparation and storage (methods 1, 2 and 3)

Using a gas–liquid chromatography (GLC) method, Nielson, Ash & Thor (1978) reported that acetate concentrations were stable in plasma/serum and standard aqueous solutions when stored for 10 days at 4 °C and 3 months at −20 °C. Repeated freezing and thawing were not found to have an effect. Akanji (1987), using an enzymatic method (method 3), found no increase in acetate when plasma was stored at 4 °C for 24 h or at −20 °C for up to 6 months.

Kveim & Bredesen (1979) reported that storage of heparinized whole blood for 30 h at 4 °C had no effect on plasma acetate concentration, although at room temperature there was a 40% increase. Plasma stored at −20 °C over 5 months showed no further change in acetate concentrations.

Tollinger, Vreman & Weiner (1979) reported that storage of whole blood at 27 °C for 2 h increased the acetate concentration (measured by GLC) relative to that observed during 2-h storage at 4 °C (38 ± 0.8 v. 29 ± 0.7 μmol/l). These workers also reported an increase in plasma acetate concentrations during storage at −20 °C (26 ± 6 v. 63 ± 4 μmol/l) for 24 h but no further increase after 30 days of storage. Some increase was also observed when plasma, with high acetate concentrations obtained during dialysis, was stored at −20 °C for 24 h. These authors considered that some acetate esters might be hydrolysed during freezing and thawing. However, the different results obtained by various workers are difficult to explain.

The measurement of acetate in tissue extracts is routinely associated with deproteinization, which removes turbidity and precipitates tissue enzymes that may cross-react in the assay. Measurement of acetate in plasma/serum has often been carried out without prior protein precipitation, e.g. in the methods of types 1a, 1b and 3. Deproteinization has not been found to have any significant effect on the results with the use of the type-3 method (Akanji, 1987).

The possible interference of other substrates in the acetate assays (e.g. acetoacetate in the sulphanilamide assay or other substrates in tissue samples on the assays involving malic dehydrogenase) can be removed by prior distillation of acetate (e.g. with Bartley's (1953) distillation procedure), or diffusion (Conway & Downey, 1950; see method 1d). No sample preparation is usually necessary for the enzymatic measurement of acetate in wine or vinegar, but dilution may be necessary. Coloured juices may be decolourized with charcoal prior to analysis. With certain types of beers, it may be necessary to remove most of the CO_2 by stirring, to prevent interference with gas bubbles. Solid foodstuffs are usually deproteinized prior to analysis.

The possible interference of acetylated compounds in enzymatic and non-enzymatic acetate assays has been repeatedly considered, although a detailed systematic assessment of the effects of a large variety of acetylated compounds in different buffers and pHs does not appear to have been carried out. Tollinger *et al.* (1979) suggested that during storage there might be an increase in plasma acetate concentrations, due to hydrolysis of acetylated compounds. Acetyl carnitine is normally found in plasma, but acetyl-CoA is not. On the other hand, acetyl-CoA is one of the most important acetylated compounds in tissues. Aqueous solutions of acetyl-CoA at pH 3–6 can be frozen for weeks without loss of activity. In alkaline solutions hydrolysis occurs rapidly, and therefore, care must be taken when acidic deproteinized samples are neutralized with strong KOH, not to render the samples alkaline (Decker, 1974). The half-life of S-acyl derivatives of saturated fatty acids with 2 to 8 carbons (Stadtman, 1957) is only 1–2 min in 0.1N NaOH at 30 °C. In general, the lower the pK_a of the acid, the more unstable is the thiol ester in alkali. There may be slow loss of activity in very acid solutions. Some acetylated compounds, e.g. acetyl adenylic acid (acetyl-AMP; Berg, 1956), are said to be hydolysed in acid pH. However, acetyl adenylic acid, which is an intermediate in the conversion of acetyl-CoA, is not released (and therefore does not accumulate) in the free form, since it is bound (like other acyl-AMPs) to the enzyme involved in the reaction (acetyl-CoA synthetase).

Discussion

The above description of methods emphasizes the multiple problems that face many of the enzymatic assays for acetate. In general, they perform well with pure solutions of acetate and with biological samples containing high concentrations of acetate. For example, for plasma acetate concentrations ranging from about 0.5 to 7.0 mmol/l a good agreement was reported between the ADP method (type-3 method) and a gas chromatographic technique (Trivin *et al.*, 1982). At the lower concentrations measured, the chromatographic technique gave lower readings relative to this enzymatic method.

Table 3.1 shows the circulating acetate concentrations obtained by various authors, who used different methods. This variability may be partly biological in origin, since various workers studied their subjects after variable periods of fasting (usually overnight fasting). Widely different results are more easily explained on methodological grounds. However, differences between two methods do not prove the superiority of one method over the other, since problems could exist with either or both methods. Nevertheless, there is concern about the large discrepancy in some of the results (e.g. the type-3 method appears to give higher results than do most other methods).

Discrepancies between enzymatic methods are more likely to occur in the analysis of biological samples with low acetate concentrations (M. Elia and G. Jennings, unpublished data). A good recovery of added acetate is not a sufficient test of the accuracy of the method. This is because non-specific reactions could co-exist, giving erroneously high and constant background results (interpreted as being acetate), without affecting recoveries of added acetate. Several examples of possible interfering substances are given in the

Table 3.1. *Concentrations of acetate (±SD or range) in the peripheral venous circulation of healthy subjects after an overnight fast, measured by different methods. Measurements in arterial blood may be substantially lower, due to utilization of acetate by peripheral limb tissues*

Method	[Acetate] (mmol/l)	Authors
Enzymatic[a]		
Type 3	0.27 ± 0.13 (male)	Trivin *et al.* (1982)
Type 3	0.31 ± 0.12 (female)	Trivin *et al.* (1982)
Type 3	0.15 ± 0.03	Smith *et al.* (1986)
Type 3	0.17 ± 0.04	Akanji *et al.* (1988)
Type 3	0.17 ± 0.03	Skutches *et al.* (1979)
Type 1a	0.065 ± 0.019	Bergmeyer & Möllering (1966)
Type 1b[b]	0.026 ± 0.012 (lean)	Seufert *et al.* (1984)
Type 1b[b]	0.029 ± 0.010 (obese)	Seufert *et al.* (1984)
Type 1b	0.065 ± 0.02	M. Elia & G. Jennings (unpublished data)
Type 1b	0–0.10 (male)	Bartelt & Kattermann (1985)
	0–0.07 (female)	Bartelt & Kattermann (1985)
Type 1d[c]	0.025–0.042	Lundquist (1962)
Gas–liquid chromatography (GLC)		
	0.051 ± 0.026	Tollinger *et al.* (1979)
	0·054 ± 0.016	Pomare *et al.* (1985)
	0.035 ± 0.007	Dankert *et al.* (1981)
	0.102 ± 0.035	Tangerman *et al.* (1983)
	0.04–0.070	Kveim & Bredesen (1979)
	<0.1–0.35	Laker & Mansell (1978)
GLC/mass spectroscopy		
	0.037 ± 0.018	Rocchiccioli *et al.* (1989)

[a] Type-3 method involves measurement of ADP formed during activation of acetate to acetyl-phosphate. Type-1 methods involve formation and measurement of acetyl-CoA (for details, see text).
[b] Measurements made on whole blood after distillation. Concentrations of acetate in whole blood are usually 80–85% of those in plasma (Nielsen *et al.*, 1978; Akanji, 1987).
[c] Mean values for transition between fasting (17 h) and fed state. The higher values were obtained in the fed state.

sections on individual methods. These fall into three general categories: enzymes, substrates and general reagents used in sample preparation.

Firstly, since multiple enzymes are used in complex assays, it not surprising that contaminating enzymes interfere with the assays. A good example is the variable contamination of some commercial preparations of acetate kinase with an enzyme that phosphorylates glucose to yield ADP and glucose-6-

phosphate. Smith *et al.* (1986) considered this enzyme to be hexokinase. Therefore, type-3 methods, which measure ADP, and the type-2b method, which measures glucose-6-phosphate, may overestimate acetate concentrations. This enzyme contamination has led some workers to remove glucose routinely from their samples prior to analysis for acetate. However, this has often not been carried out by other workers, which means that acetate concentrations have been overestimated to an uncertain degree. Furthermore, in methods that attempt to remove glucose from the sample, it is important to ensure that virtually all the glucose has been removed. If the contaminating enzyme that phosphorylates glucose is hexokinase (Smith *et al.*, 1986) and is assumed to have a low K_m for glucose (≈ 0.1 mM, as in mammals), residual glucose in the reaction mixture may have a substantial effect on the results. However, we have found that the contaminating enzyme(s) in commercial preparations of acetate kinase may have a much higher K_m for glucose. The side reaction with glucose, which leads to overestimation of acetate, may be of little signficance at high acetate concentrations, but the percentage error at low concentrations may be large, e.g. more than twofold in plasma obtained after an overnight fast (Smith *et al.*, 1986; M. Elia and G. Jennings, unpublished data).

Secondly, a variety of substrates may also interfere with the assays. For example, in type-1 methods the presence in biological samples of NAD/NADH, oxaloacetate, malate (or substrates that form them or remove them) can cause significant interference if they are present in large quantitites. In plasma, they are not normally present in sufficient quantities to cause interference. However, in some tissue samples, their concentration could be sufficiently high to cause interference, in which case extra preparatory steps (e.g. distillation or diffusion of acetate) may be necessary, making the method more complex and more time-consuming. In method 1d, a diffusion procedure is routinely recommended. The presence of variable amounts of pyruvate in biological samples is an obvious source of interference in the pyruvate kinase–lactate dehydrogenase coupling reaction in method 3, but this source of interference is eliminated by converting pyruvate to lactate (with the use of lactate dehydrogenase), prior to addition of the starter enzyme.

Thirdly, the reagents used in the assay may also interfere with the assay. The extent of the problem clearly depends on the type and amount of reagent used. For example, in methods that involve distillation or microdiffusion of acetate (see above), 4 g sodium sulphate is often used per millilitre of distillate or diffusate. In one study, anhydrous sodium sulphate (Analar grade, British Drug Houses, Poole, Dorset, UK) was found to be contaminated with about 20 nmol acetate/g (Buckley, 1974). This amounts to contamination of only

1 part/million (w/w), but 4 g contains 80 nmol, which may equal the amount of acetate present in 1 ml distillate or diffusate (e.g. plasma). Lundquist *et al.* (1961) used a different source of sodium sulphate (p.a. grade, Merck, Darmstadt, Germany) and found it to contain only 3.5 nmol/g. However, even this may be too much when dealing with samples that have low concentrations of acetate. Reagents may produce erroneously low results by inhibiting the enzymes involved in kinetic assays (e.g. residual perchlorate in the cyclic assay – method 2b). Inhibitors present in biological samples may produce similar effects in kinetic methods (e.g. see method 2b).

The specificity of enzymatic assays can be improved either by using uncontaminated enzymes that specifically react with the test substance, or by using a purer solution of the test substance. The volatility of acetate provides an important means of separating it from most other interfering substances present in biological samples. Therefore, it should be possible to test the accuracy of various enzymatic methods by comparing results obtained on the biological sample with those obtained after distillation or diffusion of acetate (with appropriate correction of recovery, which can be readily done using [^{14}C]acetate). However, it is remarkable how little work along these lines has been carried out to rigorously test the accuracy and validity of many enzymatic methods described by various authors.

The choice of enzymatic method depends on at least three considerations. First, the sensitivity of the method is an important consideration. This is because the sensitivity of different methods varies by as much as one to two orders of magnitude (compare method 2b with 1d), and therefore only some are suitable for measuring low acetate concentrations, such as those found in normal plasma after an overnight fast. Methods 1a, b and c can measure as little as 10–15 nmol in a standard 3-ml cuvette, but the use of fluorimetry can detect as little as 1 nmol (Guynn & Veech, 1974). The cyclic enzymatic assay of Buckley & Williamson (1977) can measure 2.5 nmol/cuvette without the use of fluorimetery.

Second, it is possible to automate several of the enzymatic methods, but some are more difficult to automate than others. For example, it is easy to automate method 3, which requires a single enzyme, and more difficult to automate method 1, which requires two sequential additions of 'starter' enzymes. Although some commercial autoanalysers are able to cater for this requirement, others are not. Methods that require distillation or diffusion of acetate (e.g. method 1c) are obviously difficult to automate.

Third, some methods require enzymes such as CoA transferase (method 1c) or acyl phosphate–hexose phosphotransferase, which are not commercially available. This limits the use of the methods to only a few researchers. The use of a commercial kit (Boehringer Mannheim kit 148261) that uses acetyl-CoA synthetase to activate acetate directly to acetyl-CoA (method 1b) has two important advantages over methods that form acetyl-CoA via acetyl phosphate (method 1a). One of these is that fewer enzymes are used (two fewer if LDH is included in method 1a), which means that the risk of enzyme contamination is reduced. The other is that the K_m of acetyl-CoA synthetase for acetate (method 1b) is much higher (e.g. the enzyme from beef-heart mitochondria has a K_m for acetate of 8×10^{-4} M (Webster, 1965)) than that of acetate kinase for acetate (K_m 3×10^{-1} M (Rose, 1955)), which is used in method 1a. This means that the reaction in method 1b can proceed faster or can be undertaken with less enzyme. This reduces the risk of enzyme contamination and makes extrapolation more accurate when drift is present. The affinity of acetate-CoA-transferase for acetate (method 1c; K_m 7×10^{-3} M) (Schulmann & Wood, 1971) is intermediate between that of acetate kinase and acetyl-CoA synthetase.

Several of the enzymatic methods have the advantage over GLC methods, in that multiple automated assays can be carried out simultaneously. On the other hand, the GLC methods can provide quantitative information about other SCFA, such as butyrate and propionate, which are of biological interest. Theoretically, it should be possible to measure other individual SCFA by enzymatic techniques, but according to current thinking, this would require specific activation of individual SCFA (e.g. to CoA or phosphorylated derivatives) and/or subsequent specific coupling reactions. Unfortunately, the currently available enzymes and methods are not specific enough for this purpose.

References

Akanji, A. O. (1987). Measurement of plasma acetate in humans with reference to diabetes, dietary composition and bowel function. D Phil thesis, University of Oxford, Oxford.

Akanji, A. O., Ng, L. & Humphreys, S. (1988). Plasma acetate levels in response to intravenous fat or glucose/insulin infusions in diabetic and non-diabetic subjects. *Clinical Chemistry Acta*, **178**, 85–94.

Ballard, F. J., Filsell, O. H. & Jarrett, G. (1972). Effects of carbohydrate on lipogenesis in sheep. *Biochemical Journal*, **126**, 193–200.

Bartelt, U. & Kattermann, R. (1985). Enzymatic determination of acetate in serum. *Journal of Clinical Chemistry and Clinical Biochemistry*, **23**, 879–81.

Bartley, W. (1953). An effect of bicarbonate on the oxidation of pyruvate by kidney homogenates. *Biochemical Journal*, **53**, 305–12.

Berg, P. (1956). Acyl adenylates: the synthesis and properties of adenyl acetate. *Journal of Biological Chemistry*, **222**, 1015–23.

Bergmeyer, H. U. & Möllering, H. (1966). Enzymatische Bestimmung von Acetat. *Biochemical Zeitschrift*, **344**, 167–89.

Bergmeyer, H. U. & Möllerung, H. (1974). Acetate: determination with preceding indicator reaction. In *Methods of Enzymatic Analysis*, 2nd edn, vol. 3, ed. H. U. Bergmeyer, pp. 1566–74. Weinheim: Verlag Chemie; New York, London: Academic Press.

Bratton, A. C. & Marshall, E. K. (1939). A new coupling component for sulphanilamide determination. *Journal of Biological Chemistry*, **128**, 537–50.

Bücher, T. (1974). Über ein phosphatübertragendes Garungsferment. *Biochimica et Biophysica Acta*, **1**, 292–314.

Buckel, W. & Eggerer, H. (1965). Zur optischen Bestimmung von Citrat-Synthase und von Acetyl-coenzym A. *Biochemische Zeitschrift*, **343**, 29–43.

Buckley, B. M. (1974). Aspects of neonantal metabolism. D Phil thesis, University of Oxford, Oxford.

Buckley, B. M. & Williamson, D. H. (1977). Origins of blood acetate in the rat. *Biochemical Journal*, **168**, 539–45.

Conway, E. J. & Downey, M. (1950). Microdiffusion methods. Determination of acetic acid in biological fluids. *Biochemical Journal*, **47**, IV.

Coppack, S. W., Frayn, K. N., Humphreys, S. M., Whyte, P. L. & Hockaday, D. R. (1990). Arteriovenous difference across human adipose tissue and forearm tissue after an overnight fast. *Metabolism*, **39**, 384–90.

Dankert, J., Zijlstra, J. B. & Wolthers, B. G. (1981). Volatile fatty acids in human peripheral and portal blood: quantitative determination by vacuum distillation and gas chromatography. *Clinica Chimica Acta*, **110**, 301–7.

Decker, K. (1974). Acetyl-coenzyme A UV-spectrophotometeric assay. In *Methods of Enzymatic Analysis*, 2nd edn, vol. 3, ed. H. U. Bergmeyer, pp. 1988–93. New York, London: Academic Press.

Frayn, K. N., Coppack, S. W., Walsh, P. E., Butterworth, H. C., Humphreys, S. M. & Pedrosa, H. C. (1990). Metabolic responses of forearm and adipose tissues to acute ethanol ingestion. *Metabolism*, **39**, 958–66.

Guynn, R. W. & Veech, R. L. (1974). Direct enzymatic determination of acetate in tissue extracts on the presence of acetate esters. *Analytical Biochemistry*, **61**, 6–15.

Holz, G. & Bergmeyer, H. U. (1974). Determination (of acetate) with acetate kinase and hydroxylamine. In *Methods of Enzymatic Analysis*, 2nd edn, vol. 3, ed. H. U. Bergmeyer, pp. 1528–32. New York, London: Academic Press.

Jorfeldt, L. & Juhlin-Dannfelt, A. (1978). The influence of ethanol on splanchnic and skeletal muscle metabolism in man. *Metabolism*, **27**, 97–106.

Juhlin-Dannfelt, A. (1977). Ethanol effects of substrate utilisation by the human brain. *Scandinavian Journal of Clinical and Laboratory Investigation*, **37**, 443–9.

Knowles, S. E., Jarrett, I. G., Filsell, O. E. & Ballard, F. J. (1974). Production and utilization of acetate in mammals. *Biochemical Journal*, **142**, 401–11.

Kveim, M. & Bredesen, J. E. (1979). A gas chromatographic method for determination of acetate levels in body fluids. *Clinica Chimica Acta*, **92**, 27–32.

Laker, M. F. & Mansell, M. A. (1978). Measurement of acetate in aqueous solutions and plasma by gas phase chromatography using a porous polymer stationary phase. *Annals of Clinical Biochemistry*, **15**, 228–32.

Lindeneg, O., Mellemgaard, J., Fabricus, J. & Lundquist, F. (1964). Myocardial utilisation of acetate, lactate and free fatty acids after ingestion of ethanol. *Clinical Science*, **27**, 427–35.

Lipmann, F. & Tuttle, L. C. (1945). A specific method for the determination of acyl phosphate. *Journal of Biochemical Chemistry*, **159**, 21–8.

Lundquist, F. (1962). Production and utilisation of free acetate in man. *Nature*, **193**, 579–81.

Lundquist, F. (1963). Acetate: determination with acetyl CoA synthetase and sulphanilamide. In *Methods of Enzymatic Analysis*, 1st edn, ed. H. U. Bergmeyer, pp. 303–4. New York: Academic Press.

Lundquist, F. (1974). Determination (of acetate) with acetyl-CoA synthetase and sulphanilamide. In *Methods of Enzymatic Analysis*, 2nd edn, vol. 3, ed. H. U. Bergmeyer, pp. 1528–37. New York, London: Academic Press.

Lundquist, F., Fugmann, U. & Rasmussen, J. (1961). A specific method for the determination of free acetate in blood. *Biochemical Journal*, **80**, 393–7.

Lundquist, F., Sestoft, L., Damgard, S. E., Clausen, J. P. & Trap-Jensen, J. (1973). Utilization of acetate in the human forearm during exercise after ethanol ingestion. *Journal of Clinical Investigation*, **52**, 3231–5.

Murthy, V. K. & Steiner, G. (1972). Hepatic acetate levels in relation to altered lipid metabolism. *Metabolism*, **22**, 81–4.

Nielsen, L. G., Ash, K. O. & Thor, E. (1978). Gas chromatographic method for plasma acetate analysis in acetate intolerance studies. *Clinical Chemistry*, **24**, 348–50.

Pearson, D. J. (1965). Source of error in the assay of acetyl coenzymes A. *Biochemical Journal*, **95**, 23–4c.

Pilz, van W. (1958). Die analytische Verwendung von Eisen (III). *Hydroxamaten Zeitschrift für Analytische Chemie*, **162**, 81–92.

Pomare, E. W., Branch, W. J. & Cummings, J. H. (1985). Carbohydrate fermentation in the human colon and its relation to acetate concentrations in venous blood. *Journal of Clinical Investigation*, **75**, 1448–54.

Rocchiccioli, N., Lepetit, N. & Bougneres, P. F. (1989). Capillary gas–liquid chromatographic/mass spectrometric measurement of plasma acetate content and (2-^{13}C) acetate enrichment. *Biomedical and Environmental Mass Spectrometry*, **18**, 816–19.

Rose, I. A. (1955). Acetate kinase of bacteria (acetokinase). *Methods of Enzymology*, **1**, 591–5.

Schulmann, M. & Wood, H. G. (1971). Determination and degradation of micro-quantities of acetate. *Analytical Biochemistry*, **39**, 505–20.

Seufert, C. D., Graf, M., Janson, G., Kuhn, A. & Soling, H. D. (1974). Formation of free acetate by isolated perfused livers from normal, starved and diabetic rats. *Biochemical and Biophysical Research Communications*, **57**, 901–9.

Seufert, C. D., Mewes, W. & Soeling, H. D. (1984). Effect of long-term starvation on acetate and ketone body metabolism in obese patients. *European Journal of Clinical Investigation*, **14**, 163–70.

Skutches, C. L., Holroyde, C. P., Myers, R. N., Paul, P. & Reichard, G. A. (1979). Plasma acetate turnover and oxidation. *Journal of Clinical Investigation*, **64**, 708–13.

Smith, R. F., Humphries, S. & Hockaday, T. D. R. (1986). The measurement of plasma acetate by a manual or automated technique on diabetic and non-diabetic subjects. *Annals of Clinical Biochemistry*, **23**, 285–91.

Soodak, M. (1948). An enzymatic micromethod for determination of acetic acid (abstract). *Federation Proceedings*, **7**, 190–1.

Soodak, M. M. (1957). An enzymatic micromethod for the determination of acetate. In *Methods in Enzymology*, Vol. III, ed. S. P. Colowick & N. O. Kaplan, pp. 266–9. New York: Academic Press.

Stadtman, E. R. (1957). Preparation and assay of acyl coenzyme A and other thiol esters; use of hydroxylamine. *Methods in Enzymology*, **3**, 931–4.

Stegink, L. D. (1967). Micro-enzymic method for the quantitative analysis of acetyl groups in proteins and peptides. *Analytical Biochemistry*, **20**, 502–16.

Tangerman, A., van Schaik, A., Meuwese-Arends, M. T. & van Tongeren, J. H. M. (1983). Quantitative determination of C_2–C_8 volatile fatty acids in human serum by vacuum distillation and gas chromatography. *Clinica Chimica Acta*, **133**, 341–8.

Tollinger, C. D., Vreman, H. J. & Weiner, M. W. (1979). Measurement of acetate in human blood by gas chromatography; effects of sample preparation, feeding and various diseases. *Clinical Chemistry*, **25**, 1787–90.

Trivin, C., Lenoir, F., Bretaudiere, J. P. & Sachs, C. (1982). Enzymatic determination of acetate in serum or plasma using a centrifugal fast analyser. *Clinica Chimica Acta*, **121**, 43–50.

Webster, L. T. (1965). Studies of the acetyl coenzyme A synthetase reaction. II Crystalline acetyl coenzyme A synthetase. *Journal of Biological chemistry*, **240**, 4158–63.

4

Biochemistry and microbiology in the rumen

R. J. WALLACE

Introduction

The rumen is the best known of the anaerobic gut ecosystems and is unique in the depth in which microbiological aspects of its fermentation have been studied in relation to their physiological and nutritional impact on the host animal. Its fermentation differs from that of the hindgut in non-ruminants in many respects. The substrates of the fermentation are different: animals without foregut fermentation digest and absorb many of the easily digested nutrients before the digesta pass to the microbial fermentation; in the ruminant, all nutrients are exposed to microbial attack before they become subject to digestion by host enzymes. The microbial populations are different: fermentation in the mammalian hindgut is dominated by bacteria, with relatively few instances where other organisms such as anaerobic fungi are significant; the rumen contains similar bacteria, but also large numbers of ciliate protozoa and a smaller number of anaerobic fungi. The nutritional role of the fermentation is also different: short-chain fatty acids (SCFA) produced in the rumen are the animal's principal energy source, and the microbial cells formed during fermentation its main source of amino acids; in non-ruminants, the role of SCFA is smaller, and the microbial cells are not immediately available to provide a source of amino acids.

In many other respects the rumen fermentation differs from that of the hindgut. However, the similarities are arguably much greater than the differences. Both involve the conversion of polysaccharides and proteins to SCFA by mainly anaerobic micro-organisms in an environment where oxygen is present at low concentrations. A wide range of carbohydrates is broken down and simplified so that the sugars can enter the Embden–Meyerhof–Parnas glycolytic pathway. The purpose of all these converging pathways is to provide sugar phosphates that will then be converted to phosphoenol-pyruvate (PEP) and pyruvate and form ATP for growth. The diverging

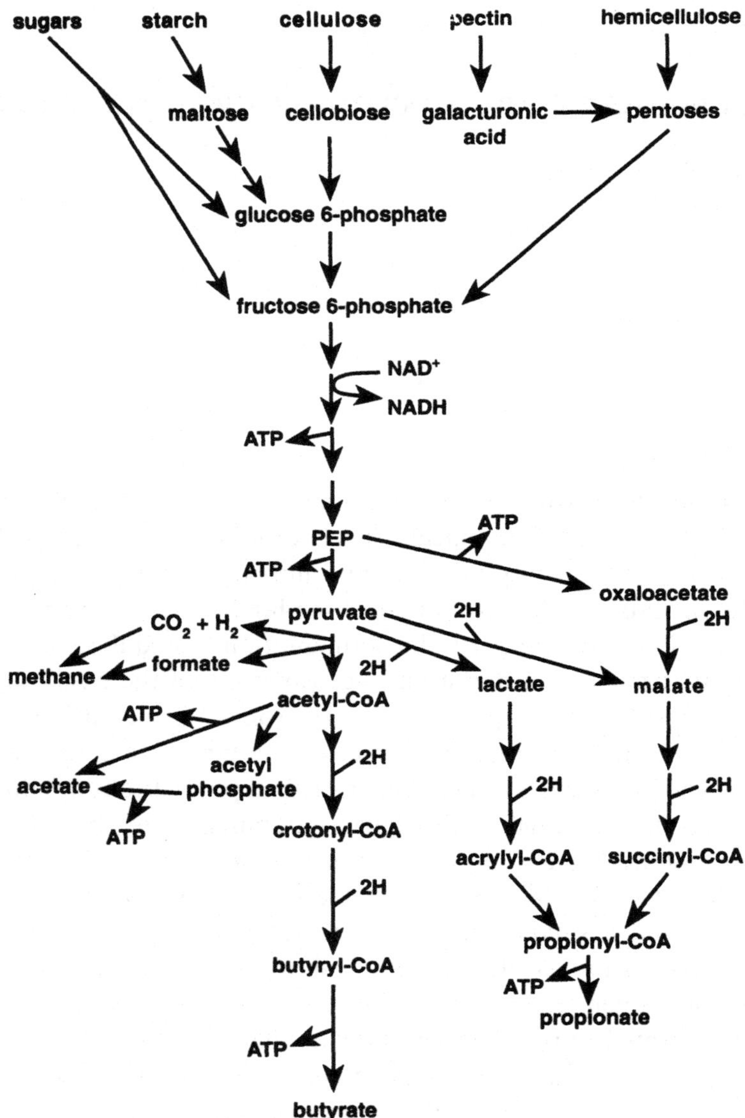

Fig. 4.1. The main metabolic pathways in rumen micro-organisms.

pathways from PEP and pyruvate onwards effectively operate to regenerate NAD^+ from the NADH formed during glycolysis, and thereby to allow the fermentation to continue. Since quantities of oxygen are limited, the rumen and gut micro-organisms resolve the metabolic problem by using internal redox couples, which ultimately lead to the formation of SCFA and methane. The overall process is summarized in Fig. 4.1.

Rumen micro-organisms

A huge variety of micro-organisms exists in the rumen. Ciliate protozoa, flagellate protozoa, yeasts, anaerobic fungi, bacteria, mycoplasmas and bacteriophages have all been observed or isolated. In terms of biomass, metabolic activity and number, the bacteria are usually predominant and always make up a substantial proportion of the total population. Numbers of ciliate protozoa are more than 10^3 times less than the bacteria, but their large size means that they can form over 50% of the biomass. On the other hand, numbers of ciliates are sometimes small and they may even be absent. The biomass of anaerobic fungi is more difficult to determine, because it is so intimately associated with the feed. Despite increasingly sophisticated calculations relating total fungi to the numbers of zoospores (France, Theodorou & Davies, 1990), which can be counted readily, the best estimate of biomass remains that of 8% made by Orpin and based on chitin measurements (Orpin & Joblin, 1988). The other microbial families are less predominant, although they may be quite numerous: more than 26 different morphotypes of bacteriophages have been observed in numbers up to 10^8/ml (Klieve & Bauchop, 1988).

Bacteria

Rumen bacteria (Table 4.1) are mainly mesophilic, chemo-organotrophic, strictly anaerobic eubacteria (Stewart & Bryant, 1988). About 10^{10}–10^{11} bacteria are present per gram of rumen digesta. The principal genera are *Prevotella*, *Butyrivibrio*, *Selenomonas*, *Ruminobacter*, *Fibrobacter* and *Ruminococcus*. *Eubacterium*, *Treponema*, *Anaerovibrio*, *Wolinella*, *Megasphaera*, *Streptococcus*, *Succinimonas*, *Succinivibrio* and *Veillonella* are also significant. *Methanobrevibacter ruminantium* is usually the main representative of the archaebacteria.

Therefore, the bacterial population of the rumen contains similar, but not the same, organisms as does the human gut. The taxonomy is very weak, however. Five years ago, *Bacteroides* would have been said to be predominant, but it has since been shown that none of the main rumen isolates are true *Bacteroides*. They are only distant cousins of 'true' gut *Bacteroides*, such as *B. fragilis*, *B. thetaiotaomicron*, and so on (Shah & Collins, 1990; Mannarelli *et al.*, 1991). *Bacteroides amylophilus* was reclassified as *Ruminobacter amylophilus* (Stackebrandt & Hippe, 1986), *Bacteroides ruminicola* became *Prevotella ruminicola* (Shah & Collins, 1990), and *Bacteroides succinogenes* was renamed *Fibrobacter succinogenes* (Montgomery, Flesher & Stahl, 1988). Other genera

Table 4.1. *Properties of predominant rumen bacteria*

	Substrates	Product[a]	Cell-wall type[b]	Ionophore sensitivity
Anaerovibrio lipolytica	lipids, lactate	A, P, S	–	resistant
Butyrivibrio fibrisolvens	hemicellulose, cellodextrins	F, B, L, H_2	+	sensitive
Fibrobacter succinogenes	cellulose	F, A, S	–	adaptively resistant
Lachnospira multiparus	pectin, sugars	F, A, L	+	sensitive
Megasphaera elsdenii	sugars, lactate	A, P, B, H_2	–	resistant
Methanobrevibacter ruminantium	$CO_2 + H_2$, formate	CH_4	–	resistant
Prevotella ruminicola	xylan, cellodextrins, sugars	F, A, S	–	resistant
Ruminobacter amylophilus	starch	F, A, S	–	resistant
Ruminococcus albus	cellulose, cellobiose	F, A, E, H_2	+	sensitive
Ruminococcus flavefaciens	cellulose, xylan	F, A, S, H_2	+	sensitive
Selenomonas ruminantium	sugars, lactate, succinate	A, P, L	–	resistant
Streptococcus bovis	starch, sugars	L	+	sensitive
Veillonella parvula	lactate, succinate	A, P, H_2	–	resistant

[a] CO_2 is produced by all species except *M. ruminantium.* A, acetate; B, butyrate; E, ethanol; F, formate; L, lactate; P, propionate; S, succinate.

[b] Gram-positive or Gram-negative cell wall morphology. This does not always correspond to the appearance of bacteria in Gram-stained smears. For example, *B. fibrisolvens* has a Gram-positive cell-wall structure, but the wall is very thin and stains Gram-negative.

will undoubtedly be reclassified as more molecular techniques are applied to the rumen ecosystem.

Protozoa

The ciliate protozoa in the rumen comprise two main families. The more numerous is usually the Ophryoscolecidae, which are motile, anaerobic organisms ranging in size from 20 to 500 (usually 50–100) μm. The cilia on these organisms are restricted to tufts located mainly near the oesophagus; their function is the propulsion of food particles into the oesophagus. The other protozoa are the so-called 'holotrichs', belonging to the order Vestibuliferida. In these organisms the cilia cover their whole surface and provide the rapid propulsion through rumen fluid that is so spectacular when fresh samples are viewed microscopically. At least 17 genera of Ophryoscolecidae are found commonly in the rumen, and up to 15 holotrichs (Williams & Coleman, 1992). Most of the protozoal species are unique to the rumen.

In terms of their metabolic activity, the ciliates possess all of the main activities of the bacteria except for methanogenesis. In addition, they ingest and digest bacteria. Indeed, the breakdown of bacteria by protozoa depresses the total microbial growth yield from the fermentation (Demeyer & Van Nevel, 1979), which has major consequences for animals in which protein flow is critically low (Preston & Leng, 1986).

Fungi

The zoospores of the anaerobic fungi of the rumen were originally misclassified as flagellate protozoa. It was only when Orpin investigated the possibility that fungi were present that it was realized that these organisms were in fact strictly anaerobic fungi, with most of the biomass present as rhizoids infiltrating fibrous plant tissue (Orpin & Joblin, 1988). Rumen anaerobic fungi are phycomycetes, related to aquatic fungi. Their classification continues to change, but is based primarily on their morphology, specifically the number of sporangia per fruiting body and the number of flagella per zoospore. The most studied species is *Neocallimastix frontalis.*

Biochemistry

Polysaccharide breakdown

Cellulolysis is carried out by relatively few species. The rumen bacteria, *F. succinogenes*, *Ruminococcus flavefaciens* and *Ruminococcus albus*, attach closely to plant fibre during digestion (Chesson & Forsberg, 1988). Their cellulases are either cell-associated or present in membranous 'blebs' secreted from the bacterial cell once it has attached. *F. succinogenes* is highly pleomorphic and moulds itself closely to the contours of the fibre. The ruminococci retain their coccal morphology and have a more extensive glycocalyx, which they use for attachment. A secondary population capable of digesting the products, such as cellodextrins, of the initial breakdown is typified by *Butyrivibrio fibrisolvens* and *P. ruminicola.*

Cellulase activity has been found in *Epidinium ecaudatum caudatum*, *Eremoplastron bovis*, *Ostracodinium obtusum bilobum* and *Eudiplodinium maggii* among the rumen protozoa (Coleman, 1985), and cellulolysis is a property of all the rumen fungi examined in detail (Orpin & Joblin, 1988). The protozoa make an extremely significant contribution to cellulolysis by the mixed population, up to 70% in some cases (Coleman, 1986), but, because of the difficulty of growing these organisms axenically, relatively little work has been done on their cellulases.

Xylan and hemicellulose are degraded by the cellulolytic bacteria, plus *P. ruminicola* and *B. fibrisolvens*, by most protozoal species, and by the anaerobic fungi (Chesson & Forsberg, 1988). Pectin is digested by bacteria and protozoa, but not fungi. Starch is engulfed by protozoa, which can help stabilize rumen fermentation, by protecting the starch from more rapid bacterial degradation (Williams & Coleman, 1992). Starch is digested by many bacterial species, including *Ruminobacter amylophilus*, *Streptococcus bovis*, *Succinimonas amylolytica*, *Selenomonas ruminantium*, *B. fibrisolvens* and *Eubacterium ruminantium* (Chesson & Forsberg, 1988). The protozoal species with the highest amylase activity are *E. bovis*, *Diploplastron affine*, *Ophryoscolex caudatus* and *Polyplastron multivesiculatum*.

SCFA production from pyruvate

Acetate is formed from acetyl-CoA, which is derived from pyruvate. It used to be assumed, based on a few enzyme surveys, that acetate and ATP were released by a phosphotransacetylase via acetyl phosphate as intermediate. However, detailed studies with *S. ruminantium* suggest that pyruvate is converted to acetyl-CoA by pyruvate–ferredoxin oxidoreductase, and then converted to acetate by an enzyme which does not form acetyl phosphate (Michel & Macy, 1990). The enzyme also deacylates succinyl-CoA and propionyl-CoA. The precise mechanism of pyruvate oxidation to acetyl-CoA probably varies from organism to organism according to which electron acceptor is used (Russell & Wallace, 1988). Whether the new deacylating enzyme is widespread has not been established. Ciliate protozoa have membranous organelles called hydrogenosomes which convert pyruvate into acetate and hydrogen (Williams & Coleman, 1992).

Propionate is generated by both the randomizing (succinyl-CoA) and non-randomizing (acrylyl-CoA) pathways in the rumen. Both pathways dispose of the same number of reducing equivalents and lead to the formation of ATP. In the randomizing pathway, pyruvate (or PEP) is converted to malate (or oxaloacetate), then dehydrated to fumarate, which is reduced to succinate. This is a symmetrical intermediate, so any label at C-2 becomes equivalent to that at C-3, and the propionate ultimately produced is labelled at both C-2 and C-3. The final stages of propionate production entail the formation of succinyl-CoA, a vitamin B_{12}-dependent mutase reaction, a decarboxylation, and finally hydrolysis of the CoA ester in an ATP-yielding reaction. The non-randomizing pathway proceeds via lactate to lactyl-CoA, then acrylyl-CoA, which is reduced to propionyl-CoA. None of the intermediates is symmetrical, therefore, and the position of label in C-2 or C-3 of pyruvate is retained.

The two main propionate producers are *S. ruminantium* and *Megasphaera elsdenii*, which use the randomizing and non-randomizing pathways, respectively. Both species ferment lactate as well as hexoses. It was estimated from labelling studies that $>80\%$ of the lactate in the rumen was fermented by *M. elsdenii* (Counotte, Lankhorst & Prins, 1983). *S. ruminantium* produces propionate from glucose and lactate. However, *M. elsdenii* only produces propionate from lactate, but not glucose – a lactate racemase is induced during growth on lactate which enables the conversion of both L- and D-lactate to lactyl-CoA (Hino & Kuroda, 1993); the enzyme is not induced during growth on glucose, which means that the D-lactate potentially formed by the action of D-lactate dehydrogenase on pyruvate is not converted to L-lactate, the substrate for lactyl-CoA synthase.

The main butyrate-producing organism in the rumen is *B. fibrisolvens*, which uses thiolase, β-hydroxybutyryl-CoA dehydrogenase, crotonase, crotonyl-CoA reductase, phosphate butyryl transferase and finally butyrate kinase, thus effectively condensing two molecules of acetyl-CoA into butyrate (Miller & Jenesel, 1979). Ciliate protozoa seem to use similar mechanisms (Williams, 1986).

Despite the anaerobic nature of the ecosystem, rumen micro-organisms make extensive use of electron transport-linked phosphorylation to generate ATP, by mechanisms involving a variety of electron carriers and probably in some cases by using novel compounds. For example, *R. amylophilus* conserves energy by electron transfer-linked phosphorylation, despite not having any of the normally recognized electron carriers (Wetzstein, McCarthy & Gottschalk, 1987). The electron acceptors in the rumen are mostly metabolites, such as fumarate, generated intracellularly. Rumen fluid has a high capacity for oxygen utilization, and substantial amounts of oxygen enter the rumen. Bacteria and protozoa are approximately equally responsible for oxygen consumption (Ellis, Williams & Lloyd, 1989). There is no indication of whether energy is conserved by oxygen consumption, but it is clear that the concentrations of O_2 found in the rumen (up to 3 μM) can influence the stoichiometry of fermentation by protozoa. Acetate, H_2 and CO_2 formation by *Polyplastron multivesiculatum* was suppressed by O_2 (Ellis *et al.*, 1991).

The mechanisms by which ciliate protozoa form SCFA have not been examined in detail. The main fermentation products are acetic and butyric acids, hydrogen and carbon dioxide. Removal of the protozoa generally results in decreased acetate and butyrate concentrations, although there are many exceptions to this general pattern (Williams & Coleman, 1992).

The anaerobic fungi use the Embden–Meyerhof–Parnas pathway to convert glucose to PEP and pyruvate, from which is formed lactate, acetate, hydrogen and carbon dioxide, with traces of formate and ethanol (Orpin & Joblin, 1988). *N. frontalis* formed significant amounts of formate, lactate, ethanol and dihydrogen as well as acetate from cellulose in pure culture; however, when a methanogen was present to remove the hydrogen, products other than acetate (and methane) became minimal (Bauchop & Mountfort, 1981).

Protein

In addition to the SCFA that arise from the metabolism of sugars, substantial amounts of SCFA are derived from amino acid breakdown. The products (mmol/l) of trypticase (15 g/l) breakdown *in vitro* were acetate, 35.7; propionate, 1.0; butyrate, 14.1; valerate, 5.4; isobutyrate, 4.3; isovalerate plus 2-methylbutyrate, 10.2 (Hino & Russell, 1985). The low propionate and high acetate and butyrate values suggest that the metabolic fate of most amino acids is acetyl-CoA and that little is converted to pyruvate, the precursor of propionate. As far as the essential amino acids are concerned, valine, leucine and isoleucine are converted to the branched-chain SCFA, isobutyrate, isovalerate and 2-methylbutyrate, by oxidative deamination and decarboxylation (Allison, 1970). These acids are present in rumen fluid at concentrations usually less than 5 mM, and they would rarely amount to more than about 5% of the total SCFA.

Three main sources of protein are substrates for microbial proteases in the rumen. The most abundant is dietary protein, which is broken down at a rate that depends on its particle size, solubility and degree of secondary and tertiary structure. Much protein is recycled within the rumen, because of extensive microbial lysis. Several factors cause lysis, but the most important quantitatively is predation of bacteria by ciliate protozoa. The third source of protein is secretions by the host animal. Rumen epithelial tissue, unlike gut cells lower down the tract, produce little mucus, but large quantities of mucoprotein are secreted in saliva. These proteins are fairly resistant to proteolysis, because of their degree of glycosylation (Nugent *et al.*, 1983).

Table 4.2. *Production of propionate from cellulose as the result of cross-feeding. The initial concentration of cellulose was 0.1%*

	Fermentation products (mM)			
	Succinate	Propionate	Acetate	Formate
Fibrobacter succinogenes (cellulolytic)	6.5	0	5.3	1.9
Selenomonas ruminantium (non-cellulolytic)	0	0	0	0
F. succinogenes + *S. ruminantium*	0	8.5	5.4	1.7

From Scheifinger & Wolin (1973).

Microbial physiology and ecology

It is clear from inspection of Table 4.1 that individual species of rumen micro-organisms growing in pure culture form many fermentation products that are not found, or occur only occasionally and transiently, in the rumen. These compounds include lactate, succinate, ethanol, formate and hydrogen. The most obvious reason that these compounds do not appear in the mixed fermentation is cross-feeding; they can be utilized by other species. However, there are more complex reasons. The products that are formed in pure culture under rapid growth conditions may be quite different from those produced *in vivo* in the mixed population.

Cross-feeding

Lactate is metabolized by the rumen bacteria, *Veillonella parvula*, *S. ruminantium* and *M. elsdenii*, to form propionate. It is also metabolized by ciliate protozoa, whose contribution must be significant, because lactic acid concentrations are generally higher in defaunated animals than in faunated animals (Williams & Coleman, 1992). Succinate is utilized by *S. ruminantium*, forming propionate, and so propionate can be produced indirectly from cellulose breakdown via the utilization of succinate formed by the primary producer (Table 4.2).

Formate and hydrogen are special cases of cross-feeding. They are used either by methanogens or by organisms that can link the utilization of hydrogen to electron transport and ATP formation in other ways. *Wolinella succinogenes* is a special example that relies on electron transport linked to hydrogen or formate oxidation for growth (Stewart & Bryant, 1988). Other species can also use hydrogen, but the higher affinity of the methanogens for hydrogen generally means that most of the hydrogen flux is to methane (Henderson, 1980).

Cross-feeding also occurs in substrate utilization. Although relatively few species are responsible for the primary breakdown of polysaccharides, a much more diverse population is present. Because hydrolysis occurs extracellularly, it is possible for many species to compete for the soluble oligosaccharides and sugars produced by the primary hydrolysers.

Regulatory mechanisms

Certain products may be formed in pure culture *in vitro* simply because of the rich nature of the medium and the rapid growth rate that can be supported. The best-known example is *S. ruminantium*, which produces lactate at a high growth rate (μ) but switches to acetate and propionate production below $\mu = 0.2$/h (Fig. 4.2). The regulatory mechanism appears to be a combination of positive co-operativity on the binding of pyruvate by lactate dehydrogenase as its concentration increases (Wallace, 1978) and hyperbolic sensitivity of the competing enzyme, pyruvate–ferredoxin oxidoreductase, to pyruvate concentration (Melville, Michel & Macy, 1988). The products formed by *S. bovis* showed a similar sensitivity to growth rate. At high μ, lactate was the sole product, whereas ethanol and acetate were produced as μ fell below 0.2/h (Russell & Baldwin, 1979). Its lactate dehydrogenase is also

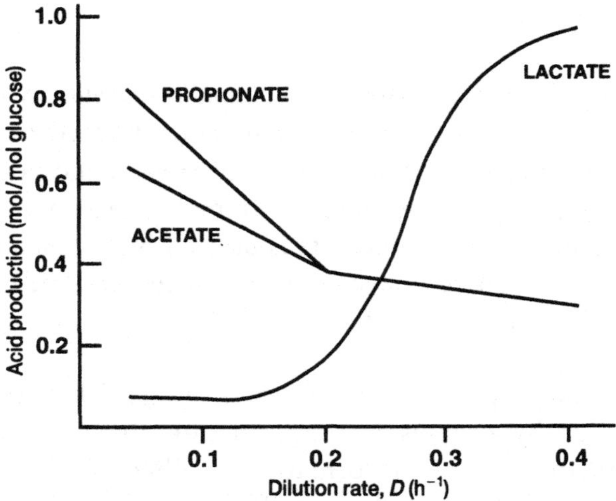

Fig. 4.2. Switch in fermentation products by *S. ruminantium* at different growth rates (from Wallace, 1978).

Table 4.3. *An example of the influence of H_2 transfer on fermentation stoichiometry.* Wolinella succinogenes *removed H_2 produced by* Ruminococcus albus

	Fermentation product (mol/mol hexose)	
	Ethanol	Acetate
R. albus	0.69	0
R. albus + *W. succinogenes*	1.31	2.00

From Iannotti *et al.* (1973).

regulated, but by fructose 1,6-bisphosphate rather than by pyruvate (van Gylswyk, 1977). The liquid dilution rate of rumen contents is usually around 0.1/h or less, so the products formed at low growth rates might be expected to predominate *in vivo*. Indeed, the low rates of lactate turnover measured by Mackie, Gilchrist & Heath (1984) suggest that the main reason lactate is not usually present in rumen fluid is that it is not formed, rather than that it is subject to cross-feeding.

Hydrogen transfer

Hydrogen transfer is a specialized case of cross-feeding (Wolin & Miller, 1988). Hydrogen is formed by many species of bacteria in pure culture, in conjunction with other reduced products. The hydrogen accumulates in the culture fluid in a way that never occurs *in vivo*, because of the activity of the methanogens and other hydrogen-utilizing organisms. As the hydrogen accumulates, the formation of more hydrogen becomes thermodynamically unfavourable, and the electrons must be disposed of in alternative products, such as ethanol. However, in the mixed culture of the rumen, the ethanol would never need to be formed as an alternative electron-sink product. An example of the phenomenon in defined mixed culture is given in Table 4.3.

Dietary effects

The composition of the diet has a major influence on the fermentation that takes place in the rumen. Unless rumen dysfunction occurs, acetate remains the most abundant SCFA in rumen fluid, but its production varies from up to 80% (mol/mol SCFA) in a roughage ration to about 60% when the animal receives concentrate. In this case, propionate increases to 20–25% of the total from a proportion of perhaps 10–15% on the roughage diet. The increased propionate production is presumed to result from a proliferation of propionate-producing sugar and starch utilizers (Table 4.1). Small changes in fermentation can have profound effects on the nutrition of the host animal, but it can be argued that it is remarkable, when one considers how changes in diet can completely transform the microbial population (Dehority & Orpin, 1988), how the fermentation products change so little.

Dysfunction and manipulation

Lactic acidosis

Rapid transformation from a roughage to a concentrate diet, or the excessive consumption of a starchy diet, can cause severe disruption to the rumen fermentation, called lactic acidosis or grain overload (Dawson & Allison, 1988). SCFA are produced rapidly from the starch, overloading the pH control exerted by saliva and absorption of the acids. The rumen pH falls to about 5.5, preventing the growth of many of the predominant rumen anaerobes, especially the cellulolytic species. *S. bovis*, which is more resistant to low pH, begins to predominate, producing lactic acid until the pH falls below 4.5, at which point even *S. bovis* cannot be sustained (Russell & Dombrowski, 1980). Lactobacilli take over, more lactate is formed, the pH continues to fall, and death of the animal frequently occurs.

Bloat

Bloat is caused by a disruption of the normal fluidity of rumen digesta. The physical properties of the fluid enable both the liquid and gaseous products of fermentation to be removed efficiently. In bloating animals, materials derived either from the plant or from bacterial polysaccharides cause a foam in the rumen, from which gas can no longer escape. Once more, the condition is frequently fatal (Dawson & Allison, 1988).

Antimicrobial feed additives

The production of propionate rather than acetate or butyrate is conventionally considered to be desirable, because propionate is glucogenic (for the host animal), whereas the other acids are not. Several microbial feed additives are available that enhance propionate production. These include the ionophores, monensin, lasalocid, salinomycin and several others, and the peptide antibiotic, avoparcin. Gram-positive species are sensitive to monensin, whereas Gram-negative bacteria are usually resistant (Table 4.1; Chen & Wolin, 1979). Thus the propionate-producing organisms, *S. ruminantium*, *V. parvula* and *M. elsdenii*, will be enriched. The increased propionate production is probably only a small part of the mode of action by which antimicrobial feed additives enhance ruminant growth, however. Protein metabolism is also affected (Newbold, Wallace & McKain, 1990), and direct effects of the ionophore on the animal itself cannot be eliminated (Rogers *et al.*, 1991).

References

Allison, M. J. (1970). Nitrogen metabolism of ruminal microorganisms. In *Physiology of Digestion and Metabolism in the Ruminant*, ed. A. T. Phillipson, pp. 456–73. Newcastle: Oriel Press.

Bauchop, T. & Mountfort, D. O. (1981). Cellulose fermentation by a rumen anaerobic fungus in both the absence and presence of rumen methanogens. *Applied and Environmental Microbiology*, **42**, 1103–10.

Chen, M. & Wolin, M. J. (1979). Effect of monensin and lasalocid-sodium on the growth of methanogenic and rumen saccharolytic bacteria. *Applied and Environmental Microbiology*, **38**, 72–7.

Chesson, A. & Forsberg, C. W. (1988). Polysaccharide degradation by rumen microorganisms. In *The Rumen Microbial Ecosystem*, ed. P. N. Hobson, pp. 251–84. London: Elsevier Applied Science.

Coleman, G. S. (1985). The cellulase content of 15 species of entodinomorphid protozoa, mixed bacteria and plant debris isolated from the ovine rumen. *Journal of Agricultural Science, Cambridge*, **104**, 349–60.

Coleman, G. S. (1986). The distribution of carboxymethylcellulase between fractions taken from the rumens of sheep containing no protozoa or one of five different protozoal populations. *Journal of Agricultural Science, Cambridge*, **106**, 121–7.

Counotte, G. H. M., Lankorst, A. & Prins, R. A. (1983). Role of the DL-lactic acid as an intermediate in rumen metabolism of dairy cows. *Journal of Animal Science*, **56**, 1222–35.

Dawson, K. A. & Allison, M. J. (1988). Digestive disorders and nutritional toxicity. In *The Rumen Microbial Ecosystem*, ed. P. N. Hobson, pp. 445–59. London: Elsevier Applied Science.

Dehority, B. A. & Orpin, C. G. (1988). Development of, and natural fluctuations in, rumen microbial populations. In *The Rumen Microbial Ecosystem*, ed. P. N. Hobson, pp. 151–83. London: Elsevier Applied Science.

Demeyer, D. I. & Van Nevel, C. J. (1979) Effect of defaunation on the metabolism of rumen micro-organisms. *British Journal of Nutrition*, **42**, 515–24.

Ellis, J. E., McIntyre, P. S., Saleh, M., Williams, A. G. & Lloyd, D. (1991). Influence of CO_2 and low concentrations of O_2 on fermentative metabolism of the rumen ciliate *Polyplastron multivesiculatum*. *Applied and Environmental Microbiology*, **57**, 1400–7.

Ellis, J. E., Williams, A. G. & Lloyd, D. (1989). Oxygen consumption by ruminal microorganisms: protozoal and bacterial contributions. *Applied and Environmental Microbiology*, **55**, 2583–7.

France, J., Theodorou, M. K. & Davies, D. (1990). Use of zoospore concentrations and life cycle parameters in determining the population of anaerobic fungi in the rumen ecosystem. *Journal of Theoretical Biology*, **147**, 413–22.

Henderson, C. (1980). The influence of extracellular hydrogen on the metabolism of *Bacteroides ruminicola*, *Anaerovibrio lipolytica* and *Selenomonas ruminantium*. *Journal of General Microbiology*, **119**, 485–91.

Hino, T. & Kuroda, S. (1993). Presence of lactate dehydrogenase and lactate racemase in *Megasphaera elsdenii* grown on glucose or lactate. *Applied and Environmental Microbiology*, **59**, 255–9.

Hino, T. & Russell, J. B. (1985). Effect of reducing-equivalent disposal and NADH/NAD on deamination of amino acids by intact rumen microorganisms and their cell extracts. *Applied and Environmental Microbiology*, **50**, 1368–74.

Iannotti, E. I., Kafkewitz, D., Wolin, M. J. & Bryant, M. P. (1973). Glucose fermentation products of *Ruminococcus albus* grown in continuous culture with *Vibrio succinogenes*: changes caused by interspecies transfer of H_2. *Journal of Bacteriology*, **114**, 1231–40.

Klieve, A. V. & Bauchop, T. (1988). Morphological diversity of ruminal bacteriophages from sheep and cattle. *Applied and Environmental Microbiology*, **54**, 1637–41.

Mackie, R. I., Gilchrist, F. M. C. & Heath, S. (1984). An *in vivo* study of ruminal microorganisms influencing lactate turnover and its contribution to volatile fatty acid production. *Journal of Agricultural Science, Cambridge*, **103**, 37–51.

Mannarelli, B. M., Ericsson, L. D., Lee, D. & Stack, R. J. (1991). Taxonomic relationships among strains of the anaerobic bacterium *Bacteroides ruminicola* determined by DNA and extracellular polysaccharide analysis. *Applied and Environmental Microbiology*, **57**, 2975–80.

Melville, S. B., Michel, T. A. & Macy, J. M. (1988). Regulation of carbon flow in *Selenomonas ruminantium* grown in glucose-limited continuous culture. *Journal of Bacteriology*, **170**, 5305–11.

Michel, T. A. & Macy, J. M. (1990). Purification of an enzyme responsible for acetate formation from acetyl coenzyme A in *Selenomonas ruminantium*. *FEMS Microbiology Letters*, **68**, 189–94.

Miller, T. L. & Jenesel, S. E. (1979). Enzymology of butyrate formation by *Butyrivibrio fibrisolvens*. *Journal of Bacteriology*, **138**, 99–104.

Montgomery, L., Flesher, B. A. & Stahl, D. A. (1988). Transfer of *Bacteroides succinogenes* (Hungate) to *Fibrobacter* gen. nov. as *Fibrobacter succinogenes* comb. nov. and description of *Fibrobacter intestinalis* sp. nov. *International Journal of Systematic Bacteriology*, **38**, 430–5.

Newbold, C. J., Wallace, R. J. & McKain, N. (1990). Effects of the ionophore tetronasin on nitrogen metabolism by ruminal microorganisms *in vitro*. *Journal of Animal Science*, **68**, 1103–9.

Nugent, J. H. A., Jones, W. T., Jordan, D. J. & Mangan, J. L. (1983). Rates of proteolysis in the rumen of the soluble proteins casein, fraction I (18S) leaf protein, bovine serum albumin and bovine submaxillary mucoprotein. *British Journal of Nutrition*, **50**, 357–68.

Orpin, C. G. & Joblin, K. N. (1988). The rumen anaerobic fungi. In *The Rumen Microbial Ecosystem*, ed. P. N. Hobson, pp. 129–50. London: Elsevier Applied Science.

Preston, T. R. & Leng, R. A. (1986). *Matching Livestock Production Systems to Available Resources.* Addis Ababa: International Livestock Centre for Africa.

Rogers, M., Jouany, J. P., Thivend, P. & Fontenot, J. P. (1991). Comparative effects of feeding and duodenal infusion of monensin or digestion in sheep. *Canadian Journal of Animal Science*, **71**, 1125–33.

Russell, J. B. & Baldwin, R. L. (1979). Comparison of maintenance energy expenditures and growth yields among several rumen bacteria grown on continuous culture. *Applied and Environmental Microbiology*, **37**, 537–43.

Russell, J. B. & Dombrowski, D. B. (1980). Effect of pH on the efficiency of growth by pure cultures of rumen bacteria in continuous culture. *Applied and Environmental Microbiology*, **39**, 604–10.

Russell, J. B. & Wallace, R. J. (1988). Energy yielding and consuming reactions. In *The Rumen Microbial Ecosystem*, ed. P. N. Hobson, pp. 185–215. London: Elsevier Applied Science.

Scheifinger, C. C. & Wolin, M. J. (1973). Propionate formation from cellulose and soluble sugars by combined cultures of *Bacteroides succinogenes* and *Selenomonas ruminantium. Applied Microbiology*, **26**, 789–95.

Shah, H. N. & Collins, M. D. (1990). *Prevotella*, a new genus to include *Bacteroides melaninogenicus* and related species formerly classified in the genus *Bacteroides. International Journal of Systematic Bacteriology*, **40**, 205–8.

Stackebrandt, E. & Hippe, H. (1986). Transfer of *Bacteroides amylophilus* to a new genus *Ruminobacter* gen. nov. *Systematic and Applied Microbiology*, **8**, 204–7.

Stewart, C. S. & Bryant, M. P. (1988). The rumen bacteria. In *The Rumen Microbial Ecosystem*, ed. P. N. Hobson, pp. 21–75. London: Elsevier, Applied Science.

Van Gylswyk, N. O. (1977). Activation of NAD-dependent lactate dehydrogenase in *Butyrivibrio fibrisolvens* by fructose 1,6-diphosphate. *Journal of General Microbiology*, **99**, 441–3.

Wallace, R. J. (1978). Control of lactate production by *Selenomonas ruminantium*: homotropic activation of lactate dehydrogenase by pyruvate. *Journal of General Microbiology*, **107**, 45–52.

Wetzstein, H. G., McCarthy, J. E. G. & Gottschalk, G. (1987). The membrane potential in a cytochrome-deficient species of *Bacteroides*: its magnitude and mode of generation. *Journal of General Microbiology*, **133**, 73–83.

Williams, A. G. (1986). Rumen holotrich ciliate protozoa. *Microbiological Reviews*, **50**, 25–49.

Williams, A. G. & Coleman, G. S. (1992). *The Rumen Protozoa.* New York: Springer-Verlag.

Wolin, M. J. & Miller, T. L. (1988). Microbe–microbe interactions. In *The Rumen Microbial Ecosystem*, ed. P. N. Hobson, pp. 343–59. London: Elsevier Applied Science.

5

Short-chain fatty acids in the hindgut

G. BREVES AND K. STÜCK

Introduction

For many years it was assumed that the major function of the hindgut was to conserve water and certain electrolytes. It has now been well established that, in addition, high-fibre diets are substantially metabolized by hindgut microbes, and the basic principles of this microbial metabolism are similar to those which have been described for the rumen. The major end products of microbial carbohydrate fermentation are acetate, propionate and butyrate, and to a lesser extent isobutyrate, valerate and isovalerate, which arise from amino acids. Measurements of the end products of microbial metabolism have been carried out on a large number of different species and the potential role of external factors influencing the rate of fermentation and the molar proportions of short-chain fatty acids (SCFA) have been determined. The aim in this chapter is to review experimental studies on SCFA in the hindgut contents of different species, to critically discuss the suitability of SCFA concentrations as quantitative indicators of fermentation rate and to consider the extent to which SCFA may be utilized by the host animal.

SCFA concentrations in the hindgut

Dietary carbohydrates that are not degraded enzymatically in the small intestine are the predominant substrates for anaerobic fermentation. Because of its high microbial concentration and anaerobic environment, the hindgut is the major site for SCFA production in non-ruminant species (Bugaut, 1987; Bergman, 1990). However, microbial metabolism may to a lesser extent also take place in the upper gastrointestinal tract.

The highest microbial SCFA production is found in the caecum, followed by the colonic contents (Hintz, Schryver & Stevens, 1978; Bugaut, 1987). The composition of the microbial population, their metabolic activity and thus the production rate of fermentation and products may be substantially influenced by changes in dietary composition, level of feed intake, ambient temperature and methodological factors, such as time interval between food intake and sampling of hindgut contents (Stevens, 1988). These factors of variance are the major determinants for the wide range of SCFA concentrations in hindgut contents, which have been shown to vary between 30 and 240 mM in different species (Bergman, 1990).

In all species acetate is the primary SCFA, and in many the proportion of propionate is higher than that of butyrate (see Tables 5.1–5.4, below). Lesser amounts of other SCFA may also be present (Stevens, 1978). Symbiotic microbial fermentation in the hindgut is a digestive strategy that has been adopted by all mammals (Bergman, 1990). Little is known about microbial hindgut fermentation in the intestinal tract of lower vertebrates such as reptiles, amphibians and fishes or in invertebrates such as insects. Indigenous micro-organisms have been detected in the digestive tract of these species, but their function remains for the most part unkown. Evidence for endosymbiosis in the gut of the tropical herbivorous surgeonfish was found by Fishelson, Montgomery & Myrberg (1985), but the role of endogenous micro-organisms is unclear.

Amphibians and reptiles

Bacterial populations from the intestines of various species of amphibians have been investigated. Gossling, Loesche & Nace (1982) found acetogenic and butyrogenic microbes in the large intestines of non-hibernating and hibernating leopard frogs (*Rana pipiens*) that had been caught in their natural habitat. Analysis of the flora indicated a similarity to that found in mammals. Hibernation resulted in a temporary reduction and a qualitative change of flora, possibly due to lower bacterial growth rates of hibernation temperatures. Throughout their life span, common iguanas are herbivores that depend upon a microbial fermentation system in their hindgut, because they swallow their food without chewing (Pough, 1973; Troyer, 1982). Newborn iguanas receive the complex microflora from direct contact with older iguanas (Troyer, 1982).

Insects

With regard to insects, hindgut metabolism has been most intensively studied in termites (McBee, 1989). The nutritional symbiosis between wood-eating termites and their intestinal cellulose-digesting microbes supplies the termites with SCFA as their source of energy (Breznak & Pankratz, 1977; Breznak, 1982; Nalepa, 1991; Thorne, 1991).

Cockroaches also contain a diverse bacterial flora in their hindgut (Bracke, Cruden & Markovetz, 1979; Nalepa, 1991; Thorne, 1991). Microbes in the hindgut of cockroach species contain cellulose-producing bacteria (Cruden & Markovetz, 1979), but the obligatory role of these cellulolytic activities for the nutrition of cockroaches is not fully understood (Cruden & Markovetz, 1984).

Klug & Kotarski (1980) investigated the bacterial hindgut colonization of larvae of aquatic craneflies. Most of the bacteria which could be isolated were facultatively anaerobic.

Aquatic herbivores

Herbivorous teleosts (*Oreochromis mossambicus*) were studied by Titus & Ahearn (1988). Along the full length of the fish intestine they found increasing acetate concentrations from 3 to 18 mM. Substantially higher SCFA concentrations between 156 and 207 mM were detected in the hindgut of the green turtle (Bjorndal, 1979). In this study the molar proportions of butyrate were higher than those of propionate, which may have been the result of the seagrass diet being low in soluble carbohydrates, or the result of differential SCFA absorption rates. It was estimated that in these animals approximately 15% of the daily energy demand was met by hindgut fermentation. The pattern of SCFA concentrations in the caecum and colon of the green turtle is similar to that of the dugong (Murray *et al.*, 1977) and the West Indian manatee, *Trichechus manatus* (Burn & Odell, 1987), which are also seagrass consumers. The SCFA concentrations in the caecum and large intestine of the dugong and manatee ranged from 183 to 236 mM and from 221 to 307 mM, respectively (Table 5.1).

Birds

Studies on the composition of hindgut contents have been performed in a variety of bird species (Table 5.2). In fowls and geese SCFA concentrations in hindgut contents were 27–34 μmol/g wet weight and 15–70 mM, respectively (Clemens, Stevens & Southworth, 1975*a*; Savory & Knox, 1991). Moss & Parkinson (1972) compared different segments of the intestinal tract of wild grouse and found that SCFA concentrations ranged from 35 to 41 mM and were similar in contents from both the caecum and lower small intestine. In both segments, molar proportions of butyrate were higher than those of propionate. Substantially higher SCFA concentrations of about 95 mM were determined in caecal contents of the hoatzin, a neotropical leaf-consuming

Table 5.1. *SCFA concentrations in the intestinal tract of aquatic herbivores*

	Bowel segment	SCFA concentration (mM)	SCFA proportions (%) (acetate : propionate : butyrate)	Reference
Herbivorous teleost	Upper	2.7–14.6 (acetate)	—	Titus & Ahearn (1988)
	Middle	6.2–17.3 (acetate)	—	
	Lower	11.7–18.2 (acetate)	—	
Green turtle	Caecum	156	93 : 2 : 6	Bjorndal (1979)
	Anterior colon	191	83 : 2 : 15	
	Middle colon	20	78 : 8 : 14	
	Rectum	62	71 : 11 : 18	
Dugong	Caecum	183	57 : 17 : 25	Murray *et al.* (1977)
	Colon	236	50 : 17 : 32	
West Indian manatee (*Trichechus manatus*)	Caecum	221	53 : 15 : 30	Burn & Odell (1987)
	Colon	307	57 : 14 : 27	

Table 5.2. *SCFA concentrations in the intestinal tract of birds and arboreal folivores*

	Bowel segment	SCFA concentration	SCFA proportions (%) (acetate : propionate : butyrate)	Reference
Fowl	Caecum	27–34 μmol/g wet wt	72 : 22 : 16	Savory & Knox (1991)
Goose	Colon/caecum	15–70 mM	—	Clemens *et al.* (1975*a*)
Red grouse	Caecum	35–41 mM	61 : 12 : 22	Moss & Parkinson (1972)
Hoatzin	Caecum	95 mM	77 : 9 : 14	Grajal *et al.* (1989)
Greater glider,				
captive	Caecum/colon	36 mM	75 : 14 : 9	Foley *et al.* (1989)
wild	Caecum	70 mM	63 : 22 : 13	
Brushtail possum	Caecum/colon	75 mM	75 : 17 : 7	Foley *et al.* (1989)

bird (Grajal *et al.*, 1989). Measurements of SCFA production rates were made in the caecum of two different ptarmigan species. In the rock ptarmigan, collected in Alaska, between 30 and 34 mmol SCFA were produced daily, with the highest levels in July and November/December, the result of seasonal changes in feed supply. The seasonal differences, however, were not significant. In comparison, in the caecum of the willow ptarmigan, the SCFA production rate was lower by about 50% (Gasaway, 1976*a*,*b*).

Rodents and rabbits

Numerous studies on hindgut metabolism have been carried out in rodents such as mice, rats and guinea pigs and in rabbits (Table 5.3). In many studies the concentration ranges of SCFA were found to be between 100 and 150 mM, with approximately 70% as acetate, 20% as propionate and 10% as butyrate. The effects of dietary components, fibre contents and fibre sources such as guar gum, gum arabic, pectin and cellulose on hindgut metabolism have been investigated extensively (Hove & King, 1979; McKay & Eastwood, 1983; McLean Ross *et al.*, 1984; Tulung, Rémésy & Demigné, 1987; McIntyre *et al.*, 1991). Diurnal variations of caecal SCFA could only be detected in rabbits when the animals were fed once daily, whereas relatively constant SCFA concentrations were measured when the animals were fed *ad libitum* (Parker & McMillan, 1976). In addition to the concentrations of SCFA, their production rates were measured in some studies. When the nutrition of mole rats was changed from sweet potatoes to carrots, the caecal SCFA production rate increased from 91 μmol/h to 139 μmol/h (Buffenstein & Yahav, 1991). In rabbits, no significant differences in caecal SCFA production rates could be detected when dietary crude fibre contents were increased. With values around 43 mmol/day for acetate, 6 mmol/day for propionate and 18 mmol/day for butyrate, the actual production rates in the caecum were similar for both the low- and the high-fibre diet (Hoover & Heitmann, 1972). In guinea pigs a similar range of about 54 mmol/day of overall SCFA production rates was measured in the caecum (Sakaguchi *et al.*, 1985). In the caecum of wild porcupines the mean SCFA concentrations ranged around 0.51 mmol/g dry weight with molar proportions for acetate, propionate and butyrate of 74%, 12% and 14%, respectively (Johnson & McBee, 1967).

Dogs

In dogs, the effects of feeding and fasting on SCFA concentrations in caecal and colonic contents were investigated (Table 5.4). Within 12 h after feed

Table 5.3. *SCFA concentrations in the intestinal tract of rodents and rabbits (Lagomorpha)*

	Bowel segment	SCFA concentration	SCFA proportions (%) (acetate:propionate:butyrate)	Reference
Mouse	Caecum	125 mmol/kg	59:11:29	Høverstad *et al.* (1985)
Rat	Caecum	130–140 mM	63:26:10	Tulung *et al.* (1987)
Wild rabbit	Caecum	368 (day), 317 (night) μmol/g dry wt	Day, 82:4:13; night, 85:3:12	Henning & Hird (1972)
	Proximal colon	291 (day), 226 (night) μmol/g dry wt	—	
	Rectum	228 (day), 43 (night) μmol/g dry wt	—	
Guinea pig	Caecum	96 mM	71:16:13	Sakaguchi *et al.* (1985)
Porcupine	Caecum	0.51 mmol/g dry wt	74:12:14	Johnson & McBee (1967)

Table 5.4. *SCFA concentrations in the intestinal tract of dogs, pigs, large ungulates and primates*

	Bowel segment	SCFA concentration (mM)	SCFA proportions (%) (acetate:propionate:butyrate)	Reference
Dog	Caecum/colon	140	—	Herschel *et al.* (1981)
Pig	Caecum	100–140	52:38:10	Bach Knudsen *et al.* (1991)
	Proximal colon	80–130	53:34:10	
	Distal colon	20–65	66:24:11	
Equine	Caecum	118	85:10:3	Mackie & Wilkins (1988)
	Colon	115		
Elephant	Caecum	138	63:20:15	Clemens & Maloiy (1982)
	Colon	65–148	72:16:9	
Rhinoceros	Caecum	144	79:14:6	Clemens & Maloiy (1982)
	Colon	53–81	70:16:11	
Hippopotamus	Colon	28–35	75:16:5	Clemens & Maloiy (1982)
Baboon	Caecum	160	—	Clemens & Phillips (1980)
	Colon	90–150	—	
Sykes monkey	Caecum	160	—	Clemens & Phillips (1980)
	Colon	130	—	

intake, SCFA concentrations were found to be around 140 mM, with no significant differences between the caecum and the colon. After a fasting period of 47 h, SCFA concentrations decreased to 90–100 mM and were substantially lower than in those animals that received no feed for 12 or 24 h (Herschel *et al.*, 1981). When dogs were kept on a meat diet, SCFA concentrations in caecal and colonic contents were found to be higher than in the caecum of ponies that were fed a carbohydrate-rich diet. This may have resulted from changes in distribution volume due to changes in the volume of the large intestine (Stevens, 1988). SCFA could also have originated from α-amylase-indigestible protein-linked carbohydrates in the meat diet and from the walls of desquamated gastrointestinal cells, which could provide a substantial source (Stevens, 1978).

Pigs

With respect to all livestock species, pigs are most commonly used for studying production, concentration and absorption of SCFA in the hindgut (Table 5.4). A wide concentration range between 100 and 130 mM in hindgut contents has been reported, with an average of 65% present as acetate, 25% as propionate and 10% as butyrate (Argenzio & Southworth, 1974; Clemens, Stevens & Southworth, 1975*b*; Kim, Benevenga & Grummer, 1978; Fleming, Fitch & Chansler, 1989). Concentrations and molar proportions of individual SCFA were found to vary in response to many dietary factors, such as level and source of neutral detergent fibre (NDF), crude fibre contents and the ratio of enzymatically degradable carbohydrates to crude fibre (Stanogias & Pearce, 1985; Fleming *et al.* 1989; Bach Knudsen *et al.*, 1991).

Large ungulates

As in pigs, SCFA are the predominant end products of microbial fermentation in the hindgut of horses. From different studies caecal SCFA concentrations tended to be higher (97–118 mM) than those in the colon (26–115 mM). Mean molar proportions were 85, 10 and 3% for acetate, propionate and butyrate, respectively (Kern *et al.*, 1974; Argenzio, 1975; Mackie & Wilkins, 1988).

In a comparative approach, Clemens & Maloiy (1982) studied digestive functions in different large ungulates. Whilst the elephant and rhinoceros are typical hindgut fermenters, the hippopotamus ferments primarily within its complex forestomach system. Therefore, hindgut SCFA concentrations were found to be higher in the elephant and rhinoceros (53–148 mM) than in the hippopotamus (28–35 mM) (Table 5.4).

Primates

Studies in captive sub-human primates indicate that caecal SCFA concentrations in the herbivorous Sykes monkey averaged 160 mM and were similar to those in the omnivorous baboon, when the animals were kept on the same diet (Clemens & Phillips, 1980). Milton & McBee (1983) measured SCFA production rates in the wild howler monkey under natural feeding conditions. They measured production rates of 2.5–3.4 μmol/g wet weight caecal contents/min for acetate, 0.1–0.3 for propionate and 0.02–0.03 for butyrate. Therefore, the molar proportions were substantially shifted towards acetate (Table 5.4).

SCFA as quantitative indicators of microbial fermentation

From measurements of SCFA concentrations in hindgut contents, a quantitative estimate of the rate of microbial fermentation has often been attempted. Although increased SCFA concentrations were found in response to an increased intake of fibre in a number of experimental studies, quantitative changes in the rate of microbial fermentation do not necessarily result in alterations of SCFA concentrations. This is mainly due to the fact that the determination of the actual SCFA concentration is influenced not only by the production rate, but also by changes in the rate of absorption or the distribution volume, i.e. the fluid volume of hindgut contents. It has been demonstrated in different studies in pigs that fluid volumes within the upper hindgut significantly increase when the percentage of dietary cellulose or crude fibre is increased (Farell & Johnson, 1970; Breves *et al.*, 1993). Therefore, it must be concluded that the SCFA production rate has to be measured directly in order to quantify the rate of microbial fermentation.

Different experimental techniques have been introduced to measure SCFA production rates quantitatively under *in vivo* conditions and most of these methods have been established in ruminants. In the rumen, both single injection and the continuous infusion technique of either radioactively or ^{13}C-labelled SCFA have been applied to calculate SCFA production rates (Sheppard, Forbes & Johnson, 1959; Gray, Jones & Pilgrim, 1960; Leng & Leonard, 1965; Leng & Brett, 1966; Breves *et al.*, 1987). These methods have also been applied for measuring SCFA production in the large intestine of rabbits, ponies, horses and pigs (Glinsky *et al.*, 1976; Parker, 1976; Kenelly, Aherne & Sauer, 1981; Ford & Simmons, 1985). With the use of ^{13}C-labelled acetate in a pig model, the mean acetate production rate was found to increase from 27.4 mmol/h to 56.2 mmol/h when the dietary crude fibre content was raised from 5.1% to 18.3%. Similar changes were recorded for propionate by the application of ^{13}C-labelled propionate (Breves *et al.*, 1993). The major advantage of the continuous technique is that the rate of interconversion between the individual SCFA can be determined.

Endogenous SCFA utilization

With respect to endogenous energetic utilization of SCFA, an important question is whether there are any limiting factors for SCFA absorption across the hindgut wall. From experiments in growing pigs, it has been demonstrated that the continuous intracaecal infusion of acetate, propionate or butyrate at a daily rate exceeding the physiological production rate by more than 100% did not result in any increase of faecal SCFA excretion, thus confirming the high absorptive capacity of the hindgut wall (Gädeken, Breves & Oslage, 1989; Breves *et al.*, 1993). With respiration chamber results for assessment of energy balance, these infusion experiments were used to calculate the efficiency of energy utilization of each individual SCFA in intermediary metabolism. This ranged between 65 and 71%, with no significant differences between acetate, propionate and butyrate (Gädeken *et al.*, 1989). These results were slightly higher than those from Jentsch, Schiemann & Hoffmann (1968) and slightly lower than those from Roth, Kirchgessner & Müller (1988). Therefore, energy utilization of SCFA tends to be lower than energy utilization of starch, as a typical carbohydrate digested enzymatically in the small intestine (Schiemann, Hoffmann & Nehring, 1961). The intermediary SCFA utilization is the physiological basis for the potential contribution of hindgut fermentation to basal metabolic rate, which may vary over a wide range when different species are compared (for review, see Rechkemmer, Rönnau & v. Engelhardt, 1988).

References

Argenzio, R. A. (1975). Functions of the equine large intestine and their interrelationship in disease. *Cornell Veterinarian*, **65**, 303–30.

Argenzio, R. A. & Southworth, M. (1974). Sites of organic acid production and absorption in gastrointestinal tract of the pig. *American Journal of Physiology*, **228**, 454–60.

Bach Knudsen, K. E., Jensen, B. B., Andersen, J. O. & Hansen, I. (1991). Gastrointestinal implications in pigs of wheat and oat fractions. *British Journal of Nutrition*, **65**, 233–48.

Bergman, E. N. (1990). Energy contributions of volatile fatty acids from the gastrointestinal tract in various species. *Physiological Reviews*, **70**, 567–90.

Bjorndal, K. A. (1979). Cellulose digestion and volatile fatty acid production in the green turtle, *Chelonia mydas*. *Comparative Biochemistry and Physiology*, **63A**, 127–33.

Bracke, J. W., Cruden, D. L. & Markovetz, A. J. (1979). Intestinal microbial flora of the American cockroach, *Periplaneta americana* L. *Applied and Environmental Microbiology*, **38**, 945–55.

Breves, G., Schulze, E., Sallmann, H. P. & Gädeken, D. (1993). The application of ^{13}C-labelled short chain fatty acids to measure acetate and propionate production rates in the large intestines. Studies in a pig model. *Zeitschrift für Gastroenterologie*, **31**, 179–82.

Breves, G., Schulze, E., Sallmann, H. P. & Höller, H. (1987). Sodium (1-^{13}C)acetate as a label for measuring acetate production rate in the rumen of sheep. *Journal of Veterinary Medicine*, **A34**, 698–702.

Breznak, J. A. (1982). Intestinal microbiota of termites and other xylophagous insects. *Annual Review of Microbiology*, **36**, 323–43.

Breznak, J. A. & Pankratz, H. S. (1977). *In situ* morphology of the gut microbiota of wood-eating termites (*Reticulitermes flavipes* (Kollar) and *Coptotermes formosanus* (Shiraki)). *Applied and Environmental Microbiology*, **33**, 406–26.

Buffenstein, R. & Yahav, S. (1991). The effect of diet on microfaunal population and function in the caecum of a subterranean and naked mole-rat, *Heteracephalus glaber*. *British Journal of Nutrition*, **65**, 249–58.

Bugaut, M. (1987). Occurrence, absorption and metabolism of short chain fatty acids in the digestive tract of mammals. *Comparative Biochemistry and Physiology*, **86B**, 439–72.

Burn, D. M. & Odell, D. K. (1987). Volatile fatty acid concentrations in the digestive tract of the West Indian manatee, *Trichechus manatus*. *Comparative Biochemistry and Physiology*, **88B**, 47–9.

Clemens, E. & Phillips, B. (1980). Organic acid production and digesta movement in the gastrointestinal tract of the baboon and sykes monkey. *Comparative Biochemistry and Microbiology*, **66A**, 529–32.

Clemens, E. T. & Maloiy, G. M. O. (1982). The digestive physiology of three East African herbivores: the elephant, rhinoceros and hippopotamus. *Journal of Zoology, London*, **198**, 141–56.

Clemens, E. T., Stevens, C. E. & Southworth, M. (1975*a*). Sites of organic acid production and pattern of digesta movement in the gastrointestinal tract of geese. *Journal of Nutrition*, **105**, 1341–50.

Clemens, E. T., Stevens, C. E. & Southworth, M. (1975*b*). Sites of organic acid production and pattern of digesta movement in the gastrointestinal tract of swine. *Journal of Nutrition*, **105**, 759–68.

Cruden, D. L. & Markovetz, A. J. (1979). Carboxymethyl cellulose decomposition by intestinal bacteria of cockroaches. *Applied and Environmental Microbiology*, **38**, 369–72.

Cruden, D. L. & Markovetz, A. J. (1984). Microbial aspects of the cockroach hindgut. *Archives of Microbiology*, **138**, 131–9.

Farell, D. J. & Johnson, K. A. (1970). Utilization of cellulose by pigs and its effects on caecal function. *Animal Production*, **14**, 209–17.

Fishelson, L., Montgomery, W. L. & Myrberg, A. A. (1985). A unique symbiosis in the gut of tropical herbivorous surgeonfish (Acanthuridae: Teleostei) from the Red Sea. *Science*, **229**, 49–51.

Fleming, S. E., Fitch, M. D. & Chansler, M. W. (1989). High-fibre diets: influence on characteristics of cecal digesta including short-chain fatty acid concentrations on pH. *American Journal of Clinical Nutrition*, **50**, 93–9.

Foley, W. J., Hume, I. D. & Cork, S. J. (1989). Fermentation in the hindgut of the greater glider (*Petauroides volans*) and the brushtail possum (*Trichosurus vulpecula*) – two arboreal folivores. *Physiological Zoology*, **62**, 1126–43.

Ford, E. J. H. & Simmons, H. A. (1985). Gluconeogenesis from caecal propionate in the horse. *British Journal of Nutrition*, **53**, 55–60.

Gädeken, D., Breves, G. & Oslage, H. J. (1989). Efficiency of energy utilization of intracaecally infused volatile fatty acids in pigs. In *Energy Metabolism of Farm Animals*, Pudoc Publication No. 43, pp. 115–18. Wageningen: EAAP.

Gasaway, W. C. (1976*a*). Seasonal variation in diet, volatile fatty acid production and size of the cecum of rock ptarmigan. *Comparative Biochemistry and Physiology*, **53A**, 109–14.

Gasaway, W. C. (1976*b*). Volatile fatty acids and metabolizable energy derived from cecal fermentation in the willow ptarmigan. *Comparative Biochemistry and Physiology*, **53A**, 115–21.

Glinsky, M. J., Smith, R. M., Spiers, H. R. & Davis, C. L. (1976). Measurement of volatile fatty acids production rates in the caecum of the pony. *Journal of Animal Science*, **42**, 1465–70.

Gossling, J., Loesche, W. J. & Nace, G. W. (1982). Large intestine bacterial flora of nonhibernating and hibernating leopard frogs (*Rana pipiens*). *Applied and Envronmental Microbiology*, **44**, 59–66.

Grajal, A., Strahl, S. D., Parra, R., Dominguetz, M. G. & Heher, A. (1989). Foregut fermentation in the hoatzin, a neotropical leaf-eating bird. *Science*, **245**, 1236–8.

Gray, E. V., Jones, G. B. & Pilgrim A. F. (1960). The rates of production of volatile fatty acids in the rumen. *Australian Journal of Agriculture Research*, **11**, 383–8.

Henning, S. J. & Hird, F. J. R. (1972). Diurnal variations in the concentrations of volatile fatty acids in the alimentary tracts of wild rabbits. *British Journal of Nutrition*, **27**, 57–64.

Herschel, D. A., Argenzio, R. A., Southworth, M. & Stevens, C. E. (1981). Absorption of volatile fatty acid, Na, and H_2O by the colon of the dog. *American Journal of Veterinary Research*, **42**, 1118–24.

Hintz, H. F., Schryver, H. F. & Stevens, C. E. (1978). Digestion and absorption in the hindgut of nonruminant herbivores. *Journal of Animal Science*, **46**, 1803–7.

Hoover, W. H. & Heitmann, R. N. (1972). Effects of dietary fibre levels on weight gain, cecal volume and volatile fatty acid production in rabbits. *Journal of Nutrition*, **102**, 375–80.

Hove, E. L. & King, S. (1979). Effects of pectin and cellulose on growth, feed efficiency, and protein utilization, and their contribution to energy requirement and cecal VFA in rats. *Journal of Nutrition*, **109**, 1274–8.

Høverstad, T., Midtvedt, T. & Bohmer, T. (1985). Short-chain fatty acids in intestinal content of germfree mice monocontaminated with *Escherichia coli* or *Clostridium difficile*. *Journal of Gastroenterology*, **20**, 373–80.

Jentsch, W., Schiemann, R. & Hoffmann, L. (1968). Modellversuche mit Schweinen zur Bestimmung der energetischen Verwertung von Alkohol, Essig- und Milchsäure. *Archiv für Tierernährung*, **18**, 352–7.

Johnson, J. L. & McBee, R. H. (1967). The porcupine cecal fermentation. *Journal of Nutrition*, **91**, 540–6.

Kenelly, J. J., Aherne, F. X. & Sauer, W. C. (1981). Volatile fatty acid production in the hindgut of swine. *Canadian Journal of Animal Science*, **61**, 349–61.

Kern, D. L., Slyter, L. L., Leffel, E. C., Weaver, J. M. & Oltjen, R. R. (1974). Ponies vs. steers: microbial and chemical characteristics of intestinal ingesta. *Journal of Animal Science*, **38**, 559–64.

Kim, K.-I., Benevenga, J. & Grummer, R. H. (1978). Lactase activity and VFA production in the cecum and colon of pigs fed a corn–soy or 40% whey diet. *Journal of Animal Science*, **46**, 1648–57.

Klug, M. J. & Kotarski, S. (1980). Bacteria associated with the gut tract of larval stages of the aquatic cranefly *Tipula abdominalis* (Diptera; Tipulidae). *Applied and Environmental Microbiology*, **40**, 408–16.

Leng, R. A. & Brett, D. J. (1966). Simultaneous measurements of the rates of production of acetic, propionic and butyric acids in the rumen of sheep on different diets and the correlation between production rates and concentrations of these acids in the rumen. *British Journal of Nutrition*, **20**, 541–52.

Leng, R. A. & Leonard, G. J. (1965). Measurement of the rates of production of acetic, propionic and butyric acids in the rumen of sheep. *British Journal of Nutrition*, **19**, 469–84.

Mackie, R. I. & Wilkins, C. A. (1988). Enumeration of anaerobic bacterial microflora of the equine gastrointestinal tract. *Applied and Environmental Microbiology*, **54**, 2155–60.

McBee, R. H. (1989). Hindgut fermentations in nonavian species. *The Journal of Experimental Zoology Supplement*, **3**, 55–60

McIntyre, A., Young, G. P., Taranto, T., Gibson, P. R. & Ward, P. B. (1991). Different fibres have different regional effects on luminal contents of rat colon. *Gastroenterology*, **101**, 1274–81.

McKay, L. F. & Eastwood, M. A. (1983). The influence of dietary fibre on caecal metabolism in the rat. *British Journal of Nutrition*, **50**, 679–84.

McLean Ross, A. H., Eastwood, M. A., Brydon, W. G., Busuttil, A. & McKay, L. F. (1984). A study of the effects of dietary gum arabic in the rat. *British Journal of Nutrition*, **51**, 47–56.

Milton, K. & McBee, R. H. (1983). Rates of fermentative digestion in the howler monkey, *Alouatta palliata* (primates: Ceboidea). *Comparative Biochemistry and Physiology*, **74A**, 29–31.

Moss, R. & Parkinson, J. A. (1972). The digestion of heather (*Calluna vulgaris*) by red grouse (*Lagopus lagopus scoticus*). *British Journal of Nutrition*, **27**, 285–98.

Murray, R. M., March, H., Heinsohn, G. E. & Spain, A. V. (1977). The role of the midgut caecum and large intestine in the digestion of sea grasses by the dungong (mammalia: Sirenia). *Comparative Biochemistry and Physiology*, **56A**, 7–10.

Nalepa, C. A. (1991). Ancestral transfer of symbionts between cockroaches and termites: an unlikely scenario. *Proceedings of the Royal Society, London, Series B*, **246**, 185–9.

Parker, D. S. (1976). The measurement of production rates of volatile fatty acids in the caecum of the conscious rabbit. *British Journal of Nutrition*, **36**, 61–70.

Parker, D. S. & McMillan, R. T. (1976). The determination of volatile fatty acids in the caecum of the conscious rabbit. *British Journal of Nutrition*, **35**, 365–71.

Pough, F. H. (1973). Lizard energetics and diet. *Ecology*, **54**, 837–44.

Rechkemmer, G., Rönnau, K. & v. Engelhardt, W. (1988). Fermentation of polysaccharides and absorption of short chain fatty acids in the mammalian hindgut. *Comparative Biochemistry and Physiology*, **90A**, 563–8.

Roth, F. X., Kirchgessner, M. & Müller, H. L. (1988). Energetische Verwertung von intracaecal infundierter Essig- und Propionsäure bei Sauen. *Journal of Animal Physiology and Animal Nutrition*, **59**, 211–17.

Sakaguchi, E., Becker, G., Rechkemmer, G. & v. Engelhardt, W. (1985). Volume, solute concentrations and production of short-chain fatty acids in the caecum and upper colon of the guinea pig. *Zeitschrift für Tierphysiologie, Tierernährung und Futtermittelkunde*, **54**, 276–85.

Savory, C. J. & Knox, A. I. (1991). Chemical composition of caecal contents in the fowl in relation to dietary fibre level and time of day. *Comparative Biochemistry and Physiology*, **100A**, 739–43.

Schiemann, R. Hoffmann, L. & Nehring, K. (1961). Die Verwertung reiner Nährstoffe. 2. Mitteilung: Versuche mit Schweinen. *Archiv für Tierernährung*, **11**, 265–83.

Sheppard, A. J., Forbes, R. M. & Johnson, B. C. (1959). Rate of acetic acid production in the rumen determined by isotope dilution. *Proceedings of the Society for Experimental Biology and Medicine*, **101**, 715–17.

Stanogias, G. & Pearce, G. R. (1985). The digestion of fibre by pigs. 2. Volatile fatty acid concentrations in large intestine digesta. *British Journal of Nutrition*, **53**, 531–6.

Stevens, C. E. (1978). Physiological implications of microbial digestion in the large intestine of mammals: relation to dietary factors. *American Journal of Clinical Nutrition*, **31**, S161–8.

Stevens, C. E. (1988). *Comparative Physiology of the Vertebrate Digestive System*, ed. C. E. Stevens, pp. 159–88. Cambridge: Cambridge University Press.

Thorne, B. L. (1991). Ancestral transfer of symbionts between cockroaches and termites: an alternative hypothesis. *Proceedings of the Royal Society of London, Series B*, **246**, 191–5.

Titus, E. & Ahearn, G. A. (1988). Short-chain fatty acid transport in the intestine of a herbivorous teleost. *Journal of Experimental Biology*, **135**, 77–94.

Troyer, K. (1982). Transfer of fermentative microbes between generations in an herbivorous lizard. *Science*, **216**, 540–2.

Tulung, B., Rémésy, C. & Demigné, C. (1987). Specific effects of guar gum or gum arabic on adaptation of cecal digestion to high fibre diets in the rat. *Journal of Nutrition*, **117**, 1556–61.

6

Microbiological aspects of the production of short-chain fatty acids in the large bowel

G. T. MACFARLANE AND G. R. GIBSON

Introduction

The human colon is increasingly being recognized as a major organ of digestion through the activities of its resident microbiota. Bacterial mass constitutes approximately 55% of solids in the large bowel (Stephen & Cummings, 1980), giving viable counts in faeces that range from 10^{11} to 10^{13}/g dry weight (Finegold, Sutter & Mathisen, 1983). Although many hundreds of different bacterial species can be isolated from the gut, a relatively small number of groups predominate, including the bacteroides, bifidobacteria, eubacteria, clostridia, and a variety of anaerobic Gram-positive cocci belonging to the genera *Ruminococcus*, *Peptococcus*, *Peptostreptococcus* and *Streptococcus*. The bacteroides alone can account for up to 30% of the total anaerobe count (Macy & Probst, 1979), and the bifidobacteria as much as 25% (Mitsuoka, 1984; Scardovi, 1986). Whilst there are undoubtedly marked interindividual variations in the composition of the gut microbiota, in general most persons within the same racial and socioeconomic groups harbour similar cell-population densities and generic distributions of bacteria in their colons.

The large bacterial mass and multiplicity of different species present in the large bowel provide the organ with considerable metabolic diversity and potential, rivalling that of the liver. This chapter deals with one of the most significant aspects of bacterial metabolism in the gut – that of fermentation and the production of short-chain fatty acids (SCFA). In the context of the human large intestine, the term 'fermentation' is loosely used to describe the great variety of reactions and the overall metabolic processes involved in the anaerobic breakdown and partial mineralization of organic matter. Quantitatively, SCFA are the major end products of fermentation and it is the purpose here to discuss the nutritional, ecological and physiological factors that affect their synthesis.

Table 6.1. *Source and composition of some polymerized carbohydrates fermented by intestinal bacteria*

Substrate	Source	Major constituents	Structure
Starch	Cereals, roots, tubers, legumes	D-Glucose	$\alpha(1 \rightarrow 4)$- and $\alpha(1 \rightarrow 6)$-linked glucan
Arabinogalactan	Plant cell walls	D-Galactose, L-Arabinose	$\beta(1 \rightarrow 4)$- or $\beta(1 \rightarrow 3)$-linked galactose backbone with a α-linked arabinose side chains
Pectin	Fruits, plant cell walls	D-Galacturonic acid, L-arabinose, D-galactose, L-rhamnose	$\beta(1 \rightarrow 4)$-linked galacturonic acid backbone with arabinose and rhamnosyl insertions or linear $\alpha(1 \rightarrow 4)$ galacturonic acid homo-polymer
Xylan	Plant cell walls	D-Xylone, L-arabinose	$\beta(1 \rightarrow 4)$-linked xylose with α-linked arabinose side chains
Guar gum	Cluster beans, food additives	L-Arabinose, D-galactose, L-rhamnose, D-glucuronic acid	$\beta(1 \rightarrow 4)$-linked mannan with α-linked galactose branches
Cellulose	Plant cell walls	D-Glucose	$\beta(1 \rightarrow 4)$-linked glucan
Raffinose, stachyose	Cereals, legumes, tubers	D-Galactose, D-glucose	$\alpha(1 \rightarrow 6)$-linked galactosaccharides
Fructo-oligosaccharides	Artichokes, onions, burdock	D-Fructose, D-glucose	$\beta(2 \rightarrow 1)$-linked fructose terminating with glucose $\alpha(1 \rightarrow 2)$ linked to fructose
Mucopolysaccharides (heparin, chondroitin sulphate, hyaluronic acid)	Epithelial cells, meat	Hexosamine and uronic acid sulphate esters	Acidic glycosaminoglycans composed of either D-glucosamine or D-galactosamine and uronic acids such as D-glucuronic acid or L-iduronic acid
Mucins	Saliva, gastric, biliary, pancreatic and respiratory secretions, small and large intestinal secretions	Neuraminic acid, galactose, hexosamines, L-fucose	Protein core with attached oligo-saccharide side chains consisting of varying combinations of galactose, fucose, *N*-acetylglucosamine, *N*-acetyl galactosamine and neuraminic acid

Data from Degnan, 1993.

Fermentation substrates

The large intestine typically receives about 1.5 kg of material from the small bowel every day. Most of this is water and is rapidly absorbed; the remainder consists of various dietary components that have escaped digestion in the small bowel, together with a range of host-derived materials (see Table 6.1).

Substrates from the diet

Many different types of substrate enter the colon in a variety of forms, including unabsorbed sugars and sugar alcohols, oligosaccharides, chitin and aminosugars. The major substrates, however, are polysaccharides, of which resistant starch is quantitatively the most important, accounting for about 8–40 g/day (Englyst & Cummings, 1987). Non-starch polysaccharides (cellulose, hemicelluloses, pectins, gums) from plant cell walls contribute somewhere in the region of 8–18 g/day of fermentable substrate in Western populations (Englyst *et al.*, 1988, 1989; Bingham, Pett & Day, 1990). With respect to organic nitrogen-containing compounds, free amino acids do not enter the large bowel in significant amounts, but dietary protein and peptides contribute between 3 and 9 g/day (Gibson, Sladen & Dawson, 1976; Chacko & Cummings, 1988).

Substrates of endogenous origin

Exfoliated epithelial cells from the small and large bowel, pancreatic enzymes (proteases, lipases, amylase, nucleic acid hydrolases), mucins and other gastrointestinal-tract secretions (e.g. glycosidases, immunoglobulins), together with the recycling of dead bacterial cells, fall into this category. The contribution that these substances make to fermentation is considerably more difficult to assess than that from the diet. However, between 4 and 6 g of pancreatic proteases (Kuknal, Adams & Preston, 1965) and 2–3 g of small-intestinal mucins (Stephen, Haddad & Phillips, 1983) may enter the colon on a daily basis.

The availability of host-derived substrates undoubtedly varies from person to person, and intraindividually may be affected on a day-to-day basis by factors such as illness, exocrine pancreatic activity, rate of turnover of the gastrointestinal epithelium and rate of mucin formation by goblet cells. Given that, for example, colonic epithelial cells have a half-life of about 6 days (Christensen, 1991), host tissues must be a significant source of fermentable substrate for intestinal bacteria. In view of the fact that the majority of bacterial fermentation products formed in the colon are absorbed and metabolized by the host, a major purpose of the organ is clearly the reclamation of energy, as well as the more traditionally recognized functions of water and solute absorption.

Breakdown of polymers by intestinal bacteria

As observed above, the gut microbiota depends for its existence on an exceptionally diverse range of polymerized carbon sources. Many bacteria are able to synthesize a wide variety of cell-bound and extracellular hydrolytic enzymes (polysaccharidases, glycosidases, proteases, peptidases) that are able to digest polymeric substances and make the component sugars and amino acids available for fermentation. The majority of these enzymes, such as the amylases that are also able to hydrolyse resistant starches, the enzymes that degrade plant cell walls and certain classes of protease have no host counterparts and are unique to the colon (Englyst, Hay & Macfarlane, 1987; Macfarlane *et al.*, 1988). Although the large bowel as a whole is a carbon-limited environment in which there is intense competition amongst bacteria for survival, the degradation of a highly complex polymerized substance is in many ways a co-operative process, which depends on the participation of a multiplicity of enzymes produced by many different bacteria.

Anatomical considerations

The structure of the large intestine affects substrate availability in its various anatomical regions. The proximal colon receives digesta from the small bowel and is comparatively rich in fermentable carbohydrates, whereas, as a result of bacterial action, these substrates become depleted as gut contents reach the distal bowel (see Fig. 6.1). As is discussed below, this can have profound effects on fermentation reactions.

Carbohydrate fermentation

Carbohydrate fermentations by human colonic anaerobes consist of a series of energy-yielding reactions that do not involve respiratory chains, in which molecular oxygen serves as the terminal electron acceptor. In these processes, the organic electron acceptor is itself a product of the substrate being oxidized, and the difference in redox potential between the substrate and products determines the amount of ATP that can be formed. In some fermentations, ATP is produced from substrate-level phosphorylation reactions, whereas respiratory chains may be involved in others.

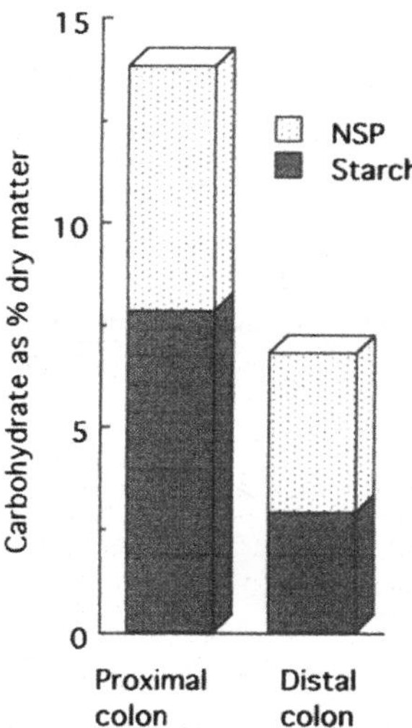

Fig. 6.1. Carbohydrate availability in different regions of the colon. NSP, non-starch polysaccharides. (J. H. Cummings, unpublished data.)

With the exception of bifidobacteria, the majority of saccharolytic anaerobes in the large intestine use the Embden–Meyerhof–Parnas pathway to ferment carbohydrates. An overview of the major routes of carbohydrate dissimilation together with the principal metabolic products and their associated bacteria is given in Fig. 6.2.

Fermentation reactions are regulated by the need to maintain redox balance through the reduction and reoxidation of pyridine nucleotides and ferrodoxins. Pyruvate and acetyl-CoA are important branch points in anaerobic metabolism (see Fig. 6.2). Fermentation pathways that are branched allow bacteria greater metabolic flexibility and enable them to adapt rapidly to change in their local microenvironment, such as substrate depletion or the introduction of new substrates. They also permit the organisms to adjust more finely the thermodynamic efficiency of substrate catabolism.

Fermentation in the colon

Figure 6.3 shows that in both the proximal and distal colons, acetate, propionate and butyrate are the main products of fermentation (Cummings *et al.*, 1987). However, a variety of other acidic and neutral metabolites, including lactase, ethanol, succinate and hydrogen, are formed to varying degrees by different types of bacteria. They function as electron sinks and are produced to maintain redox balance during fermentation, by facilitating the

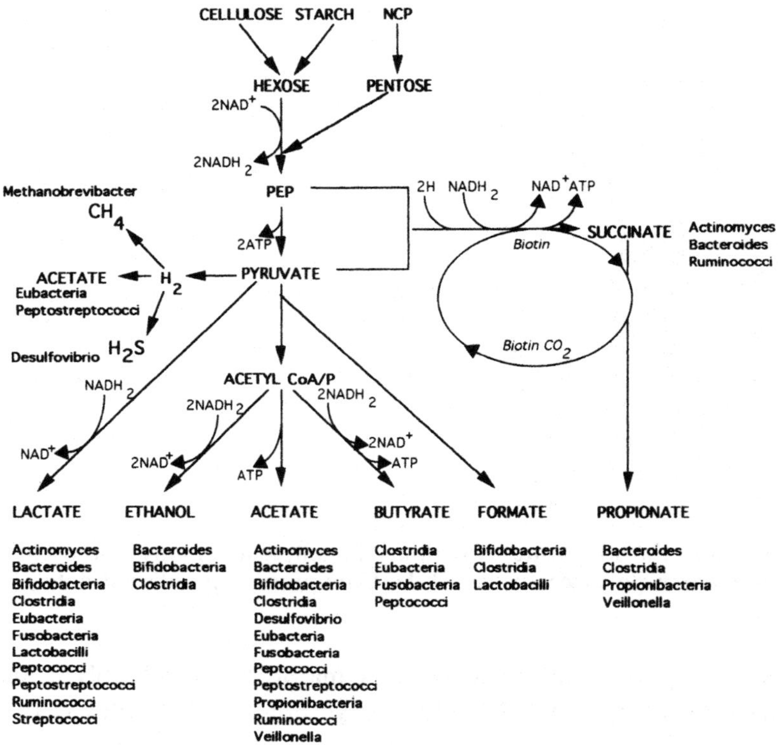

Fig. 6.2. Overview of major pathways of carbohydrate metabolism in the large intestine and the principal fermentation products formed by individual groups of anaerobic bacteria. NCP (non-cellulosic polysaccharides) include pectins and hemicelluloses. Propionate is shown as being produced by the succinate pathway, since few species in the human colon form this metabolite using the acrylate pathway.

regeneration of oxidized pyridine nucleotides (see Fig. 6.2). With the possible exceptions of hydrogen and ethanol, these fermentation intermediates do not accumulate in the healthy gut, because they serve as substrates and electron donors for cross-feeding bacteria, which convert them to SCFA.

Measurements of SCFA in gut contents taken from persons who had died suddenly show that molar ratios of acetate, propionate and butyrate are very similar in the proximal and distal colons (Fig. 6.3). This probably reflects the relative absorptive capabilities of the mucosa in these areas of the gut, and does not imply that fermentation reactions are similar. When contents from different regions of the colon are incubated *in vitro*, in the absence of exogenous substrate, significant quantitative and qualitative differences are

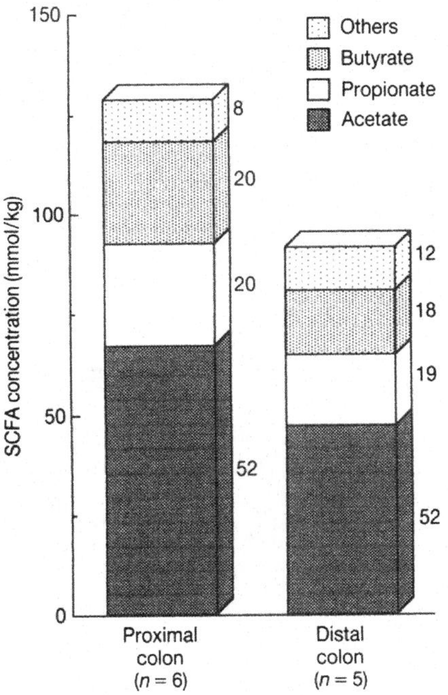

Fig. 6.3. SCFA concentrations in different locations in the colon and their respective molar ratios. 'Others' includes branched-chain fatty acids, valerate and caproate. Results are from Cummings *et al.* (1987).

observed in the patterns of SCFA produced (Fig. 6.4) that reflect differing substrate availabilities.

Control of carbohydrate metabolism

A wide range of factors influence fermentation reactions in the colon. Important amongst them is the chemical composition of the substrate. For example, Englyst *et al.* (1987) showed that starch fermentation principally yielded acetate and butyrate, whereas acetate alone was the main product when pectin and xylan were fermented by gut bacteria. Other studies have shown that lactate is an important intermediate of starch fermentation, but not of the fermentation of non-starch polysaccharides (Macfarlane & Englyst, 1986; Etterlin *et al.*, 1992).

The redox state of the substrates determines to some degree the metabolic pathways through which they are catabolized. This has been shown in studies with *Clostridium butyricum* (Crabbendam *et al.*, 1987), which could not utilize mannitol as sole carbon source, because it was unable to dispose of the excess

Table 6.2. *Influence of carbohydrate availability and growth rate on relative molar ratios of fermentation products formed by three species of human colonic bacteria grown in continuous culture*

	Dilution rate/h	Generation time (h)	Fermentation product molar ratio						
			Formate	Acetate	Propionate	Butyrate	Succinate	Lactate	Ethanol
Bifidobacterium breve[a]									
Carbon-limited	0.10	6.9	32	59	—	—	—	ND	8
	0.45	1.5	29	60	—	—	—	ND	10
Carbon-excess	0.09	7.7	ND	70	—	—	—	25	3
	0.60	1.2	ND	68	—	—	—	25	6
Bacteroides ovatus[b]									
Carbon-limited	0.06	11.6	—	58	33	—	9	ND	—
	0.19	3.6	—	53	8	—	39	ND	—
Carbon-excess	0.06	11.6	—	49	15	—	31	5	—
	0.19	3.6	—	49	11	—	36	4	—
Clostridium perfringens[c]									
Carbon-limited	0.04	17.3	—	74	—	17	6	3	—
	0.16	4.3	—	80	—	8	ND	12	—
Carbon-excess	0.04	17.3	—	49	—	12	5	35	—
	0.16	4.3	—	18	—	3	ND	80	—

[a] B. A. Degnan & G. T. Macfarlane, unpublished data.
[b] From Macfarlane & Gibson (1991).
[c] From Allison & Macfarlane (1989).
ND, not detected; dash indicates 'not applicable'.

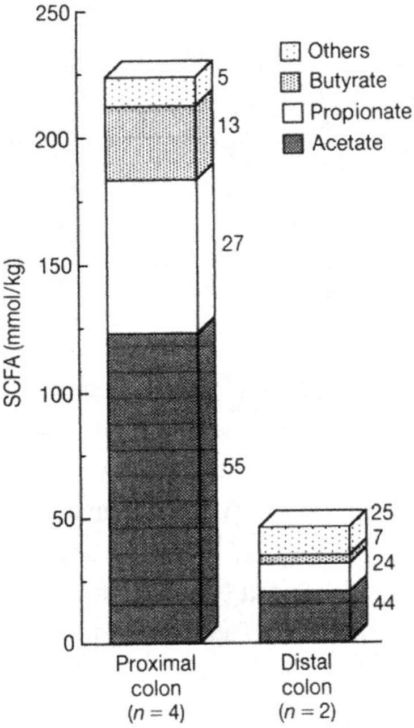

Fig. 6.4. Amounts and relative molar ratios of SCFA produced from endogenous substrates during incubation *in vitro* of gut contents under anaerobic conditions for 48 h. Others include BCFA, valerate and caproate. (G. T. Macfarlane & G. R. Gibson, unpublished data.)

reducing power generated during the fermentation. However, if acetate was also present, it could be used as an electron sink for the production of butyrate, and the sugar alcohol could be fermented.

Ecological factors also play a role. Since different bacteria produce different fermentation products (Fig. 6.2), the relative numbers of individual species and their substrate preferences affect the amounts and types of products that are formed.

The quantity of substrate that is available for fermentation influences the way that it is utilized. This is demonstrated in Table 6.2, which shows three separate studies where intestinal bacteria were grown in chemostats under carbon-limited or carbon-excess conditions at different growth rates. In the case of *Bifidobacterium breve*, growth rate had little effect on fermentation product formation, but marked differences were evident in the distribution of fermentation products as a result of carbohydrate availability. During carbohydrate limitation, formate and acetate were the principal end products of metabolism, whereas when carbohydrate was in excess, lactate and acetate predominated. These observations are explained by the fact that the bacterium used lactate as an electron sink to dispose of excess reducing power when the substrate supply was plentiful, whilst metabolism was directed towards energy generation when substrate was limiting. A similar inverse relationship between lactate and formate production has been reported to occur with *Lactobacillus casei* during growth in carbon-limited chemostats, but, unlike the bifidobacterium, the phenomenon was growth-rate dependent (DeVries *et al.*, 1970).

In the experiments with *Bacteroides ovatus*, growth rate and carbon availability affected fermentation. Acetate synthesis was maximal during carbohydrate-limited growth as a result of the need to optimize ATP formation. The other fermentation acids formed by *B. ovatus* were succinate and propionate (see Fig. 6.2). By producing succinate, the bacterium disposes of excess reducing equivalents formed in glycolysis, and, in addition, the oxidation of fumerate to succinate produces extra ATP via a primitive electron-transport system. Propionate is formed by decarboxylation of succinate; this reaction serves to regenerate biotin–carbon dioxide, which is used to convert C3 acids to C4 acids in the succinate pathway. Under conditions of carbohydrate excess, acetate and succinate were the major end products of fermentation irrespective of growth rate, whereas acetate and propionate predominated at low growth rates during carbohydrate limitation. These reactions are influenced by intracellular pCO_2, which is dependent on carbohydrate availability. When sufficient carbon dioxide is present, there is a reduced requirement to decarboxylate succinate, and this acid is therefore produced in preference to propionate.

The studies with *Clostridium perfringens* demonstrated that high substrate concentrations resulted in lower acetate and increased lactate production. The bacteria maximized energy gain during carbohydrate-limited growth by producing more ATP from acetyl phosphate, but when substrate was in excess, the decrease in acetate production reduced the efficiency of energy transduction, whilst providing for a high rate of carbon flow through the cell by using lactate as an electron sink. In this species, these reactions were controlled at the level of pyruvate.

Increasing glucose concentrations can shift the pattern of fermentation from production of acidic metabolites towards neutral products, such as alcohols in some bacteria, including *Clostridium bifermentans*, *C. sporogenes* and *Peptostreptococcus anaerobius* (Turton, Drucker & Ganguli, 1983).

Carbohydrate fermentation in some bacteria can be affected by the presence of inorganic electron acceptors such as nitrate, which act as electron sinks and enable some gut anaerobes to increase the yield of ATP from their substrates, by producing more oxidized fermentation products. This is typically manifested in an increase in acetate and a reduction in propionate, butyrate and lactate synthesis (Allison & Macfarlane, 1988, 1989).

SCFA from amino acid fermentation

Substrates and products

Although carbohydrate availability varies markedly in different regions of the large bowel, substantial levels of proteins and peptides are present throughout the length of the gut (Macfarlane, Cummings & Allison, 1986). Because the colon is a strongly proteolytic environment (Macfarlane *et al.*, 1988), these substrates are extensively digested by many species that ferment amino acids (Macfarlane & Allison, 1986). Large populations of these bacteria occur in the large intestine (see Table 6.3); many do not, or only weakly, ferment carbohydrates.

Fermentation of amino acids by human colonic anaerobes consists of a series of oxidative, transamination and reductive reactions, in which a wide variety of electron acceptors are used; these include α-keto acids, other amino acids, unsaturated fatty acids and hydrogen (Barker, 1981). Quantitatively, SCFA are the predominant organic end products of dissimilatory amino acid metabolism in the colon, accounting for about 30% of the total on a weight basis (Macfarlane & Allison, 1986). Some common amino acid substrates and their SCFA products are shown in Table 6.3.

As a group, the amino-acid fermenting clostridia have been extensively studied. They are nutritionally versatile and many species simultaneously ferment pairs of amino acids in Stickland reactions, where one amino acid acts as the electron donor and the other functions as the electron acceptor. Some common Stickland-reaction substrates and products are shown in Table 6.4. In general, branched-chain and aromatic amino acids usually serve as the electron donors in these reactions.

Less is known of the metabolism of other amino-acid-fermenting anaerobes that inhabit the colon. However, lysine is a major energy source for *Fusobacterium nucleatum*, which converts the substrate to equimolar amounts of acetate and butyrate by the 3-keto, 6-aminohexanoate pathway (Barker, Kahn & Hedrick, 1982). This bacterium is able to ferment nine different amino acids, either singly or in combination, although acetate and butyrate are always the principal fermentation products (Loesche & Gibbons, 1968). *F. nucleatum* can also ferment glucose to lactate and formate, but carbohydrate fermentation appears to occur independently and has no effect on amino-acid

Table 6.3. *Substrates and SCFA products formed by amino-acid-fermenting bacteria that occur in the human large intestine*

Bacteria	Approximate numbers in faeces ($\log_{10}$/g dry wt)[a]	Amino-acid substrate	Major fermentation acid product	Reference
Clostridia	9.8	Glycine	Acetate	Barker (1981)
		Alanine	Propionate	Gottschalk (1986)
			Acetate	Barker (1981)
		Threonine	Propionate, acetate	Elsden & Hilton (1978)
		Valine	Isobutyrate	Elsden & Hilton (1978)
		Leucine	Isovalerate	Elsden & Hilton (1978)
		Isoleucine	2-Methylbutyrate	Elsden & Hilton (1978)
		Glutamate	Acetate, butyrate	Barker (1981)
		Lysine	Acetate, butyrate	Barker, Kahn & Hedrick (1982)
Fusobacterium nucleatum	No information	Lysine	Acetate, butyrate	Loesche & Gibbons (1968)
Fusobacteria	8.4	Glutamate	Acetate, butyrate	Barker (1981)
Porphyromonas asaccharolytica	9.6	Aspartate	Acetate, succinate	Wong, Dyer & Tribble (1977)
Acidaminococcus fermentans	8.5	Glutamate	Acetate, butyrate	Rogosa (1969)
Peptococci	10.0	Glutamate	Acetate, butyrate	Barker (1981)

[a] Data from Finegold, Sutter & Mathisen (1983).

Table 6.4. *Common electron donors and acceptors involved in Stickland reactions*

Electron donor	Electron acceptor	Products
Isoleucine	Tryptophan	2-Methylbutyrate, carbon dioxide, ammonia, indolepropionate
Leucine	Proline	Isovalerate, carbon dioxide, ammonia, 5-aminovalerate
Phenylalanine	Leucine	Phenylacetate, carbon dioxide, ammonia, isocaproate
Alanine	Glycine	Acetate, carbon dioxide, ammonia

metabolism. Acetate and butyrate are also the major SCFA produced from glutamate fermentation, irrespective of whether the methylaspartate pathway, used by the majority of clostridia, or the hydroxyglutamate pathway, used by fusobacteria, peptococci and *Acidaminococcus*, are employed. The formation of propionate by clostridia occurs during fermentation of alanine via the acrylate pathway (Gottschalk, 1986) or from threonine, in reactions involving threonine dehydrase and keto acid dehydrogenases (Elsden & Hilton, 1978).

Factors affecting fermentation of amino acids

Other than substrate availability, the ecological and physiological factors that influence SCFA production from amino acids in the colon are unclear. However, the relative numbers and activities of proteolytic and amino-acid-fermenting bacteria will affect how proteins are degraded. From a physiological viewpoint, the partial pressure of dihydrogen may be significant. This gas is an important product of alanine, leucine, glutamate and valine metabolism (Barker, 1981; Nagase & Matsuo, 1982) and its concentration may determine the types of fermentation that can occur. This is because some reactions, for example, glutamate fermentation by *Acidaminobacter hydrogenoformans*, can only occur at low pH_2 (Stams & Hansen, 1984). Therefore, some amino-acid fermentations can potentially inhibit the operation of others in the large bowel. In practice, these inhibitory effects are likely to be diminished under certain circumstances by the activities of hydrogenotrophic species, such as the sulphate-reducing, methanogenic and acetogenic bacteria.

Other factors that may affect amino-acid fermentation include pH, which controls decarboxylation/deamination reactions, and carbohydrate availability, since glucose has been reported to inhibit the process in some clostridia (Saissac, Raynard & Cohen, 1948; Turton *et al.*, 1983) and *Megasphaera elsdenii* (Allison, 1978). *In vitro* fermentation studies have shown that gut bacteria produce different types and amounts of SCFA from different protein substrates, such as collagen, bovine serum albumin and casein (Macfarlane & Allison, 1986). These observations can to some extent be explained in terms of the relative amino-acid compositions of the test substrates, since, as can be seen in Tables 6.3 and 6.4, different amino acids are fermented to different end products. The situation is of course more complex, because amino-acid composition determines protein structure. This, together with the peptide-bond specificities of individual bacterial proteases and peptidases, has a major effect on the way proteins are broken down (Gibson *et al.*, 1989).

Interestingly, in the protein fermentation experiments described above, free amino acids did not accumulate to any significant extent in the fermenters, indicating that depolymerization reactions were the rate-limiting steps in mobilization of proteins for fermentation.

Host characteristics, such as colonic transit time, are important factors affecting protein fermentation. Studies *in vivo* and *in vitro* have shown that extended gut transit times resulted in more substrate becoming available to the bacteria (Cummings *et al.*, 1979; Macfarlane *et al.*, 1989).

Contribution of protein to SCFA production

Acetate, propionate and butyrate and the branched-chain fatty acids (BCFA), isobutyrate, 2-methylbutyrate and isovalerate are the major SCFA formed during the breakdown of organic nitrogen-containing compounds by human intestinal bacteria (Macfarlane *et al.*, 1992). Whilst many saccharolytic anaerobes form small amounts of BCFA during growth, amino-acid-fermenting species generate these metabolites as major end products of metabolism. Isobutyrate, isovalerate and 2-methylbutyrate are the respective reduced carbon skeletons of the branched-chain amino acids valine, leucine and isoleucine. Isocaproate is a comparatively minor BCFA in the colon and is formed by the oxidation of leucine.

It has already been seen (Fig. 6.3) that BCFA constitute a relatively small component of the SCFA pool in the large bowel; however, they do increase as a proportion of total SCFA in the distal colon. The increased production of these metabolites by bacteria in the distal gut is more evident in Fig. 6.5, which shows that BCFA formation is between three and four times higher in digesta taken from this region than in samples from the proximal gut, during incubations *in vitro*, in the absence of externally added substrates.

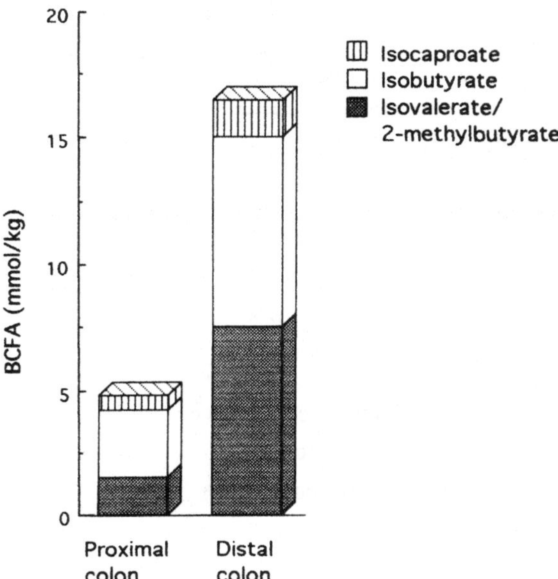

Fig. 6.5. Amounts of BCFA produced from endogenous substrates during incubation *in vitro* of gut contents under anaerobic conditions for 48 h. (G. T. Macfarlane & G. R. Gibson, unpublished data.)

The occurrence of BCFA in colonic contents has been used to estimate the contribution of protein to SCFA production in the large intestine (Macfarlane *et al.*, 1992). In this work, fermentations *in vitro* indicated that BCFA constituted approximately 20% of total SCFA produced from protein. Because the concentrations of SCFA and BCFA in the gut were known, it was calculated that 17% of SCFA in the proximal bowel and 38% in the distal region were products of amino-acid fermentation. By measuring arterial/venous differences in patients undergoing emergency surgery, the daily production of BCFA by the colon was estimated to be 11.1 mmol, which would require the digestion of approximately 12 g of protein. These data demonstrated that although carbohydrate fermentation predominates as a source of SCFA in the large intestine as a whole, the metabolism of proteinaceous materials becomes quantitatively more significant in the distal bowel.

Quantitation of SCFA production in the colon

Major difficulties arise in quantifying SCFA production in the large bowel, due largely to the inaccessibility of the proximal colon and portal vein in

Table 6.5. *Factors that affect SCFA production from polysaccharides and proteins by bacteria in the large intestine*

Chemical composition of the fermentable substrate
Amount of substrate available
Physical form of the substrate, including particle size, solubility and association with indigestible complexes such as lignins, tannins and silica
Types of bacteria present
Ecological factors, including competitive and co-operative interactions between bacteria
Rate of depolymerization of the substrate
Substrate specificities and catabolite regulatory mechanisms of individual gut species
Fermentation strategies of substrate-utilizing bacteria
pH of gut contents, particularly in the proximal colon
Availability of inorganic electron acceptors
Colonic transit time

healthy individuals. Since over 90% of SCFA formed in the colon are absorbed, measurements of these anions in faeces tell us very little. Nevertheless, two indirect methods have been used based on assessment of substrate availability and portal blood measurements in victims of sudden death, and persons undergoing emergency surgery for abdominal wounds (Cummings, Gibson & Macfarlane, 1989).

Estimations based on the availability of fermentable substrates in the diet gave an approximate value of 250 mmol/day (range 150–450), although this method underestimated the true production rate, since it could not take into consideration fermentation substrates of endogenous origin. Values derived from SCFA concentrations in portal blood gave a higher mean value of 377 mmol/day (range 50–700).

Conclusions

Although the principal fermentation pathways employed by the majority of gut bacteria are relatively well understood, it is certainly not clear how the metabolic activities of several hundred different species interact to produce the typical patterns of fermentation products that are observed in the large intestine. In view of the complexity of colonic ecosystems, this is hardly surprising. However, the numerically and metabolically predominant bacterial populations must have a major influence on the overall course of fermentation, which, as we have seen, differs both quantitatively and qualitatively in the proximal and distal colons. This is primarily determined by relative substrate availabilities, but may also reflect more subtle changes in the composition of the microflora and in the absorptive capacities of the colon itself.

It is evident that SCFA production is affected by many different though interacting factors, of which some of the more prominent are shown in Table 6.5. Host factors as well as more straightforward microbiological considerations are clearly important determinants of SCFA formation, and they undoubtedly make it more difficult to manipulate fermentation reactions *in vivo* or the composition of the microflora, through simple dietary modification. Whether this is possible or even desirable in the long term is an important question that requires serious consideration, in view of the current enthusiasm for stimulating the growth and activities of bacteria that are perceived to be 'beneficial'.

References

Allison, C. & Macfarlane, G. T. (1988). Effect of nitrate on methane production and fermentation by slurries of human faecal bacteria. *Journal of General Microbiology*, **134**, 1397–405.

Allison, C. & Macfarlane, G. T. (1989). Dissimilatory nitrate reduction by *Propionibacterium acnes*. *Applied and Environmental Microbiology*, **55**, 2899–903.

Allison, M. J. (1978). Production of branched-chain volatile fatty acids by certain anaerobic bacteria. *Applied and Environmental Microbiology*, **35**, 872–7.

Barker, H. A. (1981). Amino acid degradation by anaerobic bacteria. *Annual Review of Biochemistry*, **50**, 23–40.

Barker, H. A., Kahn, J. M. & Hedrick, L. (1982). Pathway of lysine degradation in *Fusobacterium nucleatum*. *Journal of Bacteriology*, **152**, 201–7.

Bingham, S. A., Pett, S. & Day, K. C. (1990). NSP intake of a representative sample of British adults. *Journal of Human Nutrition and Dietetics*, **3**, 339–44.

Chacko, A. & Cummings, J. H. (1988). Nitrogen losses from the human small bowel: obligatory losses and the effect of physical form of food. *Gut*, **29**, 809–15.

Christensen, J. (1991). Gross and microscopic anatomy of the large intestine. In *The Large Intestine: Physiology, Pathophysiology and Disease*, ed. S. F. Phillips, J. H. Pemberton & R. G. Shorter, pp. 13–35. New York: Raven Press.

Crabbendam, P. M., Streekstra, H., Teixeira de Mattos, M. J. & Neijssel, O. M. (1987). The effect of the degree of reduction of the carbon source on fermentation patterns. In *Proceedings of the 4th European Congress on Biotechnology*, vol. 1, ed. O. M. Neijssel, R. R. van der Meer and K. C. A. M. Luyben, p. 546. Amsterdam: Elsevier Science Publishers.

Cummings, J. H., Gibson, G. R. & Macfarlane, G. T. (1989). Quantitative estimates of fermentation in the hind gut of man. *Acta Veterinaria Scandinavica*, **86**, 76–82.

Cummings, J. H., Hill, M. J., Bone, E. S., Branch, W. J. & Jenkins, D. J. A. (1979). The effect of meat protein and dietary fiber on colonic function and metabolism. II. Bacterial metabolites in feces and urine. *American Journal of Clinical Nutrition*, **32**, 2094–101.

Cummings, J. H., Pomare, E. W., Branch, W. J., Naylor, C. P. E. & Macfarlane, G. T. (1987). Short chain fatty acids in human large intestine, portal, hepatic and venous blood. *Gut*, **28**, 1221–7.

Degnan, B. A. (1993). Transport and metabolism of carbohydrates by anaerobic gut bacteria. PhD thesis. Cambridge University, Cambridge.

DeVries, W., Kapteijn, W. M. C., van der Beek, E. G. & Stouthamer, A. H. (1970). Molar growth yields and fermentation balances of *Lactobacillus casei* L3 in batch cultures and in continuous cultures. *Journal of General Microbiology*, **63**, 333–45.

Elsden, S. R. & Hilton, M. G. (1978). Volatile acid production from threonine, valine, leucine and isoleucine by clostridia. *Archives of Microbiology*, **117**, 165–72.

Englyst, H. N., Bingham, S. A., Runswick, S. A., Collinson, E. & Cummings, J. H. (1988). Dietary fibre (non-starch polysaccharides) in fruit, vegetables and nuts. *Journal of Human Nutrition & Dietetics*, **1**, 247–86.

Englyst, H. N., Bingham, S. A., Runswick, S. A., Collinson, E. & Cummings, J. H. (1989). Dietary fibre (non-starch polysaccharides) in cereal products. *Journal of Human Nutrition & Dietetics*, **2**, 253–71.

Englyst, H. N. & Cummings, J. H. (1987). Resistant starch, a 'new' food component: a classification of starch for nutritional purposes. In *Cereals in a European Context*, ed. I. D. Martin, pp. 221–33. Chichester: Ellis Horwood.

Englyst, H. N., Hay, S. & Macfarlane, G. T. (1987). Polysaccharide breakdown by mixed populations of human faecal bacteria. *FEMS Microbiology Ecology*, **95**, 163–71.

Etterlin, C., McKeown, A., Bingham, S. A., Elia, M., Macfarlane, G. T. & Cummings, J. H. (1992). D-Lactate and acetate as markers of fermentation in man. *Gastroenterology*, **102**, A551.

Finegold, S. M., Sutter, V. L. & Mathisen, G. E. (1983). Normal indigenous intestinal flora. In *Human Intestinal Microflora in Health and Disease*, ed. D. J. Hentges, pp. 3–31. London: Academic Press.

Gibson, S. A. W., McFarlan, C., Hay, S. & Macfarlane, G. T. (1989). Significance of microflora in proteolysis in the colon. *Applied and Environmental Microbiology*, **55**, 679–83.

Gibson, J. A., Sladen, G. E. & Dawson, A. M. (1976). Protein absorption and ammonia production: the effects of dietary protein and removal from the colon. *British Journal of Nutrition*, **35**, 61–5.

Gottschalk, G. (1986). *Bacterial Metabolism*, 2nd edn. Berlin: Springer-Verlag.

Kuknal, J., Adams, A. & Preston, F. (1965). Protein producing capacity of the human exocrine pancreas. *Surgery*, **162**, 67–73.

Loesche, W. J. & Gibbons, R. J. (1968). Amino acid fermentation by *Fusobacterium nucleatum*. *Archives of Oral Biology*, **13**, 191–201.

Macfarlane, G. T. & Allison, C. (1986). Utilization of protein by human gut bacteria. *FEMS Microbiology Ecology*, **38**, 19–24.

Macfarlane, G. T., Allison, C., Gibson, S. A. W. & Cummings, J. H. (1988). Contribution of the microflora to proteolysis in the human large intestine. *Journal of Applied Bacteriology*, **64**, 37–46.

Macfarlane, G. T., Cummings, J. H. & Allison, C. (1986). Protein degradation by human intestinal bacteria. *Journal of General Microbiology*, **132**, 1647–56.

Macfarlane, G. T., Cummings, J. H., Macfarlane, S. & Gibson, G. R. (1989). Influence of retention time on degradation of pancreatic enzymes by human colonic bacteria grown in a 3-stage continuous culture system. *Journal of Applied Bacteriology*, **67**, 521–7.

Macfarlane, G. T. & Englyst, H. N. (1986). Starch utilisation by the human large intestinal microflora. *Journal of Applied Bacteriology*, **60**, 195–201.

Macfarlane, G. T. & Gibson, G. R. (1991). Co-utilization of polymerized carbon sources by *Bacteroides ovatus* grown in a two-stage continuous culture system. *Applied and Environmental Microbiology*, **51**, 1–6.

Macfarlane, G. T., Gibson, G. R., Beatty, E. & Cummings, J. H. (1992). Estimation of short-chain fatty acid production from protein by human intestinal bacteria based on branched-chain fatty acid measurements. *FEMS Microbiology Ecology*, **101**, 81–8.

Macy, J. M. & Probst, I. (1979). The biology of gastrointestinal bacteroides. *Annual Review of Microbiology*, **33**, 561–94.

Mitsuoka, T. (1984). Taxonomy and ecology of bifidobacteria. *Bifidobacteria Microflora*, **3**, 11–28.

Nagase, M. & Matsuo, T. (1982). Interactions between amino acid degrading bacteria and methanogenic bacteria in anaerobic digestion. *Biotechnology and Bioengineering*, **24**, 2227–39.

Rogosa, M. (1969). *Acidaminococcus* gen.nov., *Acidaminococcus fermentans* sp.nov., anaerobic Gram-negative diplococci using amino acids as the sole energy source for growth. *Journal of Bacteriology*, **98**, 756–66.

Saissac, R., Raynard, M. & Cohen, G.-N. (1948). Variation du type fermentaire des bactéries anaérobies du groupe de *Cl. sporogenes*, sous l'enfluence du glucose. *Annals de l'Institut Pasteur*, **75**, 305–9.

Scardovi, V. (1986). Genus *Bifidobacterium*. In *Bergey's Manual of Systematic Bacteriology*, vol. 2, ed. N. S. Mair, pp. 1418–34. New York: Williams & Wilkins.

Stams, A. J. M. & Hansen, T. A. (1984). Fermentation of glutamate and other compounds by *Acidaminobacter hydrogenoformans* gen.nov. sp.nov., an obligate anaerobe isolated from black mud: studies with pure cultures and mixed cultures with sulfate-reducing and methanogenic bacteria. *Archives of Microbiology*, **137**, 329–37.

Stephen, A. M. & Cummings, J. H. (1980). The microbial contribution to human faecal mass. *Journal of Medical Microbiology*, **13**, 45–56.

Stephen, A. M., Haddad, A. C. & Phillips, S. F. (1983). Passage of carbohydrate into the colon. Direct measurements of humans. *Gastroenterology*, **85**, 589–95.

Turton, L. J., Drucker, D. B. & Ganguli, L. A. (1983). Effect of glucose concentration in the growth medium upon neutral and acidic fermentation end-products of *Clostridium bifermentans*, *Clostridium sporogenes* and *Peptostreptococcus anaerobius*. *Journal of Medical Microbiology*, **16**, 61–7.

Wong, J. C., Dyer, J. K. & Tribble, J. L. (1977). Fermentation of L-aspartate by a saccharolytic strain of *Bacteroides melaninogenicus*. *Applied and Environmental Microbiology*, **33**, 69–73.

7

Reductive acetogenesis in animal and human gut

M. DURAND AND A. BERNALIER

Acetate is the major fatty acid produced by intestinal-tract fermentation. The two main pathways responsible for acetate production are oxidative and reductive.

The oxidative pathway requires interspecies transfer of hydrogen. Molecular hydrogen is produced by the oxidation of reduced cofactors generated during bacterial glycolysis. However, a high partial pressure of hydrogen impairs the regeneration of reduced cofactors. The rumen and some other ecosystems harbour hydrogen-using bacteria, such as methanogens, which use hydrogen as rapidly as it is formed (Wolin & Miller, 1983).

The reductive pathway (referred to as acetogenesis) requires the presence of micro-organisms that reduce two moles of carbon dioxide (CO_2) to one mole of acetate. This pathway has been clearly demonstrated in sewage and some anaerobic bacterial ecosystems, such as lake sediments. The biochemical processes involved were recently reviewed by Wood & Ljungdahl (1990) and Ragsdale (1991). Most metabolic studies have been made on a few selected species, *Clostridium thermoaceticum*, *Clostridium formicoaceticum* and *Acetobacterium woodii*. The majority of acetogens isolated to date are able to undertake two types of acetogenesis, the heterotrophic process (homoacetate fermentation of multicarbon compounds) and autotrophic acetogenesis (from one-carbon compounds). Oxidative and reductive reactions are coupled in heterotrophic acetogenesis. One hexose equivalent produces two acetates by the oxidative pathway and a third is formed by the reduction of previously released CO_2. In the autotrophic system exogenous CO_2 and molecular hydrogen (H_2) are coupled in an energy yielding reaction:

$$2CO_2 + 4H_2 \rightarrow CH_3COOH + 2H_2O$$

Carbon dioxide is first reduced to methyltetrahydrofolate (CH_3—H_4 folate), then acetyl-CoA is synthesized from CH_3—H_4 folate, CO_2 or CO and CoA

Table 7.1. *Main characteristics of H_2/CO_2-using acetogenic bacteria isolated from the digestive tract*

Isolates	Original source	Cell type[a]	Endospore formation	Guanine + cytosine (%)	Optimal temperature °C	Optimal pH	End products of organic substrate fermentation	References
Acetonema longum	Termite	−	+	51.5	30–33	7.8	Acetate + butyrate	Kane & Breznak (1991)
Clostridium mayombei	Termite	+	+	25.6	33	7.3	Acetate	Kane *et al.* (1991)
Sporomusa termitida	Termite	−	+	48.6	30	7.2	Acetate + (propionate)[b]	Breznak *et al.* (1988)
Acetomaculum ruminis	Bovine rumen	+	−	32–36	38	6.8	ND	Greening & Leedle (1989)
Eubacterium limosum	Sheep rumen Human faeces	+	−	49	39	7.2	Acetate + butyrate	Genthner *et al.* (1981); cited by Wolin & Miller (1983); Genthner & Bryant (1987)
Un-named strain	Deer rumen	−	+	52.9	ND	ND	Acetate	Rieu-Lesme *et al.* (1993)
Peptostreptococcus productus	Human faeces	+	−	45	37	6.8	Acetate + lactate, succinate, H_2	Lorowitz & Bryant (1984); Geerligs *et al.* (1987)

[a] +, Gram-positive; −, Gram-negative.
[b] Occasionally produced.
ND, not determined.

with a bound carbon monoxide intermediate formed by carbon monoxide dehydrogenase.

Acetogenic bacteria utilizing H_2/CO_2 have also been found in the digestive tracts of termites, ruminants and humans and there have been a few reports on the significance of acetogenesis in the gut. This chapter reviews the most recent data on the bacteriological, metabolic and quantitative aspects of acetogenesis in the animal gut.

Bacteriology

The enumeration, enrichment and isolation of most acetogenic bacteria have been performed with H_2/CO_2 as energy substrates. The principal acetogenic bacteria isolated from the gut are shown in Table 7.1. A Gram-positive non-motile coccus has been isolated from the cetacean colon (Wilmarth, Boone & Mah, 1985). Therefore, hydrogenotrophic acetogenesis is a property of several distantly related taxa of anaerobic bacteria, including both Gram-positive and Gram-negative genera (see Table 7.1).

Acetogens have generally been enumerated by the method that uses the most probable number. The termite (Kane & Breznak, 1991) and cetacean gut (Wilmarth *et al.*, 1985) contain 10^6 acetogenic bacteria/g of fluid content. In the rumen of cattle, a high number of H_2/CO_2 acetogens (10^7–10^8/g wet content) have been found (Greening & Leedle, 1989), whereas the sheep rumen and pig hindgut contain fewer acetogenic species (below 10^6/g wet content) (J. Doré *et al.*, unpublished data). J. Doré *et al.* (personal communication) have observed that the number of acetogens in human faeces seems to be inversely related to the number of methanogens and can be as high as 10^8/g fresh faeces in some non-methanogenic individuals.

All hindgut acetogenic bacteria are obligate anaerobes and grow only in oxygen-free media. The optimal temperature and pH for growth depend on the origin of the strain (see Table 7.1). Nutritional requirements also vary according to the isolate. For example, *Clostridium mayombei* and *Peptostreptococcus productus* require yeast extract for growth with H_2/CO_2 and CO, while *Eubacterium limosum* needs biotin, Ca-D-pantothenate and lipoic acid. In addition, Na^+ (10 mM) increases the synthesis of acetate from H_2/CO_2 by *P. productus* and stimulates the growth of *E. limosum*. The growth of some other strains can also be stimulated by adding clarified rumen fluid (5–10% v/v), yeast extract or trypticase (0.2–10% w/v).

Acetogenic bacteria can metabolize a wide range of substrates, including sugars, sugar-alcohols, alcohols and organic and amino acids. The substrate spectrum varies according to the strain. The regulation of metabolism differs

Table 7.2. *Effect of adaptation to different carbohydrates and of methanogenesis inhibition on $^{13}CO_2$ incorporation into acetate by washed bacterial suspensions*

WBS origin	Treatment	CH_4 produced (mM)	H_2 utilized (mM)	Labelled acetate in total acetate (%)	References
Adaptation to carbohydrates					
Human faeces	Lactulose	Trace	67	24.4	M. Durand *et al.* (unpublished data)
	Starch	50	160	10.9	
Inhibition of methanogenesis					
Pig hindgut	−BES	118	379	17.0	De Graeve, *et al.* (1994)
	+BES	Trace	158	51.0	
Human faeces	−BES	101	382	4.3	Bernalier *et al* (1993)
	+BES	Trace	208	29.6	
	−BES	0	235	31.4	Bernalier *et al.* (1993)
	+BES	0	225	35.8	

BES, bromoethane sulphonic acid.

from one strain to another. *S. termitida* can grow myxotrophically, i.e. by the simultaneous use of H_2/CO_2 and organic compounds for energy (Breznak & Blum, 1991), whereas glucose apparently represses the ability of *E. limosum* to use other substrates (methanol, H_2/CO_2, CO and isoleucine) (Genthner & Bryant, 1987).

Most species use H_2/CO_2 to form acetate as the sole fermentation product, but *E. limosum* also produces butyrate. The fermentation profile is wider when some of the bacteria are grown with organic substrates as energy sources (see Table 7.1). It is significant that some acetogens can be H_2-producers rather than H_2-consumers when they grow heterotrophically (see Table 7.1).

Acetogenic activity in gut contents

Studies on the stoichiometry of fermentation in the gut of termites (Breznak & Switzer, 1986), in the hindgut of several mammals (Demeyer & De Graeve, 1991; Stévani *et al.*, 1991) and in the human large intestine (Wolin & Miller, 1983) suggest that acetogenesis could be a substantial source of acetate in some situations. Clear evidence for this was first found by Prins & Lankhorst (1977), who showed that the synthesis of acetate from $^{14}CO_2$ and H_2 occurred in the caecum of rodents. Experiments measuring the incorporation of labelled [^{14}C]- or [^{13}C]CO_2 into acetic, and sometimes butyric acids, further demonstrated that acetogenesis can occur in the gut of various species. Homogenates of the gut of the termite *Reticulitermes flavipes* fix $^{14}CO_2$ into acetate, whilst methanogenesis is very low (Breznak & Switzer, 1986). Maximal rates measured under hydrogen for wood- and grass-feeding termites were 5–6 μmol acetate formed/g termite per h (Brauman *et al.*, 1992).

The rumen of adult cattle and sheep incorporate little labelled CO_2 into acetate (Prins & Lankhorst, 1977; Stévani *et al.*, 1991). However, reductive acetogenesis occurred in newborn lambs aged 24 h, but disappeared with the establishment of methanogens at 48 h of age (Doré *et al.*, 1992).

Methanogenic rat caecal suspensions (Lajoie *et al.*, 1988) and pig-hindgut washed bacterial suspensions (WBS) (De Graeve *et al.*, 1990) formed significant amounts of acetate from $^{13}CO_2$ and H_2. The rate of acetogenesis in the pig (6.3 μmol/g wet hindgut content per h) (De Graeve *et al.*, 1994) was similar to that for rats (6–8.5 μmol/g wet caecal content/h) found by Prins and Lankhorst (1977).

Lajoie *et al.* (1988) demonstrated significant acetate production from H_2 and $^{13}CO_2$ in incubations of human faecal suspensions harbouring low concentrations of methanogens ($<10^8$/g dry weight of faeces). These findings have recently been confirmed by Bernalier *et al.* (1993; see Table 7.2).

During culturing, addition of exogenous molecular hydrogen to the gas phase greatly enhanced the incorporation of labelled carbon dioxide into acetate and sometimes also butyrate in inocula other than those from the rumen. Hydrogen also had the same effect in pig WBS in the presence of exogenous carbohydrate (17–35 mM hexose equivalent; De Graeve *et al.*, 1994). Molecular hydrogen seems therefore to be a more appropriate source of electrons than are other electron donors, such as reduced cofactors, for gut acetogens.

Experiments with labelled carbon dioxide have provided information on the pathways of acetogenesis in the gut. In most studies the label was equally distributed between the methyl and carboxyl atoms, except in the study of De Graeve *et al.* (1990) with pig WBS, where the carboxyl group was slightly more heavily labelled (57% of the total). Nuclear magnetic resonance (NMR) spectroscopy of ^{13}C has shown that all acetate isotopomers (1-^{13}C, 2-^{13}C and 1, 2-$^{13}C_2$) are always present. The double-labelled molecules are probably markers of the autotrophic pathway in which exogenous carbon dioxide and molecular hydrogen are coupled, whereas the monolabelled acetates reflect the homoacetate fermentation of multicarbon compounds. The presence of methyl-monolabelled acetate may also indicate that the C_1 of the third acetate is formed by transcarboxylation from pyruvate, as shown by the equation proposed by Ragsdale (1991) for *Clostridium thermoaceticum*:

$$CH_3\text{—}CO\text{—}COO^- + CH_3\text{—}H_4\text{ folate} + 2HSCoA \rightarrow 2CH_3\text{—}CO\text{—}SCoA + H_4\text{ folate} + H_2O$$

Doubly labelled molecules accounted for 57 to 65% of the total label in the termite gut (Breznak & Switzer, 1986) as well as in rat and human faecal suspensions (Lajoie *et al.*, 1988), but monolabelled acetate predominated (55–70% of total) in the pig (De Graeve *et al.*, 1990, 1994) and human WBS (Bernalier *et al.*, 1993). Therefore, both autotrophic and heterotrophic pathways occur simultaneously in the animal gut, but the factors that favour one or other processes are not yet clearly known.

Competition between acetogenesis and other hydrogenotrophic activities

An inverse relationship between acetogenesis and methanogenesis has been shown in the termite (Brauman *et al.*, 1992), in human and rat faecal suspensions (Lajoie *et al.*, 1988), in human faecal WBS (Bernalier *et al.*, 1993), and in human faeces (Gibson *et al.*, 1990). Inhibition of methanogenesis with the specific methane inhibitor, bromoethane sulphonic acid, stimulates $^{13}CO_2$

incorporation into acetate in methanogenic WBS of the pig and human (see Table 7.2). Nevertheless, consumption of molecular hydrogen remains lower than in the presence of methanogenesis (see Table 7.2).

However, competition with sulphate-reducing bacteria is much less well documented. The addition of sulphate to cattle caecal flora *in vitro* depressed acetogenesis slightly, but in a concentration-dependent manner in both the presence and the absence of molecular hydrogen (Demeyer & De Graeve, 1991). With pig flora, the addition of sulphate (10.6 mM) in the presence of hydrogen reduced methanogenesis and [^{13}C]acetate production from $^{13}CO_2$ by more than half in two trials out of four (De Graeve *et al.*, 1994).

In energetic terms, competition for molecular hydrogen should favour sulphate reducers first, then methanogens, and finally acetogens ($\Delta G^{0\prime}$ = -152.2, -131 and -95 kJ/mol, respectively). The greater competitiveness of methanogens than acetogens is probably also partly due, as suggested by Breznak & Kane (1990), to the fact that the H_2 threshold for homoacetogenesis is much higher (10 to 100 times) than for methanogenesis, though some acetogens have K_m values for H_2 close to those of methanogens (e.g. *S. termitida*). It is likely that, even when molecular hydrogen is abundant in the gas phase, a high number of methanogens will maintain the concentration of dissolved hydrogen at a level too low for active stimulation of acetate synthesis. The fluctuating response to the addition of sulphate may also be due to differing metabolic features of the sulphate-reducing bacteria present in individual inocula, as shown for isolates from healthy and colitic individuals (Gibson, Cummings & Macfarlane, 1991).

However, ecological factors, such as a moderately low pH, may give a competitive advantage to acetogens. Gibson *et al.* (1990) observed that acetogenesis was maximal at a lower pH (pH 6.5) than methanogenesis and sulphate reduction (pH -7.5). Human faecal flora grown in continuous culture and adapted on fermentable oligosaccharides produced a lower pH than when grown on complex carbohydrates. This favoured acetogenesis rather than methanogenesis (M. Durand *et al.*, unpublished data; see Table 7.2), However, an even lower pH (<5.0), in conjunction with lactic acid fermentation, greatly reduced acetogenesis (Ducros *et al.*, 1993). The nutritional versatility of acetogenic bacteria and the ability of some species to obtain energy mixotrophically could be another factor in favour of acetogenesis.

Quantitative aspect of acetogenesis

One-third of acetate produced in wood-feeding termites may be derived from H_2/CO_2, and this process can support one-third of the animal's daily energy need (Breznak & Kane, 1990).

In methanogenic rumen contents, calculation of the hydrogen balance between production (2A + P + 4B + 3V; where A = acetate, P = propionate, B = butyrate and V = valerate) and utilization (2P + 2B + 4V + L + 4M + H_2; L = lactate and M = methane) gives values for hydrogen utilization/production of 80–100% (Demeyer & De Graeve, 1991). This calculation, together with the above results showing very small amounts of $^{13}CO_2$ incorporation, demonstrate that acetogenesis from H_2/CO_2 is quantitatively negligible in the rumen.

Conversely, hydrogen recovery is much lower (50–70%) in incubations of hindgut contents from several mammals (cattle, horses, rabbits, pigs) (Demeyer & De Graeve, 1991; Stévani *et al.*, 1991). From the hydrogen unaccounted for, Demeyer & De Graeve (1991) estimated that about 10% of the total acetate and butyrate formed were derived from CO_2 reduction in cattle and pig hindgut. This value might be an underestimate in view of the $^{13}CO_2$ incorporation data obtained in pigs (De Graeve *et al.*, 1990; and see Table 7.2). As 980 mmol of total acetate can be absorbed into the pig portal vein daily (Giusi-Perier, Fiszlewicz & Rérat, 1989), 100–200 mmol acetate, depending on the amount of H_2 released, could be derived from H_2/CO_2 in this species.

Wolin & Miller (1983), taking into account the high proportion of acetate observed in the faeces of non-methanogenic human subjects, suggested that in some subjects the equation of homoacetate fermentation ($C_6H_{12}O_6 \rightarrow 3CH_3COOH$) should be used in place of the equation proposed for methanogenic subjects ($C_6H_{12}O_6 \rightarrow 2CH_3COOH + CH_4 + CO_2$). Accordingly, acetogenesis would represent 26% of the total acetate produced. Similar values (17–26%) have been calculated from the stoichiometry of end-products obtained in continuous cultures of low methanogenic faeces (Duncan & Henderson, 1990). Data for $^{13}CO_2$ incorporation by non-methanogenic faecal WBS, in the presence of H_2 gas, corroborate these estimations (see Table 7.2). This would indicate that 50–70 mmol can be formed daily from H_2/CO_2, assuming that about 280 mmol of total acetate is absorbed into the human portal vein (Cummings *et al.*, 1987). However, the greatest difference of H_2 equivalents measured *in vivo* between methanogenic and non-methanogenic individuals was about 1 l (Christl *et al.*, 1992). When there is little hydrogen uptake by sulphate-reducing bacteria, this corresponds to only 10 mmol acetate formed daily from H_2/CO_2. Nevertheless, this last calculation included the whole large intestine, whereas it is likely that acetogenesis occurs principally in the proximal colon, where the pH is lower and considerable amounts of molecular hydrogen are produced from rapidly fermentable substrates. Acetogenesis could also occur in the proximal colon of methanogenic human subjects, as methane is mainly produced in the distal large intestine (Flourié *et al.*, 1991).

In conclusion, it has been clearly shown that the formation of acetate from H_2/CO_2 can be an active process in the animal gut. However, its relation to other hydrogenotrophic activities at various sites of the mammalian large intestine must be further investigated before its quantitative implications for short-chain production can be precisely known. This process is of great interest for the host (gain of energy in animals and reduction of fermentation gas in humans) and for the environment (reduction of methane release). A better knowledge of the bacteria involved and of their physiological, metabolic and genetic characteristics will be required before any deliberate attempt at acetogenesis stimulation is envisaged.

References

Bernalier, A., Douaneau, E., Cordelet, C., Beaumatin, P., Durand, M. & Grivet, J. P. (1993). Competition for hydrogen between methanogenesis and hydrogenotrophic acetogenesis in human colonic flora studied by ^{13}C NMR. *Proceedings of the Nutritional Society*, **52**, 118A.

Brauman, A., Kane, M. D., Labat, M. & Breznak, J. A. (1992). Genesis of acetate and methane by gut bacteria of nutritionally diverse termites. *Science*, **257**, 1384–7.

Breznak, J. A. & Blum, J. S. (1991). Mixotrophy in the termite gut acetogen, *Sporomusa termitida. Archives of Microbiology*, **156**, 105–10.

Breznak, J. A. & Kane, M. D. (1990). Microbial H_2/CO_2 acetogenesis in animal guts: nature and nutritional significance. *FEMS Microbiology Reviews*, **87**, 309–13.

Breznak, J. A. & Switzer, J. M. (1986). Acetate synthesis from H_2 plus CO_2 by termite gut microbes. *Applied and Environmental Microbiology*, **52**, 623–30.

Breznak, J. A., Switzer, J. M. & Seitz, H. J. (1988). *Sporomusa termitida* sp. nov., an H_2/CO_2-utilizing acetogen isolated from termites. *Archives of Microbiology*, **150**, 282–8.

Christl, S. U., Murgatroyd, P. R., Gibson, G. R. & Cummings, J. H. (1992). Production, metabolism, and excretion of hydrogen in the large intestine. *Gastroenterology*, **102**, 1269–77.

Cummings, J. H., Pomare, E. W., Branch, W. J., Naylor, C. P. E. & Macfarlane, G. T. (1987). Short chain fatty acids in human large intestine, portal, hepatic and venous blood. *Gut*, **28**, 1221–7.

De Graeve, K. G., Grivet, J. P., Durand, M., Beaumatin, P., Cordelet, C., Hannequart, G. & Demeyer, D. (1994). Competition between reductive acetogenesis and methanogenesis in the pig large-intestinal flora. *Journal of Applied Bacteriology*, **76**, 55–61.

De Graeve, K. G., Grivet, J. P., Durand, M., Beaumatin, P. & Demeyer, D. (1990). NMR study of $^{13}CO_2$ incorporation into short-chain fatty acids by pig large-intestinal flora. *Canadian Journal of Microbiology*, **36**, 579–82.

Demeyer, D. I. & De Graeve, K. (1991). Differences of stoichiometry between rumen and hindgut fermentation. *Advances in Animal Physiology and Animal Nutrition*, **22**, 50–61.

Doré, J., Rieu-Lesme, F., Fonty, G. & Gouet, P. (1992). Preliminary study of non-methanogenic hydrogenotrophic microflora in the rumen of new-born lambs. *Annales de Zootechnie*, **41**, 82.

Ducros, V., Durand, M., Beaumatin, P., Hannequart, G., Cordelet, C. & Grivet, J. P. (1993). Adaptation to two doses of lactulose by human colonic flora in continuous culture. *Proceedings of the Nutritional Society*, **52**, 156A.

Duncan, A. J. & Henderson, C. (1990). A study of the fermentation of dietary fibre by human colonic bacteria grown *in vitro* in semi-continuous culture. *Microbial Ecology in Health and Disease*, **3**, 87–98.

Flourié, B., Pellier, P., Florent, C., Marteau, P., Pochart, P. & Rambaud, J. C. (1991). Site and substrates for methane production in human colon. *American Journal of Physiology*, **260**, G752–7.

Geerligs, G., Aldrich, H. C., Harder, W. & Diekert, G. (1987). Isolation and characterization of a carbon monoxide utilizing strain of the acetogen *Peptostreptococcus productus*. *Archives of Microbiology*, **148**, 305–13.

Genthner, B. R. S. & Bryant, M. P. (1987). Additional characteristics of one-carbon-compound utilization by *Eubacterium limosum* and *Acetobacterium woodii*. *Applied and Environmental Microbiology*, **53**, 471–6.

Genthner, B. R. S., Davis, C. L. & Bryant, M. P. (1981). Features of rumen and sewage sludge strains of *Eubacterium limosum*, a methanol- and H_2–CO_2-utilizing species. *Applied and Environmental Microbiology*, **42**, 12–9.

Gibson, G. R., Cummings, J. H. & Macfarlane, G. T. (1991). Growth and activities of sulphate-reducing bacteria in gut contents of healthy subjects and patients with ulcerative colitis. *FEMS Microbiology Ecology*, **86**, 103–12.

Gibson, G. R., Cummings, J. H., Macfarlane, G. T., Allison, C., Segal, I., Vorster, H. H. & Walker, A. R. P. (1990). Alternative pathways for hydrogen disposal during fermentation in the human colon. *Gut*, **31**, 679–83.

Giusi-Perier, A., Fiszlewicz, M. & Rérat, A. (1989). Influence of diet composition on intestinal volatile fatty acid and nutrient absorption in unanesthetized pigs. *Journal of Animal Science*, **67**, 386–402.

Greening, R. C. & Leedle, J. A. Z. (1989). Enrichment and isolation of *Acetitomaculum ruminis* gen. sp. nov.: acetogenic bacteria from the bovine rumen. *Archives of Microbiology*, **151**, 399–406.

Kane, M. D., Brauman, A. & Breznak, J. A. (1991). *Clostridium mayombei* sp. nov., an H_2/CO_2 acetogenic bacterium from the gut of the African soil-feeding termite, *Cubitermes speciosus*. *Archives of Microbiology*, **156**, 99–104.

Kane, M. D. & Breznak, J. A. (1991). *Acetomema longum*, gen. nov. sp. nov., an H_2/CO_2 acetogenic bacterium from the termite, *Pterotermes occidentis*. *Archives of Microbiology*, **156**, 91–8.

Lajoie, S. F., Bank, S., Miller, T. L. & Wolin, M. J. (1988). Acetate production from hydrogen and [^{13}C]carbon dioxide by the microflora of human feces. *Applied and Environmental Microbiology*, **54**, 2723–7.

Lorowitz, W. H. & Bryant, M. P. (1984). *Peptostreptococcus productus* strain that grows rapidly, with CO as the energy source. *Applied and Environmental Microbiology*, **47**, 961–4.

Prins, R. A. & Lankhorst, A. (1977). Synthesis of acetate from CO_2 in the cecum of some rodents. *FEMS Microbiology Letters*, **1**, 255–8.

Ragsdale, S. W. (1991). Enzymology of the acetyl-CoA pathway of CO_2 fixation. *Critical Reviews in Biochemistry and Molecular Biology*, **26**, 261–300.

Rieu-Lesme, F., Fonty, G., Gouet, P. & Doré, J. (1993). Isolation and characterization of hydrogen oxidizing acetogenic bacteria in the rumen of deer. *Nutrition Clinique et Métabolisme*, **7**, 165.

Stévani, J., Durand, M., De Graeve, K., Demeyer, D. & Grivet, J. P. (1991). Degradative abilities and metabolisms of rumen and hindgut microbial ecosystems. In *Hindgut '91*, ed. T. Sakata & R. L. Snipes, pp. 123–35. Tokyo: Senshu University Press.

Wilmarth, K. R., Boone, D. R. & Mah, R. A. (1985). Hydrogen-utilizing bacteria in the colon of cetaceans. *Annual Meeting of the American Society for Microbiology*, **109**, 164.

Wolin, M. J. & Miller, T. L. (1983). Carbohydrate fermentation. In *Human Intestinal Microflora in Health and Disease*, ed. D. J. Hentges, pp. 147–65. New York: Academic Press.

Wood, H. G. & Ljungdahl, G. (1990). Autotrophic character of the acetogenic bacteria. In *Variations in Autotrophic Life*, ed. J. M. Shively & L. L. Barton, pp. 201–50. London: Academic Press.

8

Flow dynamics of digesta and colonic fermentation

I. D. HUME

Introduction

The extent of fermentation in the mammalian gastrointestinal tract is dependent on the size and composition of the microbial population, the substrates presented to the microbes and the time that microbes are in contact with the substrate. Therefore control of digesta retention in the fermentative region(s) of the gut is of central importance in quantitative aspects of microbial fermentation, and therefore of the production of short-chain fatty acids (SCFA).

In humans the principal site of microbial fermentation is the colon; the caecum is small (Fig. 8.1(*a*)). We are therefore typical 'colon fermenters' (Hume & Warner, 1980), along with other hominoids (the apes), equids (horses, zebras), tapirs, rhinos, elephants, wombats, dugongs and pigs (Hume & Sakaguchi, 1991). Although there is no ideal animal model of the human colon on account of the large differences in colonic anatomy among mammals, the pig is probably the closest. However, although similar in body size, pigs differ from humans in their greater hindgut capacity (48% of total gut capacity versus 17% in humans), in part because of added caecal size (15% of total gut capacity) (Fig. 8.1(*b*)) and thus their greater capacity for microbial fermentation of fibre (Van Soest *et al.*, 1983).

Rats are not a model of choice for the human colon, because the patterns of digesta flow and SCFA production in their hindgut differ so markedly from the human condition. The principal site of digesta retention and microbial fermentation in the rat is the caecum, not the colon (Fig. 8.1(*c*)). Rats are therefore 'caecum fermenters' (Hume & Warner, 1980), as also are mice and other rodents, rabbits and other lagomorphs, some small monkeys (e.g. tamarins, marmosets), and four groups of marsupials that feed more-or-less exclusively on *Eucalyptus* foliage. This includes the koala (Hume, 1982).

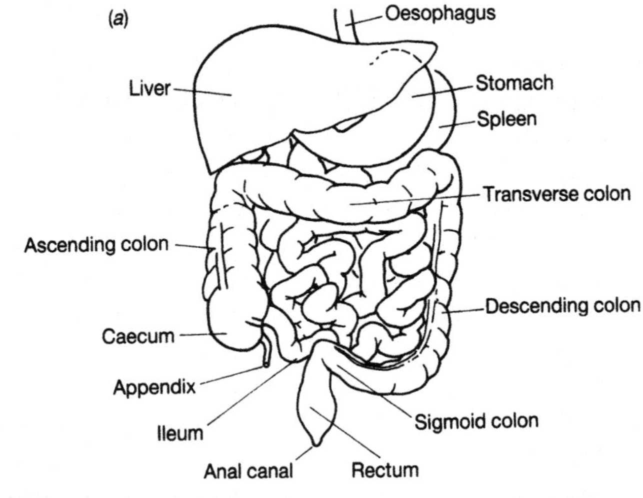
(a)
Oesophagus
Liver
Stomach
Spleen
Transverse colon
Ascending colon
Descending colon
Caecum
Appendix
Ileum
Sigmoid colon
Anal canal
Rectum

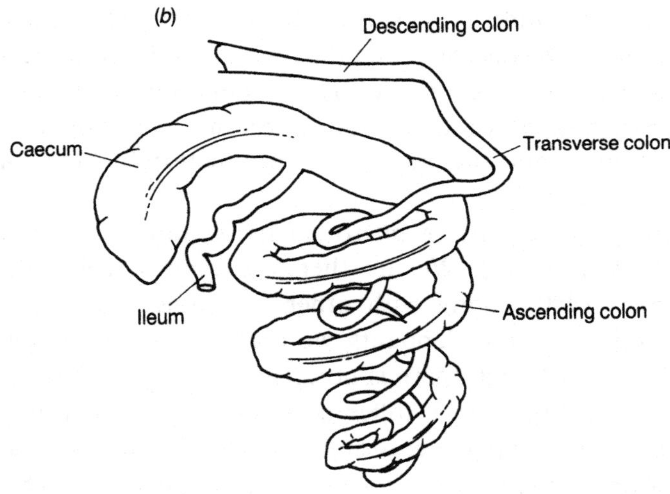
(b)
Descending colon
Caecum
Transverse colon
Ileum
Ascending colon

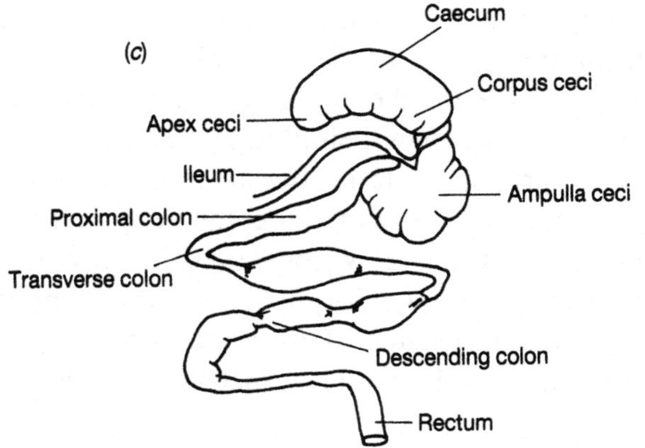
(c)
Caecum
Corpus ceci
Apex ceci
Ileum
Ampulla ceci
Proximal colon
Transverse colon
Descending colon
Rectum

With few exceptions, caecum fermenters are small (<10 kg body mass), while colon fermenters are generally large (>10 kg body mass). These two distinctly different digestive strategies among the hindgut fermenters are discussed by Hume (1989) and Hume & Sakaguchi (1991).

Structure and motility of the human colon

The human colon is short, only 1.0–1.5 m in length (Christensen, 1989), and can be divided into ascending colon, transverse colon, descending colon and sigmoid colon (Fig. 8.1(*a*)). In more herbivorous colon fermenters, including the pig, the colon is much longer and is consequently often arranged in a spiralling coil (Fig. 8.1(*b*)) (Stevens, 1988). In these animals the terms ascending, transverse and descending colon are not as applicable, and the terms proximal colon and distal colon are widely used. The proximal colon and first part of the distal colon develop from the embryonic midgut, while the rest of the distal colon develops from the embryonic hindgut. The proximal colon is the main region of microbial fermentation, and is distinguished from the distal colon by the generally smaller diameter and more segmented appearance of the latter. The distal colon is the main region of absorption of water and electrolytes and formation of faeces. In humans the ascending colon and transverse colon are more-or-less equivalent to the proximal colon.

The human colon is haustrated throughout most of its length. Haustration results from the organization of most of the outer longitudinal muscle layer into three thick bands called taeniae. The longitudinal muscle layer is present between the taeniae but is very thin (Christensen, 1989). Contractions of the circular muscle layer between the taeniae form semilunar folds internally, which manifest themselves externally as haustra. The semilunar folds or contraction rings form, disappear and reform with no constant relationship to the position of fixed points on the colon wall. Waves of contraction of the circular muscles move digesta both caudally (peristalsis) and orally (antiperistalsis).

In the proximal colon of most, if not all mammals, the dominant motor activity is antiperistalsis. These movements are involuntary, and serve to churn and mix the digesta. Compared with motions in the small intestine, colonic motions are slow and recur at long intervals. This makes it difficult

◄

Fig. 8.1. Gross morphology of the hindgut of the human (*a*) (from Lacy, 1991), pig (*b*) (from de Lahunta & Habel, 1986) and rat (*c*) (from Stevens, 1988).

to appreciate their complexity fully in short-term studies (Christensen, 1989). In the cat proximal colon, antiperistaltic contractions begin about 7 cm distal to the apex of a tiny caecum, and move toward the caecum at 1–2 cm/s. These contractions are about 1 cm apart, and occur at frequencies of 5 or 6 cycles/min (Elliott & Barclay-Smith, 1904). The extensive mixing and prolonged residence of digesta observed in the cat proximal colon also occur in the proximal colon of humans.

In the distal colon there is co-ordinated peristalsis, which drives the digesta caudally. The digesta stimulate such contractions by distension of the colon. In the sigmoid colon and rectum in humans the main activity is a strong contraction that empties the colon. These contractions are excited by stimulation of the pelvic nerves of the autonomic nervous system.

An additional type of contraction of the colon results in sudden mass movement of colonic contents distally by a series of infrequent large movements, known as mass movements or mass peristalsis (Holdstock *et al.*, 1970). The segmental contractions described above disappear before mass movement occurs, in both donor and recipient regions of the colon, but the exact nature of the wall contraction that produces mass movement is not clear.

In the human hindgut, the caecum and the sigmoid colon are seen as major points in the delay of digesta transit from mouth to anus (Christensen, 1989).

Flow dynamics of digesta in mammalian herbivores

Excretion patterns of indigestible markers have been used extensively by comparative digestive physiologists in order to determine how and where digesta are retained for microbial fermentation in several mammalian herbivores (Stevens, 1988). In colon fermenters the mean retention time of particle markers (i.e. the average time taken for digesta markers to traverse the entire gastrointestinal tract) exceeds that of fluid markers (Hume, 1989). This separation of digesta phases results from the way in which fluid is squeezed through a matrix of large particles by peristaltic contractions of the colon wall. In other words, the haustrations of the colon wall selectively retain large particles. Antiperistaltic contractions in the proximal colon result in delay in the transit of both digesta phases. Sellers *et al.* (1982) identified a pacemaker area for retropulsion events at the pelvic flexure of the equine ventral colon. In the human colon there appear to be three distinct segments of electrical control activity (Sarna *et al.*, 1980).

The pattern of marker excretion in colon fermenters (i.e. the mean retention time of particles is longer than that of fluid) is very different from the patterns found in caecum fermenters, in which there is either no significant difference between the mean retention time of fluid and particle markers, or the mean retention time of fluid exceeds that of particles (Hume & Sakaguchi, 1991). The structural and functional basis for these very different marker excretion patterns is best understood through the application of chemical reactor theory (Levenspiel, 1972) to the digestive system.

Application of chemical reactor theory to the intestines

Chemical reactor theory was first applied to animal guts by Penry & Jumars (1987) in their analysis of the digestive systems of marine deposit feeders. It has since been applied to the digestive systems of mammalian herbivores by Hume (1989) and Alexander (1991). Chemical reactors are classified on the basis of (1) whether input is discontinuous or continuous, and (2) whether reactants are brought together with or without mixing (Levenspiel, 1972). Three types of chemical reactors are applicable to the vertebrate intestine: plug-flow reactors, continuous-flow stirred-tank reactors, and modified plug-flow reactors (Hume, 1989).

Plug-flow reactors

Plug-flow reactors feature the continuous, orderly flow of material through a usually tubular reaction vessel (Fig. 8.2(*a*)). In ideal plug-flow reactors (i.e. those that can be described accurately by simple equations), material does not mix along the flow axis, although there is perfect radial mixing. Consequently, at steady state (when there is no variation with time at any point along the reactor) there is a continuous decrease in reactant concentrations from inlet along the reactor to outlet, and a continuous increase in concentrations of products. Plug-flow reactors are best represented in the vertebrate gut by the small intestine, even though we know that flow in the small intestine is not continuous and that there is some, though limited, axial mixing. Plug flow provides the greatest rate of digestive product formation in the minimum of time and volume under most conditions (Penry & Jumars, 1987), although the extent of digestion may be low unless the reactants (substrates) are easily digested.

Continuous-flow stirred-tank reactors

These reactors are characterized by continuous material flow through a usually spherical reaction vessel of minimal volume (Fig. 8.2(*b*)). The reactant

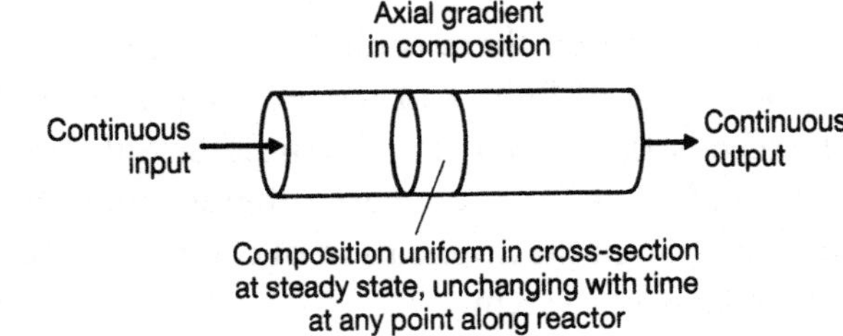

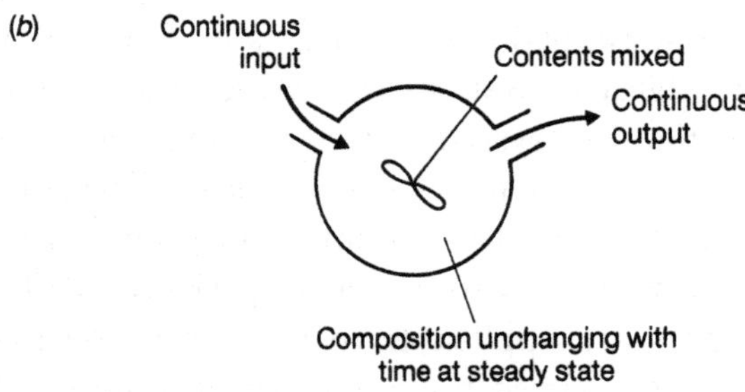

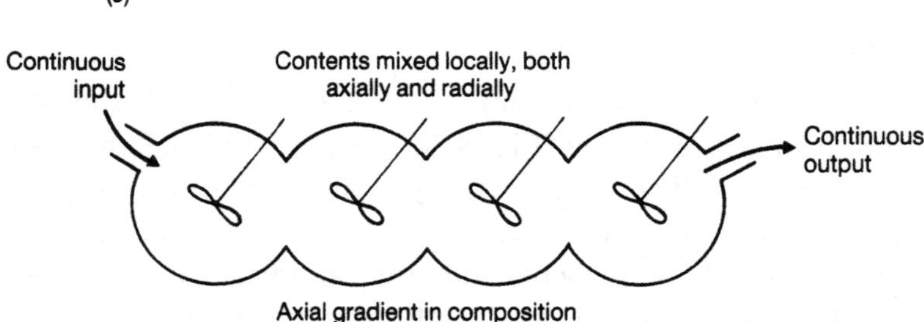

Fig. 8.2. Diagrams of an ideal plug-flow reactor (*a*), a continuous-flow stirred-tank reactor (*b*) and a modified plug-flow reactor (*c*).

concentration is diluted immediately upon entry into the vessel by material recirculating in the reactor. This reduces the reaction rate, so that the rate of digestion is lower than in plug-flow reactors, but conversion (i.e. extent of reaction) can be high if material flow is low enough. In the vertebrate gut, stirred-tank reactors are best represented by diverticulae such as the fore-stomach of foregut fermenters and the caecum. Retention times of digesta in these regions are prolonged. Long retention times in the caecum are caused by antiperistaltic contractions of the proximal colon and of the caecum itself (Hume, 1989).

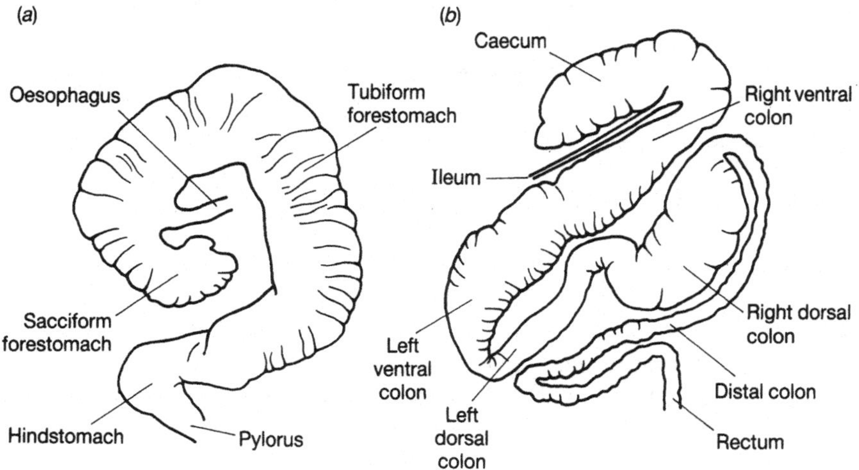

Fig. 8.3. The kangaroo forestomach (*a*) and the equine hindgut (*b*) as examples of modified plug-flow reactors. Modified from Hume & Sakaguchi (1991).

Modified plug-flow reactors

When several stirred-tank reactors are connected in series, the flow characteristics of the system are intermediate between those of a stirred-tank reactor and those of a plug-flow reactor (Fig. 8.2(*c*)). As the number of stirred-tank reactors in series increases, the reactor system becomes more and more like a plug-flow reactor (Penry & Jumars, 1987). Hume (1989) identified two vertebrate systems that were best described as 'modified plug-flow reactors': the tubiform forestomach of large kangaroos (Langer, Dellow & Hume, 1980), and the proximal colon of colon fermenters (Fig. 8.3). In this hybrid reactor system there is substantial axial as well as radial mixing, yet incoming reactants are not immediately mixed with the entire contents of the reactor vessel. In kangaroos, Dellow (1979) observed radiographically that there was effective localized mixing of contrast medium with digesta, but contrast medium did not mix with the entire contents of the forestomach. Rather, marked digesta were transported slowly along the length of the tubiform forestomach so that after 6 h, in the frequently fed animal, newly ingested food was not marked with previously administered contrast medium.

Production of SCFA in modified plug-flow reactors

Lack of mixing of digesta within a single pool in tubiform fermentation systems such as the colon makes it difficult to estimate rates of fermentation.

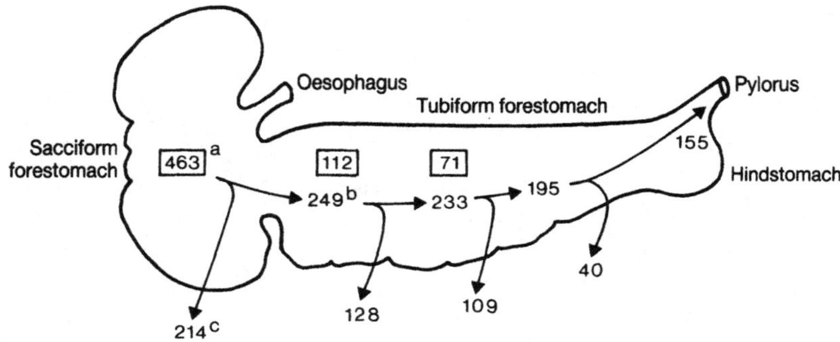

Fig. 8.4. Net production (a), absorption (c) and flow (b) of short-chain fatty acids (mmol/day) in the stomach of the wallaby *Thylogale thetis* (red-necked pademelon). From Dellow, Nolan & Hume (1983).

The most useful method for measuring rates of production of SCFA *in vivo* is by isotope dilution. However, this technique relies on rapid and uniform mixing of the infused labelled SCFA (such as [^{14}C]acetate) with the entire digesta pool (Leng & Leonard, 1965; Weston & Hogan, 1968). The requirement is readily satisfied in sacciform fermentation systems that function as stirred-tank reactors, such as the reticulorumen, but not in tubiform systems that operate as modified plug-flow reactors.

To date only one study of SCFA production based on isotope dilution in a modified plug-flow reactor gut has been reported. In that study, Dellow, Nolan & Hume (1983) treated the wallaby forestomach as four stirred-tank reactors in series (Fig. 8.4). The first stirred-tank reactor, or primary mixing pool, was the sacciform forestomach; the other three were successive sections of the tubiform forestomach. Animals were infused into the sacciform forestomach with a solution containing [^{14}C]acetate and the inert fluid marker[^{51}Cr]EDTA for 48 h, then slaughtered and the contents from each of the four forestomach segments and from the hindstomach (the region of hydrochloric acid secretion) were analysed for ^{51}Cr activity, specific radioactivity of acetate, total SCFA concentrations, and proportions of the individual acids (mainly acetate, propionate, butyrate and valerate). By assuming (1) no reversal of flow from the hindstomach to the forestomach, or from any of the three pools in the tubiform forestomach to a preceding pool, and (2) that the 'infusion rate' into any of these pools was the product of the rate of flow of fluid (estimated from ^{51}Cr activities) and the level of labelled acetate, Dellow *et al.* (1983) were able to calculate for each pool the net production rate of acetate, its flow to the next pool, and by difference its net apparent absorption from that pool (Fig. 8.4). This showed that the ratio

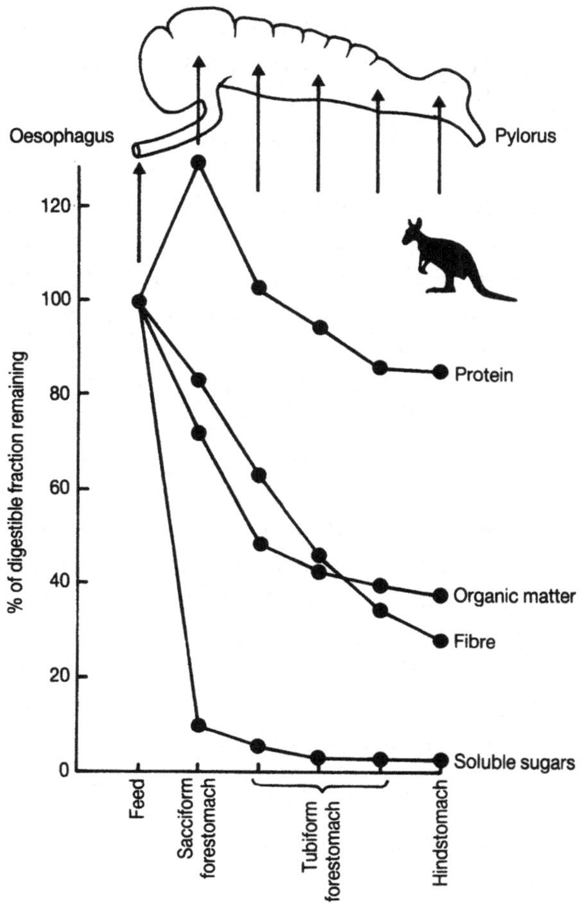

Fig. 8.5. Disappearance of digestible components of chopped lucerne hay along the stomach of the eastern grey kangaroo (*Macropus giganteus*). From Dellow & Hume (1982).

of total SCFA production to the intake of digestible organic matter was similar in the two species of wallabies examined, and also similar to published estimates for ruminants. It also showed that the rate of fermentation decreased along the length of the wallaby forestomach, which reflected the rapid disappearance of soluble carbohydrate in the sacciform and upper tubiform regions (Fig. 8.5), and the decreasing rate of apparent loss of organic matter along the tubiform forestomach (Dellow & Hume, 1982). That is, as digesta move through this gastric region the microbes are increasingly reliant on fibre as their principal substrate.

Most other estimates of rates of SCFA production in modified plug-flow reactor systems in the gut have been based on fermentation rates measured *in vitro*. This approach suffers in that it underestimates fermentation rates *in vivo* by a factor of up to four in the forestomach (Hume, 1977). This is because there is necessarily a lag from the time the animal last consumed food until the incubation commences, during which time a lot of soluble substrates disappear. There is also the problem of negative feedback by fermentation end-products on the fermentation process within the glass vessel, and exhaustion of available substrate within the vessel. The problem is likely to be less severe in the hindgut than in the forestomach, because most of the soluble substrates will have been digested in the small intestine anyway (Hume, 1982). Nevertheless, it still means that SCFA production rates measured *in vitro* cannot be directly compared with estimates made *in vivo* (Whitelaw *et al.*, 1970).

However, despite this limitation, there is little reason to doubt that comparisons made *in vitro* between fermentation sites and between animal species are valid (Dellow *et al.*, 1983). Therefore, Hume (1977) was able to show that SCFA production was much faster in the forestomach of wallabies and sheep then in the hindgut, and that, on a common diet, production rates were faster in the wallaby forestomach (a modified plug-flow reactor) than in the ruminant forestomach (a stirred-tank reactor). The last observation is entirely consistent with predictions based on chemical reactor theory.

Production of SCFA in the colon

Fermentation rates have been reported in three non-human colon fermenters: the horse, the pig and the wombat. In the horse, Argenzio, Southworth & Stevens (1974*b*) estimated SCFA production rates in the hindgut by a slaughter technique similar in several aspects to that described above for the wallaby forestomach. Fluid flow along the digestive tract was estimated from inert marker concentrations in animals slaughtered at intervals after they were given a pulse dose of the marker in the feed (Argenzio *et al.*, 1974*a*). With the assumption that there was no retrograde flow of fluid in the colon, flow rates of SCFA were calculated from fluid flows and SCFA concentrations. These, together with rates of absorption from each region of the hindgut (caecum, ventral colon, dorsal colon and small colon) estimated *in vitro*, were then used to calculate SCFA production during each time interval between measurements. Production rates in all hindgut regions were highest in the first 4–8 h after feeding, and during this period production rates were highest in the caecum and ventral colon and lowest in the small or distal colon.

In the pig, an *in vitro* study by Rose, Hume & Farrell (1987) indicated that SCFA production rates in the hindgut were highest in the caecum and proximal colon, and declined along the length of the colon of both domestic and feral pigs. On a diet of 25% neutral-detergent fibre, the pig's total SCFA production in the hindgut accounted for 20% of the intake of digestible energy (i.e. energy absorbed). Argenzio & Southworth (1974) had previously demonstrated selective retention of large-particle markers (1-cm and 2-cm plastic chips) in the pig, presumably mainly in the colon, compared with a fluid marker (polyethylene glycol 4000) and a small (2-mm) particle marker.

The wombats are the only marsupial colon fermenters; they feed on grasses and sedges, which are often high in fibre content. Their hindgut consists of a colon that is 60–80% of total digestive tract capacity, but it has only a vestigial caecum (Barboza & Hume, 1992*a*). SCFA production rates measured *in vitro* were highest in the proximal colon, and declined by about 50% along the length of the colon. The energy derived from SCFA absorbed from the colon was 30–33% of digestible energy intake in captive animals (Barboza & Hume, 1992*b*).

All three colon fermenters described in this section share the following features:

(1) The mean retention time of particle markers exceeds that of fluid (and small-particle) markers.
(2) The principal site of digesta retention appears to be the proximal colon.
(3) Digesta composition changes along the colon, particularly in content of water, nitrogen and some fibre components (see, e.g. Barboza & Hume, 1992*a*), and usually but not necessarily SCFA as well.
(4) SCFA produced in the hindgut make a substantial contribution (20–33%) to energy absorbed from the digestive tract.
(5) SCFA production rates are highest in the proximal colon (and caecum if present), and decline along the length of the colon toward the rectum.
(6) The molar proportion of acetate tends to increase along the colon, while that of propionate and butyrate decreases. This reflects both a more rapid absorption of longer chain-length SCFA (Stevens, 1988) and a change in the substrate fermented towards more and more refractory fibrous components of the digesta.

All of these features are those of modified plug-flow reactors.

Implications for the human colon

Given the difficulties in working invasively with humans, it is not surprising that quantitative data on SCFA production in the human colon are extremely limited. However, a number of indirect approaches have yielded results that are consistent with predictions based on chemical reactor theory. For instance, Cummings, Gibson & Macfarlane (1989) showed that in sudden-death victims, total SCFA concentrations were highest in the caecum, and declined progressively toward the distal colon, while pH was lowest in the caecum and highest in the distal colon. Together these results suggest that fermentation rate was greatest in the right or ascending colon, where substrate availability was likely to be greatest.

The only estimate of the rate of SCFA production appears to have been *in vitro*, using human faecal inocula with different substrates in mixed batch culture. Production was equivalent to 7.5 mmol SCFA/g polysaccharide utilized (Englyst, Hay & Macfarlane, 1987), only a little less than *in vivo* estimates of 9–10 mmol/g organic matter fermented in the wallaby forestomach (Dellow *et al.*, 1983) and 8.3 in the ruminant forestomach (Czerkawski, 1978). How this *in vitro* estimate relates to actual rates of production in the human colon is not known. Based on *in vitro* estimates, together with other approaches, such as arteriovenous differences across the gut of surgical patients, Cummings *et al.* (1989) concluded that in people on Western diets, SCFA absorbed from the gut were equivalent to 3–9% of the total energy requirement.

Until estimates of SCFA production made in *in vivo* become available, it will continue to be difficult to quantify and further characterize human colonic fermentation. To this end the approach used *in vivo* by Dellow *et al.* (1983) in the wallaby forestomach may be applicable if multilumen catheters could be inserted into the human colon. This would make possible continuous infusion of non-radioactively labelled [^{13}C]acetate and [Cr]EDTA at the level of the ileocolonic junction.

Provided that free fluid could be drawn into the catheter for sampling, the colon could be treated as a number of stirred-tank reactors, the number depending on the number of lumens in the catheter.

The type of information arising from this *in vivo* approach is likely to be important, not only because SCFAs are an energy substrate, but also because there is a growing body of evidence that SCFA are important anions involved in the maintenance of electrochemical gradients across the hindgut wall, particularly in the distal colon (Stevens, 1988). It is also becoming clear that SCFA (especially butyrate) play important roles in contractile responses of the colon wall (Yajima, 1985), and in the maintenance and repair of epithelial tissue (Roediger, 1991; Rombeau, 1991). Perhaps most importantly, dietary fibre, the principal microbial substrate entering the human colon (Cummings *et al.*, 1989), plays a central role in stimulating colonic motility and thus in maintaining normal flow dynamics of digesta in the colon.

References

Alexander, R. McN. (1991). Optimization of gut structure and diet for higher vertebrate herbivores. *Philosophical Transactions of the Royal Society, London*, **B333**, 249–55.

Argenzio, R. A., Lowe, J. E., Pickard, D. W. & Stevens, C. E. (1974*a*). Digesta passage and water exchange in the equine large intestine. *American Journal of Physiology*, **226**, 1035–42.

Argenzio, R. A. & Southworth, M. (1974). Sites of organic acid production and absorption in gastrointestinal tract of the pig. *American Journal of Physiology*, **228**, 454–60.

Argenzio, R. A., Southworth, M. & Stevens, C. E. (1974*b*). Sites of organic acid production and absorption in the equine gastrointestinal tract. *American Journal of Physiology*, **226**, 1043–50.

Barboza, P. S. & Hume, I. D. (1992*a*). Digestive tract morphology and digestion in the wombats (Marsupialia, Vombatidae). *Journal of Comparative Physiology*, **B162**, 552–60.

Barboza, P. S. & Hume, I. D. (1992*b*). Hindgut fermentation in the wombats – two marsupial grazers. *Journal of Comparative Physiology*, **B162**, 561–6.

Christensen, J. (1989). Colonic motility. In *Handbook of Physiology, Section 6: The Gastrointestinal System*, vol. 1, ed. J. D. Wood & S. G. Schultz, pp. 939–73. Bethesda: American Physiological Society.

Cummings, J. H., Gibson, G. R. & Macfarlane, G. T. (1989). Quantitative estimates of fermentation in the hind gut of man. *Acta Veterinaria Scandinavica*, **86** (Suppl.), 76–82.

Czerkawski, J. W. (1978). Reassessment of efficiency of synthesis of microbial matter in the rumen. *Journal of Dairy Science*, **61**, 1261–73.

de Lahunta, A. & Habel, R. E. (1986). Intestines. In *Applied Veterinary Anatomy*, pp. 246–56. Philadelphia: W. B. Saunders.

Dellow, D. W. (1979). Physiology of digestion in the macropodine marsupials. PhD thesis, University of New England, Armidale, Australia.

Dellow, D. W. & Hume, I. D. (1982). Studies on the nutrition of macropodine marsupials. IV. Digestion in the stomach and the intestine of *Macropus giganteus, Thylogale thetis* and *Macropus eugenii*. *Australian Journal of Zoology*, **30**, 767–77.

Dellow, D. W., Nolan, J. V. & Hume, I. D. (1983). Studies on the nutrition of macropodine marsupials. V. Microbial fermentation in the forestomach of *Thylogale thetis* and *Macropus eugenii*. *Australian Journal of Zoology*, **31**, 433–43.

Elliott, T. R. & Barclay-Smith, E. (1904). Antiperistalsis and other muscular activities of the colon. *Journal of Physiology, London*, **31**, 272–304.

Englyst, H. N., Hay, S. & Macfarlane, G. T. (1987). Polysaccharide breakdown by mixed populations of human faecal bacteria. *FEMS Microbiological Ecology*, **95**, 163–71.

Holdstock, D. J., Misiewicz, J. J., Smith, T. & Rowlands, E. N. (1970). Propulsion (mass movement) in the human colon and its relationship to meals and somatic activity. *Gut*, **11**, 91–9.

Hume, I. D. (1977). Production of volatile fatty acids in two species of wallaby and in sheep. *Comparative Biochemistry and Physiology*, **56A**, 299–304.

Hume, I. D. (1982). *Digestive Physiology and Nutrition of Marsupials*. Cambridge: Cambridge University Press.

Hume, I. D. (1989). Optimal digestive strategies in mammalian herbivores. *Physiological Zoology*, **62**, 1145–63.

Hume, I. D. & Sakaguchi, E. (1991). Patterns of digesta flow and digestion in foregut and hindgut fermenters. In *Physiological Aspects of Digestion and Metabolism in Ruminants*, ed. T. Tsuda, Y. Sasaki & R. Kawashima, pp. 427–51. San Diego: Academic Press.

Hume, I. D. & Warner, A. C. I. (1980). Evolution of microbial digestion in mammals. In *Digestive Physiology and Metabolism in Ruminants*, ed. Y. Ruckebusch & P. Thivend, pp. 665–84. Lancaster: MTP Press.

Lacy, E. R. (1991). Functional morphology of the large intestine. In *Handbook of Physiology*, section 6, *The Gastrointestinal System*, vol. IV, *Intestinal Absorption and Secretion*, ed. M. Field, R. A. Frizzell & S. G. Schultz, pp. 121–94. Bethesda, MD: American Physiological Society.

Langer, P., Dellow, D. W. & Hume, I. D. (1980). Stomach structure and function in three species of macropodine marsupials. *Australian Journal of Zoology*, **28**, 1–18.

Leng, R. A. & Leonard, G. J. (1965). Measurement of the rates of production of acetic, propionic and butyric acids in the rumen of sheep. *British Journal of Nutrition*, **19**, 469–84.

Levenspiel, O. (1972). *Chemical Reaction Engineering*, 2nd edn. New York: Wiley.

Penry, D. L. & Jumars, P. A. (1987). Modeling animal guts as chemical reactors. *American Naturalist*, **129**, 69–96.

Roediger, W. E. (1991). Cellular metabolism of short-chain fatty acids in colonic epithelial cells. In *Short-chain Fatty Acids: Metabolism and Clinical Importance*, report of the tenth Ross Conference on Medical Research, ed. A. F. Roche, pp. 67–71. Columbus, OH: Ross Laboratories.

Rombeau, J. L. (1991). Uses of short-chain fatty acids in experimental postoperative conditions. In *Short-chain Fatty Acids: Metabolism and Clinical Importance*, report of the tenth Ross Conference on Medical Research, ed. A. F. Roche, pp. 93–6. Columbus, OH: Ross Laboratories.

Rose, C. J., Hume, I. D. & Farrell, D. J. (1987). Fibre digestion and volatile fatty acid production in domestic and feral pigs. In *Recent Advances in Animal Nutrition in Australia 1987*, ed. D. J. Farrell, pp. 347–60. Armidale, Australia: University of New England Press.

Sarna, S. K., Bardakjian, B. L., Waterfall, W. E. & Lind, J. F. (1980). Human colonic electrical control activity (ECA). *Gastroenterology*, **78**, 1526–36.

Sellers, A. F., Lowe, J. E., Drost, C. J., Rendano, V. T., George, J. R. & Roberts, M. C. (1982). Retropulsion–propulsion in equine large colon. *American Journal of Veterinary Research*, **43**, 390–6.

Stevens, C. E. (1988). *Comparative Physiology of the Vertebrate Digestive System*. Cambridge: Cambridge University Press.

Van Soest, P. J., Jeraci, J., Foose, T., Wrick, K. & Ehle, F. (1983). Comparative fermentation of fibre in man and other animals. In *Fibre in Human and Animal Nutrition*, Bull. 20, ed. G. Wallace & L. Bell, pp. 75–80. Auckland: Royal Society of New Zealand.

Weston, R. H. & Hogan, J. P. (1968). The digestion of pasture plants by sheep. I. Ruminal production of volatile fatty acids by sheep offered diets of ryegrass and forage oats. *Australian Journal of Agricultural Research*, **19**, 419–32.

Whitelaw, F. G., Hyldgaard-Jensen, J., Reid, R. S. & Kay, M. G. (1970). Volatile fatty acid production in the rumen of cattle given an all-concentrate diet. *British Journal of Nutrition*, **24**, 179–95.

Yajima, T. (1985). Contractile effect of short-chain fatty acids on the isolated colon of the rat. *Journal of Physiology, London*, **368**, 667–78.

9

Transport of short-chain fatty acids in the ruminant forestomach

G. GÄBEL

Introduction

The ruminant forestomach is a large fermentation chamber compartmentalized into reticulum, rumen and omasum. It allows for microbial digestion of carbohydrates and synthesis of proteins and vitamins prior to entry to the parts of the gastrointestinal tract common to all mammals. Ingested carbohydrates are almost completely broken down and metabolized to the three major short-chain fatty acids (SCFA), acetate, propionate and butyrate, and the gases, carbon dioxide, methane and molecular hydrogen (Fahey & Berger, 1988). Fermentation of carbohydrates to SCFA is essential for the energy balance of ruminants. The total available SCFA can account for up to 80% of the animal's energy requirements (Bergman, 1990). However, to meet the demand, SCFA produced in the forestomach must be absorbed into the bloodstream to be available for use by the tissues. Various studies have indicated that most of the SCFA produced in the forestomach are absorbed directly and are not transported to distal parts of the gastrointestinal tract.

The absorptive function of the forestomach is not restricted to SCFA. Sodium, chloride, magnesium, and NH_3/NH_4^+ are transferred from the contents of the forestomach to the blood, and HCO_3^- secretion has also been demonstrated. Furthermore, there are strong indications that transport processes of these solutes are influenced by SCFA. Some studies have suggested that calcium and potassium may also be absorbed in the forestomach (Scott, 1967; Grace, Ulyatt & Macrae, 1974; Rahnema & Fontenot, 1990). However, to the author's knowledge, interrelations between K^+, Ca^{2+} and SCFA absorption have not been studied to date.

In this chapter, the literature is reviewed and data are presented from our own studies, describing the absorptive capacity of the forestomach with regard to SCFA. Suggested explanations for the underlying transport mechanisms are then discussed. Lastly, the interactions between the transport of

SCFA and bicarbonate, sodium, chloride, magnesium, and NH_3/NH_4^+ are described.

Methods used to study absorption

Absorption may be measured *in vivo* (a) by determining the net disappearance of unlabelled or radioactively labelled SCFA from a (temporarily) isolated reticulorumen filled with artificial buffer fluids; (b) by calculating the difference between the SCFA production rate and the liquid passage rate, as measured by infusion of radioactively labelled SCFA together with non-absorbable markers; and (c) by analysis of arterial and portal blood together with measurement of portal blood flow. However, the last method underestimates absorption from the forestomach, since the SCFA are metabolized to a considerable extent in forestomach epithelia (see below). Intraepithelial metabolism may also be a source of error in *in vitro* studies, if transport rates are determined on the basis of the appearance of radioactively labelled SCFA, since this procedure does not differentiate between SCFA themselves and their metabolic products. This problem has been partially circumvented by the measurement of concentration changes of unlabelled SCFA and the calculation of both the disappearance on one side of the tissue and the appearance on the other side (Stevens & Stettler, 1966*a*,*b*; Stevens & Stettler, 1967).

Capacity for absorbing SCFA

General significance of the forestomach

In regularly fed (i.e. not food-deprived) animals, SCFA are the major anions in the forestomach contents. However, the total and individual concentrations of SCFA are highly variable, depending on the time after feeding and the type of diet. Concentrations are found in the range of 60–160 mmol/l with 40–75% acetate, 17–47% propionate and 7–18% butyrate (Annison, Hill & Lewis, 1957; Sutton, 1980; Sharp, Johnson & Owens, 1982; Gäbel, 1988). Since the concentration of total SCFA in portal blood is usually lower than 3.5 mmol/l (Harmon *et al.*, 1985; Reynolds & Huntington, 1988), there is a great concentration gradient ($>17:1$) and, consequently, an effective driving force for SCFA transfer from the lumen to the blood.

Each of the *in vivo* methods mentioned above showed that nearly all the SCFA produced are directly absorbed in the reticulorumen and omasum.

Outflow from the forestomach and absorption in the distal part of the gastrointestinal tract play only a minor role. Therefore, the amount of SCFA appearing in the abomasum, the compartment distal to the omasum and similar to the stomach of monogastric animals, is consistently lower than 12% of the amount produced in the reticulorumen (Yang & Thomas, 1965; Engelhardt & Hauffe, 1975; Edrise & Smith, 1979; Peters *et al.*, 1990*a*,*b*; Peters, Shen & Robinson, 1992).

Various attempts have been made to evaluate the contribution of the omasum to the overall absorption of SCFA. In small ruminants (goats and sheep), a comparison between the reticulorumen and the omasum revealed that the first probably accounts for the greater part of total SCFA absorption (Engelhardt & Hauffe, 1975). In steers, the omasum may play a greater role, as was suggested by studies of Peters *et al.* (1990*a*). Propionate disappearance from the reticulorumen was 40–57% of the amount produced. Of the propionate that left the reticulorumen, 93–97% disappeared prior to entry to the duodenum (Peters *et al.*, 1990*a*).

Influence of diet

Diets providing extremely high levels of easily fermentable carbohydrates are recommended to cover the energy requirements of high-producing ruminants such as dairy cows and beef cattle. This type of diet increases the production rate and the intraluminal concentration of SCFA (Sutton, 1980). However, ruminants can effectively adapt the absorptive ability of the reticulorumen in response to variations in the amounts of SCFA available for absorption.

Various studies using the washed reticulorumen technique have shown that adapting the animals to energy-rich diets (i.e. increasing step by step the amount of concentrates over a period of several weeks) causes an increase of up to fourfold in the clearance rate of SCFA (Table 9.1). This functional adaptation is mainly due to morphological alterations in the rumen epithelium, with an increase in size of papillae and the number of (absorbing) epithelial cells (Dirksen *et al.*, 1984). As for the factors triggering the proliferative changes, hormones released by SCFA circulating in the blood (insulin, glucagon) are thought to play a major role (Gálfi, Neogrády & Sakata, 1991; see also Chapter 19 in this book).

By decreasing the energy intake via food deprivation, the capacity of the reticulorumen for SCFA is drastically decreased (Table 9.1). However, the underlying mechanisms are not yet clearly understood (Marek, 1991).

Table 9.1. *Influence of diet on the capacity of the forestomach to absorb short-chain fatty acids as determined in studies with the temporarily isolated and washed reticulorumen*

Diet	Net disappearance (mmol/h)			Clearance[a] (l/h)			Animal	Reference
	Acetate	Propionate	Butyrate	Acetate	Propionate	Butyrate		
100% hay	—	—	—	3.2	3.6	4.4	Cow	Thorlacius & Lodge (1973)
62–93% concentrate	—	—	—	5.1	5.9	6.3		
100% hay	162	72	54	2.5	3.1	3.8	Cow	Dirksen *et al.* (1984)
81% concentrate	552	264	162	10.6	12.2	15.4		
100% hay	20.4	10.9	2.9	0.54	0.64	0.71	Sheep	Gäbel *et al.* (1991*a*; and unpublished data)
81% concentrate	36.4	21.4	5.5	1.01	1.42	1.56		
Hay *ad libitum*	28.3	24.1	16.9	1.11	1.23	1.45	Sheep	Marek (1991)
Food deprivation (48 h)	12.2	13.1	9.5	0.46	0.61	0.82		

[a] The amount of SCFA absorbed per unit time divided by the mean concentration.

Mechanisms of SCFA transport

Influence of pH and concentration

To get an initial idea of whether SCFA are absorbed in an undissociated (HSCFA) and/or in a dissociated form ($SCFA^-$), various investigators have tested the influence of lumen pH on the absorption rate. Altering the pH in a physiological range led to a strong change in the concentration of undissociated acids but to only a slight change in the concentration of the dissociated acids. However, as shown in Table 9.2, even strong pH-dependent increases of HSCFA concentration led to only a small increase in the net luminal (mucosal) disappearance or clearance of SCFA. On the other hand, a threefold increase in acetate concentration with no change in pH (thus increasing both HSCFA and $SCFA^-$), approximately doubled the net disappearance of acetate and propionate from the lumen (Stevens & Stettler, 1966*a*; Weigand, Young & McGilliard, 1972). These studies indicate that the rate of absorption is not primarily determined by the luminal concentration of undissociated acids.

Influence of chain length and metabolism

If SCFA are mainly absorbed in the lipid-soluble, undissociated form, then absorption should correlate with their ability to permeate across artificial lipid membranes. According to a review of Walter & Gutknecht (1986), the ability of propionate to permeate through egg phosphatidylcholine decane bilayers is 5.1 times that of acetate, and the ability of butyrate is 2.7 times the propionate coefficient. As shown in Table 9.1 the differences are not fully reflected in the relative clearance rates. In solutions with a physiological pH, the clearance of propionate is 1.11–1.41 times that of acetate, and butyrate clearance is, at maximum, 1.35 times that of propionate. This indicates that absorption is not primarily determined by lipid solubility.

Numerous studies *in vitro* and *in vivo* have demonstrated the extensive metabolism of the main SCFA by the rumen epithelium (Stevens, 1970; Weekes, 1974; Weigand, Young & McGilliard, 1975; Beck, Emmanuel & Giesecke, 1984; Bergman, 1990). On the basis of these findings, it can be calculated that up to 90% of *n*-butyrate taken up into the cell is metabolized by the rumen epithelium to ketone bodies and carbon dioxide. Up to 50% of propionate may be metabolized to give rise to lactate, carbon dioxide and amino acids. Acetate metabolism in the sheep rumen epithelium was found to be up to 30%.

Table 9.2. *Influence of luminal (mucosal) pH on the absorption of short-chain fatty acids (SCFA)*

Luminal pH	HSCFA concentration ratio[a]	Acetate	Propionate	Butyrate	Type of study	Reference
6.0	1:8.6	—	196	—	*In vivo*, washed and isolated reticulorumen (calves)[b]	Weigand *et al.* (1972)
4.8		—	315	—		
6.6	1:11	3.2	3.6	4.4	*In vivo*, washed and isolated reticulorumen (cows)[c]	Thorlacius & Lodge (1973)
5.5		3.6	6.5	10.9		
6.8	1:63	0.75	0.90	1.15	*In vivo*, washed and isolated reticulorumen (sheep)[c]	Sündermann (1986; and unpublished data)
4.6		1.41	2.42	2.65		
7.4	1:9.8	6.5	14.1	18.3	*In vitro*, isolated sheets of rumen mucosa (cows)[d]	Stevens & Stettler (1966*a*)
6.4		12.9	18.1	25.8		

[a] Concentration ratio of undissociated short-chain fatty acids (HSCFA) was calculated by applying the Henderson–Hasselbach equation assuming a pK value of 4.79.
[b] Measured disappearance (mmol/h) of SCFA.
[c] Measured clearance (l/h) of SCFA.
[d] Measured disappearance (μmol/cm^2) of SCFA.

Therefore, the relative metabolic rate seems to increase in the same order as the clearance rate, i.e. *n*-butyrate > propionate > acetate. Furthermore, it has been shown that the absorption rate depends on the metabolic activity of the epithelium. Tissue anoxia (causing inhibition of metabolism) decreased the net SCFA disappearance on the lumen side (Stevens & Stettler, 1966*a*). Thus, the chain length-related differences in absorption may be due to the fact that the three main SCFA are metabolized to a different extent and that SCFA metabolism, in turn, influences absorption.

In view of the findings that the effects of chain length and pH are much smaller than expected (and may also be explained by secondary mechanisms such as metabolism), it can be concluded that processes other than non-ionic diffusion must be involved in SCFA absorption from the reticulorumen.

Interaction with bicarbonate

SCFA-dependent bicarbonate accumulation in artificial reticulorumen fluids has been repeatedly described (Masson & Phillipson, 1951; Ash & Dobson, 1963; Gäbel, Bestmann & Martens, 1991*a*). According to the models presented for the colon (Engelhardt & Rechkemmer, 1983; see also Chapter 10 in this book), coupling between SCFA and HCO_3^- can either be due to a process capable of exchanging $SCFA^-$ for intracellularly delivered bicarbonate, or be due to carbon dioxide originating from the intracellular metabolism of SCFA. In the latter case, CO_2 is subsequently catalysed to HCO_3^- and delivered into the lumen. The existence of an $SCFA^-/HCO_3^-$ exchange is suggested by the finding that mucosal addition of 4,4′-diisothiocyanatostilbene-2,2′-disulphonic acid (DIDS), an inhibitor of anion exchange mechanisms, decreased the mucosa-to-serosa flux of [^{14}C]propionate across isolated sheets of sheep rumen mucosa (G. Gäbel, T. Crönert & H. Martens, unpublished data).

Coupling between SCFA absorption and HCO_3^- secretion helps to keep the intraluminal contents alkaline, a process that may become more important if the animals are fed energy-rich diets. This type of diet usually tends to decrease the intraluminal pH, since SCFA production is increased while saliva production is decreased (Kaufmann, Hagemeister & Dirksen, 1980; Sutton, 1980). However, adapting the animals to energy-rich diets was shown to lead to an increase of SCFA-dependent HCO_3^- secretion (Gäbel *et al.*, 1991*a*), which may at least partly compensate for the H^+ gain by the increased SCFA production and by the decreased inflow of buffer with the saliva.

Interaction with sodium

Due to the enormous salivary secretion of sodium bicarbonate, which is 10 to 30 times that of non-herbivores of comparable body weight (Erdman, 1988; Gürtler, 1989), there is a high inflow of sodium into the reticulorumen. Almost half of the sodium secreted with the saliva can be reabsorbed within the forestomach (Dobson, 1959). The rate of sodium absorption may at least partly depend on the availability of SCFA, since it has been demonstrated that SCFA stimulate mucosal-to-serosal and net transport of Na^+ across isolated rumen mucosa (Gäbel, Vogler & Martens, 1991*b*).

SCFA-induced stimulation of sodium transport can be almost completely abolished by amiloride (Gäbel *et al.*, 1991*b*), an inhibitor of Na^+/H^+ exchange (Benos, 1982). This has led to the assumption that the enhancement of Na^+ transport results from activation of Na^+/H^+ exchange on the luminal side of the rumen epithelum (Gäbel *et al.*, 1991*b*). Activation of Na^+/H^+ exchange, in turn, is probably due to intracellular acidification after transmembrane inflow of SCFA.

There are at least two possible mechanisms to explain how SCFA acidify the cytosol. They are outlined in Fig. 9.1. First, transmembrane permeation of undissociated acids may lead to a direct H^+ gain in the cytosol. Second, the exchange of dissociated acids with bicarbonate will supply weaker bases ($SCFA^-$ instead of HCO_3^-) to the intracellular compartment with a consequently reduced buffer capacity and thus a higher intracellular H^+ concentration. However, the effects of SCFA on intracellular pH have not yet been determined and therefore this theory provides only a tentative explanation. The stimulatory effect of SCFA on sodium transport suggests that interactions might also occur in the opposite direction, i.e. Na^+ or the Na^+/H^+ exchange might influence the transport of SCFA. However, recent studies *in vitro* on isolated sheep rumen epithelia failed to demonstrate an inhibitory effect of amiloride on the mucosal-to-serosal flux of [^{14}C]propionate or [^{14}C]acetate (G. Gäbel, T. Crönert & H. Martens, unpublished data). From these studies, it can be concluded that SCFA transport probably does not depend on the activity of the Na^+/H^+ exchange, although the exchange is stimulated by SCFA.

Interaction with chloride

From ion replacement and inhibitor studies, it was concluded that chloride absorption across the rumen may interfere with the secretion of bicarbonate, due to the presence of Cl^-/HCO_3^- exchange in the apical membrane

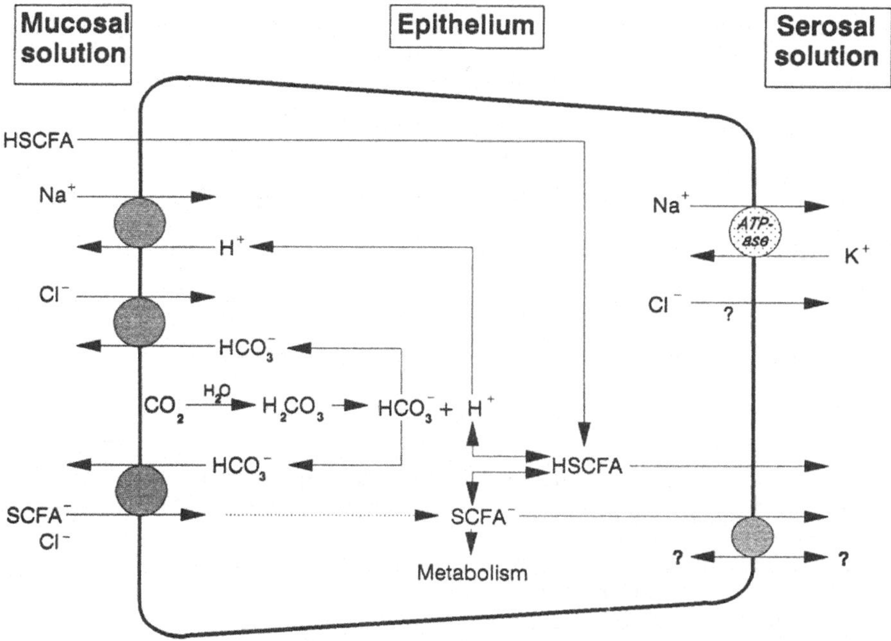

Fig. 9.1. Tentative model delineating the mechanisms of the absorption of short-chain fatty acids (SCFA) and their interactions with bicarbonate, sodium and chloride. HSCFA, undissociated acids; $SCFA^-$, dissociated acids.

(Emanovic *et al.*, 1976; Würmli, Wolffram & Scharrer, 1987; Martens, Gäbel & Strozyk, 1991*a*). However, chloride can probably also interact with SCFA transport. By using the washed reticulorumen technique, T. Kramer, H. Gürtler & G. Gäbel (unpublished data) demonstrated that substitution of chloride with gluconate increased the absorption of acetate, propionate and butyrate, a finding that was confirmed in *in vitro* studies with isolated rumen epithelia (Table 9.3). Furthermore, the interaction between chloride and SCFA was reciprocal. A mucosal (luminal) increase of SCFA concentration diminished the net disappearance of chloride *in vivo* (Marek, 1991) and the mucosal-to-serosal flux of chloride *in vitro* (Table 9.3)

Figure 9.1 illustrates a tentative model to explain the interactions between chloride and SCFA. The simplest explanation would be that chloride and SCFA anions can bind to the same external binding site of the anion-exchange mechanism. A second possibility is the existence of parallel Cl^-/HCO_3^- and $SCFA^-/HCO_3^-$ exchange mechanisms. Replacement of chloride by anions with a low affinity to the external binding site of the Cl^-/HCO_3^- exchange

Table 9.3. *Reciprocal influence of chloride and propionate transport (mean ± SEM) in isolated and short-circuited rumen mucosa of sheep*

Mucosal concentration (mM)	Mucosal-to-serosal flux (nmol/cm^2/h)		Observations
	Propionate[a]	Chloride[b]	(n)
Chloride			
4	76 ± 9		13
44	48 ± 8*		13
Propionate			
2		517 ± 41	12
112		269 ± 38**	12

[a] Determined from appearance of ^{14}C-labelled propionate not corrected for metabolism; 1 mM unlabelled propionate was present on both sides of the tissue. The serosal chloride concentration was 4 mM.
[b] Unlabelled chloride (4 mM) was present on both sides of the tissue. The serosal propionate concentration was 2 mM.
* $p < 0.05$; ** $p < 0.01$.
G. Gäbel, T. Crönert and H. Martens, unpublished data.

would then lead to diminished extrusion of HCO_3^- from the cell, and thus an increase in the amount of bicarbonate intracellularly available for exchange with $SCFA^-$. Nevertheless, further studies are needed to clarify the significance of anion-exchange mechanisms in forestomach epithelia.

Interaction with magnesium

There is compelling evidence that magnesium absorption from the forestomach is essential for the animal's Mg^{2+} balance and that impairment of absorption may contribute to the signs of hypomagnesaemic tetany (Field & Munro, 1977; Horn & Smith, 1978; Martens & Rayssiguier, 1980).

Mainly to elucidate the pathophysiology of hypomagnesaemic tetany, an attempt was made to characterize the influence of SCFA on Mg^{2+} transport. Increasing luminal (mucosal) SCFA concentration stimulated net Mg^{2+} absorption in the temporarily isolated and washed reticulorumen (Martens & Rayssiguier, 1980) and in isolated sheets of rumen epithelium (Martens, Leonhard & Gäbel, 1991*b*).

With regard to the underlying mechanisms of SCFA-induced stimulation of Mg^{2+} transport, magnesium absorption has been shown to be active (Martens & Rayssiguier, 1980) and probably partly due to $Mg^{2+}/2H^+$

exchange in the apical membrane of the epithelium (Martens *et al.*, 1991*b*). The underlying mechanism of SCFA-induced stimulation of Mg^{2+} transport would then be comparable to the influence of SCFA on Na^+/H^+ exchange, i.e. inflow of undissociated acids or exchange of HCO_3^- for $SCFA^-$, subsequent acidification of the cytosol and activation of the $Mg^{2+}/2H^+$ exchange (Martens *et al.*, 1991*b*).

Interaction with NH_3/NH_4^+

Significant quantities of NH_3/NH_4^+ are produced in the reticulorumen by microbial breakdown of proteins and of compounds containing non-protein nitrogen (NPN). Intraruminal NH_3/NH_4^+ concentration varies between 1.5 and 15 mmol/l in animals receiving protein-N, but it can increase up to 45 mmol/l if the animals are fed high amounts of easily fermentable NPN compounds, such as urea (Bolduan *et al.*, 1972). Driven by the concentration gradient between the reticulorumen and blood (Hogan, 1961), a large proportion of NH_3/NH_4^+ not used by the microbes permeates directly through the forestomach wall. However, the rate of NH_3/NH_4^+ transfer is not determined solely by the concentration gradient; it can also be influenced by SCFA. It has been demonstrated that the NH_3/NH_4^+ disappearance from the isolated and washed reticulorumen increased if the SCFA concentration was elevated (Hogan, 1961; Bödeker *et al.*, 1991).

Bödeker *et al.* (1990, 1991) suggested that reciprocal titrating processes might explain the interactions between ammonia and SCFA. In the normal range of ruminal pH, SCFA and ammonia are predominantly present as ions in the rumen fluid. It may be assumed that NH_4^+ donates its proton to $SCFA^-$ and that NH_3 and HSCFA diffuse through the epithelium (Bödeker *et al.*, 1991). As a further possibility, SCFA-dependent HCO_3^- secretion may provide HCO_3^- for NH_4^+ titration and lead to a constant NH_3 concentration at the absorptive surface (Bödeker *et al.*, 1990).

Summary and conclusions

SCFA production in the forestomach supplies ruminants with a significant proportion of their energy requirements. However, to meet the animal's energy demand fully, high SCFA production has to be accompanied by a high rate of absorption. It can be shown that most of the SCFA produced in the reticulorumen are absorbed directly. Studies on the mechanism of SCFA transport have suggested that, in addition to non-ionic diffusion, an anion exchange mechanism operating as $SCFA^-/HCO_3^-$ exchange in the apical membrane of the tissue is likely to play a physiological role in the reticulorumen.

As well as their direct involvement in supplying energy to the animal, SCFA may indirectly support the supply of minerals such as Na^+ and Mg^+, since the absorption of these solutes is stimulated by SCFA. This implies that a decreased production of SCFA (e.g. as a result of a reduced intake of carbohydrates) may eventually contribute to hyponatraemia and hypomagnesaemia, as was suggested by Martens *et al.* (1991*b*) and Holtenius & Dahlborn (1990).

References

Annison, E. F., Hill, K. J. & Lewis, D. (1957). Studies on the portal blood of sheep: 2. absorption of volatile fatty acids from the rumen of the sheep. *Biochemical Journal*, **33**, 592–9.

Ash, R. W. & Dobson, A. (1963). The effect of absorption on the acidity of rumen contents. *Journal of Physiology*, **169**, 39–61.

Beck, U., Emmanuel, B. & Giesecke, D. (1984). The ketogenic effect of glucose in rumen epithelium of ovine (*Ovis aries*) and bovine (*Bos taurus*) origin. *Comparative Biochemistry and Physiology*, **77B**, 517–21.

Benos, D. J. (1982). Amiloride: a molecular probe of sodium transport in tissues and cells. *American Journal of Physiology*, **242**, C131–C145.

Bergman, E. N. (1990). Energy contribution of volatile fatty acids from the gastrointestinal tract in various species. *Physiological Reviews*, **70**, 567–90.

Bödeker, D., Shen, Y., Kemkowski, J. & Höller, H. (1991). Influence of short-chain fatty acids on ammonia absorption across the rumen wall in sheep. *Experimental Physiology*, **77**, 369–76.

Bödeker, D., Winkler, A. & Höller, H. (1990). Ammonia absorption from the isolated reticulo-rumen of sheep. *Experimental Physiology*, **75**, 587–95.

Bolduan, G., Blödow, S., Voigt, J., Piatkowski, B. & Steger, H. (1972). Die Wirkung verschiedener Stickstoffquellen auf die Pansenfermentation sowie die Harnstoff- und Ammoniakkonzentration des Blutserums von Rindern. *Archiv für Tierernährung*, **22**, 137–48.

Dirksen, G., Liebich, H. G., Brosi, G., Hagemeister, H. & Mayer, E. (1984). Morphologie der Pansenschleimhaut und Fettsäureresorption beim Rind – bedeutende Faktoren für Gesundheit und Leistung. *Zentralblatt für Veterinärmedizin A*, **31**, 414–30.

Dobson, A. (1959). Active transport through the epithelium of the reticulo-rumen sac. *Journal of Physiology*, **146**, 235–51.

Edrise, B. M. & Smith, R. H. (1979). Absorption and secretion in the omasum of the young steer. *Annales de Recherches Vétérinaires*, **10**, 354–5.

Emanovic, D., Harrison, F. A., Keynes, R. D. & Rankin, J. C. (1976). The effect of acetazolamide on ion transport across isolated sheep rumen epithelium. *Journal of Physiology*, **254**, 803–12.

Engelhardt, W. von & Hauffe, R. (1975). Funktionen des Blättermagens bei kleinen Hauswiederkäuern IV. Resorption and Sekretion von Elektrolyten. *Zentralblatt für Veterinärmedizin* **22**, 363–75.

Engelhardt, W. von & Rechkemmer, G. (1983). Absorption of inorganic ions and short-chain fatty acids in the colon of mammals. In *Intestinal Transport*, ed. M. Gilles-Ballien & R. Gilles, pp. 26–45, Berlin, Heidelberg: Springer-Verlag.

Erdman, R. A. (1988). Dietary buffering requirements of the lactating dairy cow: a review. *Journal of Dairy Science*, **71**, 3246–66.

Fahey, G. C. Jr & Berger, L. L. (1988). Carbohydrate nutrition of ruminants. In *The Ruminant Animal. Digestive Physiology and Nutrition*, ed. D. C. Church, pp. 269–97. New Jersey: Prentice-Hall, Englewood Cliffs.

Field, A. C. & Munro, C. S. (1977). The effect of site and quantity on the extent of absorption of Mg infused into the gastro-intestinal tract of sheep. *Journal of Agricultural Science, Cambridge*, **89**, 365–71.

Gäbel, G. (1988). Natrium- und Chloridtransport im Pansen von Schafen: Mechanismen und ihre Beeinflussung durch intraruminale Fermentationsprodukte. Habilitationsschrift, Tierärztliche Hochschule Hannover.

Gäbel, G., Bestmann, M. & Martens, H. (1991*a*). Influences of diet, short-chain fatty acids, lactate and chloride on bicarbonate movement across the reticulo-rumen wall of sheep. *Journal of Veterinary Medicine*, **38**, 523–9.

Gäbel, G., Vogler, S. & Martens, H. (1991*b*). Short-chain fatty acids and CO_2 as regulators of Na^+ and Cl^- absorption in isolated sheep rumen mucosa. *Journal of Comparative Physiology B*, **161**, 419–26.

Gálfi, P., Neogrády, S. & Sakata, T. (1991). Effects of volatile fatty acids on the epithelial cell proliferation of the digestive tract and its hormonal mediation. In *Physiological Aspects of Digestion and Metabolism in the Ruminant*, ed. T. Tsuda, Y. Sasaki & R. Kawashima, pp. 49–59. San Diego: Academic Press.

Grace, N. D., Ulyatt, M. J. & Macrae, J. C. (1974). Quantitative digestion of fresh herbage by sheep. III. The movement of Mg, Ca, P, K and Na in the digestive tract. *Journal of Agricultural Science, Cambridge*, **82**, 321–30.

Gürtler, H. (1989). Die Physiologie der Verdauung und Resorption. In *Lehrbruch der Physiologie der Haustiere*, 5th edn, ed. E. Kolb, pp. 196–366. Stuttgart: Gustav Fischer Verlag.

Harmon, D. L., Britton, R. A., Prior, R. L. & Stock, R. A. (1985). Net portal absorption of lactate and volatile fatty acids in steers experiencing glucose-induced acidosis or fed a 70% concentrate diet ad libitum. *Journal of Animal Science*, **60**, 560–9.

Hogan, J. P. (1961). The absorption of ammonia through the rumen of the sheep. *Australian Journal of Biological Science*, **14**, 448–60.

Holtenius, K. & Dahlborn, K. (1990). Water and sodium movements across the ruminal epithelium in feed and food-deprived sheep. *Experimental Physiology*, **75**, 57–67.

Horn, J. P. & Smith, R. H. (1978). Absorption of magnesium by the young steer. *British Journal of Nutrition*, **40**, 473–84.

Kaufmann, W., Hagemeister, H. & Dirksen, G. (1980). Adaptation to changes in dietary composition, level and frequency of feeding. In *Digestive Physiology and Metabolism in Ruminants*, ed. Y. Ruckebusch & P. Thivend, pp. 587–602. Lancaster: MTP Press.

Marek, M. (1991). Resorption von kurzkettigen Fettsäuren und Elektrolyten aus dem Retikulorumen von Schafen: Beeinflussung durch Nahrungsentzug und intraruminale Infusion von Natrium-*n*-Butyrat. Doctoral thesis, Freie Universität, Berlin.

Martens, H., Gäbel, G. & Strozyk, B. (1991*a*). Mechanism of electrically silent Na and Cl transport across the rumen epithelium of sheep. *Experimental Physiology*, **76**, 193–14.

Martens, H., Leonhard, S. & Gäbel, G. (1991*b*). Minerals and digestion: exchanges in the digestive tract. In *Rumen Microbial Metabolism and Ruminant Digestion*, ed. J. P. Jouany, pp. 199–216. Paris: INRA Editions.

Martens, H. & Rayssiguier, Y. (1980). Magnesium metabolism and hypomagnesemia. In *Digestive Physiology and Metabolism in Ruminants*, ed. Y. Ruckebusch & P. Thivend, pp. 447–66. Lancaster: MTP Press.

Masson, M. J. & Phillipson, A. T. (1951). The absorption of acetate, propionate and butyrate from the rumen of sheep. *Journal of Physiology*, **113**, 189–206.

Peters, J. P., Shen, R. Y. W. & Chester, S. T. (1990*a*). Propionic acid disappearance from the foregut and small intestine of the beef steer. *Journal of Animal Science*, **68**, 3905–13.

Peters, J. P., Shen, R. Y. W. & Robinson, J. A. (1992). Disappearance of acetic acid from the bovine reticulorumen at basal and elevated concentrations of acetic acid. *Journal of Animal Science*, **70**, 1509–17.

Peters, J. P., Shen, R. Y. W., Robinson, J. A. & Chester, S. T. (1990*b*). Disappearance and passage of propionic acid from the rumen of the beef steer. *Journal of Animal Science*, **68**, 3337–49.

Rahnema, S. H. & Fontenot, J. P. (1990). Effects of intravenous infusion of high levels of potassium and sodium on mineral metabolism in sheep. *Journal of Animal Science*, **68**, 2833–8.

Reynolds, P. J. & Huntington, G. B. (1988). Portal absorption of volatile fatty acids and L(+)-lactate by lactating Holstein cows. *Journal of Dairy Science*, **71**, 124–33.

Scott, D. (1967). The effect of potassium supplements upon the absorption of potassium and sodium from the sheep rumen. *Quarterly Journal of Experimental Physiology*, **52**, 382–91.

Sharp, W. M., Johnson, R. R. & Owens, F. N. (1982). Ruminal VFA production with steers fed whole or ground corn grain. *Journal of Animal Science*, **55**, 1505–14.

Stevens, C. E. (1970). Fatty acid transport through the rumen epithelium. In *Physiology of Digestion and Metabolism in the Ruminant*, ed. A. T. Phillipson, pp. 101–12. Newcastle upon Tyne: Oriel Press.

Stevens, C. E. & Stettler, B. K. (1966*a*). Factors affecting the transport of volatile fatty acids across rumen epithelium. *American Journal of Physiology*, **210**, 365–72.

Stevens, C. E. & Stettler, B. (1966*b*). Transport of fatty acids mixtures across rumen epithelium. *American Journal of Physiology*, **211**, R264–R271.

Stevens, C. E. & Stettler, B. K. (1967). Evidence for active transport of acetate across bovine rumen epithelium. *American Journal of Physiology*, **213**, 1335–9.

Sündermann, M. (1986). Untersuchungen über den Einfluß energiereicher Fütterung auf Transportvorgänge der Pansenwand. Doctoral thesis, Tierärztliche Hochschule Hannover.

Sutton, J. D. (1980). Digestion and end-product formation in the rumen from production rations. In *Digestive Physiology and Metabolism in Ruminants*, ed. Y. Ruckebusch & P. Thivend, pp. 587–602, Lancaster: MTP Press.

Thorlacius, S. O. & Lodge, G. A. (1973). Absorption of steam-volatile fatty acids from the rumen of the cow as influenced by diet, buffers, and pH. *Canadian Journal of Animal Science*, **53**, 279–88.

Walter, A. & Gutknecht, J. (1986). Permeability of small nonelectrolytes through lipid bilayer membranes. *Journal of Membrane Biology*, **90**, 207–17.
Weekes, T. E. C. (1974). The *in vitro* metabolism of propionate and glucose by the rumen epithelium. *Comparative Biochemistry and Physiology*, **49B**, 393–406.
Weigand, E., Young, J. W. & McGilliard, A. D. (1972). Extent of propionate metabolism during absorption from the bovine ruminoreticulum. *Biochemical Journal*, **126**, 201–9.
Weigand, E., Young, J. W. & McGilliard, A. D. (1975). Volatile fatty acid metabolism by rumen mucosa from cattle fed hay or grain. *Journal of Dairy Science*, **58**, 1294–300.
Würmli, Wolffram, S. & Scharrer, E. (1987). Inhibition of chloride absorption from the sheep rumen by nitrate. *Journal of Veterinary Medicine A*, **34**, 476–9.
Yang, M. G. & Thomas, J. W. (1965). Absorption and secretion of some organic and inorganic constituents and the distribution of these constituents throughout the alimentary tract of young calves. *Journal of Nutrition*, **87**, 444–58.

10

Absorption of short-chain fatty acids from the large intestine

W. v. ENGELHARDT

Introduction

Short-chain fatty acids (SCFA), mainly acetate, propionate and butyrate, are produced in the large intestine in substantial amounts, are absorbed and subsequently utilized by the animal as a substrate of energy metabolism. The energy contribution of SCFA to the basal metabolic rate of the host animal has been calculated for guinea-pigs as 31% (Sakaguchi *et al.*, 1985), rabbits 40% (Marty & Vernay, 1984), pigs 30–76% (Stevens, Argenzio & Clemens, 1980; Bugaut, 1987), ponies 33% (Stevens *et al.*, 1980) and rock hyraxes 87% (Rübsamen, Hume & Engelhardt, 1982; Eloff & van Hoven, 1985).

It is remarkable that the study of electrolyte transport in the large intestine has proceeded for more than 30 years, yet only recently has attention been given to the role of SCFA, the major anions in the hindgut. Mechanisms involved in the transport of SCFA in the large intestine have been the source of controversy. Some of the findings are contradictory and interpretations are manifold. Factors repeatedly not taken into account are marked species differences, obvious segmental differences and the wide diversity of methods used.

SCFA, especially butyrate, are metabolized to different extents in the mucosa of the large intestine (Wirthensohn, 1980; Hatch & Geaghan, 1989; see Chapter 22). Therefore, SCFA that disappear from the lumen do not necessarily all arrive in the blood. In studies *in vivo* and *in situ*, the disappearance of SCFA from the perfused intestinal segment is usually determined. In most *in vitro* experiments with isolated epithelia, the appearance of SCFA on the other side of the mucosa, not the disappearance from the luminal or serosal side, is measured. Experiments *in vitro* are mostly performed under short-circuit current conditions with equal electrolyte concentrations on both sides of the epithelium; such experimental conditions are rather different from those found under natural circumstances. More recently data have been reported for uptake of SCFA into apical or basolateral membrane vesicles. It is therefore not unexpected that these different methodological approaches, and, moreover, studies with different intestinal segments from various species, have led to controversial findings. Problems in interpretation of data from *in vitro* as well as vesicle studies also arise from difficulties with the viability of tissue preparations and the fact that they are removed from neural and hormonal controls. Therefore, to assess findings on SCFA transport critically, it is important to consider the methods used in the different experiments. In absorption studies the following terms are used:

For *in vivo* and *in situ* perfusion studies: absorption, absorption rate, clearance of luminal solution (expression for permeability);
For *in vitro* studies: unidirectional fluxes, mucosal-to-serosal fluxes (J_{ms}^{SCFA}), serosal-to-mucosal fluxes (J_{sm}^{SCFA}) and the calculated difference between these two fluxes (J_{net}^{SCFA});
For membrane vesicle studies: uptake into vesicles.

The literature on SCFA transport has been comprehensively reviewed up to 1985 by Bugaut (1987), and recently some aspects of transport mechanisms were discussed by Rechkemmer (1991) and Titus & Ahearn (1992). In this review I concentrate mainly on more recent findings. Although precise mechanisms whereby SCFA are absorbed in the large intestine are not known with certainty, with reservations some conclusions are possible. Mechanisms and factors affecting SCFA transport are discussed and a model is suggested for transcellular SCFA transport across guinea-pig caecum and proximal and distal colon.

Concentration dependence

SCFA absorption is rapid in the hindgut. *In vivo* and *in situ* absorption rates in colonic segments increase linearly with increases in concentrations of SCFA in perfusion solutions (humans: Ruppin *et al.*, 1980; guinea-pigs: Rechkemmer & Engelhardt, 1988; rat caecum: Fleming, Choi & Fitch, 1991; turkey caecum: Sudo & Duke, 1980). Most of the results agree that in the large intestine the main route of SCFA transport is non-saturable. In perfusion studies in the guinea-pig, absorption of acetate increased linearly up to 120 mmol/l in both the proximal and the distal colon (Rechkemmer & Engelhardt, 1988). This corresponds to findings from similar perfusion studies for propionate in the guinea-pig caecum and proximal colon (Oltmer, 1993; Oltmer & Engelhardt, 1994) and for butyrate in the guinea-pig proximal colon (Bouley, 1978).

However, for propionate in the distal colon of the guinea-pig, Oltmer & Engelhardt (1994) recently observed an indication of saturation at physiological SCFA concentrations.

When SCFA concentrations were increased to 25 mmol/l in *in vitro* experiments under short-circuit conditions, undirectional fluxes and net fluxes for acetate, propionate and butyrate increased linearly in guinea-pig caecum and proximal and distal colon (Engelhardt & Rechkemmer, 1992). When propionate concentrations were increased to 60 mmol/l, both J_{ms}^{Pr} and J_{sm}^{Pr} increased linearly in the rabbit proximal colon, whilst J_{net}^{Pr} was not changed (Sellin & DeSoignie, 1990).

pH dependence

According to the pH-partition hypothesis, the undissociated lipid-soluble acid is able to permeate biological membranes easily. In normal colonic contents, depending on pH, only 0.1 to 5% of SCFA are present in the undissociated form. Because of this, one would expect an increase in SCFA absorption with a decrease in luminal pH. Such an effect was shown for the colon of several species (Bugaut, 1987), although the effect was mostly unexpectedly small. A decrease of perfusate pH from 7.4 to 6.4 increased the rate of SCFA absorption in the dog and pig colon, and this was associated with a parallel increase in the rate of Na^+ absorption (Crump, Argenzio & Whipp, 1980; Herschel *et al.*, 1981). This effect of pH on Na^+ absorption was not seen in the absence of SCFA in the pig colon (Crump *et al.*, 1980). Sellin & DeSoignie (1990) reduced the pH from 7.4 to 6.8 *in vitro* on both sides of an isolated epithelium of the rabbit proximal colon and showed an increase in J_{ms}^{Pr} and J_{sm}^{Pr} but no change in J_{net}^{Pr}.

However, clearance rates of SCFA in the guinea-pig colon did not change significantly when the pH in the luminal solution was decreased from 8.1 to 5.6 (Rechkemmer & Engelhardt, 1988), or from pH 7.4 to 6.3 (Oltmer & Engelhardt, 1994). Only at pH 5.3 was clearance increased in the distal colon, but the increase was much smaller than predicted by the pH-partition hypothesis (Rechkemmer & Engelhardt, 1988). Similarly, lowering the pH from 7.2 to 5.5 in the human large intestine had no effect on SCFA absorption rates (McNeil, Cummings & James, 1978). In the rat caecum, SCFA absorption rates were not affected by altering the pH in the luminal infusion between 5.4 and 7.4 (Fleming *et al.*, 1991). Absorption rates from the guinea-pig caecum were even higher from a perfusion solution at pH 7.4, compared to pH 6.3 (Oltmer & Engelhardt, 1994). The pH of large bowel contents is usually in the range of pH 5.8 to 7.8.

The unexpected independence of SCFA absorption from pH can be attributed to a microclimate of constant pH at the luminal surface of the colon (Rechkemmer *et al.*, 1986); pH in the microclimate region is close to neutral and largely independent of changes in bulk luminal pH. However, pH in the microclimate depends substantially on the presence of bicarbonate (A. K. Genz and R. Busche, unpublished data). Thus, lowering the pH in large-intestinal contents would not result in an increase in the amount of undissociated SCFA at the luminal cell surface of the mucosa. In the rat and human colon, a constant surface pH of approximately 6.5 was measured (McNeil, Ling & Wager, 1987). In the hen colonic mucosa, the surface pH was 6.27, and after incubation with propionate (7 and 40 mmol/l) it increased to pH 6.47 and 6.56, respectively (Holtug, McEwan & Skadhauge, 1992*b*). These authors concluded that the calculated SCFA concentration in the acid microclimate was not responsible for the Michaelis– Menten-like kinetics of butyrate transport observed across the hen colon (Holtug, 1989). The decrease in acidity was explained by the removal of a proton by the SCFA absorption process.

In the distal colon of the guinea-pig, the pH in the microclimate dropped when the luminal pH reached values below 5.5. At a luminal pH of 5.3, clearance rates of SCFA in the distal colon have been shown to increase significantly (Rechkemmer & Engelhardt, 1988). Under conditions of marked colonic luminal acidification, as may be present in carbohydrate malabsorption (Holtug *et al.*, 1992*a*), SCFA induced reversible injury to the porcine colon (Argenzio & Meuten, 1991). Such injury could be explained by an unphysiologically rapid uptake of the undissociated SCFA into the colonic mucosa from the bathing solution at pH below 5.0. Conclusions concerning the physiological regulatory effects of SCFA, deduced from experiments with a luminal pH as low as 4.1 (Squires *et al.*, 1992), should therefore be interpreted with care.

It has repeatedly been suggested that SCFA contribute to the development of diarrhoea. However, the case against SCFA being involved in diarrhoea is strong. SCFA are the most rapidly absorbed ions in the colon, and are thus unlikely to contribute to an increase in osmostic pressure of digesta in the hindgut. A possible effect could be through changes in luminal pH, when SCFA are generated rapidly and the colonic buffering system may not be able to deal with this, as a result of which the pH will fall below 5.5. This may promote the formation of lactate (a less well absorbed anion) by the bacteria. Lactate may be important in diarrhoea due to malabsorption, especially in children and young animals.

Chain length and lipid solubility

Differences in lipid solubility of undissociated SCFA depend mainly on chain length. The olive oil–water partition coefficient has been shown to increase by a factor of 2.8 with each CH_2 group (Danielli *et al.*, 1945). Thomson & Dietschy (1981) interpreted the findings of Westergaard & Dietschy (1974) to mean that each CH_2 group increases the permeability coefficient of intestinal cell membranes for SCFA by a factor of 1.58.

In practice, findings about the influence of chain length on the permeability of the hindgut mucosa to SCFA mostly do not follow this prediction. Dawson, Holdsworth & Webb (1964) described a rank order of butyrate > propionate > acetate for absorption rates when a mixture of SCFA was infused into a surgically isolated segment of the human colon. In the human rectosigmoid, propionate and butyrate absorption exceeded that of acetate (Saunders, 1991). In two marsupials, SCFA were absorbed in proportion to chain length in a constant ratio of 1.0:1.2:1.3 for acetate, propionate and butyrate, respectively (Rübsamen *et al.*, 1983). In the rabbit colon, absorption of SCFA also increased with chain length (Vernay, 1986).

In many other perfusion studies no influence of chain length on SCFA absorption was found. In the perfusion studies of the entire human colon, absorption of acetate, propionate and butyrate were similar (Ruppin *et al.*, 1980). In the rat colon (Umesaki *et al.*, 1979), rat caecum (Fleming *et al.*, 1991), equine ventral colon (Argenzio *et al.*, 1977), pig colon (Argenzio & Lebo, 1980), dog colon (Herschel *et al.*, 1981), and turkey caecum (Sudo & Duke, 1980) similar rates of SCFA absorption were found for all three SCFA. In the equine caecum and colon, acetate absorption was higher compared to propionate and butyrate (Argenzio, Southworth & Stevens, 1974).

However, marked segmental differences are seen when comparing the permeability characteristics of the various sections of the guinea-pig large intestine. Acetate permeability (clearance) is higher in the proximal colon than in the caecum and distal colon. Butyrate permeability, on the other hand, is lowest in the caecum, followed by the proximal colon, and is highest in the guinea-pig distal colon (Luciano *et al.*, 1984; Rechkemmer & Engelhardt, 1988; Engelhardt & Rechkemmer, 1992; Oltmer, 1993; Rechkemmer & Engelhardt, 1993; Oltmer & Engelhardt, 1994). Also in the guinea-pig distal colon, J_{ms}^{SCFA} increased with chain length ($J_{ms}^{Bu} > J_{ms}^{Pr} > J_{ms}^{Ac}$), although no such dependence was seen in the caecum, although a small increase was observed in the proximal colon (Fig. 10.1; Engelhardt & Rechkemmer, 1992; Engelhardt *et al.*, 1993). It is apparent therefore that partitioning between oil and water for SCFA is very different from the functioning of large intestinal permeability

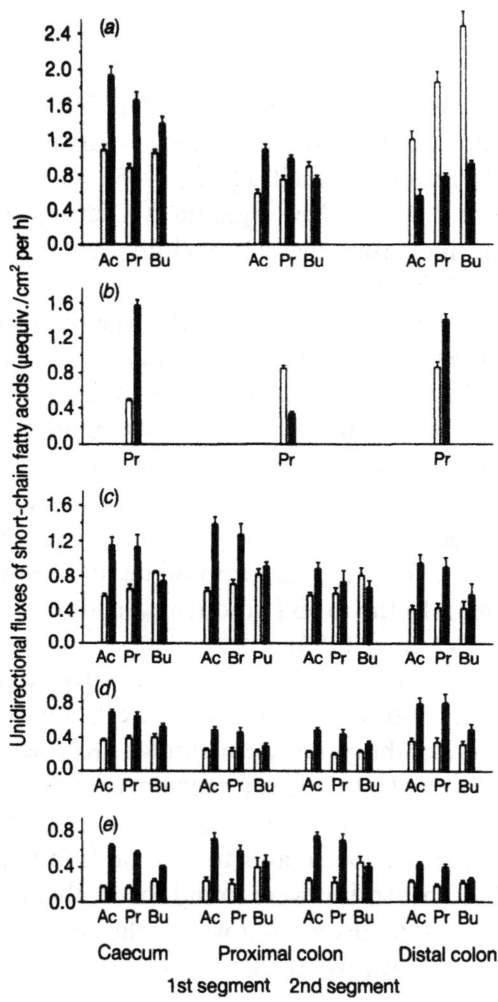

Fig. 10.1. Mucosal-to-serosal (white bars) and serosal-to-mucosal (black bars) unidirectional fluxes for acetate (Ac), propionate (Pr) and butyrate (Bu) across caecal and colonic segments under short-circuit current conditions. All experiments were performed under similar experimental conditions. Short-chain fatty acid concentrations on both sides of the stripped mucosa were 10 mM. Data for (*a*) guinea-pig, from Engelhardt & Rechkemmer (1992); (*b*) rat, from Rösel (1994); (*c*) pig, (*d*) sheep, from W. v. Engelhardt (unpublished data); Engelhardt *et al.*, 1994*b*; and (*e*) pony, from Engelhardt *et al.* (1992).

in guinea-pigs. This indicates the possibility of higher anion permeability in the intestinal membranes compared with that in lipid bilayers.

Experiments were performed under similar experimental conditions with segments of the large intestine of different animal species, and unidirectional fluxes of SCFA were measured (Fig. 10.1). It is interesting to note that, except for the guinea-pig distal colon, J_{ms}^{SCFA} increased only slightly with chain length in all segments of the other mammals. Species differences were obvious; segmental heterogeneity was more pronounced in the guinea-pig and rat, and less in the pig, sheep and pony (Fig. 10.1). In the rabbit caecum, J_{ms}^{Ac} was nearly three times higher than J_{ms}^{Pr}; in the rabbit distal colon, J_{ms}^{Ac} was about 30% higher than J_{ms}^{Ac} of the caecum (Hatch, 1987).

Comparative studies of the lipid composition of apical and basolateral cell membranes of the enterocytes from various segments of the large intestine may help to get a better understanding of the different SCFA transport characteristics.

Paracellular pathway

From studies of the permeability of acetate, propionate and butyrate, it was speculated that SCFA anions might be transported via a paracellular pathway, mainly in the leakier proximal colon, and much less in the tighter distal colon of the guinea-pig (Luciano *et al.*, 1984). An *in vivo* lumen-negative transepithelial potential difference would favour anion transport from the lumen to blood. From measurements of diffusion potential, it was concluded that a considerable part of SCFA transport in the proximal colon of the guinea-pig was due to SCFA anion diffusion (Rönnau, Guth & Engelhardt, 1989). However, *in vitro* clamping of the equine colon at 0 or 40 mV (blood positive) did not alter unidirectional SCFA fluxes (Argenzio *et al.*, 1977; Argenzio, 1988), and thus a barrier to diffusion of the dissociated SCFA anion across the paracellular pathway was postulated. Other evidence against paracellular transport of ionized SCFA comes from voltage clamping experiments that showed no influence of clamping on SCFA transport in all segments of the guinea-pig hindgut (Engelhardt & Rechkemmer, 1992).

These findings clearly indicate that no major paracellular transport of SCFA anions is present and agree with the observation that SCFA transport is independent of bulk water flow (Argenzio, Miller & Engelhardt, 1975; Argenzio & Whipp, 1979; Cummings, 1981). Paracellular flux of SCFA anions may, however, occur when transepithelial conductance is markedly increased by certain secretory stimuli in the pig colon (Argenzio & Whipp, 1983; Argenzio & Meuten, 1991), *in vitro* under Na^+-free conditions in the caecum of the guinea-pig (Engelhardt *et al.*, 1993) and after inhibition of the intercellular carbonic anhydrase in the distal colon of the guinea-pig (W. v. Engelhardt, unpublished data).

Proton antiport systems in the applied membrane

SCFA are weak acids with pK_a values of 4.75, 4.87 and 4.81 for acetate, propionate, and butyrate, respectively. As calculated from the Henderson–Hasselbalch relationship, 95 to 99.9% of the SCFA are present in the dissociated form at the physiological pH (pH 6–8) of the large intestine. A major route of SCFA absorption is by passive diffusion of the protonated form across epithelial cell membranes (Engelhardt *et al.*, 1989; Soergel *et al.*, 1989). According to the pH partition hypothesis, the apical membrane should be crossed many orders of magnitude more rapidly by the undissociated form of SCFA than by the dissociated fraction (Rechkemmer, 1991).

For non-ionic diffusion, SCFA anions have to be protonated. H^+ ions may be gained at the apical membrane by the amiloride-sensitive Na^+–H^+ exchange, or by the ouabain-sensitive K^+–H^+ ATPase that is present in the apical membrane of the distal colon. Inhibition of Na^+–H^+ exchange at the apical membrane of guinea-pig caecum and proximal colon diminished J_{ms}^{SCFA} by 35 and 30–50%, respectively (Engelhardt *et al.*, 1993). In the rabbit proximal colon, net propionate absorption was improved in the presence of adrenaline, which is known to stimulate Na^+–H^+ exchange (Sellin & DeSoignie, 1990). In the distal colon of the guinea-pig there is no amiloride-sensitive Na^+–H^+ exchange. However, a K^+–H^+ ATPase is present in the apical membrane of the guinea-pig distal colon and can be inhibited by ouabain (Rechkemmer & Engelhardt, 1993). Inhibition of K^+–H^+ ATPase in the guinea-pig distal colon diminished J_{ms}^{SCFA} by 60–80%; J_{sm}^{SCFA} was not affected (Engelhardt *et al.*, 1993). We conclude from these studies that in the guinea-pig caecum about 35%, in the proximal colon 30–50% and in the distal colon 60–80% of SCFA are absorbed in the lipid-soluble undissociated form.

Preliminary studies with and without inhibition of the apical proton antiport systems using tissues from the large intestine of rats (Rösel, 1994), sheep and pigs (W. v. Engelhardt *et al.*, unpublished data) indicate that the portion of SCFA that is transported from the lumen to the blood in the protonated form may be somewhat smaller in other animals compared to the guinea-pig; in these species most of the SCFA may be absorbed as anions.

Intracellular pH

SCFA transport from lumen to blood could be influenced considerably by an intermediate compartment of either lower or higher pH with the boundaries of the compartment having different permeabilities for ionized or non-ionized

SCFA. Protonated SCFA entering colonocytes would dissociate, thereby exposing cells to large loads of protons. Lowering of intracellular pH (pH_i), when large amounts of SCFA are absorbed, could facilitate the exit of undissociated SCFA across the basolateral membrane.

Addition of butyrate to the luminal side of the colonic tumor cell line HT29cl.19A (Busche *et al.*, 1993) or to the mucosa of guinea-pig large intestine (R. Busche & W. v. Engelhardt, unpublished data) did not alter the pH_i. Even after the inhibition of the apical Na^+–H^+ exchange with mucosal amiloride (caecum) or of the apical K^+–H^+ ATPase with mucosal ouabain (distal colon of guinea-pig) the pH_i did not change when butyrate was added to the luminal solution. However, addition of butyrate to the serosal side caused a significant decrease of pH_i in both these tissues, followed by a rapid regulation of pH_i towards the initial values. This regulation of pH_i was inhibited by amiloride and by 5-(*N*-methyl-*N*-isobutyl)-amiloride (MIA) at the serosal side in HCO_3^--free solution. Na^+-free solutions at the serosal side, but not at the mucosal side, also decreased pH_i and the pH_i was sensitive to changes of pH of the serosal solution and insensitive to changes of pH at the luminal side (R. Busche and W. v. Engelhardt, unpublished data). This indicates that the Na^+–H^+ exchange mechanism in the basolateral membrane, not in the apical membrane, regulates pH_i.

We conclude that, due to an effective pH_i regulation mechanism in the basolateral membrane, SCFA absorption does not change the pH_i of enterocytes in the large intestine.

Role of bicarbonate and $SCFA^-$–HCO_3^- exchange

SCFA that are not transported by non-ionic diffusion are transported in the dissociated form. Transepithelial transport of SCFA anions in guinea-pig large intestine (Engelhardt & Rechkemmer, 1992) and the equine large intestine (Argenzio *et al.*, 1977) is non-electrogenic. Therefore, SCFA anions have to be absorbed by anion exchange or by co-transport with a cation. A relationship between SCFA absorption and bicarbonate secretion has frequently been observed. It has been shown in a number of studies that HCO_3^- accumulates in the lumen of the large intestine in proportion to SCFA absorption, e.g. in the horse (Argenzio *et al.*, 1977), pig (Argenzio & Whipp, 1979), sheep (Rübsamen & Engelhardt, 1981), rat (Umesaki *et al.*, 1979), and human (McNeil *et al.*, 1978; Ruppin *et al.*, 1980). HCO_3^- secretion in the perfused rat colon was nearly doubled in the presence of butyrate (Roediger & Moore, 1981; Roediger *et al.*, 1986). Partial replacement of chloride by

SCFA resulted in a significantly higher bicarbonate secretion in the proximal colon and in a change from bicarbonate absorption to secretion in the distal guinea-pig colon (Rechkemmer & Engelhardt, 1982). In the presence of 10 mM propionate in the luminal solution in the guinea-pig caecum, HCO_3^- secretion was three times higher than in a propionate-free solution (T. Yajima & W. v. Engelhardt, unpublished data).

In Ussing-chamber experiments, HCO_3^--free solutions reduced J_{ms}^{Pr} in the caecum and in the guinea-pig proximal colon, and subsequent intracellular carbonic anhydrase inhibition caused a further decrease (Engelhardt *et al.*, 1994*a*). Pretreatment of the tissue with carbonic anhydrase inhibitor has been shown significantly to reduce J_{ms}^{Pr} in the caecum and proximal colon of the guinea-pig (Engelhardt *et al.*, 1994*a*), in the distal colon of the guinea-pig (W. v. Engelhardt, unpublished data) and in the rabbit caecum (Hatch, 1987). Carbonic anhydrase may be important in supplying hydrogen ions for non-ionic diffusion as well as HCO_3^- for an $SCFA^-$–HCO_3^- exchange. Whether an apical membrane-bound rather than a cytosolic carbonic anhydrase is involved should be evaluated. Carbonic anhydrase activity is high in hindgut mucosa (Carter & Parsons, 1970; Lönnerholm, 1977; Lacy & Colony, 1985; Charney *et al.*, 1986).

Recent studies with apical membrane vesicles of the rat distal colon (Mascolo, Rajendran & Binder, 1991) and human colon (Harig *et al.*, 1990) provided further evidence for an $SCFA^-$–HCO_3^- exchange. An outward HCO_3^- gradient significantly stimulated butyrate uptake into apical membrane vesicles of the rat distal colon (Mascolo *et al.*, 1991). This process was saturable (K_m for butyrate uptake 26.9 mM) suggesting the presence of an anion (butyrate–HCO_3^-) exchange. Recently Reynolds *et al.* (1991) also showed an HCO_3^--gradient-stimulated butyrate uptake into basolateral membrane vesicles from the rat distal colon, again evidence for a buyrate–HCO_3^- exchange. This exchange in the basolateral membrane was sensitive to 4,4′-diisothiocyanostilbene-2,2′-disulphonic acid (DIDS), whereas DIDS had no effect on HCO_3^--stimulated butyrate uptake into apical vesicles. Studies with apical and basolateral vesicles from fish intestine (Titus & Ahearn, 1992) suggested specific $SCFA^-$–HCO_3^--antiport mechanisms for both these membranes. However, these two exchange mechanisms in the apical and basolateral membranes have different binding affinity sites for bicarbonate as well as for SCFA.

All these findings support the view that in addition to non-ionic diffusion a considerable amount of SCFA is transported via an $SCFA^-$–HCO_3^- exchange. These exchangers in the apical and basolateral membrane may have different transport characteristics.

Unequal mucosal-to-serosal and serosal-to-mucosal fluxes of SCFA

Under physiological conditions SCFA are almost exclusively present in only luminal fluid (about 100 mmol/l in all mammals studied so far (Engelhardt & Rechkemmer, 1983*b*)), whereas concentrations in peripheral blood are very low at about 1 mmol/l. Therefore, serosal-to-mucosal fluxes are of no significance under *in vivo* conditions. On the other hand, *in vitro* studies under short-circuit conditions with equal SCFA concentrations on both sides of the mucosa may help to understand mechanisms involved in transepithelial SCFA transport. Under such conditions higher serosal-to-mucosal fluxes are mostly present ($J_{sm}^{SCFA} > J_{ms}^{SCFA}$), resulting in a calculated secretory flux (Fig. 10.1). This is the case for guinea-pig caecum and proximal colon (except for butyrate; Fig. 10.1) as well as for the rabbit caecum (Hatch, 1987) and rabbit proximal colon (Sellin & DeSoignie, 1990). However, after adrenaline stimulation and also in HCO_3^--free solutions at pH 6.8 (but not at pH 7.4) J_{ms}^{Pr} was higher than J_{sm}^{Pr} resulting in a net propionate absorptive flux (Sellin & DeSoignie, 1990). In the distal colon of the guinea-pig and in the proximal colon of the rat, basal J_{sm}^{SCFA} was smaller than J_{ms}^{SCFA}, resulting in a considerable net absorptive flux. Unidirectional fluxes for butyrate were similar in the proximal colon of the guinea-pig and pony, and in the pig caecum (Fig. 10.1).

In the caecum and proximal colon of the guinea-pig, the higher J_{sm}^{SCFA} compared to J_{ms}^{SCFA} seems to be coupled to a transmembrane Na^+ gradient generated by the basolateral Na^+–K^+ ATPase. Inhibition of the basolateral Na^+–K^+ ATPase with serosal ouabain or incubation of the epithelium in a Na^+-free solution abolished J_{net}^{SCFA} in the proximal colon and largely reduced J_{net}^{SCFA} in the caecum (Engelhardt *et al.*, 1993). Similarly, in the rabbit proximal colon, serosal ouabain entirely blocked an adrenaline-stimulated increase in J_{ms}^{Pr}, resulting in zero J_{net}^{Pr} (Sellin & DeSoignie, 1990). Ouabain injected into the mesenteric artery and into the luminal solution diminished SCFA absorption in the aboral part of the rabbit proximal colon by approximately 50% (Vernay, 1986).

On the other hand, in the guinea-pig distal colon, the higher J_{ms}^{SCFA} compared to J_{sm}^{SCFA} was independent of Na^+ and was related to the activity of the apical K^+–H^+ ATPase. When the K^+–H^+ ATPase was inhibited by mucosal ouabain, J_{ms}^{SCFA} was similar to J_{sm}^{SCFA}. Therefore, the net absorptive flux in the distal colon under short-circuit conditions is primarily caused by hydrogen ion supplied from the K^+–H^+ ATPase in the apical membrane (Engelhardt *et al.*, 1993).

The functional polarity of epithelial cells is partly reflected in different lipid compositions of the apical and basolateral membrane. Most brush-border membranes contain more cholesterol than do the basolateral membranes (Brasitus, 1983; Brasitus & Keresztes, 1983; Brasitus & Dudeja, 1988) rendering the apical membrane less fluid. This difference could bring an intrinsic asymmetry to the cellular lipid diffusion barriers with regard to weak electrolyte partitioning (Rechkemmer, 1991). Differences in membrane fluidity may also contribute to the observed segmental differences of SCFA fluxes. Using filipin as a marker for membrane cholesterol content, Luciano, Konitz & Reale (1989) determined about twice as many filipin–cholesterol complexes in the brush-border of the guinea-pig proximal colon than in the distal colon, indicating a greater lipid fluidity of the membrane in the distal colon. Additionally, the microvilli of the enterocytes in the guinea-pig proximal colon were shorter than in the distal colon (Luciano *et al.*, 1989).

A further explanation for the asymmetric behaviour of unidirectional fluxes could be the different properties of transport mechanisms in the apical and basolateral membranes. In vesicles from apical and basolateral membranes of the fish intestine, significantly different properties of the $SCFA^-$–HCO_3^- antiport mechanisms were described (Titus & Ahearn, 1992).

SCFA absorption and sodium transport

An interaction between SCFA and Na^+ transport has been observed repeatedly in *in vivo* studies with the perfused colon: in the rat (Umesaki *et al.*, 1979; Lutz & Scharrer, 1991), human (Ruppin *et al.*, 1980; Roediger & Moore, 1981), pig (Argenzio & Whipp, 1979), dog (Herschel *et al.*, 1981), sheep (Rübsamen & Engelhardt, 1981), goat (Argenzio *et al.*, 1975) and guinea-pig caecum and proximal colon (not distal colon) (Engelhardt & Rechkemmer, 1983*a*; Oltmer, 1993). Quantitative relations are, however, different between the species. In the rabbit colon (Vernay, 1986) as well as in the human colon (Roediger & Moore, 1981) sodium absorption was several times higher than SCFA absorption. Absorption of Na^+ was twice SCFA absorption in the rat colon (Umesaki *et al.*, 1979), whereas in the colon of the dog (Herschel *et al.*, 1981) and goat (Argenzio *et al.*, 1975), both were absorbed at approximately the same rate. In the cranial portion of the pony colon (Argenzio *et al.*, 1977) and colon of the pig (Argenzio & Whipp, 1979), Na^+ was absorbed considerably less than were SCFA. Replacing sodium with choline resulted in decreased absorption of SCFA from the colon of rat (Umesaki *et al.*, 1979) and sheep (Rübsamen & Engelhardt, 1981). Aldosterone stimulated sodium and butyrate absorption in the rabbit proximal colon (Vernay & Marty, 1984). In the proximal colon of the pig, J_{ms}^{Bu} increased with sodium concentration but in the distal colon stimulation was less and proprionate even inhibited sodium absorption (Holtug, Rasmussen & Mortensen, 1992*c*).

The most likely interaction between SCFA and sodium is thought to be the recycling of hydrogen ions. Transport of un-ionized acid into the cell could drive Na^+–H^+ exchange and thus stimulate sodium absorption. However, there are several inconsistencies in this model. Net Na^+ absorption is not stimulated by SCFA *in vivo* or *in vitro* in the proximal colon of the pony (Argenzio *et al.*, 1977). Argenzio (1988) proposed that this lack of stimulation may be due to the apparent absence or suppression of Na^+–H^+ exchange in the apical membrane under basal conditions. In two marsupials, also, no interrelationship between Na^+ and SCFA absorption was found (Rübsamen *et al.*, 1983). A significant reduction of sodium absorption in the presence of SCFA was observed in the rabbit caecum (Leng, 1978) and, in the presence of propionate, in the pig distal colon (Holtug *et al.*, 1992*c*). Acetate and butyrate stimulated sodium absorption in the proximal, not in the distal, colon of rats (Lutz & Scharrer, 1991). In the pig colon *in vivo*, acetate in luminal perfusion media (pH 7.4) significantly reduced sodium absorption (Crump *et al.*, 1980). However, if the pH was lowered to 6.4, SCFA caused an increase in sodium absorption.

Under short-circuit conditions, J^{Na}_{ms} and J^{Na}_{sm} across the mucosa of the guinea-pig caecum and proximal colon were not significantly affected, whether 10 mM propionate was present or not (W. v. Engelhardt, unpublished data). Neither acetate nor propionate significantly altered J^{Na}_{net} in the rabbit caecum (Hatch, 1987). In the proximal colon of cattle, J^{Na}_{net} was diminished in the absence of SCFA; in the distal colon, SCFA had no effect on J^{Na}_{net} (Diernaes *et al.*, 1993). Also in the equine colon and caecum, under *in vitro* conditions, acetate decreased net sodium transport (Argenzio *et al.*, 1977), and in the avian caecum no stimulation of Na^+ flux was observed (Grubb, 1991).

These findings on the interrelationship between SCFA and sodium absorption are conflicting. To my mind these data indicate that the electroneutral Na^+ absorption may stimulate SCFA absorption and not substantially vice versa; SCFA absorption may not, or only very slightly, affect Na^+ transport. Segmental and species differences may play a role. The basolateral Na^+–H^+ exchange may conceal an effect attributed to the apical Na^+–H^+ exchange. When SCFA enter the cell by non-ionic diffusion, they rapidly dissociate. In the colonic epithelial cell line HT 29cl.19A and in the guinea-pig caecum and distal colon, the basolateral (not apical) sodium–proton exchange is turned on in response to the intracellular proton load to keep the intracellular pH constant (Busche *et al.*, 1993; R. Busche, unpublished data); sodium is then excluded from the cell by the basolateral Na^+–K^+ ATPase.

SCFA absorption and potassium absorption in the distal colon

In the rat distal colon (but not in the proximal colon) a close relationship between SCFA absorption and K^+ absorption was observed (Stingelin, Wolffram & Scharrer, 1986). Likewise, in the guinea-pig distal colon (not in the proximal colon and caecum) the interrelationship between SCFA absorption and K^+ absorption was tight (Oltmer, 1993). *In vitro*, however, under short-circuit conditions in the guinea-pig distal colon, J_{ms}^{Rb} and J_{sm}^{Rb} were not affected by the presence or absence of propionate (W. v. Engelhardt, unpublished data).

This interrelationship between SCFA and potassium absorption seems to be due to the activity of the K^+–H^+ ATPase in the apical membrane of the guinea-pig distal colon. Protonation and thus non-ionic diffusion of SCFA depend on the activity of this K^+–H^+ ATPase; but SCFA obviously do not affect the activity of this pump.

Role of chloride

Ussing-chamber flux studies do not convincingly suggest a role for Cl^- in SCFA transport. In Cl^--free solutions, J_{ms}^{Pr} in the guinea-pig distal colon was diminished, whilst no effect was observed in the caecum, and in the proximal colon J_{ms}^{Pr} was increased (W. v. Engelhardt, unpublished data). Butyrate on the other hand stimulated electroneutral Na–Cl absorption under voltage-clamp conditions in the rat distal colon (Binder & Mehta, 1989), and was explained by coupling of Na^+–H^+ and Cl^-–butyrate exchange. However, studies with apical membrane vesicles of the rat distal colon did not confirm the presence of Cl^-–butyrate exchange (Mascolo *et al.*, 1991). A stimulation of sodium absorption by SCFA occurred in the absence of chloride in the human rectum *in vivo* (McNeil, Cummings & James, 1979), but chloride was needed for this effect in the rat distal colon (Binder & Mehta, 1989). In both the rat (Umesaki *et al.*, 1979) and the pig (Argenzio & Whipp, 1979), the increased appearance of HCO_3^- in the perfused colon was a function of the concentration of SCFA but not of Cl^-.

The physiological role of chloride is unclear. It should be remembered that chloride concentrations within the colon under normal physiological conditions are far below those used in *in vitro* clamp experiments.

Model for apical and basolateral membrane properties

SCFA enter the enterocytes in the hindgut by non-ionic diffusion and in parallel through an electroneutral anion exchanger. The contribution of each

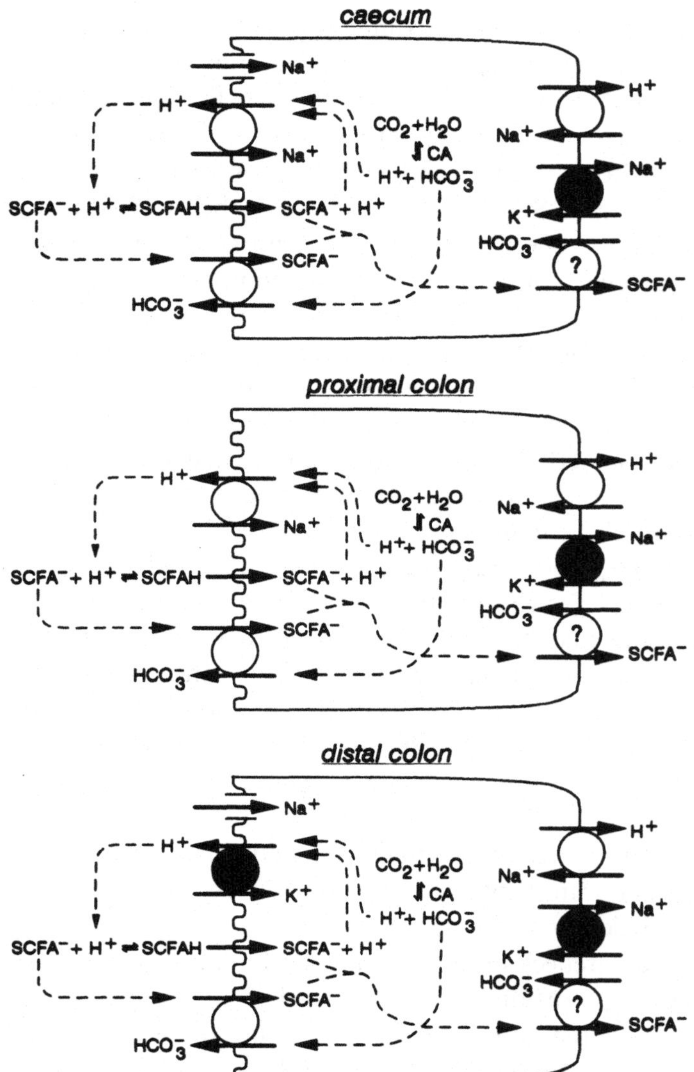

Fig. 10.2. Model for cellular mechanisms involved in absorption of short-chain fatty acids (SCFA) in the caecum and the proximal and distal colon of the guinea-pig. SCFAH, the non-ionic form; $SCFA^-$, the ionic form. This model is an extension of those suggested recently (Rechkemmer & Engelhardt, 1993; Engelhardt *et al.*, 1994*a*).

of these pathways has not yet sufficiently been determined. Significantly segmental and species differences exist.

As a result of comprehensive studies in the guinea-pig, a transport model was derived and the mechanisms involved are summarized in Fig. 10.2. In the caecum about 35%, and in the proximal colon of the guinea-pig 30–50% of SCFA may be absorbed in the protonated, non-ionic form. In the guinea-pig caecum and proximal colon, H^+ needed for the protonation of SCFA anions is available as a result of the Na^+–H^+ exchange. Luminal hydration of CO_2 to form HCO_3^- and H^+, as proposed by Engelhardt & Rechkemmer (1983*a*) and Stevens, Argenzio & Roberts (1986), does not appear to have a major effect on SCFA transport. The application of a macromolecular carbonic anhydrase inhibitor, compared with a carbonic anhydrase inhibitor that enters enterocytes easily, showed that the carbonic anhydrase involved in SCFA transport is not likely to be extracellular (Engelhardt *et al.*, 1994*a*). HCO_3^--free solutions, inhibition of intracellular carbonic anhydrase, and studies with membrane vesicles indicate that the presence of an $SCFA^-$–HCO_3^- exchange in the apical membrane and its importance for SCFA transport in the ionized form is most probable.

In the distal colon of the guinea-pig, 60–80% of SCFA are absorbed in the undissociated form. In guinea-pig distal colon, K^+–H^+ ATPase in the apical membrane provides H^+ for protonation and subsequent non-ionic diffusion of SCFA. SCFA anions may be transported via an $SCFA^-$–HCO_3^- exchange, similar to that in the caecum and proximal colon. Intracellular carbonic anhydrase is important for the availability of HCO_3^- and probably also H^+.

Mechanisms involved in the passage of SCFA across the basolateral membranes are unkown so far. There is evidence for $SCFA^-$–HCO_3^- exchange from vesicle studies in other species. In the course of SCFA absorption, pH_i in the enterocytes remains constant. Exchange of Na^+–H^+ in the basolateral membrane (not Na^+–H^+ exchange in the apical membrane) extrudes protons efficiently and regulates pH_i.

Marked species differences exist. Preliminary findings indicate that in a number of animals the portion of SCFA absorbed in the protonated form may be smaller than in the guinea-pig, especially in the distal colon. Proton secretion via the K^+–H^+ ATPase, present in the distal colon of the guinea-pig, may not play such a dominating role in other mammals.

Conclusions

Mechanisms of SCFA transport have been subject to considerable study and some controversy. SCFA absorption in the large intestine involves several transcellular processes. Paracellular transport of SCFA anions is not of significance under physiological conditions. Previously it was thought that SCFA transport in the large intestine was solely by non-ionic diffusion. However, recent studies clearly emphasize the combination of diffusion after protonation and carrier-mediated SCFA anion exchanges with bicarbonate. The proportions of transport contributed by non-ionic diffusion across the cell membranes and by the carrier-mediated component are different for different segments of the large intestine. Moreover, these are marked species differences. In addition, mechanisms of uptake into enterocytes and elimination from cells seem to be different.

SCFA transport is undoubtedly a complex process involving a number of factors and mechanisms. Many of these mechanisms are not fully understood as yet. These disparate observations indicate that a great deal more needs to be learned about transport of SCFA across the large intestine. Further research on transport mechanisms, kinetic processes, lipid composition of cell membranes and the fluidity of the apical and basolateral membrane, as well as regulatory events, will help to gain a better understanding of SCFA absorption.

References

Argenzio, R. A. (1988). Fluid and ion transport in the large intestine. In *Aspects of Digestive Physiology in Ruminants*, ed. A. Dobson & M. Dobson, pp. 140–55. Ithaca, London: Comstock Publishing Associates.

Argenzio, R. A. & Lebo, D. (1980). Ion transport by the pig colon: effects of time and anesthesia. *American Journal of Veterinary Research*, **41**, 39–45.

Argenzio, R. A. & Meuten, D. J. (1991). Short-chain fatty acids induce reversible injury of porcine colon. *Digestive Diseases and Sciences*, **36**, 1459–68.

Argenzio, R. A., Miller, N. & Engelhardt, W. v. (1975). Effect of volatile fatty acids on water and ion absorption from the goat colon. *American Journal of Physiology*, **229**, 997–1002.

Argenzio, R. A., Southworth, M., Lowe, J. E. & Stevens, C. E. (1977). Interrelationship of Na, HCO_3 and volatile fatty acid transport by equine large intestine. *American Journal of Physiology*. **233**, E469–E478.

Argenzio, R. A., Southworth, M. & Stevens, C. E. (1974). Sites of organic acid production and absorption in the equine gastrointestinal tract. *American Journal of Physiology*, **226**, 1043–50.

Argenzio, R. A. & Whipp, S. C. (1979). Inter-relationship of sodium, chloride, bicarbonate and acetate transport by the colon of the pig. *Journal of Physiology*, **295**, 365–81.

Argenzio, R. A. & Whipp, S. C. (1983). Effect of theophylline and heat-stable enterotoxin of *Escherichia coli* on transcellular and paracellar ion movement across isolated porcine colon. *Canadian Journal of Physiology and Pharmacology*, **61**, 1138–48.

Binder, H. J. & Mehta, P. (1989). Short-chain fatty acids stimulate active sodium and chloride absorption *in vitro* in the rat distal colon. *Gastroenterology*, **96**, 989–96.

Bouley, V. (1978). Der Einfluß steigender Butyratkonzentrationen auf die Resorption von Butyrat, Natrium und Wasser im proximalen Colon des Meerschweinchens. Diplomarbeit, University of Hohenheim, Stuttgart.

Brasitus, T. A. (1983). Lipid dynamics and protein–lipid interactions in rat colonic epithelial cell basolateral membranes. *Biochimica et biophysica acta*, **728**, 20–30.

Brasitus, T. A. & Dudeja, P. K. (1988). Effect of hypothyroidism on the lipid composition and fluidity of rat colonic apical plasma membranes. *Biochimica et Biophysica Acta*, **939**, 189–96.

Brasitus, T. A. & Keresztes, R. S. (1983). Isolation and partial characterization of basolateral membranes from rat proximal colonic epithelial cells. *Biochimica et Biophysica Acta*, **728**, 11–19.

Bugaut, M. (1987). Occurrence, absorption and metabolism of short chain fatty acids in the digestive tract of mammals. *Comparative Biochemistry and Physiology*, **86B**, 439–72.

Busche, R., Jeromin, A., Engelhardt, W. v. & Rechkemmer, G. (1993). Basolateral mechanisms of intracellular pH regulation in the colonic epithelial cell line HT 29 clone 19A. *Pflügers Archiv*, **425**, 219–24.

Carter, M. J. & Parsons, D. S. (1970). The carbonic anhydrase of some guinea pig tissues. *Biochimica et Biophysica Acta*, **206**, 190–2.

Charney, A. N., Wagner, J. D., Birnbaum, G. J. & Johnstone, J. N. (1986). Functional role of carbonic anhydrase in intestinal electrolyte transport. *American Journal of Physiology*, **251**, G682–G687.

Crump, M. H., Argenzio, R. A. & Whipp, S. C. (1980). Effects of acetate on absorption of solute and water from pig colon. *American Journal of Veterinary Research*, **41**, 1565–8.

Cummings, J. H. (1981). Short chain fatty acids in the human colon. *Gut*, **22**, 763–79.

Danielli, J. F., Hitchcock, M. W. S., Marshall, R. A. & Phillipson, A. T. (1945). The mechanism of absorption from the rumen as exemplified by the behaviour of acetic, propionic and butyric acids. *Journal of Experimental Biology*, **22**, 75–84.

Dawson, A. M., Holdsworth, C. D. & Webb, J. (1964). Absorption of short chain fatty acids in man. *Proceedings of the Society of Experimental Biology and Medicine*, **117**, 97–100.

Diernaes, L., Sehested, J., Møller, P. D. & Skadhauge, E. (1993). Sodium transport in the proximal and distal colon of cattle – interaction with SCFA. *Acta Veterinaria Scandinavica*, **89** (Suppl.), 105–6.

Eloff, A. K. & van Hoven, W. (1985). Volatile fatty acid production in the hindgut of *Procavia capensis*. *Comparative Biochemistry and Physiology*, **80A**, 291–5.

Engelhardt, W. v., Burmester, M., Hansen, K. & Becker, G. (1992). Transepithelialer Transport von Acetat, Propionat und Butyrat im Caecum, im proximalen und im distalen Colon von Ponys. *Pferdeheilkunde Sonderheft*, 171–4.

Engelhardt, W. v., Burmester, M., Hansen, K. & Becker, G. (1994*b*). Fluxes of propionate across caecal and colonic epithelium in sheep. *Proceedings of the Society of Nutrition Physiology*, **3**, 105.

Engelhardt, W. v., Burmester, M., Hansen, K., Becker, G. & Rechkemmer, G. (1993). Effects of amiloride and ouabain on short-chain fatty acid transport in guinea pig large intestine. *Journal of Physiology*, **460**, 455–66.

Engelhardt, W. v., Gros, G., Burmester, M., Hansen, K., Becker, G. & Rechkemmer, G. (1994*a*). Functional role of bicarbonate in propionate transport across guinea pig caecum and proximal colon. *Journal of Physiology*, **477**, 365–71.

Engelhardt, W. v., Rechkemmer, G. (1983*a*). Absorption of inorganic ions and short-chain fatty acids in the colon of mammals. In *Intestinal Transport – Fundamental and Comparative Aspects*, ed. M. Gilles-Baillien & R. Gilles, pp. 26–45. Berlin, Heidelberg, New York: Springer-Verlag.

Engelhardt, W. v. & Rechkemmer, G. (1983*b*). The physiological effects of short-chain fatty acids in the hindgut. In *Fiber in Human and Animal Nutrition*, Bulletin 20, ed. G. Wallace & L. Bell, pp. 149–55. Wellington: Royal Society of New Zealand.

Engelhardt, W. v. & Rechkemmer, G. (1992). Segmental differences of short-chain fatty acid transport across guinea pig large intestine. *Experimental Physiology*, **77**, 491–9.

Engelhardt, W. v., Rönnau, K., Rechkemmer, G. & Sakata, T. (1989). Absorption of short-chain fatty acids and their role in the hindgut of monogastric animals. *Animal Feed Science and Technology*, **23**, 43–53.

Fleming, S. E., Choi, S. Y. & Fitch, M. D. (1991). Absorption of short-chain fatty acids from the rat cecum *in vivo*. *Journal of Nutrition*, **121**, 1787–97.

Grubb, B. R. (1991). Avian cecum – role of glucose and volatile fatty acids in transepithelial ion transport. *American Journal of Physiology*, **260**, G703–G710.

Harig, J. M., Knaup, S. M., Shoshara, J., Dudeja, P. K., Ramaswamy, K. & Brasitus, T. A. (1990). Transport of *N*-butyrate into human colonic luminal membrane vesicles. *Gastroenterology*, **98**, A543.

Hatch, M. (1987). Short-chain fatty acid transport and its effects on ion transport by rabbit cecum. *American Journal of Physiology*, **253**, G171–G178.

Hatch, M. & Geaghan, J. P. (1989). Oxidative metabolism of rabbit and rat intestine with short chain fatty acids and glucose: an evaluation of data analysis. *Comparative Biochemistry and Physiology*, **92B**, 779–86.

Herschel, D. A., Argenzio, R. A., Southworth, M. & Stevens, C. E. (1981). Absorption of volatile fatty acid, Na and H_2O by the colon of the dog. *American Journal of Veterinary Research*, **42**, 1118–24.

Holtug, K. (1989). Mechanisms of absorption of short chain fatty acids – coupling to intracellular pH regulation. *Acta Veterinaria Scandinavica*, **85**, 126–33.

Holtug, K., Clausen, M. R., Hove, H., Christiansen, J. & Mortensen, P. B. (1992*a*). The colon in carbohydrate malabsorption: short-chain fatty acids, pH, and osmotic diarrhoea. *Scandinavian Journal of Gastroenterology*, **27**, 545–52.

Holtug, K., McEwan, G. T. A. & Skadhauge, E. (1992*b*). Effects of propionate on the acid microclimate of hen (*Gallus domesticus*) colonic mucosa. *Comparative Biochemistry and Physiology*, **103A**, 649–52.

Holtug, K., Rasmussen, H. S. & Mortensen, P. B. (1992*c*). An *in vitro* study of short-chain fatty acid concentrations, production and absorption in pig (*Sus scrofa*) colon. *Comparative Biochemistry and Physiology*, **103A**, 189–97.

Lacy, E. R. & Colony, P. C. (1985). Localization of carbonic anhydrase activity in the developing rat colon. *Gastroenterology*, **89**, 138–50.

Leng, E. (1978). Absorption of inorganic ions and volatile fatty acids in the rabbit caecum. *British Journal of Nutrition*, **40**, 509–19.

Lönnerholm, G. (1977). Carbonic anhydrase in the intestinal tract of the guinea-pig. *Acta Physiologica Scandinavica*, **99**, 53–61

Luciano, L., Konitz, H. & Reale, E. (1989). Localization of cholesterol in the colonic epithelium of the guinea pig: regional differences and functional implications. *Cell and Tissue Research*, **258**, 339–47.

Luciano, L., Reale, E., Rechkemmer, G. & Engelhardt, W. v. (1984). Structure of zonulae occludentes and the permeability of the epithelium to short-chain fatty acids in the proximal and the distal colon of guinea pig. *Journal of Membrane Biology*, **82**, 145–56.

Lutz, T. & Scharrer, E. (1991). Effect of short-chain fatty acids on calcium absorption by the rat colon. *Experimental Physiology*, **76**, 615–18.

Marty, J. & Vernay, M. (1984). Absorption and metabolism of the volatile fatty acids in the hindgut of the rabbit. *British Journal of Nutrition*, **51**, 265–77.

Mascolo, N., Rajendran, V. M. & Binder, H. J. (1991). Mechanism of short-chain fatty acid uptake by apical membrane vesicles of rat distal colon. *Gasroenterology*, **101**, 331–8.

McNeil, N. I., Cummings, J. H. & James, W. P. T. (1978). Short-chain fatty acid absorption by the human large intestine. *Gut*, **19**, 819–22.

McNeil, N. I., Cummings, J. H. & James, W. P. T. (1979). Rectal absorption of short-chain fatty acids in the absence of chloride. *Gut*. **20**, 400–3.

McNeil, N. I., Ling, K. L. E. & Wager, J. (1987). Mucosal surface pH of the large intestine of the rat and of normal and inflamed large intestine in man, *Gut*, **28**, 707–13.

Oltmer, S. (1993). Die Resorption von kurzkettigen Fettsäuren und Elektrolyten aus dem Caecum und Colon des Meerschweinchens. PhD thesis, School of Veterinary Medicine, Hannover.

Oltmer, S. & Engelhardt, W. v. (1994). Absorption of short-chain fatty acids from the *in situ* perfused caecum and colon of guinea pig. *Scandinavian Journal of Gastroenterology*, in press.

Rechkemmer, G. (1991). Transport of weak electrolytes. In *Handbook of Physiology, The Gastrointestinal System IV*, ed. M. Field & R. A. Frizzell, pp. 371–88. New York: Oxford University Press.

Rechkemmer, G. & Engelhardt, W. v. (1982). Absorptive processes in different colonic segments of the guinea-pig and the effects of short-chain fatty acids. In *Colon and Nutrition*, ed. R. Kasper & G. Goebell, pp. 61–7. Lancaster, Boston: MTP Press.

Rechkemmer, G. & Engelhardt, W. v. (1988). Concentration- and pH-dependence of short-chain fatty acid absorption in the proximal and distal colon of guinea pig (*Cavia porcellus*). *Comparative Biochemistry and Physiology*, **91A**, 659–63.

Rechkemmer, G. & Engelhardt, W. v. (1993). Absorption and secretion of electrolytes and short-chain fatty acids in the guinea pig large intestine. In *Ion Transport in Vertebrate Colon, Advances in Comparative and Environmental Physiology*, vol. 16, ed. W. Clauss, pp. 139–67. Heidelberg, New York: Springer-Verlag.

Rechkemmer, G., Wahl, M., Kuschinsky, W. & Engelhardt, W. v. (1986). pH-Microclimate at the luminal surface of the intestinal mucosa of guinea pig and rat. *Pflügers Archiv.*, **407**, 33–40.

Reynolds, D., Rajendran, V. M. & Binder, H. J. (1991). Butyrate transport in rat distal colon basolateral membrane vesicles: evidence for bicarbonate/butyrate exchange. *Gastroenterology*, **100**, A838.

Roediger, W. E. W., Deakin, E. J., Radcliffe, B. C. & Nance, S. (1986). Anion control of sodium absorption in the colon. *Quarterly Journal of Experimental Physiology*, **71**, 195–204.

Roediger, W. E. W. & Moore, A. (1981). Effect of short-chain fatty acid on sodium absorption in isolated human colon perfused through the vascular bed. *Digestive Diseases and Sciences*, **26**, 100–6.

Rönnau, K., Guth, D. & Engelhardt, W. v. (1989). Absorption of dissociated and undissociated short-chain fatty acids across the colonic epithelium of guinea pig. *Quarterly Journal of Experimental Physiology*, **74**, 511–19.

Rösel, E. (1994). Transportvorgänge des Dickdarmepithels bei keimfreien und konventionellen Ratten. PhD thesis, School of Veterinary Medicine, Hannover (in preparation).

Rübsamen, K. & Engelhardt, W. v. (1981). Absorption of Na, H ions and short chain fatty acids from the sheep colon. *Pflügers Archiv*, **391**, 141–6.

Rübsamen, K., Hume, I. D. & Engelhardt, W. v. (1982). Physiology of the rock hyrax. *Comparative Biochemistry and Physiology*, **72A**, 271–8.

Rübsamen, K., Hume, I. D., Foley, W. J. & Rübsamen, U. (1983). Regional differences in electrolyte, short-chain fatty acid and water absorption in the hindgut of two species of arboreal marsupials. *Pflügers Archiv*, **399**, 68–73.

Ruppin, H., Bar-Meir, S., Soergel, K. H., Wood, C. M. & Schmitt, M. G. (1980). Absorption of short-chain fatty acids by the colon. *Gastroenterology*, **78**, 1500–7.

Sakaguchi, E., Becker, G., Rechkemmer, G. & Engelhardt, W. v. (1985). Volume, solute concentrations and production of short-chain fatty acids in the caecum and upper colon of the guinea pig. *Zeitschrift für Tierphysiologie, Tierernährung und Futtermittelkunde*, **54**, 276–85.

Saunders, D. R. (1991). Absorption of short-chain fatty acids in human stomach and rectum. *Nutrition Research*, **11**, 841–7.

Sellin, J. H. & DeSoignie, R. (1990). Short-chain fatty acid absorption in rabbit colon *in vitro*. *Gastroenterology*, **99**, 676–83.

Soergel, K. H., Harig, J. M., Loo, F. D., Ramaswamy, R. & Wood, C. M. (1989). Colonic fermentation and absorption of SCFA in man. *Acta Veterinaria Scandinavica*, **86**, 107–15.

Squires, P. E., Rumsey, R. D. E., Edwards, C. A. & Read, N. W. (1992). Effect of short-chain fatty acids on contractile activity and fluid flow in rat colon *in vitro*. *American Journal of Physiology*, **262**, G813–G817.

Stevens, C. E., Argenzio, R. A. & Clemens, E. T. (1980). Microbial digestion: rumen versus large intestine. In *Digestive Physiology and Metabolism in Ruminants*, ed. Y. Ruckebush & P. Thivend, pp. 743–61. Lancaster: MTP Press.

Stevens, C. E., Argenzio, R. A. & Roberts, M. C. (1986). Comparative physiology of the mammalian colon and suggestions for animal models of human disorders. *Clinics in Gastroenterology*, **15**, 763–85.

Stingelin, Y., Wolffram, S. & Scharrer, E. (1986). Evidence for potassium/acetate cotransport in rat distal colon. In *Ion Gradient-Coupled Transport*, ed. F. Alvarado & C. H. van Os, pp. 317–20. Amsterdam: Elsevier Science Publishers.

Sudo, S. Z. & Duke, G. E. (1980). Kinetics of absorption of volatile fatty acids from the ceca of domestic turkeys. *Comparative Biochemistry and Physiology*, **67A**, 231–7.

Thomson, A. B. R. & Dietschy, J. M. (1981). Intestinal lipid absorption: major extracellular and intracellular events. In *Physiology of the Gastrointestinal Tract*, ed. L. R. Johnson, pp. 1147–220. New York: Raven Press.

Titus, E. & Ahearn, G. A. (1992). Vertebrate gastrointestinal fermentation: transport mechanisms for volatile fatty acids. *American Journal of Physiology*, **262**, R547–R553.

Umesaki, Y., Yajima, T., Yokokura, T. & Mutai, M. (1979). Effect of organic acid absorption on bicarbonate transport in rat colon. *Pflügers Archiv*, **379**, 43–7.

Vernay, M. (1986). Colonic absorption of inorganic ions and volatile fatty acids in the rabbit. *Comparative Biochemistry and Physiology*, **83A**, 775–84.
Vernay, M. & Marty, J. (1984). Absorption and metabolism of butyric acid in rabbit hind gut. *Comparative Biochemistry and Physiology*, **77A**, 89–96.
Westergaard, H. & Dietschy, J. M. (1974). Delineation of the dimensions and permeability characteristics of the two major diffusion barriers to passive mucosal uptake in the rabbit intestine. *Journal of Clinical Investigation*, **54**, 718–32.
Wirthensohn, K. (1980). Der Stoffwechsel kurzkettiger Fettsäuren im Colonepithel des Meerschweinchens und seine Bedeutung für die Natriumresorption. PhD thesis, University of Hohenheim, Stuttgart.

11

Metabolism of short-chain fatty acids in the liver

C. RÉMÉSY, C. DEMIGNÉ AND C. MORAND

Acetate, propionate and butyrate are the major end-products of the microbial metabolism of carbohydrates in the large intestine. In addition, smaller amounts of branched short-chain fatty acids (isobutyrate, isovalerate, 2-methyl-butyrate) are produced from microbial breakdown of some amino acids, mainly in the distal colon (Macfarlane & Cummings, 1991). Short-chain fatty acids (SCFA) are readily absorbed from the colon lumen (see Chapter 10). Theoretically, the rate of absorption of aliphatic monocarboxylates increases in parallel with chain length, yet butyrate is found in a lower proportion in the blood draining the large intestine than in the lumen. This reflects the fact that a large part of absorbed butyrate is metabolized by the mucosa (to carbon dioxide and ketone bodies). The mucosal metabolism of other SCFA seems quite limited: propionate utilization is low, some acetate utilization has been shown *in vitro* and it is conceivable that acetate makes a non-negligible contribution to mucosal metabolism, without noticeable changes in the rate of absorption.

SCFA concentrations in the portal vein are closely dependent on digestive fermentations (Demigné, Yacoub & Rémésy, 1986*a*). The major site of SCFA metabolism is the liver, where propionate and butyrate are almost entirely taken up, but the percentage of acetate uptake is lower (frequently less than 50%). However, due to its higher concentration in the portal vein, acetate uptake generally exceeds that of propionate or butyrate (Bergman, 1990; Rémésy, Demigné & Morand, 1992).

Acetate metabolism

Acetate uptake by the liver is proportional to portal concentrations (Buckley & Williamson, 1977; Rémésy, Demigné & Chartier, 1980) but this uptake is detectable only for concentrations higher than 0.25 mM. For lower

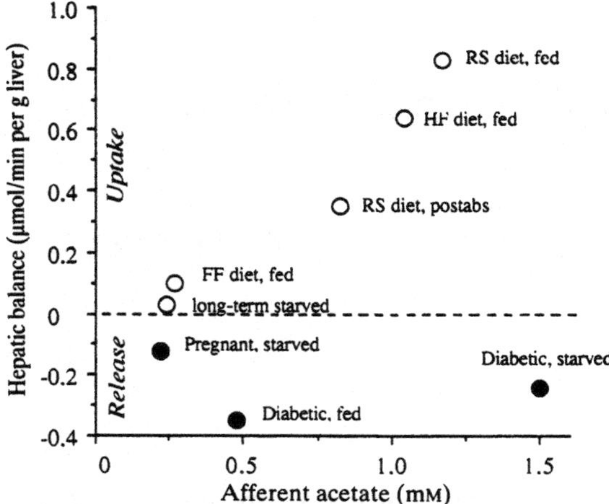

Fig. 11.1. Relationship between the hepatic balance of acetate and its afferent concentration in the rat, under different nutritional or metabolic conditions. The afferent concentration is ([portal vein] × 0.7) + ([artery] × 0.3), and the hepatic balance is ([hepatic vein] − [afferent]) × hepatic blood flow (ml/min/g liver). The example values (0.7 and 0.3) used for calculation of afferent concentration represent the respective contribution of portal vein and hepatic artery to hepatic blood flow. FF, fibre-free; HF, high-fibre; RS, resistant starch.

concentrations, a net release of acetate by the liver may be observed (Buckley & Williamson, 1977; Rémésy *et al.*, 1992). This reflects a possible futile cycle between acetate and various pools of acetyl-CoA. In fact, a direct relationship between afferent acetate and hepatic uptake is not systematically observed *in vivo*; some ketotic situations are characterized by high circulating concentrations of acetate without any significant uptake of acetate (Fig. 11.1).

Enzymes of acetate metabolism

There is a relatively high capacity for acetate activation in the liver, but it is still uncertain whether acetate activation is predominantly cytosolic or mitochondrial (Fig. 11.2). The low K_m (0.1 mM) of the cytosolic acetyl-CoA synthetase (Scholte & Groot, 1975) has long been taken as an argument that acetate activation is chiefly cytosolic. Furthermore, this is consistent with the recently reported, predominantly periportal location of the cytosolic acetyl-CoA synthetase (Knudsen *et al.*, 1992). Nevertheless, Baranyai & Blum (1989) and Crabtree, Gordon & Christie (1990) estimated that acetate activation should be essentially mitochondrial. This hypothesis implies that acetyl-CoA

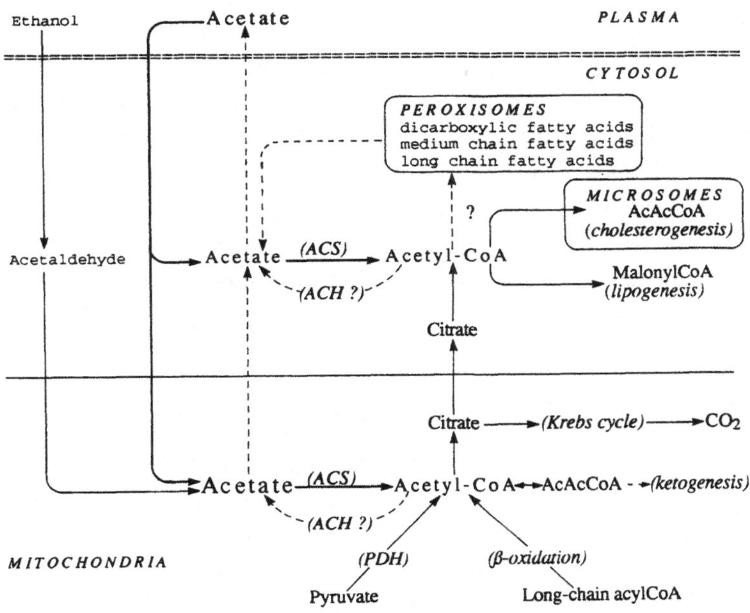

Fig. 11.2. Pathway of acetate metabolism in the liver. AcAc, acetoacetyl; ACH, acetyl-CoA hydrolase; ACS, acetyl-CoA synthetase; PDH, pyruvate dehydrogenase.

production from acetate takes place in parallel with major pathways of acetyl-CoA production (pyruvate dehydrogenase and β-oxidation).

The mitochondrial acetyl-CoA synthetase has a high K_m (≈ 10 mM) for acetate and represents a minor fraction of total acetyl-CoA synthetase activity in liver cells (Scholte & Groot, 1975). Therefore, it has been calculated that the mitochondrial enzyme has frequently to operate at its maximal theoretical rate (Crabtree *et al.*, 1990), or is activated by an unidentified factor. It was widely accepted that acetyl-CoA hydrolysis was chiefly mitochondrial (Söling & Rescher, 1985), in view of the fact that production of endogenous acetate is frequently concomitant with situations of high acetyl-CoA availability in mitochondria, such as starvation or diabetes. Nevertheless, investigations based on the evaluations of carbon fluxes between the acetate and acetyl-CoA pools in hepatocytes have underscored the role of extramitochondrial production of acetate (Baranyai & Blum, 1989; Crabtree, Souter & Anderson, 1989).

Whether acetyl-CoA hydrolysis is merely cytoplasmic or takes place in organelles is still unclear, since peroxisomes have a relatively high capacity for acetogenesis (Leighton *et al.*, 1989). This could be viewed as an 'overflow mechanism' for hydrolysis of excess acetyl-CoA generated *in situ* (for example, medium-chain fatty-acid metabolism) or, possibly, of acetyl-CoA from other pools (Hovik *et al.*, 1991). Nonetheless, acetate released by liver cells generally originates from mitochondria (long-chain fatty acids or ethanol metabolism) and there are probably, in physiological conditions, systems that limit substrate cycling between acetate and acetyl-CoA pools. Des Rosiers *et al.* (1991) have shown that the pool of mitochondrial acetyl-CoA is not isotopically homogeneous and acetyl-CoA produced from acetate seems preferentially used for citrate synthesis.

Influence of substrates and hormones on acetate metabolism

Propionate and butyrate are liable to inhibit acetate metabolism by liver cells (Demigné *et al.*, 1986*b*; Gordon & Crabtree, 1992). As shown in Fig. 11.3, acetate is readily metabolized by isolated hepatocytes under appropriate conditions; propionate at almost physiological concentrations is a potent inhibitor of acetate utilization; a net release of acetate is observed in the presence of octanoate. An inhibition of mitochondrial activation, by competition for the free CoA pool, may be invoked (Lumeng & Davis, 1973). If such an effect is relevant *in vivo*, it can probably be ascribed to propionate, since the portal concentration of butyrate is lower than that of propionate.

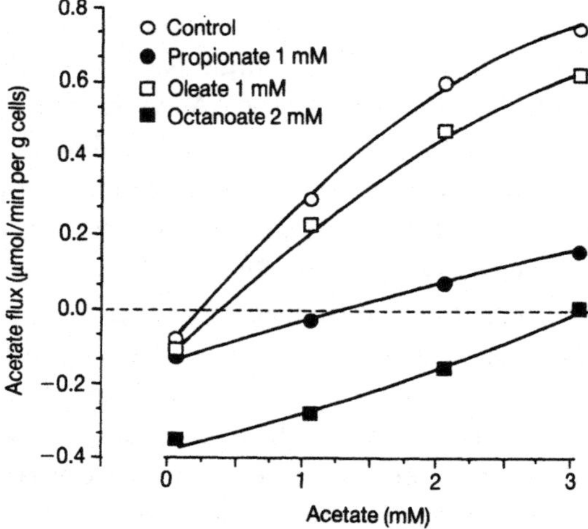

Fig. 11.3. Effect of propionate (short-chain), octanoate (medium-chain) and oleate (long-chain fatty acid) on the flux of acetate in hepatocytes isolated from fed rats, in the absence or in the presence of acetate (1, 2 or 3 mM) at the beginning of the experiment. The negative fluxes corresponded to a net release, and the positive fluxes to a net utilization.

Table 11.1. *Effect of adaptation to a high fermentable carbohydrate diet on hepatic metabolism and on the activity of key enzymes of gluconeogenesis or lipogenesis*

Dietary conditions (starch supply)	Control diet (70% wheat)	Fermentable carbohydrate diet (50% amylomaize + 20% wheat)
General metabolic parameters		
Glucose hepatic balance[a] (μmol/min/rat)	−20	+5
Total lipogenesis (μmol ^3H_2O/g liver)	47	23
Insulin, artery (mU/ml)	148	91
Enzyme activities[b] *(μmol/min/g liver)*		
Phosphoenolpyruvate carboxykinase	0.9	1.8
Acetyl-CoA carboxylase	1.3	1.0
Fatty acid synthase	0.14	0.09
ATP-citrate lyase	2.8	1.4
Acetyl-CoA synthase	0.59	0.74

[a] Negative value corresponds to a net uptake, positive value to a net release by the liver.
[b] All enzyme activities determined on cytosolic extracts.

Other substrates yielding acetyl-CoA (medium- and long-chain fatty acids) could be potential inhibitors of acetate activation, but only medium-chain fatty acids (if present in the diet) can be taken up in significant amounts by the liver during the postprandial period. Insulin has been reported to bring about an induction of cytosolic acetyl-CoA synthetase (Del Boca & Flatt, 1969; Knowles *et al.*, 1974). Accordingly, acetate activation is depressed in diabetes (Seufert *et al.*, 1974; Murthy & Steiner, 1973) and in starvation (Barth *et al.*, 1972).

However, other factors could also be involved, since a higher activity of acetyl-CoA synthetase was found in rats fed a high-resistant starch diet (characterized by high SCFA absorption) than in control animals fed a digestible starch diet with higher insulinaemia (Table 11.1). The possibility that acetyl-CoA synthetase could be inducible by SCFA themselves or by other factors connected to the development of digestive fermentations awaits further investigation. Besides direct effects of insulin on liver metabolism, microinjection of insulin into the amygdala (but not into the parietal cortex) may depress ^{14}C transfer from ^{14}C-acetate into CO_2 and alter the labelling of lipid fractions (Seto *et al.*, 1985).

Various compounds may affect acetate metabolism. Allicin, a naturally occurring sulphur compound from garlic, may act as a specific inhibitor of acetyl-CoA synthetase of various origins (Focke, Field & Lichtenthaler, 1990). Inhibitors of lipogenesis, such as (−)-hydroxycitrate (inhibitor of ATP–citrate lyase), could affect acetate metabolism if activation takes place in mitochondria (Crabtree *et al.*, 1990), but this effect has not been consistently observed (Beynen & Geelen, 1982). Some antibiotics (cycloheximide, chloramphenicol) may inhibit lipogenesis from acetate (MacNamara, Quackenbush & Rodwell, 1970). Since some of the acetate released by hepatocytes may stem from peroxisome metabolism (Hovik *et al.*, 1991), it is conceivable that drugs liable to influence the specific metabolism of these organelles (or their degree of proliferation) affect the rate of acetate release.

The metabolism of ethanol leads to the production of acetate and NADH in the liver. In human beings, even a moderate consumption of ethanol (25 g daily) corresponds to the production of 0.5 mol acetate. This value is about twice that produced from microbial fermentation of 40 g carbohydrate. Furthermore, acetate disposal from ethanol is restricted to a relatively short nyctohemeral period.

Metabolic effects of acetate

The metabolic fate of acetate and its role in the liver is connected to the general orientation of metabolism towards carbohydrate or lipid utilization. Theoretically, activation in the cytosol favours acetyl-CoA utilization for lipid biosynthesis, whereas activation in mitochondria may shift pyruvate metabolism towards gluconeogenesis (inhibition of pyruvate dehydrogenase, activation of pyruvate carboxylase).

The fact that the cytosolic acetyl-CoA synthetase seems preferentially located in the periportal zone (Knudsen *et al.*, 1992) should channel acetyl-CoA towards cholesterogenesis (essentially periportal; Li *et al.*, 1988) rather than towards lipogenesis (mainly perivenous). However, this model does not necessarily fit published data. For example, acetate actually stimulates fatty-acid synthesis but inhibits cholesterogenesis by isolated rat hepatocytes (Beynen *et al.*, 1982; Nishina & Freedland, 1990). Several investigations indicate that there is interference between acetate and lactate metabolism in the liver. Snoswell *et al.* (1982) reported inhibition of acetate metabolism (for lipogenesis, essentially) by lactate. This needs further investigation and may be metabolically relevant, since both lactate and acetate may represent important substrates in the portal vein.

In hepatocytes from fed rats, acetate depressed lactate release and increased its utilization at physiological lactate concentrations, namely about 2 mM

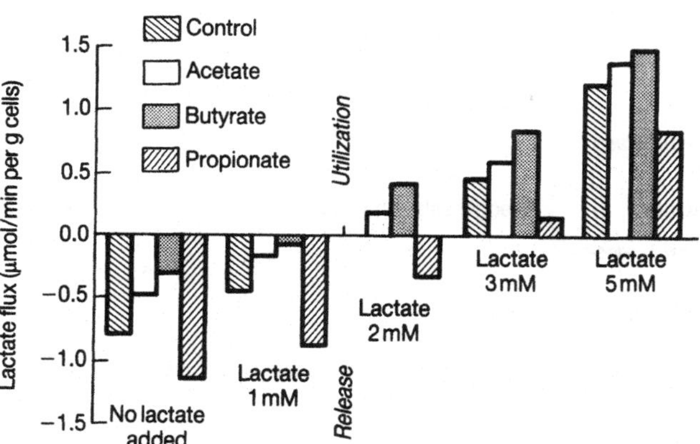

Fig. 11.4. Effects of the different short-chain fatty acids on the flux of L-lactate in hepatocytes isolated from fed rats, in the absence or the presence of L-lactate (1, 2, 3 or 5 mM) at the beginning of the experiment.

(Fig. 11.4). Fatty acids are inhibitors of glycolysis (Hue, Maisin & Rider, 1988). However, acetate has a less potent effect than butyrate, octanoate or long-chain fatty acids (Nomura *et al.*, 1983; Morand, Rémésy & Demigné, 1993).

Furthermore, acetate can stimulate gluconeogenesis from lactate (Whitton, Rodrigues & Hems, 1979). In starved rats, acetate is poorly ketogenic, in contrast to butyrate (Rémésy *et al.*, 1980), which suggests that activation of acetate to acetyl-CoA in mitochondria is relatively inefficient.

Propionate metabolism

Characteristics of propionate metabolism in liver cells

Under normal conditions, propionate is totally taken up by the liver. This process is certainly favoured by facilitated diffusion, which is efficient even in the presence of relatively low concentrations of propionate (Fafournoux, Rémésy & Demigné, 1985). The pathway of propionate metabolism in the liver is depicted in Fig. 11.5. In ruminants and guinea-pigs, propionate is activated in liver mitochondria by a specific propionyl-CoA synthetase (Ash & Baird, 1973; Groot & Scheek, 1976). In the rat, the existence of such a specific enzyme is uncertain; propionyl-CoA is probably synthesized by one or more SCFA-activating enzymes with broad substrate specificity (Barth *et al.*, 1972; Scholte & Groot, 1975). Propionyl-CoA is transformed into methylmalonyl-CoA (catalysed by the ATP-dependent propionyl-CoA carboxylase). The subsequent conversion to succinyl-CoA is mediated by a methyl-

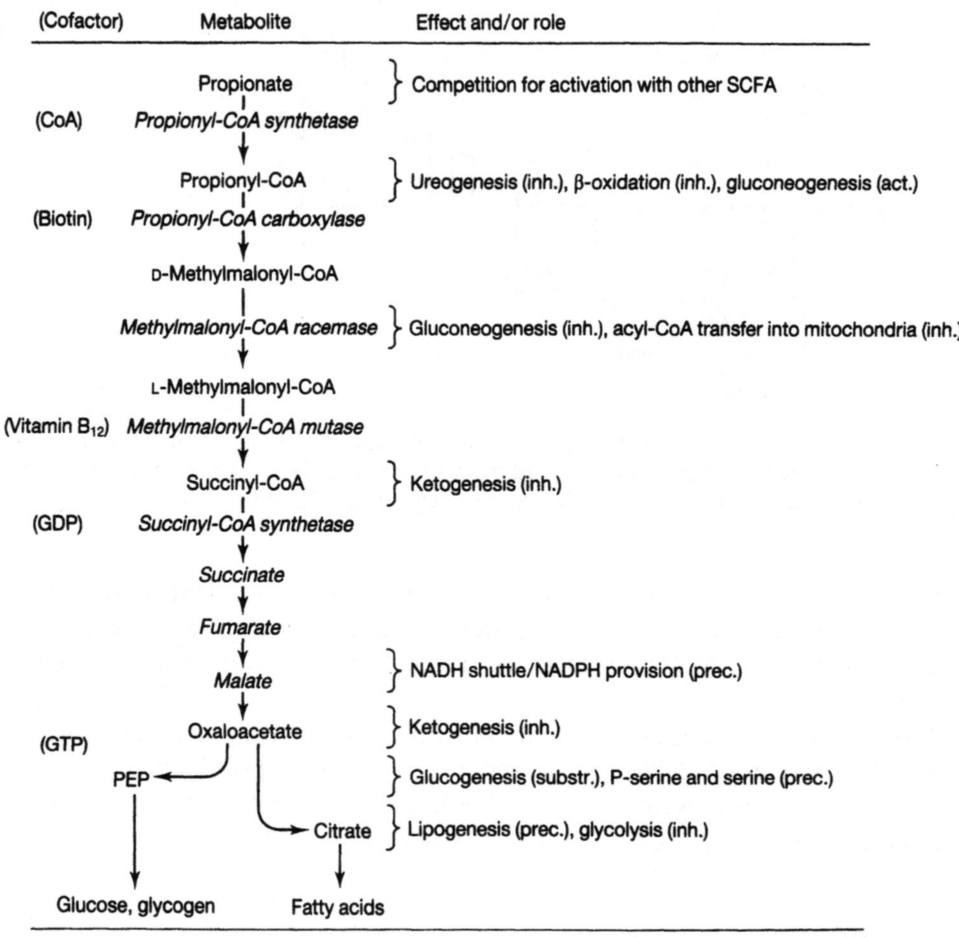

Fig. 11.5. Pathway of propionate metabolism in the liver and metabolic effects of the various intermediates of propionate metabolism. inh., inhibitor; act., activator; substr., substrate; prec., precursor; PEP, phosphoenolpyruvate.

malonyl-CoA mutase, with vitamin B_{12} as the cofactor. Propionyl-CoA and succinyl-CoA also arise from the catabolism of certain amino acids, such as valine, isoleucine, methionine and threonine. This supply is probably minor in normal subjects, compared to that of colonic propionate. In subjects with inherited disorders of propionate metabolism, in which colonic production is inhibited by metronidazole, endogenous production is still sufficient to maintain a risk of methylmalonic aciduria (Bain *et al.*, 1988; Thompson *et al.*, 1990). Propionate metabolism depends on the bioavailability of vitamin B_{12} or biotin (Chiang & Mistry, 1974). Propionate metabolism increases the requirements for vitamin B_{12}, which could be critical with dietary fibres such as pectin, which may interfere with vitamin B_{12} reabsorption during its enterohepatic cycle (Cullen & Oace, 1989*a,b*).

Effects of propionate on carbohydrate metabolism

Propionate is a very effective glucogenic substrate in most species (Bergman, 1990). However, its maximal absorption generally takes place during the late absorptive period, when gluconeogenesis is not fully active. This raises the question of the metabolic fate of propionate under such circumstances. Propionate probably constitutes a precursor for glycogen synthesis as well as, possibly, for lipid synthesis. Propionate seems to have priority over lactate for metabolism during the absorptive period (Rémésy & Demigné, 1983; Fig. 11.6). Propionate is an inhibitor of pyruvate oxidation in hepatocytes from fed rats (Brass, Fennessey & Miller, 1986; Krahenbuhl & Brass, 1991), and of gluconeogenesis from pyruvate in hepatocytes from starved rats (C. Rémésy, unpublished data). The various CoA intermediates of propionate metabolism may affect the activity of pyruvate carboxylase. The resulting effect is complex, since propionyl-CoA is an activator whereas succinyl-CoA and methylmalonyl-CoA are inhibitors of this enzyme (Barritt, Zander &

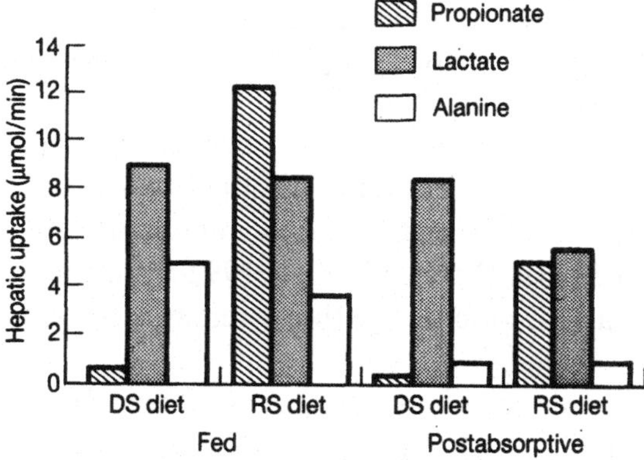

Fig. 11.6. Hepatic balance of the major 3-carbon glucogenic substrates *in vivo*. The rats were adapted for 3 weeks to semi-purified diets providing carbohydrate either as 70% digestible starch (DS diet) or as 50% amylomaize starch + 20% digestible starch (RS diet). This last diet thus contained substantial amounts of resistant starch (about 180 g/kg) which was fermented in the large intesine, resulting in a considerable production and absorption of short-chain fatty acids. The hepatic balance, for a given diet, was compared between the fed and postabsorptive period. The hepatic uptake was calculated as ([hepatic vein] − [afferent]) × hepatic blood flow.

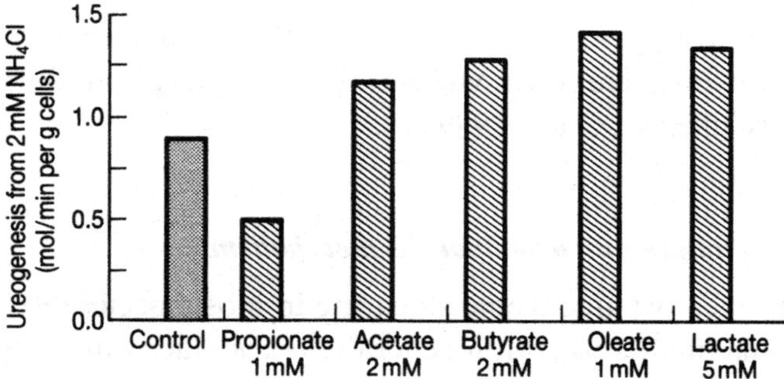

Fig. 11.7. Effects of different short-chain fatty acids on ureogenesis from ammonium choride in hepatocytes isolated from fed rats, compared to the effect of a long-chain fatty acid (oleate) or L-lactate. Control, no energy-yielding substrate added.

Utter, 1976). When there are large amounts of propionate, methylmalonyl-CoA accumulates (Corkey *et al.*, 1982), because the methylmalonyl-CoA mutase is the rate-limiting enzyme of the pathway. Propionate increases the release of lactate in hepatocytes from fed rats by increasing glycolysis (Fig. 11.4). This effect is counteracted by oleate, which suggests that propionate inhibits the production of acetyl-CoA and citrate (Patel *et al.*, 1983; Nakai *et al.*, 1991). Reversal of propionate inhibition of pyruvate utilization by octanoate is associated with a strong decrease in propionyl-CoA concentration (Krahenbuhl & Brass, 1991) and it seems likely that butyrate has similar effects on propionate metabolism.

In the rat, the contribution of propionate to gluconeogenesis depends on dietary fibre fermentation. High-fibre diets limit the fluctuations of hepatic glycogen during the dark/light cycle, owing to the delay of glucose absorption and the continuous supply of SCFA (Morand *et al.*, 1992*a*). In humans, the actual importance of propionate in glucose synthesis remains to be assessed quantitatively.

Propionate may depress the rate of ureogenesis, in contrast to acetate and butyrate, which activate it (Fig. 11.7). This has been ascribed to the inhibition by propionyl-CoA of the synthesis of *N*-acetylglutamate, which activates carbamoylphosphate synthase (Coudé, Sweetman & Nyhan, 1979). However, such an effect of propionate is difficult to examine *in vivo*, because acetyl-CoA-yielding substrates are permanently present (acetate, butyrate, long-chain fatty acids). *In vitro*, excess ammonia may inhibit propionate metabolism, or channel it towards the synthesis of amino acids rather than glucose. In the postabsorptive period, there is a progressive mobilization of protein

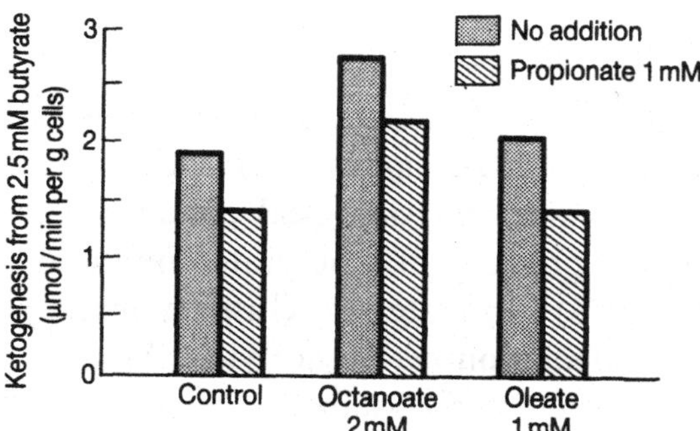

Fig. 11.8. Effect of propionate on the rate of ketogenesis from a medium-chain (octanoate) or long-chain (oleate) fatty acid, in hepatocytes isolated from rats fasted for 24 h. The data presented correspond to the rate of production of acetoacetate (AcAc) + 3-hydroxybutyrate (3-HB). The values for the 3-HB/AcAc ratio were (0.31 in control conditions, with no fatty acid added (v. 0.25 in the presence of propionate), 1.82 with octanoate as a substrate (v. 1.08 in the presence of propionate) or 1.80 with oleate as a substrate (v. 0.94 in the presence of propionate).

amino acids for gluconeogenesis. Thus, it would be interesting to assess whether propionate may contribute to protein-sparing during that period.

Propionate and lipid metabolism in the liver

Propionate may inhibit the β-oxidation of fatty acids, since propionyl-CoA leads to a 'suicide inactivation' of the FAD dehydrogenase of the short-chain acyl-CoA (Shaw & Engel, 1985). This inhibition should affect long-chain fatty acids rather than butyrate. In hepatocytes from starved rats, propionate has a potent antiketogenic effect accompanied by a depressed 3-hydroxybutyrate/acetoacetate ratio (Fig. 11.8). Part of the antiketogenic effects of propionate, besides an enhanced supply of oxaloacetate in mitochondria, could be ascribed to succinylation (using succinyl-CoA) of hydroxymethyl-glutaryl-CoA synthase (Lowe & Tubbs, 1985), a rate-limiting enzyme of the ketogenesis pathway. An inhibition of the acylcarnitine transferase I (and, therefore, of fatty acid transfer into mitochondria) by methylmalonyl-CoA was observed in liver mitochondria from sheep (Brindle, Zammit & Pogson, 1985). Such an effect could be relevant under some circumstances, such as vitamin B_{12} deficit or inherited metabolic disturbances.

Butyrate metabolism

A small percentage of plasma butyrate is bound to albumin, from 10% in the rat to 30% in the sheep (Rémésy & Demigné, 1974). Hepatic uptake of butyrate is practically total under any physiological conditions. Butyrate uptake could be facilitated by the presence of a butyrate-binding protein in the cytosol (Marioka & Ono, 1978). Butyrate is exclusively metabolized in mitochondria (carnitine-independent source of acetyl-CoA) and it is a potentially ketogenic substrate during the postabsorptive period. Butyrate activation is probably mediated by medium-chain acyl-CoA synthetase(s) (Scholte & Groot, 1975; Groot & Scheek, 1976). The subsequent dehydrogenase step is catalyzed by a specific short-chain acyl-CoA dehydrogenase (Ikeda, Okamura-Ikeda & Tanaka, 1985). In fed subjects, butyrate may represent a precursor for lipogenesis. High concentrations of butyrate inhibit propionate utilization (Demigné *et al.*, 1986*a*). Because of the provision of acetyl-CoA in mitochondria, butyrate is an effective activator of gluconeogenesis from lactate, and of ureogenesis; thus, butyrate probably thwarts some of the inhibitory effects of propionate on gluconeogenesis.

Although butyrate has various effects on cellular metabolism (see Chapter 18), specific studies on hepatic metabolism are still scarce. Butyrate activation may lead to a dramatic accumulation of pyrophosphate, which can trap the mitochondrial Ca^{2+}, especially after addition of calcium-dependent hormones (Davidson & Halestrap, 1988). More specifically, it has been shown that butyrate can modulate the expression of tyrosine aminotransferase, a highly inducible enzyme (Plesko *et al.*, 1983; Staecker & Pitot, 1988), or stimulate the synthesis and secretion of certain apolipoproteins (Kaptein, Roodenburg & Princen, 1992). Like colonocytes, hepatocytes are probably adapted to a permanent supply of butyrate, and other cell types might be more responsive to butyrate effects.

Metabolic consequences of the replacement of glucose by SCFA

Fermentation of polysaccharides in the large intestine results, for the host, in the replacement of carbohydrate by SCFA. This leads to losses (40–50%) of carbon units, and only propionate (15–35% of total SCFA) is glucogenic. It is thus important to consider the overall effects of the replacement of a proportion of glucose by SCFA. Furthermore, various soluble fibres may delay glucose absorption from digestible starch.

The utilization of resistant starch (crude potato starch or amylomaize starch) is useful to study the metabolic effects of the replacement of glucose by SCFA. In the rat, diets containing a high-amylose maize (amylomaize) starch leads to the absorption of large amounts of SCFA, especially propionate (Morand *et al.*, 1992*b*). In such conditions, propionate is the major glucogenic substrate taken up by the liver, but lactate utilization is not abolished by the high propionate availability (see Fig. 11.6). The plasma insulin level was reduced in rats fed amylomaize starch compared to control rats, and there were smaller fluctuations of plasma insulin and liver glycogen between the fed and postabsorptive period. All these metabolic characteristics indicate that hepatic metabolism is oriented towards gluconeogenesis with diets rich in fermentable carbohydrates (Demigné *et al.*, 1986*a*; Morand *et al.*, 1992*b*). In parallel, there is a decrease in the activity of enzymes for lipogenesis (especially ATP–citrate lyase). In spite of a lower insulin level, acetyl-CoA synthetase activity was slightly higher in rats fed an amylomaize starch diet (see Table 11.1).

It has been proposed that propionic acid may mediate the hypocholesterolaemic effects of some plant fibres (Chen, Anderson & Jennings, 1984). Such an effect has been obtained experimentally in rats and pigs (Thacker & Bowland, 1981; Illman *et al.*, 1988). Ide *et al.* (1978) have demonstrated that hydroxymethylglutaryl (HMG)-CoA reductase activity is reduced by medium-chain fatty acids. It is conceivable that SCFA exert similar effects on cholesterogenesis. However, with diets rich in soluble fibres, there is also an increase in faecal bile acid excretion (Ebihara & Schneeman, 1989), which tends in turn to induce the activity of HMG-CoA reductase (Mazur *et al.*, 1990). In such conditions, large amounts of SCFA appear unable to depress the activity of HMG-CoA reductase.

Since SCFA are extensively metabolized in the liver, they may constitute a carbon source for lipogenesis (when relatively low-fat diets are fed). Generally, propionate has little effect on lipogenesis from other substrates, such as lactate. *In vitro*, propionate inhibits lipogenesis (and cholesterogenesis) from acetate (Nishina & Freedland, 1990). This could merely be a reflection of the inhibition of acetate metabolism by propionate (Fig. 11.3). Wright, Anderson & Bridges (1990) also suggested that propionate may inhibit cholesterol and fatty-acid biosynthesis *in vivo*, but only with a high (extra-physiological) concentration of propionate. If gluconeogenesis is not active when propionate is metabolized, propionate itself could be used for cholesterogenesis (Fears, 1981) although the metabolic pathways are still speculative (Emmanuel & Robblee, 1984).

The lipid-lowering effect of fibre is now well-established in appropriate conditions, but neither digestive effects (by enhancing faecal excretion of steroids) nor SCFA effects alone can account entirely for the metabolic effect of fibres. In the rat, a considerable increase in bile acid excretion (with cholestyramine administration) does not necessarily depress cholesterolaemia, and additional acetate fails to mimic completely the effect of fibres (Beynen & Lemmers, 1987).

Besides fermentable polysaccharides, plant foods contain various components, such as phytosterols, flavonoids or saponins, that can affect lipid absorption or enhance the faecal excretion of bile acids (Shutler, Walker & Low, 1987). Furthermore, a variety of antioxidant products (ascorbic acid, tocopherols and tocotrienols, carotenoids, etc.), present in fruits and vegetables, may contribute to the protective effect and reinforce the beneficial effects of fibres on lipid metabolism.

Comparative aspects

It is interesting to consider SCFA metabolism in the ruminant liver. Because of the extensive breakdown of carbohydrates in the forestomach, practically no glucose is absorbed from the intestine. Ruminants rely permanently on gluconeogenesis for their glucose needs. Gluconeogenesis operates at maximal rate during the postprandial period. This permanent orientation of liver metabolism is associated with some specific features: low glucokinase activity, low lipogenic capacities in the liver, and low rate of acetate utilization.

Liver cells from ruminants have a very high capacity to remove and metabolize propionate and a relatively low capacity to metabolize buryrate, a situation opposite to that in the rat (Demigné *et al.*, 1986*b*, 1991; Bergman, 1990). *In vitro*, the yield of propionate conversion to glucose is very high (up to 80%) but it is lower when the concentration of propionate is high. However, this process is more responsive to a series of inhibitors (mainly ethanol, butyrate and ammonia) in ruminants than in rats (Demigné *et al.*, 1991). This could relate to the existence of a mitochondrial form of phosphoenolpyruvate carboxykinase in ruminants. It is well established that, in humans, gluconeogenesis is markedly inhibited by ethanol, in relation to changes in the redox state in the liver, and it seems conceivable that propionate metabolism could also be affected by ethanol. In ruminants, conditions of impaired gluconeogenesis from propionate are associated with an accumulation of malate in liver cells (Demigné *et al.*, 1991), in contrast to rats, in which there is rather an accumulation of fumarate and succinate (Nakai *et al.*, 1991). In ruminant hepatocytes, it has been shown that propionate is a potent activator of glycogen synthetase, but in omnivorous species, lactate is a more efficient activator than is propionate (Morand *et al.*, 1990, 1992*a*). In ruminant hepatocytes, propionate or butyrate stimulates ureogenesis. In contrast to the rat, there is little toxic effect of excess propionate in the ruminant, probably due to the absence of propionyl-CoA accumulation. In isolated sheep hepatocytes, propionate also elicited an accumulation of phosphoserine and serine (Demigné *et al.*, 1991) which could influence phospholipid metabolism in the liver.

Extrahepatic metabolism of SCFA

A substantial fraction of acetate from digestive fermentation is not taken up by the liver (from 30 to 80%) and the splanchnic balance of acetate is always positive, even during fasting periods (Rémésy & Demigné, 1983). Most of the extrasplanchnic tissues can metabolize acetate. Adipose tissue and mammary gland contain a cytosolic acetyl-CoA synthetase. Muscles, kidneys and the heart contain a mitochondrial acetyl-CoA synthetase (Groot & Scheek, 1976). The cytosolic localization should channel acetate towards lipogenesis, whereas the mitochondrial localization favours its utilization for energy supply in the Krebs cycle. The half-life of acetate is particularly short ($\approx$2–4 min); acetate uptake by muscles depends on its arterial concentration. Acetate apparently fails to alter energy consumption by muscles and this suggests that it may replace long-chain fatty acids as a fuel (Steffen, McKenzie & Haddy, 1982), particularly since acetate is antilipolytic (Abramson & Arky, 1968; Akanji, Bruce & Frayn, 1989). In diabetic subjects, there is a severe reduction in the peripheral utilization of acetate and an increase in systemic concentrations (Seufert *et al.*, 1974; Akanji & Hockaday, 1990). Besides its role as a fuel for various tissues, acetate has other physiological effects due to its vasodilator action (Liang & Lowenstein, 1978), but the mechanism is still uncertain (Nutting *et al.*, 1991). Only minute quantities of propionate are available for peripheral tissues and the possible physiological significance of this is still unknown.

In conclusion, even with diets containing substantial amounts of fibres, the overall contribution of SCFA to energy is relatively low in humans. Nevertheless, it must be kept in mind that SCFA are not negligible fuels for the large-intestine mucosa (butyrate) and for the liver (acetate and propionate). Furthermore, since propionate and butyrate are very rapidly taken up and metabolized by liver cells, it is conceivable that their metabolism frequently takes place in a subpopulation of hepatocytes on which they might have more potent effects.

References

Abramson, E. A. & Arky, R. A. (1968). Acute antilipolytic effects of ethyl alcohol and acetate in man. *Journal of Laboratory and Clinical Medicine*, **72**, 105–18.

Akanji, A. O., Bruce, M. A. & Frayn, K. N. (1989). Effect of acetate infusion on energy expenditure and substrate oxidation rates in non-diabetic and diabetic subjects. *European Journal of Clinical Nutrition*, **43**, 107–15.

Akanji, A. O. & Hockaday, T. D. R. (1990). Acetate tolerance and the kinetics of acetate utilization in diabetic and non diabetic subjects. *American Journal of Clinical Nutrition*, **51**, 112–18.

Ash, R. & Baird, G. D. (1973). Activation of volatile fatty acids in bovine liver and rumen epithelium. Evidence for control by autoregulation. *Biochemical Journal*, **136**, 311–19.

Bain, M. D., Jones, M., Borriello, S. P., Reed, P. J., Trecey, B. M., Chalmers, R. A. & Stacey, T. E. (1988). Contribution of gut bacterial metabolism to human metabolic disease. *Lancet*, **1**, 1078–9.

Baranyai, J. M. & Blum, J. J. (1989). Quantitative analysis of intermediary metabolism in rat hepatocytes incubated in the presence or the absence of ethanol with a substrate mixture including ketoleucine. *Biochemical Journal*, **258**, 121–40.

Barritt, G. J., Zander, G. L. & Utter, M. F. (1976). The regulation of pyruvate carboxylase activity in mammalian species. In *Gluconeogenesis: Its Regulation in Mammalian Species*, ed. R. W. Hanson & M. A. Mehlman, pp. 3–46. New York: Wiley.

Barth, C., Sladek, M. & Decker, K. (1972). Dietary changes of cytoplasmic acetyl-CoA synthetase in different rat tissues. *Biochimica et Biophysica Acta*, **260**, 1–9.

Bergman, E. N. (1990). Energy contribution of volatile fatty acids in the gastrointestinal tract in various species. *Physiological Reviews*, **70**, 567–90.

Beynen, A. C., Buechler, K., Van Der Molen, A. J. & Geelen, M. J. H. (1982). The effects of lactate and acetate on fatty acid and cholesterol biosynthesis by isolated rat hepatocytes. *International Journal of Biochemistry*, **14**, 165–9.

Beynen, A. C. & Geelen, M. J. H. (1982). Effects of insulin and glucagon on fatty acid synthesis from acetate by hepatocytes incubated with (−)-hydroxycitrate. *Endokrinologie*, **79**, 308–10.

Beynen, A. C. & Lemmers, A. G. (1987). Dietary acetate and cholesterol metabolism in rats. *Zeitschrift für Ehrnärungswissenschaft*, **26**, 79–83.

Brass, E. P., Fennessey, P. V. & Miller, L. V. (1986). Inhibition of oxidative metabolism by propionic acid and its reversal by carnitine in isolated rat hepatocytes. *Biochemical Journal*, **236**, 131–6.

Brindle, N. P. J., Zammit, V. A. & Pogson, C. I. (1985). Inhibition of sheep liver carnitine palmitoyltransferase by methylmalonyl-CoA. *Biochemical Society Transactions*, **33**, 880–1.

Buckley, B. M. & Williamson, D. H. (1977). Origin of blood acetate in the rat. *Biochemical Journal*, **166**, 539–44.

Chen, W.-J., L., Anderson, J. W. & Jennings, D. (1984). Propionate may mediate the hypocholesterolemic effects of certain soluble plant fibers in cholesterol-fed rats. *Proceedings of the Society for Experimental Biology and Medicine*, **175**, 215–18.

Chiang, G. S. & Mistry, S. P. (1974). Activities of pyruvate carboxylase and propionyl CoA carboxylase in rat tissues during biotin deficiency and restoration of the activities after biotin administration. *Proceedings of the Society for Experimental Biology and Medicine*, **146**, 21–4.

Corkey, B. E., Martin-Requero, A., Walajtys-Rode, E., Williams, R. J. & Williamson, J. R. (1982). Regulation of branched chain α-ketoacid pathway in liver. *Journal of Biological Chemistry*, **257**, 9668–76.

Coudé, F. X., Sweetman, L. & Nyhan, W. L. (1979). Inhibition by propionyl-coenzyme A of *N*-acetylglutamate synthesis in rat liver mitochondria. *Journal of Clinical Investigations*, **64**, 1544–51.

Crabtree, B., Gordon, M.-J. & Christie, S. L. (1990). Measurement of the rates of acetyl-CoA hydrolysis and synthesis from acetate in rat hepatocytes and the role of these fluxes in substrate cycling. *Biochemical Journal*, **270**, 219–25.

Crabtree, B., Souter, M.-J. & Anderson, S. E. (1989). Evidence that the production of acetate in rat hepatocytes is a predominantly cytoplasmic process. *Biochemical Journal*, **257**, 673–8.

Cullen, R. W. & Oace, S. M. (1989*a*). Fermentable dietary fibers elevate urinary methylmalonate and decrease propionate oxidation in rats deprived of vitamin B-12. *Journal of Nutrition*, **119**, 1115–20.

Cullen, R. W. & Oace, S. M. (1989*b*). Dietary pectin shortens the biological half-life of vitamin B-12 in rats by increasing fecal and urinary losses. *Journal of Nutrition*, **119**, 1121–7.

Davidson, A. M. & Halestrap, A. P. (1988). Inorganic pyrophosphate is located primarily in the mitochondria of the hepatocyte and increases in parallel with the decrease in light-scattering induced by glucogenic hormones, butyrate and ionophore A23187. *Biochemical Journal*, **254**, 379–84.

Del Boca, J. & Flatt, J. P. (1969). Fatty acid synthesis from glucose and acetate and the control of lipogenesis in adipose tissue. *European Journal of Biochemistry*, **11**, 127–34.

Demigné, C., Yacoub, C., Morand, C. & Rémésy, C. (1991). Interactions between propionate and amino acid metabolism in isolated sheep hepatocytes. *British Journal of Nutrition*, **65**, 301–17.

Demigné, C., Yacoub, C. & Rémésy, C. (1986*a*). Effects of absorption of large amounts of volatile fatty acids on rat liver metabolism. *Journal of Nutrition*, **116**, 77–86.

Demigné, C., Yacoub, C., Rémésy, C. & Fafournoux, P. (1986*b*). Propionate and butyrate metabolism in rat or sheep hepatocytes. *Biochimica et Biophysica Acta*, **874**, 535–42.

Des Rosiers, C., David, F., Garneau, M. & Brunengraber, H. (1991). Nonhomogeneous labeling of liver mitochondrial acetyl-CoA. *Journal of Biological Chemistry*, **266**, 1574–8.

Ebihara, Y. & Schneeman, B. O. (1989). Interaction of bile acids, phospholipids, cholesterol and triglyceride with dietary fiber in the small intestine of rats. *Journal of Nutrition*, **119**, 1100–6.

Emmanuel, B. & Robblee, A. R. (1984). Cholesterogenesis from propionate: facts and speculations. *International Journal of Biochemistry*, **16**, 907–11.

Fafournoux, P., Rémésy, C. & Demigné, C. (1985). Propionate transport in rat liver cells. *Biochimica et Biophysica Acta*, **818**, 73–80.

Fears, R. (1981). The contribution of the cholesterol biosynthetic pathway to intermediary metabolism and cell function. *Biochemical Journal*, **199**, 1–7.

Focke, M., Feld, A. & Lichtenthaler, H. K. (1990). Allicin, a naturally occuring antibiotic from garlic, specifically inhibits acetyl-CoA synthetase. *FEBS Letters*, **261**, 106–8.
Gordon, M.-J. & Crabtree, B. (1992). The effects of propionate and butyrate on acetate metabolism in rat hepatocytes. *International Journal of Biochemistry*, **24**, 1029–31.
Groot, P. H. & Scheek, L. M. (1976). Acyl-CoA synthetase in guinea-pig liver mitochondria. Purification and characterization of distinct propionyl-CoA synthetase. *Biochimica et Biophysica Acta*, **441**, 260–7.
Hovik, R., Brodal, B., Bartlett, K. & Osmunden, H. (1991). Metabolism of acetyl-CoA by isolated peroxisomal fractions: formations of acetate and acetoacetyl-CoA. *Journal of Lipid Research*, **32**, 993–9.
Hue, L., Maisin, &. & Rider, M. H. (1988). Palmitate inhibits liver glycolysis. Involvement of fructose 2,6-bisphosphate in the glucose/fatty acid cycle. *Biochemical Journal*, **251**, 541–5.
Ide, T., Horii, M., Yamamoto, T. & Kawashima, K. (1978). Contrasting effects of water-soluble and water-insoluble dietary fibers on bile acid conjugation and taurine metabolism in the rat. *Lipids*, **25**, 335–40.
Ikeda, Y., Okamura-Ikeda, K. & Tanaka, K. (1985). Purification and characterization of short-chain, medium-chain, and long-chain acyl-CoA dehydrogenases from rat liver mitochondria. *Journal of Biological Chemistry*, **260**, 1311–25.
Illman, R. J., Topping, D. L., McIntosh, G. H., Trimble, R. P., Storer, G. B., Taylor, M. N. & Cheng, B-Q. (1988). Hypocholesterolemic effects of dietary propionate: studies in whole animal and perfused rat liver. *Annals of Nutrition and Metabolism*, **32**, 97–107.
Kaptein, A., Roodenburg, L. & Princen, H. M. G. (1992). Butyrate stimulates the secretion of apolipoprotein (apo) A-1 and apo B100 by the human hepatoma cell line Hep G2. *Biochemical Journal*, **278**, 557–64.
Knowles, S. E., Jarrett, I. G., Filsell, O. H. & Ballard, F. J. (1974). Production and utilization of acetate in mammals. *Biochemical Journal*, **142**, 401–11.
Knudsen, C. T., Immerdal, L., Grunnet, N. & Quistorff, B. (1992). Periportal zonation of the cytosolic acetyl-CoA synthetase of male rat liver. *European Journal of Biochemistry*, **204**, 359–62.
Krahenbuhl, S. & Brass, E. P. (1991). Inhibition of hepatic propionyl-CoA synthetase activity by organic acids. Reversal of propionate inhibition of pyruvate metabolism. *Biochemical Pharmacology*, **41**, 1015–23.
Leighton, F., Bergseth, S. Rørtveit, T., Christiansen, E. N. & Bremer, J. (1989). Free acetate production by rat hepatocytes during peroxisomal fatty acid and dicarboxylic oxidation. *Journal of Biological Chemistry*, **264**, 10347–50.
Li, A. C., Tanaka, R. D., Callaway, K., Fogelman, A. M. & Edwards, P. A. (1988). Localization of 3-hydroxy-3-methylglutaryl CoA reductase and 3-hydroxy-3-methylglutaryl CoA synthase in the rat liver and in intestine is affected by cholestyramine and mevinolin. *Journal of Lipid Research*, **29**, 781–96.
Liang, C. S. & Lowenstein, J. M. (1978). Metabolic control of the circulation; effects of acetate and pyruvate. *Journal of Clinical Investigations*, **62**, 1029–38.
Lowe, D. M. & Tubbs, P. K. (1985). Succinylation and inactivation of 3-hydroxy-3-methylglutaryl-CoA synthase by succinyl-CoA and its possible relevance in the control of ketogenesis. *Biochemical Journal*, **232**, 37–42.
Lumeng, L. & Davis, J. (1973). The oxidation of acetate by liver mitochondria. *FEBS letters*, **79**, 124–6.

Macfarlane, G. T. & Cummings, J. H. (1991). The colonic flora, fermentation, and large bowel function. In *The Large Intestine: Physiology, Pathophysiology, and Disease*, ed. S. F. Phillips, J. H. Pemberton & R. G. Shorter, pp. 52–92. New York: Raven Press.

MacNamara, D. J., Quackenbush, F. W. & Rodwell, V. W. (1970). Cycloheximide and chloramphenicol: effect on rat liver acetate metabolism. *Lipids*, **5**, 146–8.

Marioka, K. & Ono, T. (1978). Butyrate-binding protein from rat and mouse liver. *Journal of Biochemistry*, **83**, 349–56.

Mazur, A., Rémésy, C., Gueux, E., Levrat, M.-A. & Demigné, C. (1990). Effects of diets rich in fermentable carbohydrates on plasma lipoprotein levels and on lipoprotein catabolism in rats. *Journal of Nutrition*, **120**, 1037–45.

Morand, C., Redon, C., Rémésy, C. & Demigné, C. (1990). Non-hormonal and hormonal control of glycogen metabolism in isolated sheep hepatocytes. *International Journal of Biochemistry*, **22**, 873–81.

Morand, C., Rémésy, C. & Demigné, C. (1992*a*). Contrôle du métabolisme du glycogène au niveau du foie. *Diabète & Métabolisme*, **18**, 87–95.

Morand, C., Rémésy, C. & Demigné, C. (1993). Fatty acids are potent modulators of lactate utilization in isolated hepatocytes from fed rats. *American Journal of Physiology*, **264**, E816–E823.

Morand, C. Rémésy, C., Levrat, M.-A. & Demigné, C. (1992*b*). Replacement of digestible wheat starch by resistant cornstarch alters splanchnic metabolism in rats. *Journal of Nutrition*, **122**, 345–54.

Murthy, V. K. & Steiner, G. (1973). Hepatic acetate levels in relation to altered lipid metabolism. *Metabolism*, **22**, 81–5.

Nakai, A., Shigematsu, Y., Saito, M., Kikawa, Y. & Sudo, M. (1991). Pathophysiologic study on methylmalonic aciduria: decrease in liver high-energy phosphate after propionate loading in rats. *Pediatric Research*, **30**, 5–10.

Nishina, P. M. & Freedland, R. A. (1990). Effects of propionate on lipid biosynthesis in isolated rat hepatocytes. *Journal of Nutrition*, **120**, 667–3.

Nomura, T., Iguchi, A. Sakamoto, N. & Harris, R. A. (1983). Effects of octanoate and acetate upon hepatic glycolysis and lipogenesis. *Biochimica et Biophysica Acta*, **754**, 315–20.

Nutting, C. W., Islam, S. I., Ye, M., Battle, D. C. & Daugirdas, J. T. (1991). The vasorelaxant effects of acetate: role of adenosine, glycolysis, lyotropism, and pH_i and Ca^{2+}. *Kidney International*, **41**, 166–74.

Patel, T. B., DeBuysere, M. S. & Olson, M. S. (1983). The effect of propionate on the regulation of the pyruvate dehydrogenase complex in rat liver. *Archives of Biochemistry and Biophysics*, **220**, 405–14.

Plesko, M. M., Hargroves, J. L., Granner, D. K. & Chalkley, R. (1983). Inhibition by sodium butyrate of enzyme induction by glucocorticoids and dibutyryl cyclic AMP. *Journal of Biological Chemistry*, **258**, 13738–44.

Rémésy, C. & Demigné, C. (1974). Determination of volatile fatty acids in plasma after ethanolic extraction. *Biochemical Journal*, **141**, 86–91.

Rémésy, C. & Demigné, C. (1983). Changes in availability of glucogenic and ketogenic substrates and liver metabolism in fed or starved rats. *Annals of Nutrition & Metabolism*, **27**, 57–70.

Rémésy, C., Demigné, C. & Chartier, F. (1980). Origin and utilization of volatile fatty acids in the rat. *Reproduction, Nutrition et Développement*, **20**, 1339–49.

Rémésy, C., Demigné, C. & Morand, C. (1992). Metabolism and utilisation of short chain fatty acids produced by colonic fermentation. In *Dietary Fibre – a*

Component of Food, ILSI Human Nutrition Reviews, ed. T. F. Schweitzer & C. A. Edwards, pp. 137–50. London: Springer-Verlag.

Scholte, H. R. & Groot, P. H. (1975). Organ and intracellular localization of short-chain acyl-CoA synthetases in rat and guinea-pig. *Biochimica et Biophysica Acta*, **409**, 283–96.

Seto, K., Saito, H. Edashige, N., Kawakami, T., Yoshimtsu, K., Horiuchi, C. & Kawakami, M. (1985). Influence of microinjection of insulin into amygdala on acetate metabolism in liver slices of rabbit. *Experimental Clinical Endocrinology*, **86**, 233–6.

Seufert, C. D., Graf, M., Janson, A., Kuhn, A. & Söling, H. D. (1974). Formation of free acetate in isolated perfused livers from normal, starved and diabetic rats. *Biochemical and Biophysical Research Communications*, **57**, 901–9.

Shaw, L. & Engel, P. C. (1985). The suicide inactivation of ox liver short chain acyl-CoA dehydrogenase by propionyl-CoA. *Biochemical Journal*, **230**, 723–31.

Shutler, S. M., Walker, A. F. & Low, A. G. (1987). The cholesterol-lowering effects of legumes II: effects of fibre, sterols, saponins and isoflavones. *Human Nutrition: Food Sciences and Nutrition*, **41F**, 87–102.

Snoswell, A. M., Trimble, R. P., Fishlock, R. C., Storer, G. B. & Topping, D. L. (1982). Metabolic effects of acetate in perfused liver. Studies on ketogenesis, glucose output, lactate uptake and lipogenesis. *Biochimica et Biophysica Acta*, **716**, 290–7.

Söling, H.-D. & Rescher, C. (1985). On the regulation of cold-labile cytosolic and mitochondrial acetyl-CoA hydrolase in rat liver. *European Journal of Biochemistry*, **147**, 111–17.

Staecker, J. L. & Pitot, H. C. (1988). The effect of sodium butyrate on tyrosine aminotransferase induction in primary cultures of normal adult rat hepatocytes. *Archives of Biochemistry and Biophysics*, **261**, 291–8.

Steffen, R. P., McKenzie, J. Z. & Haddy, F. J. (1982). The possible role of acetate in exercise hyperemia in dog skeletal muscle. *Pflügers Archiv*, **392**, 315–21.

Thacker, P. A. & Bowland, J. P. (1981). Effect of dietary propionic acid on serum lipids and lipoproteins of pig fed diets supplemented soybean meal or canula meal. *Canadian Journal of Animal Science*, **61**, 439–48.

Thompson, G. N., Walter, J. H., Bresson, J.-L., Ford, G. C., Lyonnet, S. L., Chalmers, R. A., Saudubray, J.-M., Leonard, J. V. & Halliday, D. (1990). Sources of propionate in inborn errors of propionate metabolism. *Metabolism*, **39**, 1133–7.

Whitton, P. D., Rodrigues, L. M. & Hems, D. A. (1979). Stimulation by acetate of gluconeogenesis in hepatocyte suspension. *FEBS Letters*, **98**, 85–7.

Wright, R. S., Anderson, J. W. & Bridges, S. R. (1990). Propionate inhibits hepatocyte lipid synthesis. *Proceedings of the Society for Experimental Biology and Medicine*, **195**, 26–9.

12

Effects of short-chain fatty acids on gastrointestinal motility

C. CHERBUT

Motility of the digestive tract in mammals is sensitive to the chemical and physical luminal environment. Short-chain fatty acids (SCFA) are the major anion constituents of the digestive contents in the forestomach of ruminants and in the hindgut of non-ruminant mammals. In ruminants, the motor effects of SCFA were highlighted about 20 years ago. Since then, the mechanisms of action have been elucidated. Interest in the potential physiological effects of SCFA in non-ruminants, however, has developed only recently.

In this chapter, we discuss the effects of SCFA on the motility of the gastrointestinal tract of ruminant and non-ruminant mammals, mechanisms by which the effects of SCFA are transmitted, the physiological importance of these effects, and their implications.

Modulation of gastrointestinal motility by SCFA in ruminants

Studies in cattle and sheep experiencing ruminal acidosis have indicated that SCFA modulate gastrointestinal motility in ruminants. Acidosis is caused by over-feeding of diets rich in readily fermentable carbohydrates. As a result, SCFA accumulate and ruminal pH falls (Huber, 1976). According to Dirksen's results (1970), the decrease in pH during the first 8 h of acidosis is caused by an increased production of SCFA, e.g. acetic, propionic and butyric acids, the relative proportion of which may vary. If acidosis further develops, lactic acid concentration will reach a peak 7–24 h after overfeeding, thereafter decreasing, although the pH remains low for several days. During acidosis, the cyclic contractions of the reticulorumen decrease, and finally they disappear completely. The inhibition of reticuloruminal motility can be reproduced experimentally by infusing SCFA and lactic acid into the rumen of normal sheep (Ash, 1959; Svendsen, 1973; Upton, Ryan & Leek, 1976).

The mechanisms of such action of SCFA are complex. The undissociated form of SCFA activates sensitive epithelial receptors, which are connected with vagal fibres and possibly with myenteric neurones. However, SCFA might also affect the gastric motor centres by a systemic effect or act directly on smooth muscle.

Gastrointestinal motor response to SCFA in ruminants

Effects of ruminal SCFA on rumen motility

The major effect of SCFA in ruminants appears to be the local inhibition of reticuloruminal motility. The reticuloruminal movements occur cyclically. A primary cycle starts with a biphasic contraction of the reticulum, followed by a monophasic contraction of the dorsal ruminal sac and then of the ventral ruminal sac. This cycle occurs about once every minute. A second cycle follows alternate primary cycles. It consists of a monophasic contraction of the dorsal ruminal sac and then of the ventral ruminal sac (Leek, 1983). When SCFA are infused directly into the rumen, the amplitude of the primary ruminal contractions decreases. The frequency of the secondary ruminal contractions and the strength of the reticular contractions are reduced (Svendsen, 1973; Gregory, 1987). Finally, both reticular and ruminal contractions are abolished.

Table 12.1 shows the different doses, pH and sites of infusion that have been used by the numerous workers who have studied the effects of SCFA on reticuloruminal motility. Most of these experimental infusions resulted in physiological pH and concentrations of undissociated acids within the rumen. Crichlow & Chaplin (1985) measured maximal concentrations of around 16 mM and 30 mM, respectively, of undissociated SCFA and lactic acid in sheep ruminal fluids during the inhibition of the ruminal motility caused by wheat engorgement.

Effects of SCFA in other gut segments on rumen motility

When they are infused into the abomasum, SCFA also influence reticuloruminal motility (Gregory, 1987). They reduce the strength of the ruminal contractions at an abomasal concentration of undissociated acids of 60 mM and above, and they increase the reticular motility at a concentration of about 80 mM. However, it is unlikely that such high concentrations of SCFA would occur in the abomasum. In healthy sheep, the abomasal concentration of total SCFA is only about 6 mM (Bueno *et al.*, 1972). When SCFA were infused into the rumen at a concentration of 4 M, the ruminal motility was largely inhibited, yet the abomasal concentrations of SCFA and lactic acid did not exceed 12 mM and 20 mM, respectively. Therefore, the inhibitory influence from abomasal SCFA is likely to be negligible.

SCFA and lactic acid also reduce the ruminal motility when they are infused into the duodenum (Bruce & Huber, 1973; Smith, Krishnamurti & Kitts, 1979; Gregory, 1987). The amount of SCFA that has to be delivered to the duodenum to cause a significant inhibition of the ruminal motility is at least 1 mmol/min (Table 12.1). The abomasal motility is strongly inhibited by lower concentrations of SCFA (0.4 mmol/min) in the duodenum (Gregory & Miller, 1989). It can therefore be deduced that the high concentration of SCFA required to affect the ruminal motility is unlikely to reach the duodenum, for it would inhibit the abomasal outflow.

Properties of SCFA that inhibit reticuloruminal motility

Two major parameters govern the inhibitory effect of SCFA: the concentration of undissociated acids and the structure of the molecule. The inhibition of motility by SCFA is more pronounced when the pH is lower (Ash, 1959; Crichlow & Leek, 1981). Yet the effect does not depend on the hydrogen ion per se, since introduction into the empty rumen of acidic solutions without SCFA does not affect the ruminal motility. Therefore, the presence of SCFA is required for the inhibition. The degree of inhibition increases according to the concentration of undissociated acids (Svendsen, 1973; Upton *et al.*, 1976; Leek, 1983; Crichlow & Chaplin, 1984). This concentration is controlled by both the fermentation rate and the pH. At neutral pH, SCFA are mostly dissociated, but, according to the Henderson–Hasselbalch equation, when the pH falls, the proportion of undissociated acids increases. Thus, as the production of SCFA increases, the pH goes down and the concentration of undissociated acids accordingly increases. Strong acids, such as lactic acid, make the pH very low and cause more of the total SCFA to become undissociated.

Acetic, propionic and butyric acids all inhibit reticuloruminal motility, but with different levels of efficiency (Ash, 1959; Leek, Ryan & Upton, 1978). Motor activity decreases more sharply with butyric acid than with either acetic or propionic acid, and a lower concentration of butyric acid is needed for the contractions to disappear completely (Svendsen, 1973; Gregory, 1987). Butyric acid thus appears to be the most potent SCFA to inhibit the cyclical movements of the rumen.

The action of lactic acid is more controversial. Gregory (1987) reported that, when lactic acid was infused into rumen, it was as effective as SCFA

Table 12.1. *Effects of ruminal, abomasal and duodenal infusion of short-chain fatty acids on reticuloruminal motility in the sheep*

Acid type	Concentration of total acids in the perfusate (M)	Concentration of undissociated acids in the contents (mM)	pH: In the perfusate	pH: In the contents	Effect on ruminal contractions	References
Ruminal infusion						
Acetic (C2)	0.2		5		Decreased frequency	Ash (1959)
C2	0.1–0.2		3.6–4		Complete inhibition	
Propionic (C3)	0.1–0.2		3.6–4		Similar effects to C2	
Butyric (C4)	0.1–0.2		3.6–4		More pronounced effects than C2 and C3	
Lactic	0.1–0.2		3.6–4		No effect	
Lactic	0.2		2.5		Complete inhibition	
C2	1.5		6.1		Decreased strength	Svendsen (1973)
C3	1.5		6.1		Similar effect to C2	
C4	1.5		6.1		More pronounced effect than C2 and C3	
Lactic	1		4		No effect	
Mixture, C2:C3:C4 (63:20:17)	1.5	0.7–8.1	6.1	6.2–6.7	Decreased strength Dose-related effect	
Lactic	0.15		2, 4, 6		No effect	Smith *et al.* (1979)
Lactic	0.7		2, 4, 6		No effect	
C2	4	20–85			Decreased frequency and amplitude	Gregory (1987)
C3	4	21–52			Similar effect to C2	
C4	4	14–40			More pronounced effect than C2 and C3	
Lactic	4	12–87			Similar effect to C2	
Mixture, C2:C3:C4 (65:25:10)	4	18–70			Additional effects of C2, C3 and C4	
Mixture, C2:C3:C4 (33:33:33)	4	15–35			Additional effects of C2, C3 and C4	
Mixture, C2:C3:C4:lactic	4	17–35			Additional effects of lactic to C2, C3 and C4	

Abomasal infusion						
C2	0.5	89–93		2.9	Decreased strength, increased frequency	Gregory (1987)
C3	0.5	97–102		2.8	Similar effects for all the acids	
C4	0.5	67–76		2.9		
Lactic	0.5	98–105		2.8		
Duodenal infusion						
C2	0.5 (5–10 ml/min)				No effect on ruminal motility, but inhibition of abomasal motility at 10 ml/min. Similar effects for all the acids	Gregory (1987)
C3	0.5 (5–10 ml/min)					
C4	0.5 (5–10 ml/min)					
Lactic	0.5 (5–10 ml/min)					
C2	1 (5–10 ml/min)				Strong inhibition of abomasal motility at 5 ml/min. Complete inhibition of abomasal motility, and decreased frequency and amplitude of ruminal contractions. Similar effects for all the acids	
C3	1 (5–10 ml/min)					
C4	1 (5–10 ml/min)					
Lactic	1 (5–10 ml/min)					
Lactic	0.7		2		Decreased frequency and amplitude of ruminal and abomasal contractions	Bruce & Huber (1973)
Lactic	0.15–0.7		2, 4, 6		Complete inhibition of ruminal motility at pH 2. Effect less pronounced at pH 4 and 6	Smith *et al.* (1979)

in inhibiting reticuloruminal motility, while other authors did not observe any change in ruminal motility (Svendsen, 1973; Smith *et al.*, 1979). This discrepancy may be due to the dose that was infused into the rumen. In Gregory's study, the infusion of lactic acid was four times more concentrated than that used by Svendsen and Smith *et al.* (Table 12.1). Ash (1959) showed that the effect of lactic acid depends on the concentration, since introduction of 80 mM undissociated lactic acid into the empty rumen had no effect, whereas introduction of 200 mM undissociated acid completely inhibited the ruminal motility. It can, therefore, be suggested that the threshold concentration of lactic acid for reduction of the ruminal motility may be much higher than that of SCFA.

When acetic, propionic and butyric acids are infused together, they still exert an inhibitory effect on reticuloruminal motility. The degree of inhibition can be explained by the sum of the effects of the concentrations (as undissociated acid) of each constituent acid (Gregory, 1987). The inhibitory effect of SCFA thus appears to be synergistic. Lactic acid combined with SCFA mixtures also inhibits reticuloruminal motility in an additive fashion, and may even increase the sensitivity to SCFA (Crichlow & Chaplin, 1984).

Mechanisms of inhibitory action of SCFA on reticuloruminal motility

When they are infused into the systemic circulation, SCFA abolish contractions of the reticulorumen (Le Bars *et al.*, 1954). This effect was suggested to result from a depression of the gastric motor centres. It might also involve a direct action of SCFA in the gastrointestinal wall, either on the myenteric plexus or on the smooth muscle cells, which are drained by the systemic blood flow. However, acidosis reduces the reticuloruminal motility before there is any change in pH and SCFA level in arterial and venous blood (Ash, 1959; Mullen, 1976; Crichlow & Chaplin, 1985). Therefore, it is unlikely that systemic SCFA induce the reticuloruminal states that occurs in the early stages of acidosis, but they may contribute to the inhibition after they are absorbed.

The reticuloruminal motility disappears almost immediately after SCFA are infused into the rumen (Ash, 1959; Gregory, 1987), which suggests that nervous rather than hormonal mediation is involved. The inhibition of motility has been attributed to a vagovagal reflex through excitation of epithelial receptors (Leek & Harding, 1975; Upton *et al.*, 1976).

Vagally innervated receptors, which respond to light tactile stimulation and which are excited by solutions containing suitable concentrations of sodium hydroxide, hydrochloric acid or SCFA, have been detected in the epithelium of the reticulum and rumen (Harding & Leek, 1972*a*; Leek & Harding, 1975). Similar receptors are also identified in the abomasal, pyloric and proximal duodenal mucosa (Harding & Leek, 1972*b*). Electrophysiological and histological studies suggest that the receptors are unspecialized sensory nerve endings, lying at around 150 μm below the luminal surface of the reticuloruminal epithelium and the duodenal mucosa (Leek & Harding, 1975).

The functional characteristics of these receptors can explain most of the effects of SCFA on reticuloruminal motility. The receptors are not pH-sensitive, but their activation is closely related to the titratable acidity or the level of undissociated acids in the rumen (Leek & Harding, 1975; Crichlow & Leek, 1986). A threshold concentration of undissociated acids is necessary to excite the receptors. This threshold ranges from 10 to 100 mM, 50% of the tested receptors responding at a concentration of 50 mM for acetic, propionic and butyric acids (Upton *et al.*, 1976; Crichlow, 1988).

Although butyric acid has repeatedly been shown to be more potent than either acetic or propionic acid in inducing ruminal stasis (Ash, 1959; Svendsen, 1973; Upton *et al.*, 1976; Gregory, 1984), the receptor's threshold concentration for this acid is not markedly different from those of acetic and propionic acids. However, butyric acid activates a higher proportion of epithelial receptors than do acetic and propionic acids (Crichlow, 1988), which could explain its greater potency in inhibiting reticuloruminal contractions. In contrast, lactic acid is not very effective in activating receptors, and the responsive receptors have a threshold of at least 200 mM (Crichlow, 1988).

Reticuloruminal motility was also inhibited in vagotomized sheep by intraruminally infused SCFA at a concentration comparable to that needed in vagus-intact sheep (Gregory, 1987). This suggests that local mechanisms may interact with the central control of reticuloruminal motility. One possible explanation might be that the epithelial acid receptors are innervated by myenteric neurones as well as by sensory vagal fibres, so that motility would be similarly affected in intact and vagotomized sheep. Such a dual innervation has been proposed for the tension receptors of the rumen (Gregory, 1984). SCFA might also affect transmission within the myenteric plexus or act directly on the smooth muscle cells. These hypotheses have to be further studied to clarify the involvement of local mechanisms in the inhibitory effect of SCFA on reticuloruminal motility.

Effects of SCFA on gastrointestinal motility in non-ruminants

In non-ruminant mammals, the physiological importance of SCFA has been highlighted only recently. Potential effects of SCFA on digestive motility were suggested less than 10 years ago, and they are not so well understood as are those in ruminants. The action of SCFA leads to different effects in the small intestine, particularly in the ileum, and in the large intestine.

Gastric and small-intestinal responses to SCFA

For many years, it has been known that acids in a meal slow gastric emptying in humans and monogastric animals. Duodenal receptors are activated by acids and inhibitory vagal reflexes are elicited (Malagelada & Azpiroz, 1989). The response of the receptors is related to the titratable acidity of duodenal contents. As far as SCFA are concerned, the threshold concentration required to slow gastric evacuation of a water meal ranges from 60 to 80 mM undissociated acids, acetic acid being the most potent stimulus (Hunt & Knox, 1969). However, a much lower level of SCFA was detected in the non-ruminant duodenum (Hoverstad *et al.*, 1985; Bernier, Adrian & Vidon, 1988). Therefore, it can be concluded that though SCFA are capable of slowing the gastric emptying, it is unlikely that they accumulate in a sufficient amount to activate the duodenal acid-sensitive receptors.

In contrast, a larger concentration of SCFA can be measured in the ileal contents (Florent *et al.*, 1985; Mortensen *et al.*, 1989). The presence of SCFA in the ileal fluid influences gastrointestinal motility. Instillation of SCFA into the ileum induced bursts of phasic contractions that rapidly migrated aborally in the dog and the human (Kamath, Hoepfner & Phillips, 1987; Kamath, Phillips & Zinsmeister, 1988), and shortened stomach-to-caecum transit time in the rat (Richardson *et al.*, 1991) as well as ileal emptying in the dog (Fich *et al.*, 1989). Intravenous injection of SCFA also elicited ileal contractions in anaesthetized rats (Yajima, 1984).

Although all the major SCFA stimulate ileal motility, there are noticeable differences among them. Potency of the acids is inversely related to the chain length (Kamath *et al.*, 1987; Richardson *et al.*, 1991). Acetic acid is more effective than propionic acid, and butyric acid is the least potent to influence small-intestinal motility. The degree of ileal stimulation also depends on acid concentration. Ileal SCFA at concentrations found in the colon (100–150 mM) induced a maximal contractile response of the dog ileum (Kamath *et al.*, 1987), and the shortest orocaecal transit time in the rat (Richardson *et al.*, 1991).

It is not clear whether the stimulatory effect of SCFA in the ileum is affected by pH. SCFA at pH 5.8 and 6.5 induced a comparable stimulation of the ileal contractions in the dog, but there was a trend toward a greater effect of SCFA at pH 7.0 than at pH 3.8 (Kamath *et al.*, 1987). Therefore, SCFA may be more efficient in the ileum when they are dissociated, which suggests that they reach their sites of action by ionic diffusion.

Conversely, SCFA do not affect the motility of the upper small intestine. In the human, intraduodenal SCFA at low (1 mM) or high concentration (100 mM) did not change the duodenojejunal motility and transit time (Masliah *et al.*, 1992). When they were infused into the systemic circulation, SCFA were still unable to modify the jejunal contractions of anaesthetized rats (Yajima, 1984). In addition, SCFA failed to affect the motility of isolated segments of the upper small intestine *in vitro* (Yokokura, Yajima & Hashimoto, 1977).

Colonic effects of SCFA

SCFA constitute the major anions of the colonic contents and their total concentration levels off at around 100–150 mM in most of the monogastric species (Cummings, 1981). As the colon is in general sensitive to its luminal environment (Christensen, 1989), it makes sense to wonder whether SCFA may influence colonic motility.

Mucosal application of SCFA on isolated segments of the rat colon evoked a tonic contraction that was sustained for about 1 min. The contractile effects were dose-dependent within a narrow range of concentrations: the colon did not respond to the stimulus below 0.02 mM, and the maximal response was attained at approximately 0.1 mM. A rising concentration of SCFA up to 10 mM did not further increase the effect (Yajima, 1985). In contrast to this result, infusion of a high concentration of a SCFA mixture (100 mM) abolished the contractile activity, and reduced the fluid flow throughout an entirely isolated rat colon *in vitro* (Squires *et al.*, 1992). Infusion of less concentrated SCFA solutions (10 mM) did not cause any change in the motility of the isolated colon.

From these results, it seems that the effect of SCFA on colonic motility should be concentration-dependent: low doses stimulate the motility, whereas high doses inhibit the contractions. This was confirmed *in vivo*. Instillation of 0.1 mM of undissociated SCFA into the sheep caecum increased the caecal motility (Svendsen, 1972). Conversely, the strength of the caecal contractions was strongly depressed following instillation of undissociated SCFA at 10 mM. When SCFA were infused at a rate of 1 mmol/h into the caecum of fasted rats, they first stimulated the colonic motility for around 30 min, and then progressively inhibited the colonic contractions (Cherbut *et al.*, 1991*a*). The stimulation could have been caused by the low amounts of SCFA at the beginning of the infusion, whereas the inhibition would result from the accumulation of higher amounts of SCFA during the infusion process.

After more than 48 h of SCFA infusion into the rat caecum, the colonic motility was still reduced, and the duration of colonic propagated propulsive contractions was significantly shorter than after infusion of saline solution. Nevertheless, this effect did not alter the transit time of colonic contents (Salvador, Cherbut, & Delort-Laval, 1993). Daily administration of antibiotics, which abolishes SCFA production in the rat digestive tract, increased the duration of the colonic propagated contractions, without changing the colonic transit time (Cherbut *et al.*, 1991*a*). Eventually, the colonic propagated contractions were also inhibited when SCFA were infused into the horse caecum (Candau & Vigroux, 1974). These results indicate that SCFA could exert an inhibitory influence on caecocolonic motility in normal conditions. The inhibition may be due to a reduction of the propagated contractions that are responsible for the mixing and propulsion of the colonic contents.

However, Flourié *et al.* (1989) did not observe any change in the motility of a dog's colonic loop when a physiological mixture of sodium salts of SCFA (108 mM) was infused. Squires *et al.* (1992) reported that the sodium salts of SCFA did not change the motility of the rat colon *in vitro*, whereas the acidic form of SCFA inhibited the contractions. The pH per se cannot account for this effect, since an acidic Krebs solution without SCFA had no effect. Therefore, it seems that SCFA must be in an undissociated form to influence the large-intestinal motility.

The effectiveness of SCFA also depends upon characteristics of the acid molecule: acetic acid was less potent than propionic acid, while butyric acid was the most effective acid to affect colonic motility (Svendsen, 1972; Yajima, 1985; Squires *et al.*, 1992; Salvador *et al.*, 1993). Thus, diet and the microbial environment of the colon, which control the relative production of the different acids, could influence the potential of colonic contents to affect colonic motility.

Mechanisms of action: hypotheses

SCFA may affect the digestive motility in non-ruminants through at least three different mechanisms: (1) SCFA could elicit nervous reflexes by activating chemosensitive receptors connected with either vagal nerves or myenteric neurones; (2) regulatory peptides could be released by SCFA, and then mediate some of their motor effects; and (3) SCFA could act directly on the tone of the intestinal smooth muscle.

Many sensory chemoreceptors have been identified in the digestive tract of monogastrics (Mei, 1985). Some might respond to SCFA and elicit nervous impulses which would in turn affect motility, as has been shown in ruminants (Leek & Harding, 1975). The existence of such SCFA-sensitive receptors in the colon of non-ruminant mammals was suggested by Yajima (1985). Comparing the contractile effect of SCFA on everted and uneverted segments of rat colon *in vitro*, the author demonstrated that SCFA must be applied to the mucosa to stimulate motility. Moreover, scraping off the mucosa or applying a local anaesthetic to the epithelial surface inhibited the response evoked by SCFA. Therefore, it seems that a sensory mechanism for SCFA could exist in or just beneath the epithelium in the rat colon. Neither the structural properties of the SCFA capable of acting as stimuli, nor the functional characteristics of the receptor have been described. The receptors may be comparable to those involved in the SCFA-induced secretory response in the rat colonic mucosa (see Chapter 13). The receptors would be activated specifically by 3–6-carbon molecules with a single carboxyl group (Yajima, 1989), which could explain the ineffectiveness of acetic acid, a 2-carbon molecule, in altering colonic contractile activity (Yajima, 1985; Squires *et al*., 1992). Nevertheless, the receptors must be different from those in the ileum, since acetic acid is the most potent acid in the ileum.

Most of the sensory chemoreceptors of the intestine, especially the acid- and alkali-receptors, are associated with vagal afferent fibres (Mei, 1985). Sakata & Engelhardt (1983) reported that a bilateral surgical vagotomy at the fundic level or a chemical sympathectomy with guanethidine abolished the colonic epithelial proliferation induced by SCFA, which indicated the possible involvement of the extrinsic nervous system. However, there is currently no experimental evidence that demonstrates the involvement of the vagus in the motor effects of SCFA in non-ruminants.

On the other hand, SCFA can influence ileal and colonic motility by local reflexes that do not require systemic control. Infusion of SCFA into an isolated ileal Thiry–Vella loop did not cause any change in motility and transit time of the intact ileum in the rat (Richardson *et al*., 1991). Moreover, general anaesthesia did not abolish the contractile effect of SCFA in the dog ileum, whereas local anaesthesia completely blocked the ileal response (Kamath & Phillips, 1988).

The neural circuits involved in the motor response of the digestive tract to SCFA were further studied pharmacologically. In the ileum, neither adrenergic nor cholinergic blockade reduced the stimulatory effect of SCFA (Kamath & Phillips, 1988). The ileal response also remained after pretreatment of dogs with blockers for serotonin receptors. In contrast to the ileal response, the colonic effect of SCFA may be mediated through a cholinergic nervous pathway. Indeed, tetrodotoxin and atropine inhibited the SCFA-induced contraction in the rat colon *in vitro*, whereas eserine enhanced it. However, hexamethonium did not block the colonic response to SCFA (Yajima, 1985). That may indicate that SCFA would act on the colonic motility through release of acetylcholine by stimulating cholinergic nerves. However, the lack of influence of hexamethonium suggests that a non-cholinergic ganglionic transmission might also be involved.

SCFA may also stimulate secretion of gastrointestinal regulatory peptides, which modulate motility. Particularly, SCFA increase the release of peptide YY (PYY) from the isolated perfused rabbit colon (Longo *et al.*, 1991). As PYY plays an important paracrine role in the regulation of gastrointestinal motility (Sheikh, 1991), it may be involved in the motor action of SCFA. The circulating level of PYY was unchanged when a bolus of SCFA was injected into the human ileum. Likewise, the systemic concentration of other intestinal peptides, such as substance P, vasoactive intestinal polypeptide, neurotensin, or glucagon, did not fluctuate during the ileal contractile activity induced by SCFA (Kamath *et al.*, 1988). However, measurements of peptides in the peripheral circulation are probably not sensitive enough to evaluate the peptidergic control mechanisms within the intestinal wall.

Surprisingly, only one work so far has investigated the effect of SCFA on contractility of the gastrointestinal smooth-muscle cell. When applied on strips of longitudinal smooth muscle isolated from the rat distal colon, 1 mM propionate had no contractile effect (Yajima, 1985). On the other hand, acetic, propionic and butyric acids, alone and in combination, caused a concentration-dependent (range 0.1–30 mM) relaxation of the smooth-muscle cells of human colonic resistance arteries (Mortensen *et al.*, 1990). Therefore, SCFA could act directly on smooth-muscle cells, but the effects would depend on the type of cell.

Physiological implications of the motor effects of SCFA in the gastrointestinal tract

Abolition of reticuloruminal motility could be a protective mechanism, as the concentrations of SCFA and lactic acid increase. The inhibition of ruminal contractions should lead to less mixing of the contents, and could thereby reduce the fermentation rate. Moreover, the absorption of lactic acid would be impaired by the stasis of the rumen. These two phenomena should prevent metabolic acidosis. However, if this feeble self-curing mechanism is insufficient, the ruminal acidity will continue to increase and will be fatal or at least give rise to complications such as metabolic acidosis, ketosis and the loss of integrity of the ruminal lining.

Stimulation of the contractile activity of the ileum and acceleration of the ileal emptying elicited by SCFA may represent protective mechanisms against colo-ileal reflux. SCFA, which are the major anions of the colonic contents, may function in the ileum in a way analogous to that of hydrochloric acid in the oesophagus. They may be chemical signals of reflux and, by stimulating ileal chemoreceptors, induce peristaltic contractions that correct or limit the extent of reflux.

The ileal SCFA may also contribute to the 'ileal brake', which is the decrease of gastric emptying induced by infusion of nutrients into the ileum (Welch, Cunningham & Read, 1988). This physiological phenomenon may be important in the normal control of nutrient absorption. When starch escapes digestion and reaches the ileum, gastric emptying is slowed, while the small-intestinal transit time is decreased (Layer, Zinsmeister & Dimagno, 1986; Kim *et al.*, 1990). It has been suggested that these effects are caused by metabolites such as SCFA, rather than by starch itself (Jain *et al.*, 1989). Ileal SCFA decrease the orocaecal transit time in the rat (Richardson *et al.*, 1991). However, their effects on gastric emptying are currently unknown.

The motor response of the colon to SCFA is still unclear, and caution is necessary in speculation on its physiological importance. At high concentration, SCFA could inhibit the colonic propagated propulsive contractions. This should result in a reduction of the mixing and propulsive movements of the colon, and may also affect the tone of the colonic wall and allow the proximal colon to accommodate larger volumes (Kamath *et al.*, 1990).

As already proposed for the ruminal effects of SCFA, the inhibition of colonic motility might be a mechanism by which the fermentation rate and the absorption of SCFA could be controlled. In normal conditions, these effects would be only slight, but they may increase with abnormal SCFA concentrations and pH in the colon, such as occurs in ulcerative colitis (Holtug, Rasmussen & Mortensen, 1988), or irritable bowel syndrome in the human (Mortensen *et al.*, 1987). SCFA may also be involved in the action of some dietary fibres that can decrease the gastrointestinal transit time in the human, although they are almost totally degraded in the colon (Cherbut *et al.*, 1991*b*).

Conclusion

SCFA, produced in the lumen of the digestive tract, modulate gastrointestinal motility both in ruminant and non-ruminant mammals. Thus, they may be considered as luminal chemical stimuli which contribute to the regulation of digestive motility. In ruminants, acid-sensitive receptors located in the epithelium of the reticulorumen mediate the action of SCFA, but their existence has only been suggested in the ileal and colonic wall of non-ruminants. The physiological, clinical and nutritional significance of the SCFA motor effects are not completely understood and deserve to be further studied. In ruminants, the inhibition of reticuloruminal motility, which occurs when SCFA are highly concentrated, might be regarded as a self-control mechanism, as the stasis leads to some reduction in fermentation rate. In the ileum of non-ruminants, SCFA might be chemical signals of a colo-ileal reflux and, by eliciting contractile activity, they might limit the extent of the reflux. Because they either stimulate or inhibit colonic contractions, SCFA might be involved in several phenomena in the colon. They might regulate the overall transit through the large intestine. They might control colonic absorption. Eventually, they might represent a self-regulating mechanism for fermentation.

References

Ash, R. W. (1959). Inhibition and excitation of reticulo-rumen contractions following the introduction of acids into the rumen and abomasum. *Journal of Physiology*, **147**, 58–73.

Bernier, J. J., Adrian, K. & Vidon, N. (1988). *Les aliments dans le tube digestif.* Paris: Doin Editeurs.

Bruce, L. A. & Huber, T. L. (1973). Inhibitory effect of acid in the intestine on rumen motility in sheep. *Journal of Animal Science*, **37**, 164–8.

Bueno, L., Goodall, E. D., Kay, R. N. & Ruckebusch, Y. (1972). On the function of the sheep's omasum. *Journal of Physiology*, **227**, 14P–15P.

Candau, M. & Vigroux, P. (1974). Sur la mécanisme de phyfermontilie caecale liée au repas chez le cheval. *Comptes Rendus de la Société de Biologie*, **168**, 893–7.

Cherbut, C., Ferré, J. P., Corpet, D. E., Ruckebusch, Y. & Delort-Laval, J. (1991*a*). Alterations of intestinal microflora by antibiotics. Effects on fecal excretion, transit time, and colonic motility in rats. *Digestive Diseases and Sciences*, **36**, 1729–34.

Cherbut, C., Salvador, V., Barry, J. L., Doulay, F. & Delort-Laval, J. (1991*b*). Dietary fibre effects on intestinal transit in man: involvement of their physicochemical and fermentative properties. *Food Hydrocolloids*, **5**, 15–22.

Christensen, J. (1989). Colonic motility. In *Handbook of Physiology*, section 6, The gastrointesinal tract, vol. 1, part 2, ed. S. G. Schultz, J. D. Wood & B. B. Rauner, pp. 939–73. Bethesda, MD: American Physiological Society.

Crichlow, E. C. (1988). Ruminal lactic acidosis: forestomach epithelial receptor activation by undissociated volatile fatty acids and rumen fluids collected during loss of reticuloruminal motility. *Research in Veterinary Science*, **45**, 364–8.

Crichlow, E. C. & Chaplin, R. K. (1984). Forestomach epithelial receptor activation by grain overload rumen fluids. *Canadian Journal of Animal Science*, **64**, 5–7.

Crichlow, E. C. & Chaplin, R. K. (1985). Ruminal lactic acidosis: relationship of forestomach motility to nondissociated volatile fatty acid levels. *American Journal of Veterinary Research*, **46**, 1908–11.

Crichlow, E. C. & Leek, B. F. (1981). The importance of pH in relation to the acid-excitation of epithelial receptors in the reticulo-rumen of sheep. *Journal of Physiology*, **310**, 60P–61P.

Crichlow, E. C. & Leek, B. F. (1986). Forestomach epithelial receptor activation by rumen fluids from sheep given intraruminal infusions of volatile fatty acids. *American Journal of Veterinary Research*, **47**, 1015–8.

Cummings, J. H. (1981). Short chain fatty acids in the human colon. *Gut*, **22**, 763–79.

Dirksen, G. (1970). Acidosis. In *Physiology of Digestion and Metabolism in the Ruminant*, ed. A. T. Phillipson, pp. 613–29. Newcastle upon Tyne: Oriel Press.

Fich, A., Phillips, S. F., Hakim, N. S., Brown, M. L. & Zinsmeister, A. R. (1989). Stimulation of ileal emptying by short-chain fatty acids. *Digestive Diseases and Sciences*, **34**, 1516–20.

Florent, C., Flourié, B., Leblond, A., Rautureau, M., Bernier, J. J. & Rambaud, J. C. (1985). Influence of chronic lactulose ingestion on the colonic metabolism of lactulose in man (an *in vivo* study). *Journal of Clinical Investigation*, **75**, 608–13.

Flourié, B., Phillips, S., Richter, H. & Azpiroz, F. (1989). Cyclic motility in canine colon: responses to feeding and perfusion. *Digestive Diseases and Sciences*, **34**, 1185–92.

Gregory, P. C. (1984). Control of intrinsic reticulo-ruminal motility in the vagotomized sheep. *Journal of Physiology*, **346**, 379–93.

Gregory, P. C. (1987). Inhibition of reticulo-ruminal motility by volatile fatty acids and lactic acid in sheep. *Journal of Physiology*, **382**, 355–71.

Gregory, P. C. & Miller, S. J. (1989). Influence of duodenal digesta composition on abomasal outflow, motility and small intestinal transit time in sheep. *Journal of Physiology*, **413**, 415–31.

Harding, R. & Leek, B. F. (1972*a*). Rapidly adapting mechanoreceptors in the reticulo-rumen which also respond to chemicals. *Journal of Physiology*, **223**, 32P–33P.

Harding, R. & Leek, B. F. (1972*b*). Gastro-duodenal receptor responses to chemical and mechanical stimuli, investigated by a 'single fibre' technique. *Journal of Physiology*, **222**, 139P–140P.

Holtug, K., Rasmussen, H. S. & Mortensen, P. B. (1988). Short chain fatty acids in inflammatory bowel disease. The effect of bacterial fermentation of blood. *Scandinavian Journal of Clinical and Laboratory Investigation*, **48**, 667–71.

Hoverstad, T., Bjorneklett, A., Fausa, O. & Midtvedt, T. (1985). Short-chain fatty acids in the small bowel bacterial overgrowth syndrome. *Scandinavian Journal of Gastroenterology*, **20**, 492–9.

Huber, T. L. (1976). Physiological effect of acidosis in feedlot cattle. *Journal of Animal Science*, **45**, 902–9.

Hunt, J. N. & Knox, M. T. (1969). The slowing of gastric emptying by nine acids. *Journal of Physiology*, **201**, 161–79.

Jain, N. K., Boivin, M., Zinsmeister, A. R., Brown, M. L. & Malagelada, J. R. (1989). Effect of ileal perfusion of carbohydrates and amylase inhibitor on gastrointestinal hormones and emptying. *Gastroenterology*, **88**, 1005–11.

Kamath, P. S., Hoepfner, M. T. & Phillips, S. F. (1987). Short-chain fatty acids stimulate motility of the canine ileum. *American Journal of Physiology*, **253**, G427–G433.

Kamath, P. S. & Phillips, S. F. (1988). Initiation of motility in canine ileum by short chain fatty acids and inhibition by pharmacological agents. *Gut*, **29**, 941–8.

Kamath, P. S., Phillips, S. F., O'Connor, M. K., Brown, M. L. & Zinsmeister, A. R. (1990). Colonic capacitance and transit in man: modulation by luminal contents and drugs. *Gut*, **31**, 443–9.

Kamath, P. S., Phillips, S. F. & Zinsmeister, A. R. (1988). Short-chain fatty acids stimulate ileal motility in humans. *Gastroenterology*, **95**, 1496–502.

Kim, B. H., Lin, H. C., Gu, Y. G., Doty, J. E. & Meyer, J. H. (1990). Gastric emptying of solid food is most potently inhibited by carbohydrate in the distal small intestine. *Gastroenterology*, **98**, A366.

Layer, P., Zinsmeister, A. R. & Dimagno, E. P. (1986). Effects of decreasing intraluminal amylase activity on starch digestion and postprandial gastrointestinal function in humans. *Gastroenterology*, **91**, 41–8.

Le Bars, H., Lebrument, J., Nitescu, R. & Simonnet, H. (1954). Recherches sur la motricité du rumen chez les petits ruminants. Actions de l'injection intraveineuse d'acides gras à courte chaîne. *Bulletin des Académies Vétérinaires Françaises*, **27**, 53–67.

Leek, B. F. (1983). Clinical diseases of the rumen: a physiologist's view. *Veterinary Record*, **113**, 10–14.

Leek, B. F. & Harding, R. H. (1975). Sensory nervous receptors in the ruminant stomach and the reflex control of reticulo-ruminal motility. In *Digestion and Metabolism in the Ruminant*, ed. I. W. McDonald & A. C. I. Warner, pp. 60–76. Armidale, Australia: University of New England Publishing Unit.

Leek, B. F., Ryan, J. P. & Upton, P. K. (1978). On the greater potency of butyric acid in inhibiting ruminant stomach (reticulo-ruminal) movements. *Journal of Physiology*, **284**, 158P–159P.

Longo, W. E., Ballantyne, G. H., Sacova, P. E., Adrian, T. E., Bilchik, A. J. & Modlin, I. M. (1991). Short-chain fatty acid release of peptide YY in the isolated perfused rabbit distal colon. *Scandinavian Journal of Gastroenterology*, **26**, 442–8.

Malagelada. J. R. & Azpiroz, F. (1989). Determinants of gastric emptying and transit time in the small intestine. In *Handbook of Physiology*, section 6, The Gastrointestinal Tract, vol. 1, part 2, ed. S. G. Schultz, J. D. Wood & B. B. Rauner, pp. 909–37. Bethesda, MD: American Physiological Society.

Masliah, C., Cherbut, C., Bruley des Varannes, S., Barry, J. L., Dubois, A. & Galmiche, J. P. (1992). Short-chain fatty acids do not alter jejunal motility in man, *Digestive Diseases and Sciences*, **37**, 193–7.

Mei, N. (1985). Intestinal chemosensitivity. *Physiological Reviews*, **65**, 211–37.

Mortensen, P. B., Andersen, J. R., Arffman, S. & Krag, E. (1987). Short-chain fatty acids and the irritable bowel syndrome: the effects of wheat bran. *Scandinavian Journal of Gastroenterology*, **22**, 185–92.

Mortensen, P. B., Heghnoj, J., Rannem, T., Rasmussen, H. S. & Holtug, K. (1989). Short-chain fatty acids in bowel contents after intestinal surgery. *Gastroenterology*, **97**, 1090–6.

Mortensen, F. V., Nielsen, H., Mulvany, M. J. & Hessov, I. (1990). Short chain fatty acids dilate isolated human colonic resistance arteries. *Gut*, **31**, 1391–4.

Mullen, P. A. (1976). Overfeeding in cattle: clinical, biochemical and therapeutic aspects. *The Veterinary Record*, **98**, 439–43.

Richardson, A., Delbridge, A. T., Brown, N. J., Rumsey, R. D. E. & Read, N. W. (1991). Short chain fatty acids in the terminal ileum accelerate stomach to caecum transit time in the rat. *Gut*, **32**, 266–9.

Sakata, T. & Engelhardt, W. v. (1983). Stimulatory effect of short-chain fatty acids on the epithelial cell proliferation in rat large intestine. *Comparative Biochemistry and Physiology*, **74A**, 459–62.

Salvador, V., Cherbut, C. & Delort-Laval, J. (1993). Role of short-chain fatty acids in digestive motor effects of dietary fibre. *Proceedings of the Nutrition Society*, **52**, 116A.

Sheikh, S. P. (1991). Neuropeptide Y and peptide YY: major modulators of gastrointestinal blood flow and function. *American Journal of Physiology*, **261**, G701–G715.

Smith, C. M., Krishnamurti, C. R. & Kitts, W. D. (1979). Effect of lactic acid administration on rumen myoelectrical activity and pressure changes in the sheep. *Canadian Journal of Animal Science*, **59**, 255–63.

Squires, P. E., Rumsey, R. D. E., Edwards, C. A. & Read, N. W. (1992). Effect of short-chain fatty acids on contractile activity and fluid flow in rat colon *in vitro*. *American Journal of Physiology*, **262**, G813–G817.

Svendsen, P. (1972). Inhibition of cecal motility in sheep by volatile fatty acids. *Nordisk Veterinaermedicin*, **24**, 393–6.

Svendsen, P. (1973). The effect of volatile fatty acids and lactic acid on rumen motility in sheep. *Nordisk Veterinaermedicin*, **25**, 226–31.

Upton, P., Ryan, J. P. & Leek, B. F. (1976). Acid as a sensory stimulus in the alimentary canal (sheep). *Irish Journal of Medical Science*, **145**, 307–8.

Welch, I., Cunningham, K. M. & Read, N. W. (1988). Effect of ileal perfusion of lipid on jejunal motor patterns after a nutrient and nonnutrient meal. *American Journal of Physiology*, **255**, G800–G806.

Yajima, T. (1984). Effect of sodium propionate on the contractile response of the rat ileum *in situ*. *Japanese Journal of Pharmacology*, **35**, 265–71.

Yajima, T. (1985). Contractile effect of short-chain fatty acids on the isolated colon of the rat. *Journal of Physiology*, **368**,, 667–78.

Yajima, T. (1989). Chemical specificity of short-chain fatty acid-induced electrogenic secretory response in the rat colonic mucosa. *Comparative Biochemistry and Physiology*, **93A**, 851–6.

Yokokura, T., Yajima, T. & Hashimoto, S. (1977). Effect of organic acid on gastrointestinal motility of rat *in vitro*. *Life Sciences*, **21**, 59–62.

13

Sensory mechanisms for short-chain fatty acids in the colon

T. YAJIMA

Introduction

Short-chain fatty acids (SCFA), in addition to their significance for energy metabolism (Bergman, 1990), are important as luminal chemical stimuli that can modify epithelial proliferation (see Chapter 19), intestinal blood flow (Bergman, 1990), motility (Cottrell & Gregory, 1991; Chapter 12) and secretion (Yajima & Sakata, 1987). The effects vary among SCFA, and are dose-dependent. Therefore, the sensory mechanisms of the gastrointestinal tract must be able to detect not only the presence of individual SCFA, but also their concentration.

Chemical sensory mechanisms in the gastrointestinal tract

Generally in sensation, stimuli are received at sensory receptors and information is then coded at the receptor and integrated into the nervous system. The chemical preabsorptive characteristics of nutrients are distinguished by sensory mechanisms in the gastrointestinal tract (Mei, 1985), which is richly innervated both by extrinsic (spinal, cranial, sympathetic and parasympathetic) and intrinsic (enteric) nerves (Costa, Furness & Llewellyn-Smith, 1987). After the coded information is integrated into the hierarchical structures of the nervous system in the gut wall, prevertebral ganglia and brain, responses are sent to the gastrointestinal tract.

In the integration of sensory information from the lumen of the gastrointestinal tract, the enteric nervous system (ENS) is more important than the central nervous system (Ewart, 1985). The ENS performs a highly sophisticated function, following the 'law of the intestine' (Bayliss & Starling, 1900), as an integrated system independent of the central nervous system (Wood, 1987; see Fig. 13.1). This might be deduced from the fact that the ENS in the gut wall has a similar number of neurones (10^8 in humans) to the spinal cord.

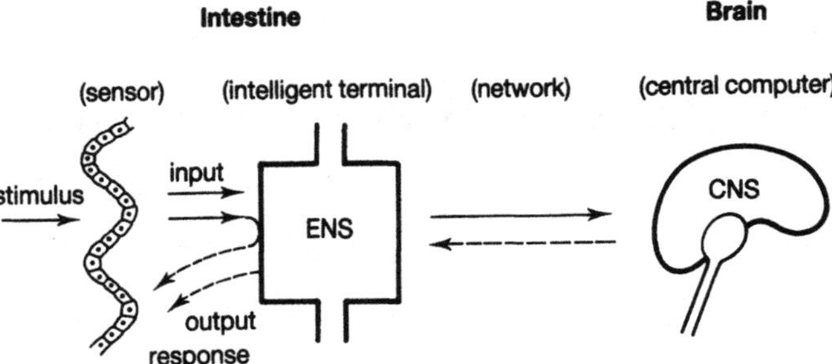

Fig. 13.1. The enteric nervous system (ENS) functions like an intelligent terminal in a computer-based system. This terminal computer integrates information from the lumen and outputs the response to the intestine. The central nerous system (CNS) also monitors the sensory information from the gut and commands the terminal computer to control the overall digestive state (Wood, 1987).

The ENS consists of three nerve plexuses, the myenteric, submucosal and mucosal plexuses (Furness & Costa, 1980). The myenteric (Auerbach's) plexus lies between the longitudinal and circular muscular layers and innervates these muscles, which have a major role in the control of motility. The submucosal (Meissner's) plexus supplies the major innervation of the mucosa and controls epithelial functions. Both plexuses have many ganglia, which are interconnected.

Effect of SCFA stimuli on gastrointestinal function

The effects of SCFA stimuli on gut motility have been extensively investigated in various animal species (see Chapter 12). However, the sensory mechanisms for luminal stimuli that cause intestinal secretion are little known. With the use of an isolated mucosal–submucosal preparation containing the submucosal nerve from the rat distal colon, it was shown that luminal SCFA stimulate Cl^- secretion via an enteric nervous reflex (Yajima, 1988). Chloride secretion is easily monitored as a change in electrical flux (short-circuit current; I_{sc}) across the tissue mounted in an Ussing chamber. In this way the colonic sensory mechanisms for SCFA may be studied *in vitro* by using the I_{sc} response as the measure.

Propionate-induced secretion of Cl^- in the colon

A transient increase in the transmural potential difference appears within a few seconds of the addition of propionate to the luminal side of the colonic

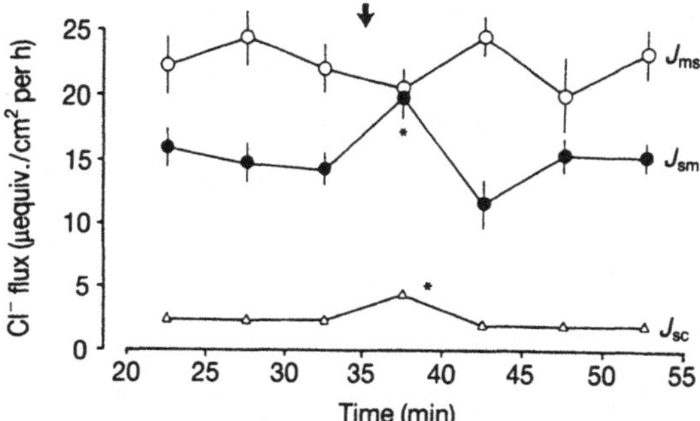

Fig. 13.2. The propionate-induced chloride (Cl^-) secretion in the rat distal colon resulted from an increase in unidirectional serosal-to-mucosal Cl^- movement (J_{sm}). The increase in short-circuit current (I_{sc}) shown in integrated I_{sc} (J_{sc}) was mainly due to Cl^-. Propionate (0.5 mM) was added to the mucosal side at the time indicated by the arrow.

mucosa of the rat distal colon *in vitro* (Yajima, 1988; Hubel & Russ, 1993). The increase in potential difference (mucosal-side negative) is primarily due to an increase in I_{sc}, which depends on chloride secretion, together with an increase in conductance (Fig. 13.2).

The I_{sc} response to propionate in the rat distal colon is dose-dependent, with a median effective dose of approximately 0.07 mM. The response reaches a maximum level at 0.2–0.5 mM. Such high sensitivity as well as the transient nature of the response to propionate is different from other luminal stimuli, such as dehydroxycholate (4–8 mM) and ricinoleate (6 mM), which also cause fluid secretion (Karlstrom *et al.*, 1986).

Comparison of the effects of different SCFA

Three other SCFA, *n*-butyrate, *n*-valerate and *n*-caproate, have the ability to increase both potential difference and I_{sc} in the rat distal colon (Yajima, 1988). The plots of response against a semi-logarithmic concentration of SCFA are sigmoid (Fig. 13.3), as are many other sensory input–output relationships (Beidler, 1971). Propionate is the most potent amongst these acids. Acetate and heptanoate have no effect up to 1 mM (Yajima, 1988, 1989).

Comparison of the effects of SCFA in different colonic regions

All rat colonic segments respond to propionate, *n*-butyrate, *n*-valerate and *n*-caproate by producing an increase in potential difference. The response to

Table 13.1. *Effect of neuroblocking agents on the intestinal secretory response to various luminal chemical stimuli. Drugs were added to the blood side before luminal addition of stimuli*

	Tetrodotoxin	Lidocaine	Hexamethonium	Atropine	Reference
Cholera toxin	+	+	+	–	Cassuto *et al.* (1983)
Na-dehydroxycholate (4 or 8 mM)	+	+	+	–	Karlstrom *et al.* (1986)
Na-ricinoleate (6 mM)	NT	+	+	–	Karlstrom *et al.* (1986)
Na-propionate (0.5 mM)	+	+	+	+	Yajima (1988); Hubel & Russ (1993)

+, Significant inhibition of secretory response; –, no effect on secretory response; NT, not tested.

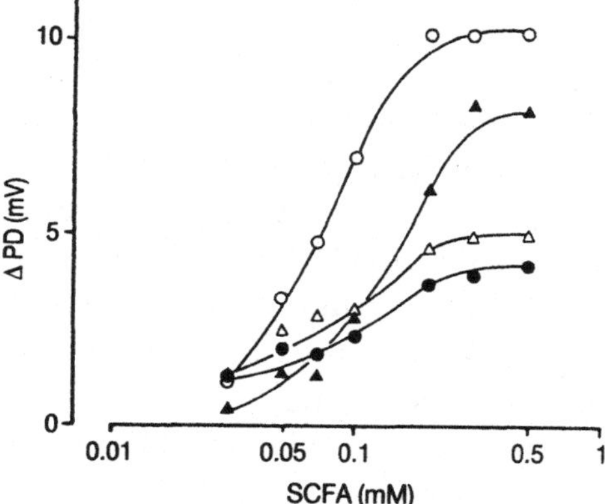

Fig. 13.3. The sigmoidal nature of the dose–response curve of change in potential difference (PD) evoked by short-chain fatty acids (SCFA) in the rat distal colon. Open circles, propionate; filled circles, butyrate; open triangles, valerate; filled triangles, caproate.

propionate is in the order proximal < middle < distal colon. Propionate also increases potential difference and I_{sc} in the distal colon of the guinea-pig (T. Yajima, unpublished data). Unlike the situation in the colon, luminal acetate as well as propionate and *n*-butyrate increase the potential difference in the rat small intestine *in vitro* (Wall *et al.*, 1976).

Secretory response mediated by an enteric nervous reflex

The enteric nerves regulate intestinal ion transport with the submucosal plexus having the most important role across the small and large intestinal mucosa (Cooke, 1987). Neuroblockers such as tetrodotoxin (TTX), hexamethonium and somatostatin diminish the propionate-induced I_{sc} increase (Yajima, 1988). Therefore, the secretory response is evidently not due to a direct action of SCFA on the electrogenic ion pump in the apical membrane of epithelial cells (Wall *et al.*, 1976), but is mediated by a neural reflex (see Table 13.1). The reflex centre may be located in the submucosal ganglia, since the tissue used in these studies contained the submucosal but not the myenteric nerve plexus.

The inhibitory action of hexamethonium, a blocker of cholinergic ganglionic transmission, on the secretory response to SCFA indicates the involvement of a cholinergic synapse in this neural reflex chain (Yajima, 1988). This participation of the cholinergic ganglionic transmission in chemoreflexes also occurs in the intestinal secretory response to cholera and *Escherichia coli* toxins, sodium dehydroxycholate and sodium ricinoleate (Table 13.1).

The reflex pathway of luminal SCFA action has been investigated pharmacologically. The failure of inhibition by 5-hydroxytryptamine (5-HT) receptor antagonists (xylamidine and metoclopramide) suggests that the response to luminal propionate is not mediated by the 5-HT_2 or 5-HT_3 receptor. The receptors for calcitonin-gene-related peptide, histamine, neuromedin U and substance-P also may not mediate the response, since the effects of propionate are not inhibited after the tissue has been desensitized to these neurotransmitters (Hubel & Russ, 1993; T. Yajima, unpublished data). Inhibition by the cyclooxygenase inhibitor, piroxicam or indomethacin, suggests that the production of prostaglandins might be involved in the reflex pathway (Hubel & Russ, 1993; T. Yajima, unpublished data). The final motor neurone in the secretory response to SCFA is cholinergic, since the TTX-sensitive response is abolished by the cholinergic muscarinic receptor antagonist, atropine (Yajima, 1988). The cholinergic nerve endings' response to luminal propionate is insensitive to conotoxin but sensitive to lidocaine (Hubel & Russ, 1993). This atropine-sensitive nature of the SCFA chemoreflex is different from atropine-insensitive sectory reflexes induced by other chemical stimuli (see Table 13.1). Non-cholinergic secretory transmitters, such as vasoactive intestinal polypeptide and substance P, might be involved in the secretory responses to cholera toxin and bile acids (Lundgren, 1988). It is still unclear why such a difference exists among stimuli in the final motor neurones.

Adaptation of SCFA-induced secretory response

Adaptation in a sensory response is characterized by a decline in response over a period when sustained stimulation is applied to a sensory receptor (Guyton, 1981). The secretory response to SCFA rapidly adapts to cumulative stimulation (see Fig. 13.4(*a*)). However, the initial response is reproduced when the tissue is washed with fresh buffer solution without stimulant between stimulations. This means that the adaptation is reversible. On the other hand, serosal application of acid has no effect on potential difference or adaptation. The adaptation occurs not only with the same acid, but also with different acids (Fig. 13.4(*b*)). Once the adaptation has been induced by butyrate or valerate, an additional application of propionate no longer produces a response. This type of adaptation is called cross-adaptation, in contrast to the former, which is known as self-adaptation.

The smaller potential-difference response of the proximal colon to SCFA (see Fig. 13.4) may be explained through continuous exposure of the luminal

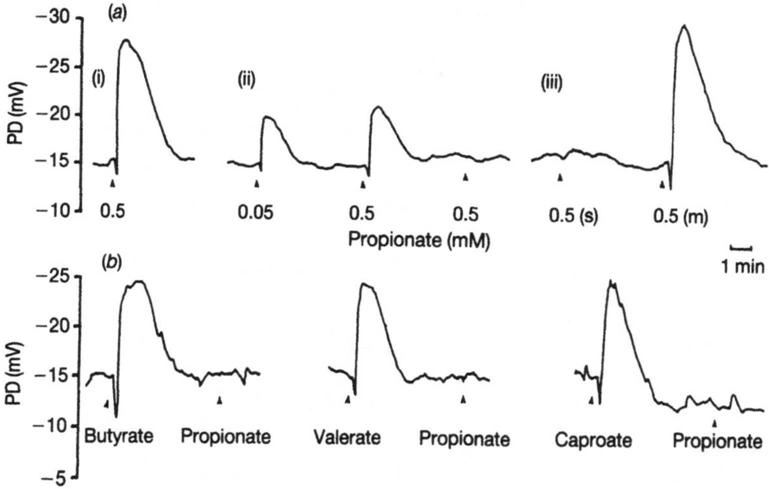

Fig. 13.4. Adaptation of potential difference (PD) change induced by short-chain fatty acids in the rat distal colon. (*a*) Self-adaptation induced by propionate: (i) control; (ii) effect of cumulative additions to the mucosal side; (iii) effect of initial addition to the serosal side (s). (*b*) Cross-adaptation: each acid was added to the mucosal side.

surface of the proximal colon to higher concentrations of SCFA than that of the distal colon (Yajima & Sakata, 1992). This view is supported by the observation that the proximal colon of germ-free rats shows a higher potential-difference response than that of a conventional rat (Yajima, 1988).

Self- and cross-adaptations are seen not only in the chemosensations of olfaction and taste (McBurney, 1987), but also in those of the gastrointestinal tract (Mei, 1985). Adaptation is considered to occur at the level of the receptor molecule in most sensory systems (Guyton, 1981). In olfactory and gustatory sensations, however, adaptations occur mostly at the level of the central nervous system. For gut chemosensitivity the mechanism of adaptation remains to be clarified.

Structural requirement for the stimulation of the secretory response

It is possible to make some suggestions about the nature of the chemoreceptor in the gastrointestinal tract, based on the chemical nature of stimulative substances and cross-adaptation. This allows us to speculate about the nature of the receptor molecule, even though it is at present unknown. For example, an intestinal amino acid receptor may be specified by its chemical structure–activity relationship; the receptor can distinguish not only ten kinds of

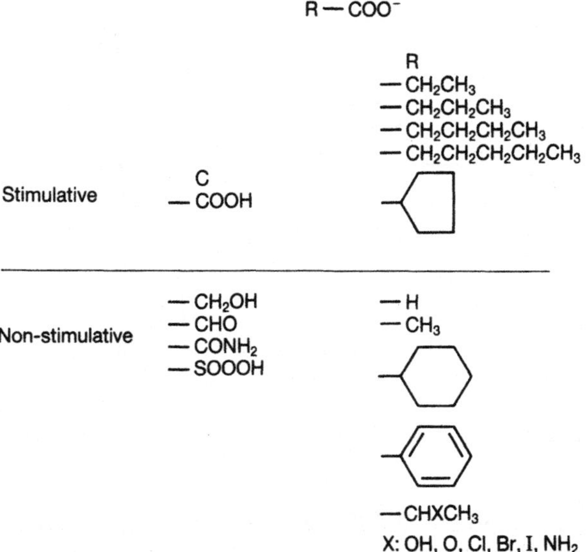

Fig. 13.5. Structural requirement for the stimulation of the secretory response in the rat distal colon.

stimulative amino acid but also L- and D-isomers of leucine (Jeanningros, 1982).

The structural requirements of the SCFA receptor of the rat colon have been specified for its stimulation of a secretory reponse by using 43 analogues of SCFA (Yajima, 1989). A definite number, three to six, of carbon atoms in SCFA is required for stimulating a secretory response, measured as a change in potential difference across the distal colon. The form of the chain can be either straight, branched or cyclic (see Fig. 13.5). These compounds generate cross-adaptation with propionate. A single carboxyl group is an essential prerequisite, since its replacement with an aldehyde, alcohol, amino or sulphonate group or addition of further carboxyl group(s) (di- or tricarboxylic acid) abolishes activity. The requirement for a single carboxyl group resembles that of the Na^+-dependent acid transport system of the renal brush border (Nord *et al.*, 1983) and acid-induced amylase release from pancreatic segments of ruminants (Katoh & Yajima, 1989). The preference for a 3–6 carbon chain is also found in the binding site of the renal monocarboxylate carrier, but not in pancreatic amylase release.

A hydrocarbon tail, especially a methylene group (—CH_2—), is necessary to stimulate a secretory response in the distal colon, since the compounds in which the methylene group has been substituted with a ketone, hydroxy or amino group lose their stimulative activity. The loss of stimulatory activity by introducing an unsaturated carbon into propionate or butyrate further supports the necessity for the methylene group in the hydrocarbon tail. These findings suggest that a more hydrophilic carbon tail impedes its affinity for the receptor molecule. Essentially similar characteristics of the SCFA receptor are found in the renal monocarboxylate transport system (Nord *et al.*, 1983) and in pancreatic amylase release (Katoh & Yajima, 1989). A more hydrophobic tail than the hydrocarbon tail may not be necessary for the receptor mechanism of SCFA and the secretory response, since halogenated monocarboxylic acids, which are more hydrophobic in nature than the parent compounds, lose their stimulatory activity. This differs from that of the renal transport system (Nord *et al.*, 1983) and pancreatic amylase release (Katoh & Yajima, 1989).

3-Chloropropionate and crotonate do not stimulate a secretory response, but are able to cross-inhibit the effect of propionate, suggesting that they have an affinity with the receptor. If such compounds and propionate are applied simultaneously to the luminal side of the rat colonic mucosa, then they will compete for the same binding site on the receptor. The concentration–response curve for propionate shifts to the right, in parallel, when 3-chloropropionate or crotonate is simultaneously added, thereby showing typical competitive inhibition (see Fig. 13.6). The competitive inhibition of propionate by these acids strongly supports the presence of an SCFA-specific receptor.

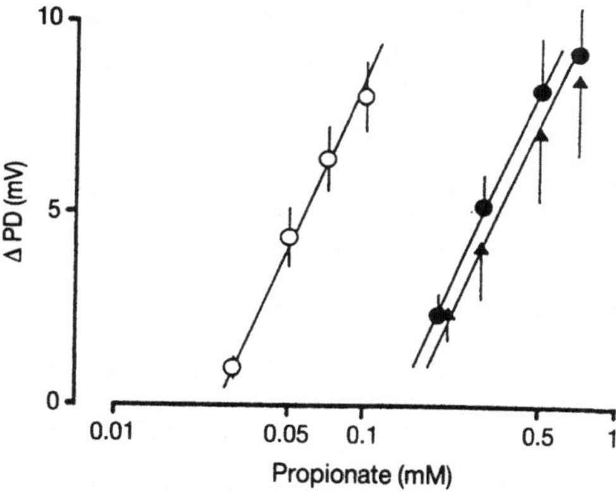

Fig. 13.6. Competitive inhibition by propionate analogue, 3-chloropropionate (filled circles), and butyrate analogue, crotonate (filled triangles), of the potential difference (PD) response to propionate in the rat distal colon. After measurement of the control response to propionate (open circles), 3-chloropropionate (0.05 mM) or crotonate (0.2 mM) and the appropriate concentration of propionate were simultaneously added to the mucosal side.

Characterization of the SCFA receptor

Specialized nerve endings and the taste-bud cell function as sensory receptors in olfactory and gustatory sensations (DeSimone *et al.*, 1984). The intestinal sensory chemoreceptors, including the SCFA receptor, have been identified functionally but not yet structurally. However, we can characterize, to a certain extent, the structure and localization of receptors in the gut wall from sensitivity to anaesthetics and the latent time of the response.

With single-fibre recording of vagal afferent neural activity, Leek and Harding (1975) measured the latent period of the response (12–50 s) and, using published diffusion coefficients for SCFA, they estimated the location of the receptor at about 150 μm from the epithelial surface of the sheep rumen. The colonic contractile and secretory responses have a shorter latency period (<10 s), suggesting that the receptor for SCFA may exist somewhere in or just below the epithelium of the rat colon (Yajima, 1985, 1988).

The serosal application of SCFA has no direct excitatory action on the nerve (Yajima, 1985) or nerve fibre; instead, SCFA act as a local anaesthetic (Hiji *et al.*, 1987). Stimuli from luminal SCFA are likely to be received at the epithelial sensory receptor (Hubel, 1985), not directly at the sensory nerve ending of the secretory reflex or the cholinergic motor neurone. Two different experiments support such a view (see Table 13.2). A short (2-min) application of procaine to the luminal surface of the isolated rat distal colon inhibits the secretory response to propionate but not to electrical field stimulation, which causes chloride secretion by a direct stimulation of the enteric nerve (Yajima, 1988). Further, the mucosal injury induced by treatment with hyperosmolar sodium sulphate or *d*-xylose on the luminal surface for 30 min markedly

Table 13.2. *Effects of luminal anaesthetic and high osmolar load on short-circuit current (I_{sc}) response to propionate in the rat distal colon*

	Response (% I_{sc} of control)			
	Na-propionate	EFS	Aminophylline	Reference
Procaine (0.5 mM)	18[a]	90		Yajima (1988)
Na-sulphate (6.0 M)	10[a]		59[a]	Hubel & Russ (1993)
d-Xylose (4.5 M)	14[a]		92	Hubel & Russ (1993)

[a] Significantly different from control.
EFS, Electrical field stimulation.

inhibits the propionate-induced secretory response (Hubel & Russ, 1993). These data support the view that the reception of luminal SCFA stimuli probably occurs on the epithelial receptor cell but not on nerve dendrites or sensory nerves projecting from just under the epithelium.

A candidate for the receptor cell is the enteroendocrine cell which contains chemical transmitters (peptide and/or amine). The morphology of these cells, i.e. the presence of cytoplasmic projections into the lumen, strongly suggests paracrine and neuroendocrine functions (Fujita & Kobayashi, 1977), in which chemical transmitters are released by luminal stimuli and act on sensory and motor nerve receptors (Fujita *et al.*, 1980; Lundgren, 1988). The sensitivity of the SCFA-induced secretory responses, both to mucosal surface anaesthesia and to mucosal injury, also support the idea that enteroendocrine cells are responsible for the sensory mechanism of luminal SCFA stimulation.

Physiological significance of colonic SCFA sensation

The physiological significance of SCFA sensation in the hindgut remains as obscure as that of other intestinal chemosensations (Mei, 1985). We may speculate that diarrhoea due to fluid secretion stimulated by bacterial toxins or bile acids is primarily protective (Hubel, 1985). However, SCFA sensation may differ from these protective phenomena, since the transient and adaptive nature of the secretory responses to SCFA hardly cause diarrhoea. The secretory response evoked by SCFA may provide a lubricant to move faeces by co-ordinating with concomitant colonic contractions evoked by SCFA (Yajima, 1985).

Conclusion

The colonic SCFA receptor has chemical specificity. The receptor probably exists on an epithelial cell that is very likely enteroendocrine. The information coded at the receptor is transmitted to the enteric nervous system and reflexively causes chloride secretion. The co-ordination between secretory and motor responses evoked by luminal SCFA might integrate colonic function; however, the physiological significance of SCFA sensation remains to be clarified. Whether information about SCFA is transmitted to the brain has not been demonstrated.

References

Bayliss, W. M. & Starling, E. H. (1900). The movements and the innervation of the large intestine. *Journal of Physiology*, **26**, 107–18.

Beidler, L. M. (1971). Taste receptor stimulation with salts and acids. In *Handbook of Sensory Physiology IV, Chemical Senses 2. Taste*, ed. L. M. Beidler, pp. 200–20. Berlin: Springer-Verlag.

Bergman, E. N. (1990). Energy contribution of volatile fatty acids from the gastrointestinal tract in various species. *Physiological Reviews*, **70**, 567–90.

Cassuto, J., Siewert, A., Jodal, M. & Lundgren, O. (1983). The involvement of intramural nerves in cholera toxin induced intestinal secretion. *Acta Physiologica Scandinavica*, **117**, 195–202.

Cooke, H. J. (1987). Neural and humoral regulation of small intestinal electrolyte transport. In *Physiology of the Gastrointestinal Tract*, 2nd edn, ed. L. R. Johnson, pp. 1307–50. New York: Raven Press.

Costa, M., Furness, J. B. & Llewellyn-Smith, I. J. (1987). Histochemistry of the enteric nervous system. In *Physiology of the Gastrointestinal Tract*, 2nd edn, ed. L. R. Johnson, pp. 1–40. New York: Raven Press.

Cottrell, D. F. & Gregory, P. C. (1991). Regulation of gut motility by luminal stimuli in the ruminant. In *Physiological Aspects of Digestion and Metabolism in Ruminants*, ed. T. Tsuda, Y. Sasaki & R. Kawashima, pp. 3–59. San Diego: Academic Press.

DeSimone, J. A., Heck, G. L., Nierson, S. & DeSimone, S. K. (1984). The active ion transport properties of canine lingual epithelia *in vitro*. *Journal of General Physiology*, **83**, 633–56.

Ewart, W.-R. (1985). Sensation in the gastrointestinal tract. *Comparative Biochemistry and Physiology*, **82A**, 489–93.

Fujita, T. & Kobayashi, S. (1977). Structure and function of gut endocrine cell. *International Review of Cytology*, **6** (Suppl.), 187–233.

Fujita, T., Muraki, S., Sato, K., Noguchi, R. & Shimoji, K. (1980). Effect of atropine and tetrodotoxin upon pancreozymin release from canine duodenum in response to luminal stimuli. *Biomedical Research*, **1**, 59–65.

Furness, J. B. & Costa, M. (1980). Types of nerves in the enteric nervous system. *Neuroscience*, **5**, 1–20.

Guyton, A. C. (1981). *Textbook of Medical Physiology*. Philadelphia: W. B. Saunders.

Hiji, Y., Miyoshi, M., Ichikawa, O. Kasagi, T. & Imoto, T. (1987). Enhancement of local anaesthesia action by organic acid salts (I): possible change of excitability in nerve fibre membrane. *Archives internationales physiologie et de biochimie*, **95**, 113–20.

Hubel, K. A. (1985). Intestinal nerves and ion transport: stimuli, reflex, and responses. *American Journal of Physiology*, **248**, G261–G273.

Hubel, K. A. & Russ, L. (1993). Mechanisms of the secretory response to luminal propionate in rat descending colon *in vitro*. *Journal of the Autonomic Nervous System*, **43**, 219–30.

Jeanningros, R. (1982). Vagal unitary response to intestinal amino acid infusions in the anesthetized cat: a putative signal for protein induced satiety. *Physiological Behavior*, **28**, 9–21.

Karlstrom, L., Cassuto, J., Jodal, M. & Lundgren, O. (1986). Involvement of the enteric nervous system in the intestinal secretion induced by sodium deoxycholate and sodium ricinoleate. *Scandinavian Journal of Gastroenterology*, **21**, 331–40.

Katoh, K. & Yajima, T. (1989). Effects of butyric acid and analogues on amylase release from pancreatic segments of sheep and goats. *Pflügers Archiv*, **413**, 256–60.

Leek, B. F. & Harding, R. H. (1975). Sensory nervous receptors in the ruminant stomach and the reflex control of reticulo-ruminal motility. In *Digestion and Metabolism in the Ruminant*, ed. I. W. McDonald & A. C. I. Warner, pp. 60–76. Armidale: the University of New England Publishing Unit.

Lundgren, O. (1988). Nervous control of intestinal fluid transport: physiology and pathophysiology. *Comparative Biochemistry and Physiology*, **90A**, 603–9.

McBurney, D. H. (1987). Taste and olfaction: sensory discrimination. In *Handbook of Physiology, Section 1; Nervous System*, vol. III, part 2, *Sensory Process*, ed. I. Darian-Smith, pp. 1097–186. Washington, DC: American Physiological Society.

Mei, N. (1985). Intestinal chemosensitivity. *Physiological Reviews*, **65**, 211–37.

Nord, E. P., Wright, S. H., Kippen, I. & Wright, E. M. (1983). Specificity of the Na^+-dependent monocarboxylic acid transport pathway in rabbit renal border membrane. *Journal of Membrane Biology*, **72**, 213–21.

Wall, M. J., Declusin, R. J., Soergel, K. H. & Baker, R. D. (1976). The effect of short chain fatty acids on transmural potential across rat small intestine *in vivo*. *Biochemica et Biophysica Acta*, **433**, 654–61.

Wood, J. D. (1987). Physiology of the enteric nervous system. In *Physiology of the Gastrointestinal Tract*, 2nd edn. ed. L. R. Johnson, pp. 67–109. New York: Raven Press.

Yajima, T. (1985). Contractile effect of short-chain fatty acids on the isolated colon of the rat. *Journal of Physiology*, **368**, 667–78.

Yajima, T. (1988). Luminal propionate-induced secretory response in the rat distal colon *in vitro*. *Journal of Physiology*, **403**, 559–75.

Yajima, T. (1989). Chemical specificity of short-chain fatty acid-induced electrogenic secretory response in the rat colonic mucosa. *Comparative Biochemistry and Physiology*, **93A**, 851–6.

Yajima, T. & Sakata, T. (1987). Influence of short-chain fatty acids on the digestive organs. *Bifidobacteria Microflora*, **6**, 7–14.

Yajima, T. & Sakata, T. (1992). Core and periphery concentration of short-chain fatty acids in luminal contents of the rat colon. *Comparative Biochemistry and Physiology*, **103A**, 353–5.

14

Effects of short-chain fatty acids on exocrine and endocrine pancreatic secretion

K. KATOH

Introduction

Recently, short-chain fatty acids (SCFA) have received attention as one of the regulators that influence exocrine and endocrine pancreatic functions (Kato, Katoh & Barej, 1991; Katoh, 1991; Croom, Bull & Taylor, 1992; Harmon, 1992). According to these reviews, which mainly discuss the pancreatic functions of ruminants, SCFA apparently exert stimulatory effects on pancreata. Because ruminants possess a unique digestive system and utilize a large amount of SCFA as their main energy source, intensive studies have been performed and the physiological relevance of SCFA has been investigated in these species. However, as SCFA are a common product of fermentation in the gastrointestinal tract of not only foregut but also hindgut fermenters (see Chapter 5), they might be widely effective on pancreatic functions in a range of other animal species as well. Indeed, SCFA stimulate exocrine secretion in non-ruminant mammalian species such as guinea-pigs, voles and rats (see Kato *et al.*, 1991).

In addition, since a functional interaction between the exocrine and endocrine pancreas (the insulin–pancreatic acinar axis) has been postulated and is supported by morphological and biochemical evidence (Williams & Goldfine, 1985), it would be rational to elucidate the responsiveness of the two functionally different parts of the pancreas to stimulation with SCFA. However, as regards the endocrine pancreas, studies of the effects of SCFA and of species differences have been mostly restricted to insulin and glucagon secretion in ruminants (Horino *et al.*, 1968; Mineo *et al.*, 1986, 1990*a,b,c*; Mineo, 1992).

In this chapter, I give an overview of current knowledge of the action of SCFA on exocrine and endocrine pancreatic secretions, and mainly focus on (1) systemic actions of SCFA; (2) relationships between the chemical structure of SCFA and their effectiveness; and (3) cellular mechanisms of action of SCFA.

Stimulatory actions of SCFA

Exocrine pancreas

Although it is known that SCFA are stimulatory for both functions of the pancreas, we must examine the involvement of the nervous and humoral systems to understand the mechanisms of action of SCFA. In particular, the location of the sites of action of SCFA, i.e. whether SCFA exist in the lumen or in the bloodstream, is critical for the mechanisms of action of SCFA. Their effects at the luminal side are generally caused by excitation of the nervous system and gastrointestinal hormone secretion, whereas those at the apical (blood) side involve not only direct actions but sometimes also excitation of the autonomic nervous system.

In humans and dogs, fatty acids with carbon chain lengths of 8 to 10 potently stimulated exocrine secretion when injected into the duodenum (Meyer, 1981). In sheep, SCFA infusion into the rumen or into the duodenum also stimulated fluid and amylase secretion (Magee, 1961; Taylor, 1962). In some animal species, the responses to duodenal fatty acid infusion may be caused by gasrointestinal hormones, because fatty acids are potent releasers of secretin and cholecystokinin from gastrointestinal endocrine cells (Meyer, 1981). However, the involvement of these two gastrointestinal hormones remains uncertain in adult ruminants, since plasma concentrations of these hormones do not change after feeding (see Kato *et al.*, 1991).

Harada & Kato (1983) found that SCFA infused into the venous blood stimulated fluid and protein (digestive enzyme) secretion from the ovine pancreas, a finding that was also confirmed in isolated lobule preparations. Since these studies were carried out, stimulatory responses to SCFA have been reported in sheep, goats, cattle, deer, guinea-pigs, voles and rats, but not yet in rabbits, mice, hamsters, pigs, cats or chickens (see Kato *et al.*, 1991). The ability to respond to SCFA stimulation is thought to be congenital, because SCFA stimulation was able to increase amylase release from pancreatic segments isolated from the fetus of goats in late gestation (K. Katoh, unpublished data).

In anaesthetized guinea pigs, an intravenous bolus injection of butyrate at 1 mmol/kg body wt enhanced fluid and amylase secretion, which was not affected by prior injection of atropine (1.4 μmol/kg body wt) or hexamethonium (40 μmol/kg body wt) (Katoh & Tsuda, 1987). However, the enhanced amylase release induced by butyrate injection at the same dose into the caecum was abolished by prior intravenous injection of atropine or hexamethonium (K. Katoh, unpublished data). These findings imply that excitation of the autonomic nervous system is involved in the enhanced exocrine secretion induced by intraluminal SCFA administration, and that intravenously administered SCFA exert a direct action on the acinar cells.

Endocrine pancreas

Administration of a large amount of SCFA into the rumen or into the venous or portal vessel stimulates insulin and glucagon secretion in sheep, goats and cows (Harmon, 1992). The mechanism of action of intravenous SCFA may be complex. The insulin secretory response induced by intravenous butyrate infusion apparently involves excitation of the autonomic nervous system in sheep (Bloom & Edwards, 1985). However, SCFA also exert a direct action on the B cell, since they stimulate insulin secretion from *in vitro* preparations such as isolated ovine islets (Hertelendy, Machlin & Kipnis, 1969) and tissue fragments (Sasaki, Weekes & Bruce, 1977). Unfortunately, there is little information concerning the mechanism of SCFA-induced glucagon secretion or the effects of SCFA on other pancreatic hormone secretions.

Structural requirements for SCFA

Exocrine pancreas

Katoh & Yajima (1989) used butyrate and its derivatives in order to elucidate their secretory effectiveness in ovine and caprine pancreatic tissue segments, and concluded that the structural requirement for SCFA as an agonist is to possess a carboxyl (—COOH) group coupled with a hydrophobic group (an aliphatic hydrocarbon chain, or a benzene or cyclohexane ring). In particular, the introduction of a hydrophilic component into the hydrophobic group markedly reduced the effectiveness of butyrate. Interestingly, succinic and phthalic acids were weak stimulants, but reduced the effective dose (ED_{50}) of butyrate when they co-existed. It is likely that dicarboxylic acids would be a useful tool for kinetic analysis of biological activities induced by SCFA.

Our group (Ohbo *et al.*, 1989; Ohbo, 1990) compared the relationships between secretory efficacy and carbon chain length in sheep and rats. Amylase release was increased with increasing carbon chain lengths in both species. The maximum response was achieved when the agonist was octanoic acid ($C_{8:0}$) in sheep and hexadecanoic acid ($C_{16:0}$) in rats. In sheep, the maximum response was reduced in response to stimulation with fatty acids of carbon chain length greater than eight. These findings suggest that the pancreata of sheep and rats respond to fatty acids with a wide range of carbon chain lengths, and imply a difference in receptive mechanisms to fatty acids among animal species. The species difference might be partly explained by differences in fatty-acid utilization as a preferred energy source.

Endocrine pancreas

The ability of SCFA to increase insulin and glucagon secretion when injected into the venous blood of sheep depends to some extent on their carbon chain length (Mineo *et al.*, 1990*a*,*c*; Mineo, 1992). The carbon number for the maximal effectiveness of SCFA was 4–5 for insulin and glucagon secretion. Additionally, isobutyrate or isovalerate was more potent than the corresponding *n*-isomers for insulin secretion, whereas this was not the case for glucagon secretion (Mineo *et al.*, 1990*a*). These findings suggest that the receptive mechanisms for SCFA in the A cell are different from those in the B cell in sheep. Structural features of SCFA for stimulating insulin and glucagon secretion seem to be similar to those for exocrine secretion in sheep (H. Mineo, unpublished data). The co-existence of carboxyl and hydrophobic groups is also fundamental for pancreatic hormone secretions.

Cellular mechanisms

Exocrine secretion

We have suggested that Ca^{2+} would be an important cellular messenger, and proposed a stimulus–secretion coupling model that was based on electrophysiological evidence and the dependency of SCFA-induced responses on the presence of Ca^{2+} in the medium for amylase release by SCFA (Katoh & Tsuda, 1984; Kato *et al.*, 1991; Katoh, 1991). Recently we tried to measure the change in cytosolic Ca^{2+} concentration ($[Ca^{2+}]_i$) in response to SCFA by fluorimetry using Fura-2 (Sigma), and found that octanoic (caprylic) acid increased $[Ca^{2+}]_i$ in ovine pancreatic acinar cells (Fig. 14.1). Stimulation with octanoic acid, which slightly increased $[Ca^{2+}]_i$ even in Ca^{2+}-free medium, considerably and rapidly increased $[Ca^{2+}]_i$ immediately after the extracellular (medium) Ca^{2+} concentration was elevated to 2.5 mM. Although broadly similar results were reproduced in response to acetylcholine stimulation, the increase in $[Ca^{2+}]_i$ induced by SCFA stimulation was more sustainable than that induced by acetylcholine. That is, acetylcholine stimulation caused a transient and sharp rise followed by a lower sustained $[Ca^{2+}]_i$ level, whereas an initial rise as shown in the response to acetylcholine stimulation was lacking in the response to SCFA. In addition, we measured membrane currents in ovine and rat acinar cells using a whole-cell patch–

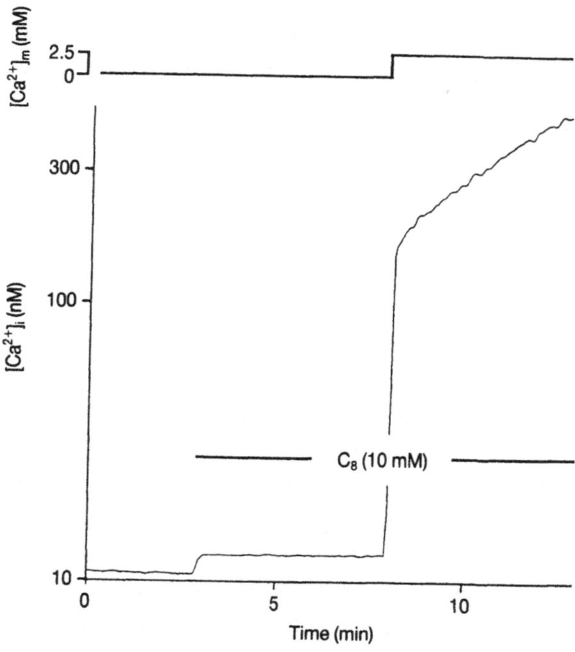

Fig. 14.1. Effects of stimulation with octanoate (C_8) and of an increase in medium $CaCl_2$ concentration on intracellular Ca^{2+} concentration ($[Ca^{2+}]_i$) of ovine pancreatic acinar cells. Cytosolic calcium concentration was measured by fluorimetry using Fura-2-loaded cells. At first the cells were incubated in a Ca-depleted medium and stimulated with octanoate (10 mM). During stimulation with octanoate, the calcium concentration in the medium was increased to 2.5 mM by addition of $CaCl_2$ solution into the cell suspension. An increase in $[Ca^{2+}]_i$ was detected on stimulation with octanoate at concentrations of more than 0.1 mM in a medium containing 2.5 mM $CaCl_2$ (not shown).

clamp configuration, and found that both SCFA and acetylcholine caused an increase in Ca^{2+}-dependent inward (Cl^-) currents (K. Katoh and M. Wakui, unpublished data). In this experiment, we tried to inject SCFA into the cytosol through a patch–clamp pipette, and found that SCFA were much less effective when applied internally than externally. These findings offer more confident support to the Ca^{2+} hypothesis for the cellular mediation of SCFA action, and imply that SCFA might be recognized on the outside of the cell membrane of pancreatic acinar cells.

To our knowledge, there is little information available concerning the existence of recognition sites for SCFA in the pancreas. Ohbo (1990), however, recently found that trypsin treatment of rat and hamster pancreatic acinar cells dramatically reduced amylase release by SCFA, while at the same time the treatment scarcely changed the responsiveness to acetylcholine. This finding implies the existence of SCFA recognition proteins which are easily inactivated by trypsin treatment.

Endocrine secretion

As mentioned above, the stimulatory effects of SCFA involve, in part, a direct action on the B cell. However, the details remain to be determined, since there are few reports available examining the cellular mechanisms.

A putative stimulus–secretion coupling model for insulin release based on findings mainly relating to the actions of long-chain fatty acids was discussed in a previous review (Katoh, 1991). The first and most important cellular step is ATP production, caused by fatty-acid oxidation as well as liberation of inositol 1,4,5-trisphosphate (IP_3) and diacylglycerol by phosphatidylinositol 4,5-bisphosphate breakdown. Adenosine triphosphate production is essential for ATP-dependent K^+ channel closure, which leads to depolarization of the cell membrane, successively activating voltage-dependent Ca^{2+}-channel opening (with an increase in Ca^{2+} influx). On the other hand, IP_3 is able to liberate Ca^{2+} from non-mitochondrial Ca^{2+} stores, such as the endoplasmic reticulum. These two cellular processes increase the cytosolic $[Ca^{2+}]_i$, which is essential for insulin release by exocytosis.

However, there is no information showing whether the action of SCFA is similar to that of the long-chain fatty acids, or why there are differences between the A cell and the B cell.

Clinical implications

Since the finding of SCFA action on islet hormone secretion in ruminants, a critical debate continued as to whether SCFA are effective at so-called 'physiological' concentrations (De Jong, 1982; and Chapter 17, this book). To elucidate SCFA actions on the secretory functions, it is necessary to simulate carefully the changes in SCFA concentrations in blood or in the gastrointestinal tract to match changes found after feeding. In this regard, a physiological role for acetate in blood would be possible in respect of exocrine pancreatic secretion in sheep. The maximal postprandial peripheral plasma concentrations of acetate, propionate and butyrate in concentrate (grain)-fed sheep have been reported to be more than 1, 0.2 and 0.03 mM, respectively, and 1 mM acetate did stimulate amylase release from ovine pancreatic tissue segments (Katoh & Tsuda, 1984).

Among the SCFA, propionate seems to be a promising candidate as one of the physiological mediators that increase insulin secretion in sheep, since plasma insulin concentrations are increased in parallel with an increasing molar ratio of propionate to acetate in the rumen that is commonly seen in concentrate-fed ruminants (Harmon, 1992). In addition, increasing levels of propionate infusion into the rumen caused a linear increase in the net insulin secretion into the portal vein (Gross *et al.*, 1990). However, the mechanism remains to be determined.

Acetate, a major SCFA and an important energy source for ruminants, showed a unique feature regarding islet hormone secretion when intravenously infused in sheep (Mineo *et al.*, 1986; Mineo, 1992) and rats (H. Mineo and T. Sakata, unpublished data). Acetate infusion at doses above 1 μmol/kg/min markedly enhanced the plasma insulin stimulation caused by glucose injection above the response to glucose injection alone (Mineo *et al.*, 1986). The acetate doses used in this study did not increase the plasma insulin concentration by themselves, although doses of more than 312 μmol/kg body wt increased the insulin concentration with no effect on glucagon in sheep (Mineo *et al.*, 1986, 1990*b*). The above synergism was also not seen in relation to glucagon secretion. Although it remains to be clarified whether the synergism for insulin secretion between SCFA and other nutrients (or metabolites) can be reproduced at the usual peripheral blood concentrations and in other animal species, the feature of acetate action mentioned above is interesting not only for endocrine but also for exocrine secretions. It will also be of interest to elucidate the recognition mechanisms of the cells, because such studies will enable us not only to clarify the biological role of SCFA but also to control SCFA action and utilization in some animal species in the future.

References

Bloom, S. R. & Edwards, A. V. (1985). Pancreatic neuroendocrine responses to butyrate in conscious sheep. *Journal of Physiology*, **364**, 281–8.

Croom, W. J., Bull, L. S. & Taylor, I. L. (1992). Regulation of pancreatic exocrine secretion in ruminants: a review. *Journal of Nutrition*, **122**, 191–202.

De Jong, A. (1982). Patterns of plasma concentrations of insulin and glucagon after intravascular and intraruminal administration of volatile fatty acids in the goat. *Journal of Endocrinology*, **92**, 357–70.

Gross, K. L., Harmon, D. L., Minton, J. E. & Avery, T. B. (1990). Effects of isoenergetic infusions of propionate and glucose on portal-drained visceral nutrient flux and concentrations of hormone in lambs maintained by total intragastric infusion. *Journal of Animal Science*, **68**, 2566–72.

Harada, E. & Kato, S. (1983). Effect of short-chain fatty acids on the secretory response of the ovine exocrine pancreas. *American Journal of Physiology*, **244**, G284–G290.

Harmon, D. L. (1992). Impact of nutrition on pancreatic exocrine and endocrine secretion in ruminants: a review. *Journal of Animal Science*, **70**, 1290–301.

Hertelendy, F., Machlin, L. & Kipnis, D. M. (1969). Further studies on the regulation of insulin and growth hormone secretion in the sheep. *Endocrinology*, **84**, 192–9.

Horino, M., Machlin, L. J., Hertelendy, F. & Kipnis, D. M. (1968). Effect of short-chain fatty acids on plasma insulin in ruminant and nonruminant species. *Journal of Endocrinology*, **83**, 118–28.

Kato, S., Katoh, K. & Barej, W. (1991). Regulation of exocrine pancreatic secretion in ruminants. In *Physiological Aspects of Digestion and Metabolism in Ruminants*, ed. T. Tsuda, Y. Sasaki & R. Kawashima, pp. 89–109. Orlando: Academic Press.

Katoh, K. (1991). The effect of short-chain fatty acids on the pancreas. In *Short-chain Fatty Acids: Metabolism and Clinical Importance* (Report of the Tenth Ross Conference on Medical Research), ed. E. Silverman, pp. 74–7. Columbus: Ross Laboratories.

Katoh, K. & Tsuda, T. (1984). Effects of acetylcholine and short-chain fatty acids on acinar cells of the exocrine pancreas in sheep. *Journal of Physiology*, **356**, 479–89.

Katoh, K. & Tsuda, T. (1987). Effects of intravenous injection of butyrate on the exocrine pancreatic secretion in guinea pigs. *Comparative Biochemistry and Physiology*, **87A**, 469–72.

Katoh, K. & Yajima, T. (1989). Effects of butyric acid and analogues on amylase release from pancreatic segments of sheep and goats. *Pflügers Archiv*, **413**, 256–60.

Magee, D. F. (1961). An investigation into the external secretion of the pancreas in sheep. *Journal of Physiology*, **158**, 132–43.

Meyer, J. H. (1981). Control of exocrine secretion. In *Physiology of Gastrointestinal Tract*, vol. 2, ed. L. R. Johnson, pp. 821–9. New York: Raven Press.

Mineo, H. (1992). Dynamic analysis of the secretion of insulin and glucagon in sheep. PhD dissertation, Tohoku University, Sendai.

Mineo, H., Kanai, M., Kato, S. & Ushijima, J. (1990*a*). Effects of intravenous injection of butyrate, valerate and their isomers on endocrine pancreatic responses in conscious sheep. *Comparative Biochemistry and Physiology*, **95A**, 411–16.

Mineo, H., Kitade, A., Kawakami, S., Kato, S. & Ushijima, J. (1990*b*). Effect of intravenous injection of acetate on the pancreas of sheep. *Research in Veterinary Science*, **48**, 310–13.

Mineo, H., Murao, R., Kato, S. & Ushijima, J. (1990*c*). Effect of intravenous injection of short-chain fatty acids on glucagon secretion in sheep. *Japanese Journal of Zootechnical Science*, **61**, 349–53.

Mineo, H., Nishimura, M., Kato, S. & Ushijima, J. (1986). The effect of intravenous infusion of acetate on glucose-induced insulin secretion in sheep. *Japanese Journal of Zootechnical Science*, **57**, 765–9.

Ohbo, M. (1990). Effects of fatty acids on the amylase release from ovine and murine pancreas. MSc dissertation, Tohoku University, Sendai.

Ohbo, M., Katoh, K. & Sasaki, Y. (1989). Effects of short-, medium- and long-chain fatty acids on amylase release from pancreatic segments of rats. *Asian–Australasian Journal of Animal Science*, **2**, 193–4.

Sasaki, Y., Weekes, T. E. C. & Bruce, J. B. (1977). Effects of glucose and butyrate on insulin release from perfused fragments of sheep pancreas. *Journal of Endocrinology*, **72**, 415–16.

Taylor, R. B. (1962). Pancreatic secretion in sheep. *Research in Veterinary Science*, **3**, 63–77.

Williams, J. A. & Goldfine, I. D. (1985). The insulin–pancreatic acinar axis. *Diabetes*, **34**, 980–6.

15

Effect of short-chain fatty acids on salivary flow in ruminants

P. NØRGAARD

Introduction

In ruminant animals, saliva is secreted principally from four major anatomically distinct pairs of glands: the parotid, inferior molar, mandibular and sublingual glands. In addition there are numerous minor salivary glands. In the first section of the gland, a primary secretion is produced, which is modified in the secretory duct, where sodium is actively reabsorbed, chlorine is passively absorbed, and potassium and bicarbonate are secreted by the ductal cells, which thus modify the primary secretion (Compton *et al.*, 1980; Cook & Young, 1989). Mixed saliva from ruminants is alkaline, with pH values of 8.1–8.5. It has a buffer capacity of 140 mequiv./l, a high phosphorus content (10–30 mM), a high bicarbonate content (100–130 mM) and a low chloride content (5–20 mM), whereas monogastric species produce saliva with a pH of 6.5–7.6 and a lower buffering capacity (Kay, 1966; Lau *et al.*, 1990).

The main function of salivary secretion in ruminants is to stabilize the pH and fluidity of the fermenting contents of the rumen, for the rumen has no secretory glands of its own. Saliva also contains surfactant and mucus, which aid in moistening and lubricating the chewed food, and help to maintain oral hygiene. The parotids plus the inferior molars, which are functionally identical glands, account for the total saliva secreted (Kay, 1966).

The secretion of the sheep's parotid gland may amount to 0.02–0.25 ml/g wet tissue/min on stimulation (Wilson & Tribe, 1963; Cook & Young, 1989). The glands secrete continuously, and the main stimuli to high flow rates during eating and ruminating behaviour include sight of the food, physical rubbing of the oral and reticular mucosae by coarse food particles, stretching of the oesophagus, cardiac orifice and reticulum, as well as chemical stimuli in the mouth and reticulorumen (Kay, 1966; Leek & Stafford, 1989). These stimuli act reflexively by way of the parasympathetic nervous system and

Table 15.1. *Review of experiments performed on the effect of short-chain fatty acids (SCFA) in mouth and oesophagus on saliva secretion*

Species	Condition	Treatment	pH	Cannulation	Rate of flow (% of control)	References
Oral mucosa						
Sheep ($n = 1$)	Anaesthesia	0.5 M SCFA	4	SP	200–400	Kay (1958*a*)
Sheep ($n = 1$)	Resting	5 ml acetic acid	2–3	SP	600	Denton (1957)
		6 ml acetic acid	4–2		100–150	
Tongue						
Sheep ($n = 3$)	Anaesthesia	Acetic acid	3	SP	100–≫100	Coats *et al.* (1956)
		0.1–0.3 M Na-acetate	7		100	
Infusion into mouth						
Sheep ($n = 3$)	Resting	0.2 M SCFA mix	3.3	RP	250	P. Nørgaard *et al.* (unpublished data)
		0.3 M SCFA mix	3.3		360	
		0.4 M SCFA mix	3.3		480	
Drinking						
Sheep ($n = 3$)	Resting	1 M acetic acid	3–4	SP	≫100	Krasusky & Krymskaya (1940)
		1 M butyric acid	3–4		≫100	
Solution through oesophagus						
Sheep ($n = 3$)	Resting	1 M acetic acid	3	SP	>100	Krasusky & Krymskaya (1940)
		1 M butyric acid	3		>100	
Inclusion into diet (500 ml/kg hay)						
Cattle ($n = 1$)	Eating	0.18 M SCFA mix	3	SRP	150	Hagemeister & Kaufmann (1970)
		0.36 M SCFA mix	3		170	
		0.36 M Na-SCFA mix	6		220	
		0.36 M Na-SCFA mix	8.3		150	

SP, cannulation of parotid duct; RP, re-entrant cannulation of parotid duct; SRP, cannulation of parotid duct and recirculation of saliva to rumen.

cause increased blood flow through the glands (Coats *et al.*, 1956; Kay, 1958*a*), thereby supporting the increased production of saliva. Stimulation of the sympathetic nerve to the gland causes the myoepithelium to contract, expelling preformed saliva from the gland, and reducing blood flow through the gland (Kay, 1958*b*).

The flow rate during a period of eating begins to decline after 5-10 min and may decrease curvilinearly to a level lower than that before the meal (Bailey & Balch, 1961*b*; Sato, Kato & Tsuda, 1976; Carter, Grovum & Greenberg, 1990). The rate of saliva secretion is related to the rate of food intake; short meals produce a higher rate of secretion and more saliva per kilogram of food eaten (Carter & Grovum, 1990).

The actual rate of saliva secretion from a single gland depends on the size of the gland and the balance between the stimulatory and inhibitory factors (Kay, 1966). General observations in this area are as follows. The rate of secretion during rest and during ruminating increases from 1 to 14 h after a long meal of forage (Bailey, 1961, 1966; Bailey & Balch, 1961*b*). The flow of parotid saliva is highly variable even during eating. At the onset of eating or during rumination the flow from one stimulated parotid gland was found to be 0.5–1.0 ml/min per kg $BW^{0.75}$ compared with 0.03–0.34 ml/min per kg $BW^{0.75}$ during resting (Bailey & Balch, 1961*b*; Kay, 1966; Hagemeister & Kaufmann, 1970; Sato *et al.*, 1976; Carter & Grovum, 1990).

The rate of total salivary flow (ml/min per kg $BW^{0.75}$) in sheep and cattle was found to be 2.0, 1.8 and 0.2–1.0 during short meals, ruminating and resting periods, respectively (Bailey & Balch, 1961*b*; Cassida & Stokes, 1986; Carter *et al.*, 1990). Total daily salivary secretion may be 8–16 l in sheep and 100–200 l in dairy cows, which is equivalent to a daily flow of 0.5–2 l/24 h per kg $BW^{0.75}$ in sheep and cattle fed a forage diet *ad libitum* (Bailey, 1961; Kay, 1966). The daily secretion is affected by intake (Kay, 1966), physical form of the diet (Wilson, 1963), length of meals (Carter & Grovum, 1990), tonicity of blood and rumen fluid (Carter & Grovum, 1990), sodium deficiency and dehydration (Denton, 1957; Compton *et al.*, 1980), drugs such as slaframine (Froetschel *et al.*, 1986), and stage of lactation (Cassida & Stokes, 1986).

Effect of SCFA in the mouth

Table 15.1 summarizes experiments on the effects of acetic, propionic and butyric acids, individually and in mixtures, on parotid secretion during anaesthesia and during rest, and on total saliva during eating. The introduction of 0.15–1 M solutions of SCFA into the mouth of sheep under general

Table 15.2. *Review of experiments performed on the effect of short-chain fatty acids (SCFA) in the reticulorumen and in blood on saliva secretion*

Species	Condition	Treatment	pH	Cannulation	Rate of flow (% of control)	References
Solutions into washed rumen						
Sheep ($n = 1$)	Anaesthesia	0.5 M acetic acid	3	SP	200–400	Kay (1958*a*)
		0.5 M propionic acid	3		200–400	
		0.5 M butyric acid	3		200–400	
		0.5 M Na-acetate	7		100	
Sheep ($n = 1$)	Anaesthesia	0.05–0.2 M acetic acid	3.8	SP	200–600	Ash & Kay (1959)
		0.05–0.2 M acetic acid	5.7		100	
		0.02–0.15 M butyric acid	3.8		200–600	
		0.02–0.15 M butyric acid	5.7		100	
		0.2 M SCFA mix	3.8		200–600	
			5.7		100	
Sheep ($n = 2$)	Resting	1 l 0.5 M acetic acid	5.0	SP	50–150	Obara *et al.* (1972*b*)
		0.9 l 0.5 M propionic acid	5.0		40–60	
		1.2 l 0.5 M butyric acid	5.0		15–20	
SCFA into rumen						
Sheep ($n = 2$)	Resting	0.25–0.5 l 0.5 M acetic acid	5.0	SP	40–80	Obara *et al.* (1967)
		0.76 l 0.5 M propionic acid	5.0	SP	40–100	
		0.2–0.5 l 0.5 M butyric acid	5.0	SP	30–100	
Cattle ($n = 4$)	Resting	0.17 M SCFA mix	5.6	Total	75–100	Bailey & Balch (1961*a*)
Cattle ($n = 3$)	Resting	Rumen acidosis	5.6–4.3	SP	50–25	Randhawa *et al.* (1981)
SCFA (0.04 mmol/kg body wt/min) for 2 h into jugularis						
Sheep ($n = 4$)	Resting	Acetic acid		SP	>100	Obara *et al.* (1972*a*)
		Butyric acid		SP	100	

SP, cannulation of parotid duct.

anaesthesia, infused together with saliva (P. Nørgaard *et al.*, unpublished data) or by inclusion in drinking water, or included in the diet, stimulates parotid saliva secretion during rest by 1.5–6 times and by 1.5–2 times during eating.

The reflex stimulation of parotid secretion by SCFA is transmitted through the parasympathetic nervous system (Comline & Kay, 1958). The introduction of 20 ml/0.5 M acetic acid sometimes increased salivary flow in anaesthetized sheep, but no effect was observed with water, 0.5 M NaCl or 0.1 M HCl (Kay, 1958*a*). The lag time from the introduction of SCFA into the mouth until increased secretion occurred was found to vary from 15 to 60 s (Ash & Kay, 1959). The stimulating effect of SCFA is related to the pH of the solution in contact with the mucosa of the mouth (Table 15.1) and the rumen (Table 15.2); SCFA solutions with pH of 5.7 or higher have no stimulating effect on parotid saliva secretion. The influence of pH on saliva secretion is parallel to the inhibitory effect on rumen movements, which is related to the concentration of undissociated SCFA (Cottrell & Gregory, 1991; Chapter 12).

Parallel to the reflex effect of SCFA on saliva secretion, a reflex stimulating effect on parotid salivary secretion is caused by lactic, tannic, formic, hydrochloric and sulphuric acids in the mouth (Krasusky & Krymskaya, 1940; Denton, 1957; Kay, 1958*a*). Solutions of NaCl, KCl, and $NaHCO_3$ in the mouth produce a less stimulating effect on parotid secretion than do SCFA. Krasusky & Krymskaya (1940) found that in contrast to a salt solution, SCFA made the saliva even more alkaline.

The stimulating effect of SCFA in the mouth during eating seems to be less than the effect during resting (Table 15.1), but this may be due to the fact that the intake of hay itself produces a strong physical stimulus on the oral mucosa and in the oesophagus, and the additional effect of SCFA might be the same as is found at rest.

Effect of SCFA in the reticulorumen

The effect of SCFA via the reticuloruminal mucosa on parotid salivary secretion and total salivary secretion (Table 15.2) is less clear than its effect in the mouth (Table 15.1). In a washed empty rumen, solutions of 0.05–0.5 M SCFA produce a significant stimulus to the sheep's parotid only at pH below 4, with parallel inhibition of rumen movements (Kay, 1958*a*; Ash & Kay, 1959). There was no response at higher rumen pH values (5.5–5.9). Dietary and artificial elevation of the concentrations of SCFA in rumen fluid to more than 0.15 M caused increased tonicity of rumen fluid and blood, decreased the pH of rumen fluid to less than 5.5 and decreased the rate of resting parotid saliva flow by 25 to 85% (Obara *et al.*, 1967) as well as that of total saliva flow (Bailey & Balch, 1961*a*; Randhawa *et al.*, 1981; Table 15.2).

More evidence (Carter & Grovum, 1990) indicates that the inhibitory effect of a high concentration of SCFA in rumen fluid may be due to the elevation of the tonicity of rumen fluid. Parotid salivary flow during rest has been found to be linearly and negatively related to the osmostic pressure of rumen fluid and of blood (Warner & Stacey, 1977; Silanikove & Tadmor, 1989). Warner & Stacey (1977) found that parotid secretion in sheep decreased as the tonicity of ruminal fluid or jugular plasma was increased by osmotic loads of various solutions into the rumen. Infusion of high-tonicity solutions into the portal vein produced a greater inhibitory effect on saliva secretion than infusion into the jugular vein. This observation supports the suggestion of a central mediator in the brain for the effect of tonicity of blood plasma on the rate of parotid saliva secretion (Carter *et al.*, 1990; Carter & Grovum, 1990).

Importance of SCFA to saliva secretion

SCFA constitute 2–10% of dry matter in silage produced by anaerobic preservation of fresh herbage (McDonald, 1981). Most of the dairy cows in northern Europe and the USA are fed silage *ad libitum* and may spend 2–5 h eating silage (Nørgaard, 1989; Reeve, 1989). According to the findings of Hagemeister & Kaufmann (1970) (Table 15.1), one might expect saliva secretion to be stimulated by SCFA in silage. In cattle, Bailey (1961) found a flow of total saliva of 2.3–2.7 ml/min per kg $BW^{0.75}$ when they were eating grass or herbage silage. The flow of saliva per kilogram hay eaten gradually decreased, and the flow of saliva per kilogram silage eaten tended to increase during a long meal. The resulting flow of saliva after a long meal of silage was less than the flow after a meal of hay and grass (Bailey & Balch, 1961*a*). Regurgitation of rumen contents during rumination also introduces SCFA into the mouth for 5–8 h daily (Nørgaard, 1989). The dietary concentration of SCFA in silage juice is 100–400 mM (McDonald, 1981) compared with 60–150 mM in regurgitated rumen content. The pH value of silage ranges from 3.8 to 5.2, and the SCFA are often together with 0.1–0.4 M lactic acid, which makes 40–80% of the SCFA undissociated, whereas the pH value of rumen contents of 5.5–7 causes only 1–10% of the SCFA to be undissociated.

A high level of nutrition, a huge intake of easily fermentable carbohydrates, large meals of silage, or poorly adapted rumen epithelium to high absorption of SCFA in industrialized dairy and beef cattle herds may lead to high concentrations of SCFA in the rumen (Dirksen, 1989). This is a major contributor to increased rumen fluid tonicity (Bergen, 1972; Bennink *et al.*,

1978; Phillip, Buchanan-Smith & Grovum, 1981; Carter & Grovum, 1990). The rate of secretion of parotid saliva during rest is negatively related to rumen tonicity in sheep and cattle at constant rumen pH and SCFA concentration (Wilson, 1963; Warner & Stacey, 1977; Silanikove & Tadmor, 1989).

It is surprising at first sight that conditions leading to an excessive accumulation of SCFA in the rumen should inhibit salivary secretion (Carter & Grovum, 1990), for ruminant saliva normally serves to stabilize the environment of the rumen ecosystem. On the other hand, inhibition of salivary secretion by accumulation of SCFA in rumen fluid may protect the ruminant from metabolic acidosis and dehydration by excessive alkaline saliva secretion.

Effect of SCFA on salivary secretion in humans

Together with lactic and citric acids, SCFA such as acetic, propionic and butyric acids are significant constituents of preserved vegetables, salads and beer. In human beings, organic acids such as citric acid have a greater stimulating effect on salivary secretion than do inorganic salts and mastication. A drop of citric acid on the human tongue immediately stimulates salivary secretion and increases the pH values and bicarbonate content of saliva (from 5 to 50 mM). In the human mouth, this has a highly protective effect on plaque pH in the mouth, thereby neutralizing acids produced by oral bacteria so that they do not dissolve tooth enamel (Meurman *et al.*, 1987; Lau *et al.*, 1990).

Acknowledgement

The author is grateful to Dr R. N. B. Kay for his critical perusal of the chapter and his valuable suggestions.

References

Ash, R. W. & Kay, R. N. B. (1959). Stimulation and inhibition of reticulum contractions, rumination and parotid secretion from the forestomach of conscious sheep. *Journal of Physiology*, **149**, 43–57.

Bailey, C. B. (1961). Saliva secretion and its relation to feeding in cattle. 3. The rate of mixed saliva in the cow during eating, with an estimate of the magnitude of the total daily secretion of mixed saliva. *British Journal of Nutrition*, **15**, 443–51.

Bailey, C. B. (1966). A note on the relationship between the rate of secretion of saliva and the rate of swallowing in cows at rest. *Animal Production*, **8**, 325–8.

Bailey, C. B. & Balch, C. C. (1961*a*). Saliva secretion and its relation to feeding in cattle. 2. The composition and rate of secretion of mixed saliva in the cow during rest. *British Journal of Nutrition*, **15**, 383–402.
Bailey, C. B. & Balch, C. C. (1961*b*). Saliva secretion and its relation to feeding in cattle. 1. Composition and rate of secretion of parotid saliva in a small steer. *British Journal of Nutrition*, **15**, 371–83.
Bennink, M. R., Tyler, T. R., Ward, G. M. & Johnson, D. E. (1978). Ionic milieu of bovine and ovine rumen as affected by diet. *Journal of Dairy Science*, **61**, 315.
Bergen, W. G. (1972). Rumen osmolality as a factor in feed intake control of sheep. *Journal of Animal Science*, **34**, 1054–60.
Carter, R. R. & Grovum, W. L. (1990). A review of the physical significance of hypertonic body fluid on feed intake and ruminal function: salivation, motility and microbes. *Journal of Animal Science*, **68**, 2811–32.
Carter, R. R., Grovum, W. L. & Greenberg, G. R. (1990). Parotid secretion patterns during meals and their relationship to the tonicity of body fluids and to gastrin and pancreatic polypeptide in sheep. *British Journal of Nutrition*, **63**, 319–27.
Cassida, K. A. & Stokes, M. R. (1986). Eating and resting salivation in early lactation in dairy cows. *Journal of Dairy Science*, **69**, 1882–92.
Coats, D. A., Denton, D. A., Goding, J. R. & Wright, R. D. (1956). Secretion by the parotid gland in sheep. *Journal of Physiology*, **131**, 13–31.
Comline, R. S. & Kay, R. N. B. (1955). Reflex secretion by the parotid gland of the sheep. *Journal of Physiology*, **129**, 55–6.
Compton, J. S., Nelson, J., Wright, R. S. & Young, J. A. (1980). A micropuncture investigation of electrolyte transport in the parotid glands of sodium-replete and sodium-depleted sheep. *Journal of Physiology*, **309**, 429–46.
Cook, D. I. & Young, J. A. (1989). Fluid and electrolyte secretion by salivary glands. In *Handbook of Physiology*, section 6: *The Gastrointestinal System*, vol. III, ed. S. G. Schultz, J. G. Forte & B. B. Raunter, pp. 1–23. Bethesda: American Physiological Society.
Cottrell, D. F. & Gregory, P. G. (1991). Regulation of gut motility by luminal stimuli in the ruminant. In *Physiological Aspects of Digestion and Metabolism in Ruminants*, ed. T. Tsuda, Y. Sasaki & R. Kawashima, pp. 3–32. San Diego: Academic Press.
Denton, D. A. (1957). The study of sheep with permanent unilateral parotid fistulae. *Quarterly Journal of Experimental Physiology*, **42**, 72–95.
Dirksen, G. (1989). *Rumen Function and Disorders Related to Production Disease.* Proceedings of the VIIth International Symposium on Production Disease in Farm Animals, pp. 350–61. Ithaca, NY: New York State College of Veterinary Medicine.
Froetschel, M. A., Croom, W. J., Hagler, W. M., Tate, L. P. & Broquist, H. P. (1986). Effects of slaframine on ruminant digestive function: resting saliva flow and composition in cattle. *Journal of Animal Sciences*, **62**, 1404–11.
Hagemeister, H. von & Kaufmann, W. (1970). Der stimulierende Effekt organischer Säuren und Saltze auf die Parotissekretion bei Wiederkäuern. *Zeitschrift für Tierphysiologie, Tierernährung und Futtermittelkunde*, **26**, 258–64.
Kay, R. N. B. (1958*a*). Continuous and reflex secretion by the parotid gland in ruminants. *Journal of Physiology*, **144**, 463–75.
Kay, R. N. B. (1958*b*). The effect of stimulation of the sympathetic nerve and of adrenaline on the flow of parotid saliva in sheep. *Journal of Physiology*, **144**, 476–89.

Kay, R. N. B. (1966). The influence of saliva on digestion in ruminants. *World Review of Nutrition and Dietetics*, **6**, 292–328.

Krasusky, V. K. & Krymskaya, W. M. (1940). Certain biological features in the work of ruminants' parotid gland. *Sechenov Journal of Physiology of the USSR*, **28**, 272–83.

Lau, K. R., Elliott, A. C., Brown, P. D. & Case, R. M. (1990). Bicarbonate transport by salivary gland acinar cells. In *Epithelial Secretion of Water and Electrolytes*, ed. A. Young & P. Y. Wong, pp. 171–87. Berlin, Heidelberg: Springer-Verlag.

Leek, B. F. & Stafford, K. J. (1989). The nervous reflex mechanisms responsible for the increased salivation occurring during rumination in sheep. *Asian Australian Journal of Animal Science*, **2**, 139–40.

McDonald, P. (1981). *The Biochemistry of Silage*. Chichester: John Wiley & Sons.

Meurman, J. H., Rytömaa, I., Kari, I., Laakso, T. & Murtomaa, H. (1987). Salivary pH and glucose after consuming various beverages, including sugar-containing drinks. *Caries Research*, **21**, 353–9.

Nørgaard, P. (1989). The influence of the physical form of the diet on chewing activity and reticulo-rumen motility in cows. *Acta Veterinaria Scandinavica*, **83** (Suppl.), 46–52.

Obara, Y., Gomi, K., Ootomo, Y. & Tsuda, T. (1967). Effects of the ruminal condition on the parotid saliva secretion of sheep. *Tohoku Journal of Agricultural Research*, **18**, 125–37.

Obara, Y., Sasaki, Y., Watanabe, S., Satoh, Y. & Tsuda, T. (1972*a*). The effect of intravenous infusion of volatile fatty acid on the parotid secretion of sheep. *Tohoku Journal of Agricultural Research*, **23**, 141–8.

Obara, Y., Watanabe, S., Satoh, Y. & Tsuda, T. (1972*b*). The effects of the administration of volatile fatty acid to the empty rumen on the parotid saliva secretion of sheep. *Tohoku Journal of Agricultural Research*, **23**, 132–40.

Phillip, L. E., Buchanan-Smith, J. G. & Grovum, W. L. (1981). Food intake and ruminal osmolality from that of the products of maize silage fermentation. *Journal of Agricultural Science, Cambridge*, **96**, 439–45.

Randhawa, S. S., Setia, M. S., Choudhuri, P. C. & Misra, S. K. (1981). Effect of preacute lactic acidosis on the physico-chemical changes in parotid saliva of cross-bred calves. *Zeitschrift für Tierphysiologie, Tierernährung und Futtermittelkunde*, **45**, 60–5.

Reeve, A. (1989). What can silage produce? An R and D view. In *Silage for Milk Production*, Occasional Symposium no. 23, ed. C. S. Mayne, pp. 31–41. Worcestershire: British Grassland Society.

Sato, H., Kato, S. & Tsuda, T. (1976). Effect of hay to concentrate ratio on parotid secretion and its sodium, potassium and phosphorus levels in sheep. *Japanese Journal of Veterinary Science*, **38**, 347–54.

Silanikove, N. & Tadmor, A. (1989). Rumen volume, saliva flow rate, and systemic fluid homeostasis in dehydrated cattle. *American Journal of Physiology*, **256**, R809–R815.

Warner, A. C. I. & Stacey, B. D. (1977). Influence of ruminal and plasma osmotic pressure on salivary secretion in sheep. *Quarterly Journal of Experimental Physiology*, **62**, 133–42.

Wilson, A. D. (1963). The effect of diet on the secretion of parotid saliva by sheep. II. Variations in the rate of salivary secretion. *Australian Journal of Agricultural Research*, **14**, 680–9.

Wilson, A. D. & Tribe, D. E. (1963). The effect of diet on the secretion of parotid saliva by sheep. 1. The daily secretion of saliva by caged sheep. *Australian Journal of Agricultural Research*, **14**, 670–9.

16

Utilization of short-chain fatty acids in ruminants

E. R. ØRSKOV

My interest in the metabolism of short-chain fatty acids (SCFA) was first aroused when as a PhD student at Reading University I was looking for a challenging subject to study. Sir Kenneth Blaxter and his colleagues (see Blaxter, 1962) had just shown that acetic acid was possibly inefficiently utilized by sheep and this provided an elegant explanation for differences in utilization of digestible energy between fibrous feeds and cereals, which had been observed by many workers and to some extent quantified by Kellner (1926). Sir Kenneth had been quick to see the importance of SCFA metabolism when its contribution to absorbed energy had been established. While his initial ideas have not altogether been proved, they have nevertheless provided the stimulus to a lot of work and to a much better understanding of energy metabolism in ruminants.[1]

It is remarkable considering the importance of SCFA as energy sources for ruminants that they were only recognized at a relatively late stage. In fact as late as 1942 Baker and other microbiologists thought that the main energy source in ruminants was bacterial polysaccharide formed during anaerobic fermentation in the rumen and that SCFA were waste products (Baker, 1942). The recognition of their importance must be attributed to the group working in Cambridge and led by Sir Joseph Barcroft (Barcroft *et al.*, 1944). They observed the quantitative importance of SCFA as fermentation end products and that they were absorbed from the rumen and indeed utilized by the host animal tissue. About 70% of energy absorbed is in the form of SCFA.

After that period many research groups took up the search to study the qualitative and quantitative importance of SCFA in ruminants. This indeed was made easier by the progress in chromatography and many laboratories were first equipped with large cumbersome steam-heated glass tubes, referred

[1] Sir Kenneth Blaxter was an intellectual giant. By standing on his shoulders it became possible to reach out a little further. Sir Kenneth died on April 18, 1992.

Table 16.1. *Effect of type of carbohydrate on molar proportion (mmol/mol) of short-chain fatty acids in the rumen of two steers receiving purified diets*

Substrate	Acetic acid	Propionic acid	Butyric acid	Higher acids
Cellulose	737	183	48	32
Starch	604	247	104	45
Starch + glucose	571	289	99	41
Sucrose	496	232	202	70
Glucose	380	223	258	139
Standard error	28	29	10	—

From Ørskov & Oltjen (1967).

to as 'the James and Martin apparatus' (James & Martin, 1952). These were later replaced by the much faster gas–liquid chromatography.

Here it is perhaps pertinent to mention the important pathways of the major SCFA produced. Acetic acid is absorbed unchanged and converted in the liver and other tissues to acetyl-CoA, which can be utilized for lipid synthesis, oxidation or other metabolic pathways. It cannot be converted to glucose or glucose precursors. Propionic acid is metabolized via methyl malonic acid to succinic acid. It can then be converted to glucose or glucose precursors. It can also be used for milk lactose synthesis or be oxidized. Butyric acid, except for being largely changed to β-hydroxybutyric acid in the rumen wall, is metabolized in a similar manner to acetic acid.

The ability rapidly to separate the different SCFA soon led to the general observation that there were considerable differences in the fermentation end products from different diets.

Table 16.1 summarizes some results that represent the general findings, namely, that fermentation of cellulose gives a much higher proportion of acetic acid than does fermentation of starch or soluble carbohydrates. Starchy diets increased the level of propionic acid. Mono- and disaccharides – glucose and sucrose – sometimes gave a very high proportion of butyric acid. This, however, was by no means consistent, particularly with diets containing starch and soluble sugars. Here the pH was also important, as that greatly influenced the microflora (Ørskov, Fraser & Gordon, 1974). An example of this is given in Table 16.2, which shows the effect of cereal processing on type of fermentation, an effect clearly associated with the change in rumen pH.

Table 16.2. *Effect of cereal processing on rumen pH and proportion of short-chain fatty acids (mol/100 mol) in sheep*

	Rumen pH	Acetic acid	Propionic acid	Higher acids
Barley, whole	6.4	52.5	30.1	17.4
Barley, rolled	5.4	45.1	45.3	9.6
Wheat, whole	5.9	52.3	32.2	15.5
Wheat, rolled	5.0	34.2	42.6	23.2
Oats, whole	6.7	65.0	18.6	16.4
Oats, rolled	6.1	52.2	37.6	10.2
Maize, whole	6.1	47.2	38.7	14.1
Maize, ground	5.2	41.3	43.2	15.5

From Ørskov *et al.* (1974).

Absorption of SCFA

Although this chapter does not deal comprehensively with absorption, it is important to establish for further understanding of utilization that SCFA are mainly absorbed in the undissociated form as the free acid. As the pH in the rumen is generally between 6 and 7 and the p*K* of the SCFA is about 4.7, most of the SCFA in the rumen are dissociated. However, the rumen wall is selectively permeable to SCFA in their undissociated form. This is important for the control of rumen pH. The saliva normally secreted would be sufficient only to neutralize about 15 to 20% of the SCFA produced, had they been absorbed in the dissociated form (see Ørskov & Ryle, 1990). Buffer is lost through liquid outflow from the rumen, but about 90% of the SCFA are absorbed through the rumen wall. The rate of absorption varies between the different SCFA and changes with pH. At low rumen pH, the absorption rate is higher for propionic and butyric acids than for acetic acid (MacLeod & Ørskov, 1984), but at higher rumen pH, 'about 7.5', acetic acid is absorbed more rapidly. It is important to recognize that the proportions of SCFA found in the rumen do not represent the proportions in which they are produced. At low rumen pH, the discrepancy can be quite large. MacLeod & Ørskov (1984) observed with intragastric infusion that the molar proportion of acetic acid in the rumen was about 10% higher than in the infusate when the rumen pH was about 5.8. These differences became very small at rumen pH around 7.0.

Utilization of SCFA

As soon as the importance of SCFA was recognized and that acetic acid constituted a large proportion of the end products of fermentation with cellulosic feeds, it was immediately thought that this might explain a phenomenon that had puzzled scientists for some years, namely that the metabolizable energy from cellulosic diets was utilized less efficiently than energy from concentrate or barley-based diets. In order to equate metabolizable energy Kellner (1926), in his feed evaluation based on starch, gave a list of correction values for roughages based on crude fibre. He attributed these differences to the work of digestion. The new knowledge of the Krebs citric cycle, which showed the dependence of acetic utilization on oxaloacetic acid generated from glucose or glucose precursors, no doubt added to this and led McClymont (1952) to put forward the hypothesis that the higher heat losses associated with roughage diets could be attributed to problems of acetic acid utilization and effectively to a lack of glucose precursors. Since only propionic acid of the major SCFA could give rise to a net synthesis of glucose, low propionic acid and high acetic acid seemed a likely explanation for the lower efficiency of roughage diets.

Here another development helped, namely, progress in cannulation techniques and progress in the development of respiration chambers. Sir Kenneth Blaxter and his colleagues at the Hannah Dairy Research Institute built several chambers and started to examine the utilization of SCFA. In a series of experiments (Armstrong *et al.*, 1957, 1958; Armstrong & Blaxter, 1957*a*,*b*) SCFA were infused singly or in mixtures into the rumens of sheep, and the changes in heat production were measured. When mixtures were infused below energy maintenance, i.e. below the amount of energy required for energy balance, they observed no difference, but above energy maintenance or when a grass hay diet was fed above maintenance, they observed that acetic acid was utilized less efficiently (33%) than propionic (56%) or butyric acids (62%). They also showed that mixtures high or low in acetic acid were utilized with differing efficiencies, suggesting a linear relationship between proportions of acetic acid and utilization of absorbed energy. This conclusion was, however, based on some miscalculation, as pointed out by Ørskov *et al.* (1979).

The differing efficiency below or above maintenance became a feature of the Agricultural Research Council (1965) feed evaluation system. The results of the work that indicated different efficiencies received immediate acceptance. Many commercial organizations started to invent methods to reduce the proportion of acetic and increase the proportion of propionic acid. Here of

Table 16.3. *Molar and energy proportions of different mixtures of short-chain fatty acids* (%)

Molar (*mmol/mol*)				
Acetic acid	75	65	55	45
Propionic acid	15	25	35	45
Butyric acid	10	10	10	10
Energy (*J/kJ*)				
Acetic acid	59	48	39	30
Propionic acid	21	33	43	53
Butyric acid	20	19	18	17

course it must be pointed out that the fermentation efficiency or capture of hydrogen is more efficient with propionic acid fermentation, as less methane is produced (Ørskov, Flatt & Moe, 1968). There were, however, several problems that did not receive immediate attention. If lack of glucose precursors gave rise to an inefficient utilization of acetic acid, then one would expect the same problem with butyric acid, which apparently was efficiently utilized. The other problem was that while the difference between acetic and propionic acids appears large, it could only explain a relatively small amount of the difference in utilization of metabolizable energy. The reason for this is that the importance of acetic acid is often overemphasized when it is expressed as molar proportion in the rumen. When it is expressed as a proportion of absorbed energy, it is far less important (see Table 16.3). The result was that even the difference as large as the one described in the previous paragraph could hardly have been detected with normal diets and could not explain the differences often observed between roughages and concentrates.

In a series of experiments (Ørskov & Allen 1966*a*,*b*,*c*; Ørskov, Hovell & Allen, 1966) in which salts of SCFA were fed to growing lambs, it was not possible to demonstrate any difference in utilization among the SCFA. Bull, Reid & Johnson (1970), using triacetin, found essentially the same results. This was later also shown by Hovell, Greenhalgh & Wainman (1976). In dairy cows, Ørskov *et al.* (1969) showed that while acetic and propionic acids resulted in differences in partition of energy between milk and body tissue insofar as propionic acid stimulated tissue synthesis and acetic acid stimulated milk production, there was no difference in heat production.

Although all the work carried out between 1960 and 1978 showed equal efficiency in the utilization of the different SCFA, it was not sufficiently convincing for the scientific community, no doubt due to the fact that the concept of inefficient utilization of acetic acid provided such an elegant explanation of the differences between roughage and concentrate. The problem of providing good data was that it was only possible to feed about 15% of absorbed energy in the form of SCFA or SCFA salts before appetite was affected and with the prevailing variability between animals it was difficult to demonstrate differences between SCFA with accuracy. Because of differences between animals, it was often difficult to detect differences in growth rate of 5–10% with statistical precision, so that it was even more difficult to estimate whether there were differences caused by the nature of the SCFA. It also had to be assumed that the added SCFA did not interfere with the utilization of the basal diet. This problem was also apparent in the original work of Blaxter and his colleagues, so it was clearly necessary to develop a new tool to provide convincing data. This difficulty led us in 1979 to develop the intragastric infusion technique (Ørskov *et al.*, 1979), which subsequently solved many problems in both protein and energy nutrition in ruminants.

The development of this technique requires a little further explanation. Two early methods invariably failed through problems of pH and/or problems of osmotic pressure. On the infusion of SCFA into the rumen the pH fell, and at pH below about 5.5 the animal suffered from acidosis and rumenitis. On the other hand, if partially neutralized SCFA were infused at a pH similar to that which was prevalent in the rumen, then the animals would suffer from alkalosis. In our trials we made both mistakes and only in exasperation asked how the animals themselves managed to do it!

As already mentioned, the SCFA are absorbed mainly in the undissociated form. Saliva keeps the rumen pH normally between 6 and 7 and saliva is lost through liquid outflow. It followed, therefore, that the amount of buffer infused should be no more than equivalent to the deficit in the normally secreted saliva, and that should be infused separately from the SCFA to allow flexible control. Saliva and SCFA are therefore infused separately into the rumen and normally protein is infused into the abomasum. With this development and the use of roughage substitutes in the rumen (in our case, plastic pan-scrubbers), it became possible to maintain nutritional status almost at levels normally achieved when the animal ate high-quality roughage, and supported a growth rate of about 1 kg/day in cattle, and milk production in excess of 20 kg/day.

The technique made it possible to nourish ruminants by complete infusion of SCFA. It was thus possible to vary the SCFA proportions at will and measure the differences, if any, in respiration chambers. A large trial involving 40 growing lambs was subsequently carried out (Ørskov *et al.*, 1979). Over the molar range of 45–85% acetic acid, the utilization was identical, as seen

Table 16.4. *Efficiency of utilization of different molar mixtures (%) of short-chain fatty acids infused into the rumen of growing lambs*

Acetic acid	85	75	65	55	45
Propionic acid	5	15	25	35	45
Butyric acid	10	10	10	10	10
Efficiency	0.59	0.61	0.61	0.57	0.64

From Ørskov *et al.* (1979).

in Table 16.4. This confirmed that differences in utilization of metabolizable energy between roughage and concentrate diets are probably not due to different products of fermentation.

A more extensive trial has recently been carried out with steers kept in respiration hoods, also with continuous infusion, but where in addition to heat production, nitrogen excretion and blood metabolites were also measured (Ørskov, MacLeod & Nakashima, 1991). The effects on blood metabolites are seen in Fig. 16.1. The level of energy infusion in the work was estimated as 1.5 times energy maintenance. Propionic acid varied reciprocally with acetic acid while the proportion of butyric acid was held constant at molar 8%. It can be seen that the breaking point occurred at around molar 80% of acetic acid or molar 12% of propionic acid. With still higher proportions of acetic acid there was clearly an elevation in β-hydroxybutyrate and free SCFA and a fall in insulin and blood glucose, all indicating a glucose deficiency. There was also an elevation in nitrogen excretion as seen in Fig. 16.2, as intermediates from protein turnover were used as glucose precursors. What was more important, however, was that the heat production decreased, due to the fact that some of the acetic acid was not oxidized, as it was excreted in the urine (Fig. 16.2). Thus there was never an elevation, but actually a significant reduction in heat production, as shown in Fig. 16.3. The response of the host animal to an excess of acetic acid was not futile cycling but excretion in the urine together with some β-hydroxybutyrate. It is worth noting, however, that this point of molar 80% acetic acid exceeds normal values, as the molar proportion even with the highest fibre diets seldom if ever exceeds 75%. This work has since been repeated at three levels of energy input (Ørskov & MacLeod, 1993), namely, 1.0, 1.5 and 2.0 times estimated maintenance energy, to see if the point of glucose deficiency differed according to level of energy infused. The result showed essentially the same breaking point regardless of energy infused, in other words the ratio of glucose precursors required appeared not to be affected by level of energy input. It

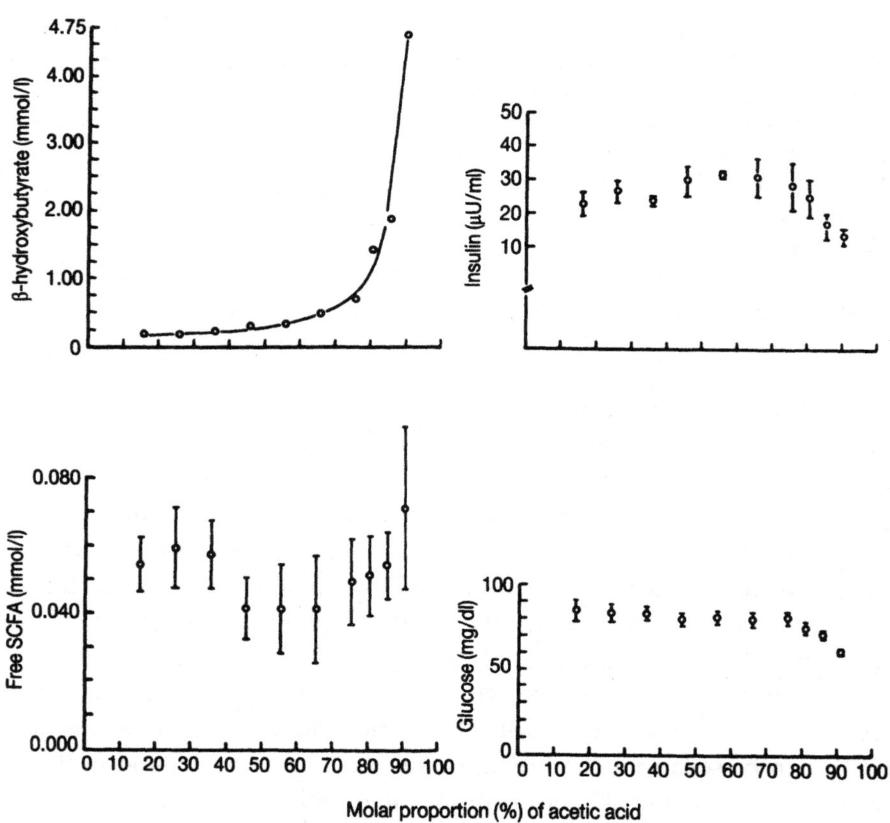

Fig. 16.1. Effects of molar proportion of acetic acid in infused mixture of short-chain fatty acids (SCFA) on plasma β-hydroxybutyrate, insulin, free SCFA and glucose.

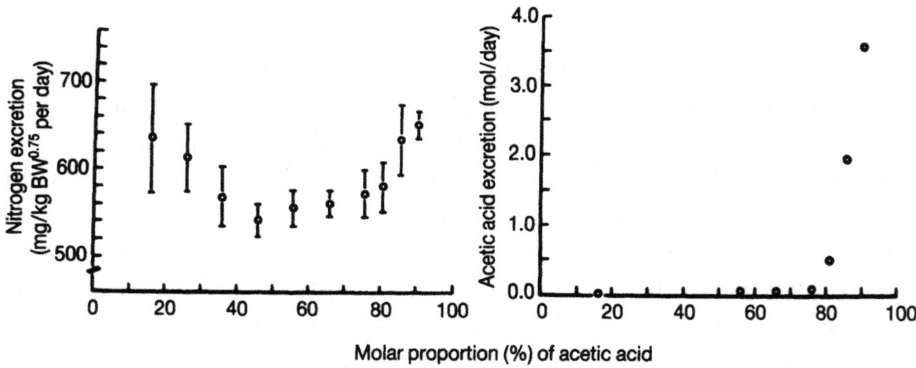

Fig. 16.2. Effect of molar proportion of acetic acid in infused mixture of short-chain fatty acids on urinary nitrogen and acetic acid excretion.

would appear therefore, that on the whole, manipulation of rumen fermentation cannot change the efficiency of utilization of SCFA.

SCFA and abnormal fat synthesis

Ørskov *et al.* (1974) observed that processed barley diets, which fermented to give a high molar proportion of propionic acid (40–45%), resulted in soft subcutaneous fat in lambs but not in cattle. The soft fat was caused by a high proportion of methyl-branched-chain fatty acids (BCFA), sometimes accounting for 10–20% of the subcutaneous fat. This problem was overcome by not processing the grain, which resulted in a decrease in the molar proportion of propionic acid (25–35%; Table 16.2). It was suggested that the deposition of abnormal amounts of BCFA in the subcutaneous fat of sheep (but not cattle) fed rations containing a high proportion of rapidly fermentable cereal was due to an inability to metabolize, via the normal route, the large amounts of propionate absorbed from the rumen. Although methylmalonyl-CoA mutase, involved in the conversion of propionate to succinate, is B_{12}-dependent, the amount of cobalt in the Rowett cereal rations should have ensured that the activity of this key enzyme was not impaired through lack of B_{12} cofactor. Since BCFA could arise through the incorporation of methylmalonate (MMA) into fatty acids in place of malonate, it was thought that mutase activity was the limiting factor in sheep. Therefore, it was argued that if propionate absorption was high enough to cause BCFA formation, then increases in plasma MMA should be detectable. However, when sheep were maintained totally by infusion (for close control over propionate input) and injected at regular intervals with vitamin B_{12}, high inputs of propionate did not increase plasma MMA nor were these BCFA produced. In fact, plasma MMA remained below 3.5 μmol/l, the normal levels for this metabolite being <5 in grazing sheep (Rice *et al.*, 1987) and <19 μmol/l in concentrate-fed sheep (O'Harte *et al.*, 1989). Plasma propionate, insulin and glucose also remained within the normal ranges, which indicated that there was no impairment in the conversion of methylmalonyl-CoA to succinyl-CoA when propionate was infused at a level equivalent to or higher than (up to molar 70%) that expected to be produced in the rumen by rapidly fermentable cereal diets.

The evidence currently available indicates that while sheep have the capacity to metabolize large amounts of propionate normally, propionate metabolism is in some way impaired in B_{12}-adequate sheep when large amounts of propionate are derived from rumen fermentation, but not when infused into the rumen. Vitamin B_{12} and a number of its α-analogues that

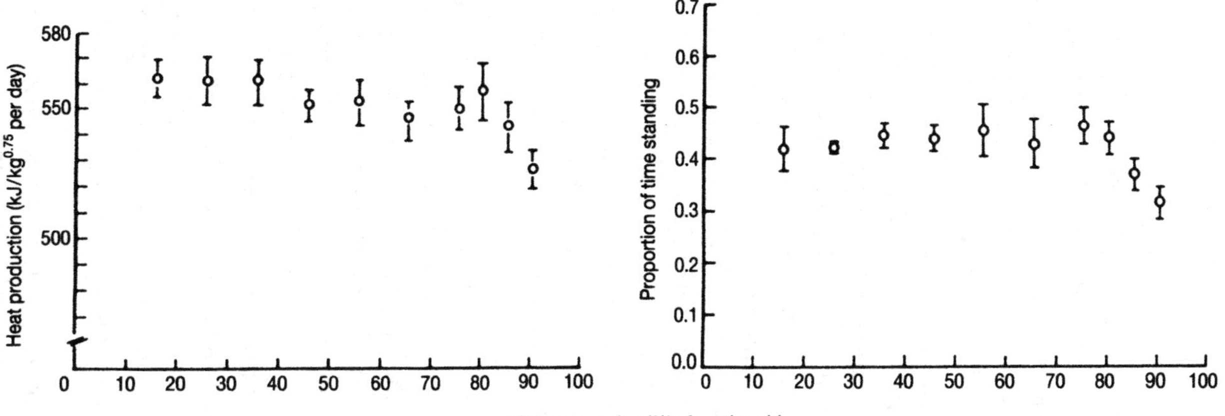

Fig. 16.3. Effect of molar proportion of acetic acid in infused mixture of short-chain fatty acids on daily heat production and time spent standing.

lack cofactor activity are synthesized by the rumen micro-organisms. It is therefore tempting to speculate that some of these analogues may be absorbed and inhibit activity of the mutase enzyme by competing with true B_{12} for the cofactor binding site on the enzyme. Although there is evidence that α-analogues are present in the plasma of both cattle and sheep (Halpin *et al.*, 1984), it is not known whether they originated in the rumen or systematically. Furthermore, it is not known whether any of the analogues in plasma are capable of inhibiting methylmalonyl-CoA mutase. Rumen production of analogues is, however, known to be greater in concentrate-fed animals compared to grazing animals. It is also interesting to note that sheep plasma contains a single B_{12} binder, transcobalamin Tc2, while cattle have Tc1 and Tc2 (Price, 1991). Both binders have an affinity for analogues as well as the true vitamin. Since Tc2 is responsible for transporting B_{12} into cells (Hall, 1979), it is possible that any analogues on this binder may also be internalized and hence influence mutase activity. The function of Tc1 remains unknown. However, since it is not involved in transporting B_{12} into cells, it may possibly have a role in binding analogues in plasma, preventing them from being carried into cells. If this were the case, it might explain why abnormal BCFA synthesis occurs in cereal-fed sheep but not in cattle.

SCFA and lactation

For maintenance and growth, recent evidence therefore suggests that, at least below molar 75–80% acetic acid in the rumen, there is unlikely to be a deficiency of glucose, as there is no elevation in β-hydroxybutyrate and free fatty acids nor a decrease in plasma insulin. For lactation some glucose is required for lactose synthesis as well, therefore a higher glucose requirement for lactating animals can be expected. However, the evidence so far suggests that if the cows are consuming sufficient feed to meet their requirement for milk production, the glucogenic energy absorbed, i.e. propionic and glucose precursors generated from the protein that is not utilized for synthesis of protein, is sufficient to meet their need. Glucose deficiency, however, can occur if body fat constitutes a very large proportion of the energy required to support lactation. This typically occurs in high-yielding cattle, such as Holstein, if they, for some reason, stop eating or if the feed quality given restricts intake to such an extent that absorbed energy falls far short of requirement. In such cases the animals will suffer from ketosis or acetonaemia. Ketosis is a common occurrence in high-yielding cows, and this is almost invariably due to animals going off feed, due to acidosis caused by high levels of concentrate feeding. At high levels of concentrate feeding, the amount of propionic acid absorbed can cause an elevation in blood insulin. Increasing concentrations of insulin stimulate most cells to take up nutrients from the blood. In lactating animals, this can deprive the mammary glands of sufficient nutrients and cause reduction in milk fat and eventually also in milk yield. Sutton (1980) demonstrated that this effect was most pronounced in dairy cows when concentrate was given twice rather than six times daily, due to diurnal peaks in propionic acid production. It is much less common when the diets are completely mixed rather than when concentrate and roughage are given separately. When milk production is stimulated by feeding protein, which is not degraded in the rumen, Ørskov, Reid & Tait (1987) showed that 10–15 kg of milk per day could be supported from body fat without any occurrence of ketosis; however, at 20 kg of milk per day from body fat, ketosis was induced.

Why are roughages used less efficiently than concentrates?

As mentioned before, Kellner thought the differences between roughages and concentrates could be explained by the so-called *Verdauungsarbeit* or 'work of digestion'. If by this we understand the work involved in eating, ruminating and standing up to eat, the difference can be explained (Ørskov & MacLeod, 1990). The biochemical efficiency of SCFA utilization measured on several occasions (Ørskov *et al.*, 1979, 1991; Ørskov & MacLeod, 1993; S. A. Chowdhury, unpublished data) is about 60%. If part of this energy is used in the physical work of eating, ruminating, walking, standing up, etc., the measured efficiency may be lower.

Another point illuminated by the technique of intragastric nutrition has been the distinction between efficiency below or above maintenance. This appears to a large extent to be due to the fact that during fasting, heat production is actually elevated. During fasting, when only fat is utilized, there is a glucose deficiency; as a result, nitrogen excretion is elevated, since some glucogenic amino acids released through protein turnover are utilized. In part due to urea synthesis, etc., heat production is high. If a small amount of glucose or even protein is infused into the abomasum of fasted ruminants, heat production actually decreases by about 10% (S. A. Chowdhury, unpublished data). The result is that from the point at which the glucose deficiency is alleviated, which occurs at about 0.2 or 0.3 times maintenance, there is no difference in the slope of efficiency of utilization of dietary energy below or above energy maintenance. The practical implication of this is that, provided a ruminant can consume about 0.2 to 0.3 times its energy maintenance, the body fat is efficiently utilized without excessive drain on protein tissue.

Ruminants evolved to utilize SCFA and within physiological limits they do so efficiently, regardless of the type of rumen fermentation.

References

Agricultural Research Council (1965). *The Nutrient Requirement of Farm Livestock. No. 2. Ruminants.* London: Her Majesty's Stationery Office.

Armstrong, D. G. & Blaxter, K. L. (1957*a*). The heat increment of steam volatile fatty acids in fasting sheep. *British Journal of Nutrition*, **11**, 247–72.

Armstrong, D. G. & Blaxter, K. L. (1957*b*). The utilization of acetic, propionic and butyric acids by fattening sheep. *British Journal of Nutrition*, **11**, 413–25.

Armstrong, D. G., Blaxter, K. L. & Graham, N. McC. (1957). The heat increment of mixtures of steam volatile fatty acids in fasting sheep. *British Journal of Nutrition*, **11**, 392–408.

Armstrong, D. G., Blaxter, K. L., Graham, N. McC. & Wainman, F. W. (1958). The utilization of the energy of two mixtures of steam volatile fatty acids by fattening sheep. *British Journal of Nutrition*, **12**, 177–88.

Baker, F. (1942). Microbial factors in the digestive assimilation of starch and cellulose in herbivora. *Nature*, **150**, 479.

Barcroft, J., McAnally, R. A. & Phillipson, A. T. (1944). Absorption of acetic, propionic and butyric acids from the alimentary canal. *Biochemical Journal*, **38**, iii.

Blaxter, K. L. (1962). *The Energy Metabolism of Ruminants.* London: Hutchinson.

Bull, L. S., Reid, J. T. & Johnson, D. R. (1970). Energies of sheep concerned with the utilization of acetic acid. *Journal of Nutrition*, **100**, 262–76.

Hall, C. A. (1979). The plasma transport of cobalamin. In *Proceedings of the Third European Symposium on Vitamin B_{12} and Intrinsic Factor*, ed. B. Zagalak & W. Friedrich, pp. 725–42. Berlin: de Gruyter.

Halpin, C. G., Harris, D. J., Caple, I. W. & Petterson, D. S. (1984). Contribution of cobalamin analogues to plasma vitamin B_{12} concentrations in cattle. *Research in Veterinary Science*, **37**, 249–51.

Hovell, F. D. DeB., Greenhalgh, J. F. D. & Wainman, F. G. (1976). The utilization of diets containing acetate salts by growing lambs as measured by comparative slaughter and respiration calorimetry, together with rumen fermentation. *British Journal of Nutrition*, **35**, 343–63.

James, A. T. & Martin, A. J. P. (1952). Gas liquid partitions chromatography. The separation and micro-estimation of volatile fatty acids from formic to dodecanoic acid. *Biochemical Journal*, **50**, 579–683.

Kellner, O. (1926). *The Scientific Feed of Animals.* London: Duckworth.

MacLeod, N. A. & Ørskov, E. R. (1984). Absorption and utilization of volatile fatty acids in ruminants. *Canadian Journal of Animal Science*, **62** (Suppl.), 354–5.

McClymont, G. L. (1952). Specific dynamic actions of acetic acid and heat increment of feeding in ruminants. *Australian Journal of Scientific Research*, **5B**, 374.

O'Harte, F. P. M., Kennedy, D. G., Blanchflower, W. J. & Rice, D. A. (1989). Methylmalonic acid in the diagnosis of cobalt deficiency in barley fed lambs. *British Journal of Nutrition*, **62**, 729–38.

Ørskov, E. R. & Allen, D. M. (1966*a*). Utilization of salts of volatile fatty acids by growing sheep. 1. Acetate, propionate and butyrate as sources of energy for young growing lambs. *British Journal of Nutrition*, **20**, 295–305.

Ørskov, E. R. & Allen, D. M. (1966*b*). Utilization of salts of volatile fatty acids by growing sheep. 2. Effect of stage of maturity and hormone implantation of volatile fatty acids as sources of energy for growth and fattening. *British Journal of Nutrition*, **20**, 509–17.

Ørskov, E. R. & Allen, D. M. (1966*c*). Utilization of salts of volatile fatty acids by growing sheep. 4. Effects of type of rumen fermentation of the basal diet on the utilization of salts of volatile fatty acids for nitrogen retention and body gains. *British Journal of Nutrition*, **20**, 519–32.

Ørskov, E. R., Flatt, W. P. & Moe, P. W. (1968). A fermentation balance approach to estimate extent of fermentation and efficiency of volatile fatty acid formation in ruminants. *Journal of Dairy Science*, **51**, 1429–35.

Ørskov, E. R., Flatt, W. P., Moe, P. W. & Munson, A. W. (1969). The influence of ruminal infusion of volatile fatty acids on milk yield and composition and on energy utilization by lactating cows. *British Journal of Nutrition*, **23**, 443.

Ørskov, E. R., Fraser, C. & Gordon, J. G. (1974). Effect of processing of cereals on rumen fermentation, digestibility, rumination time and firmness of subcutaneous fat. *British Journal of Nutrition*, **23**, 59–69.

Ørskov, E. R., Grubb, D. A., Wenham, G. & Corrigall, W. (1979). The sustenance of growing and fattening ruminants by intragastric infusion of volatile fatty acids and protein. *British Journal of Nutrition*, **41**, 553–8.

Ørskov, E. R., Hovell, F. D. DeB. & Allen, D. M. (1966). Utilization of salts of volatile fatty acids by growing sheep. 2. Effects of stage of maturity and hormone implantation on the utilization of volatile fatty acid salts as sources of energy for growth and fattening. *British Journal of Nutrition*, **20**, 307–15.

Ørskov, E. R. & MacLeod, N. A. (1990). Dietary-induced thermogenesis and feed evaluation in ruminants. *Proceedings of the Nutrition Society*, **49**, 227–37.

Ørskov, E. R. & MacLeod, N. A. (1993). Effect of level of input of different proportions of volatile fatty acids on energy utilization in growing ruminants. *British Journal of Nutrition*, **70**, 679–87.

Ørskov, E. R., McLeod, N. A. & Nakashima, Y. (1991). Effect of different volatile fatty acid mixtures on energy metabolism in cattle. *Journal of Animal Science*, **69**, 3389–97.

Ørskov, E. R. & Oltjen, R. R. (1967). Influence of carbohydrate and nitrogen sources on the rumen volatile fatty acids and ethanol of cattle fed purified diets. *Journal of Nutrition*, **93**, 222–8.

Ørskov, E. R., Reid, G. W. & Tait, A. G. (1987). Effect of fish meal on the mobilization of body energy in dairy cows. *Animal Production*, **45**, 345–8.

Ørskov, E. R. & Ryle, M. (1990). *Energy Nutrition in Ruminants*. Amsterdam, London: Elsevier.

Price, J. (1991). Demonstration of a high affinity vitamin B_{12} binder in cattle plasma and its relevance to problems in assessing cobalt/vitamin B_{12} status in the bovine. In *Proceedings of the Seventh International Symposium on Trace Elements in Man and Animals*, ed. B. Momcilovic, pp. 17–22. Zagreb: IMI.

Rice, D. A., McLoughlin, M., Blanchflower, W. J., Goodall, E. A. & McMurray, C. H. (1987). Methylmalonic acid as an indicator of vitamin B_{12} deficiency in grazing sheep. *Veterinary Record*, **121**, 472–3.

Sutton, J. D. (1980). Digestion and end product formation in the rumen from production rations. In *Digestive Physiology and Metabolism in the Ruminant*, ed. Y. Ruckebush & P. Thivend, pp. 271–80. Lancaster: MPT Press.

17

Short-chain fatty acids, pancreatic hormones and appetite control

A. DE JONG

Introduction

The mechanisms involved in the control of feeding behaviour are highly complex and are not yet clearly understood. Regulation is probably achieved by negative feedback controls, which inform the central nervous system, in particular the hypothalamus, of the nutritional state of the body (Baldwin, 1985; Woods, Taborsky & Porte, 1986). Various signals originating from the gut, caused by stretch, osmoconcentration or chemical stimuli, must be relayed to the brain, either neurally or hormonally, to be integrated with postabsorptive signals and a plethora of social factors and learned associations, to reach a satiating response. In domestic ruminants there is substantial experimental evidence for this metabolic regulation (Conrad, 1966; and for critical reviews see Grovum, 1987; Ketelaars & Tolkamp, 1991), although it has long been thought that ruminant animals have their feeding limited only by gastrointestinal fill (physical control).

Food intake in the ruminant is a composite of meals, as is the case in most mammals. Size and/or frequency of the meals determine the amount of food ingested. Many metabolites and hormones have been ascribed roles in controlling meal patterns. For a substance in the blood or rumen to fulfil such a regulatory function, ingestion of food must change the concentration of the component. Further, changes in the concentration should result in an altered food intake. Grossly unphysiological amounts of putative satiety signals, however, may trigger mechanisms that normally do not function or may cause discomfort or illness.

In this chapter, current concepts are reviewed on the role of short-chain fatty acids (SCFA) in the physiological control of voluntary food intake in ruminants. The focus is on spontaneous, rather than scheduled, meals and mainly short-term factors are considered. The role of SCFA in the regulation of food intake, and then the contribution of the major pancreatic hormones in relation to SCFA, are reviewed. The literature on SCFA and other humoral feedback systems in controlling feeding has already been reviewed (see e.g. Baile & Forbes, 1974; de Jong, 1987; Grovum, 1987; Forbes, 1992). There are also reviews about involvement of the neural mechanisms (Baldwin, 1985; Woods *et al.*, 1986), brain and gut peptides (de Jong, 1986; Silver & Morley, 1991; Rayner, 1992) and physical stimuli (Grovum, 1987; Forbes & Barrio, 1992) in appetite control.

Short-chain fatty acids

Virtually all nutrients and metabolites have been proposed as being major signals which, either in surplus or deficit, indicate satiety or hunger. The importance of SCFA in ruminant energy metabolism (see Chapter 16) would indicate that SCFA are likely to have a controlling function on food intake and, therefore, their role is discussed below.

Effects of food intake on SCFA

Blood circulation

In ruminants adapted to restricted access to feed, jugular SCFA concentrations increase rapidly during and after eating (Simkins, Suttie & Baumgardt, 1965); Evans, Buchanan-Smith & MacLeod, 1975; Theurer & Wanderley, 1987). This is not only true for acetate – quantitatively the main SCFA – but also for propionate and *n*-butyrate (de Jong, 1981*a*), the systemic levels of which are very low, due to their removal by the liver and the rumen wall. Similar findings were observed in the hepatic portal circulation (Theurer & Wanderley, 1987). Generally, both peripheral and portal SCFA increase within 15 min of starting to eat (Chase *et al.*, 1977*a*; de Jong, 1981*a*).

In the case of free-feeding, the meals are much smaller and more frequent. For instance, sheep and goats usually take 10–20 meals per day, with an average size of 50–250 g. To verify whether meals affect portal and peripheral SCFA levels in this case, a remote sampling device was used, which permits frequent blood sampling without disrupting feeding behaviour (Chase, Wangsness & Martin, 1977*b*; de Jong, 1981*b*). Neither study showed that spontaneous meals affect the peripheral or portal SCFA concentration. However, even at constant SCFA concentrations, an increased blood flow might trigger SCFA receptors. Increased portal blood flow has been observed in sheep and cattle being fed infrequently (Barnes, Comline & Dobson, 1986), but no significant rise in the net uptake of SCFA was observed in sheep after spontaneous meals (Adams & Forbes, 1982). Therefore, the onset of spontaneous meals is neither preceded nor followed by changes in blood SCFA that could transmit feedback signals.

Rumen fluid

In the absence of changes in circulating SCFA levels, the SCFA in the rumen might provide feedback cues. Here, too, in scheduled feeding, large meals induced marked increases in acetate, propionate and *n*-butyrate (see e.g. Simkins *et al.*, 1965; Robinson, Tamminga & van Vuuren, 1986), but it still remains to be seen whether spontaneous meals are related to the ruminal SCFA. However, work on cattle on high concentrate diets of equal portions at 2-h intervals (Bragg, Murphy & Davis, 1986) or at varying intervals (Sutton *et al.*, 1986) suggests that under these conditions ruminal SCFA levels are not consistently related to the meals. Moreover, ruminal SCFA in sheep fed *ad libitum* do not rise and fall with spontaneous feeding (A. de Jong, unpublished data). Therefore, a relation between spontaneous meals and ruminal SCFA appears unlikely.

Effects of SCFA infusions on food intake

If meal patterns are governed by SCFA (either in the circulation or in the rumen), feeding behaviour should be prevented or delayed by infusion of SCFA in amounts that do not greatly exceed their normal range.

Blood circulation

Intrajugular infusions of SCFA only in a few instances decreased intake (Baile & Forbes, 1974; de Jong, 1981*c*). However, the interpretation of these results is open to question, due to non-physiological conditions as regards dose, tonicity or acidity. In some studies the energy content of the SCFA may have accounted for a reduced food intake (Papas & Hatfield, 1978).

We investigated the influence of SCFA in the hepatic portal system on meal patterns in non-lactating goats having free access to a concentrate diet, where intake was recorded continuously (de Jong, Steffens & de Ruiter, 1981). Portal infusions of individual SCFA or mixtures of SCFA were given at a constant rate for 4 h and the effects on feeding behaviour and peripheral blood levels were tested. Despite the high SCFA levels reached, the infusion of acetate, propionate or butyrate failed to affect meal size, intermeal interval, latency to eating the first meal or total 4-h intake. Similarly, infusions of mixtures of these SCFA did not affect meal patterns, despite about twofold elevations in blood SCFA levels over 4 h (Tables 17.1 and 17.2). If circulating

Table 17.1. *Effect of 4-h intraportal infusions of short-chain fatty acids (SCFA) on feeding behaviour of goats (n = 5). Results expressed as mean ± SEM of the ratio of the parameter on the infusion day to that on the preinfusion day*

Treatment	Meal size	Interval length	Latency to first meal
Control	1.1 ± 0.1	1.0 ± 0.1	1.1 ± 0.1
SCFA mixture	1.1 ± 0.1	1.3 ± 0.3	1.0 ± 0.1

Adapted from de Jong (1981*c*).

Table 17.2. *Effect of 4-h intraportal infusions of short-chain fatty acids (SCFA) on blood composition of goats (n = 5). Results expressed as mean ± SEM*

		Peripheral blood concentration	
SCFA mixture	Doses (μmol/kg/min)	Preinfusion (μmol/l)	Infusion (μmol/l)
Acetate	29	452 ± 80	815 ± 181
Propionate	7	11.5 ± 2.2	23.2 ± 5.4
n-Butyrate	3	6.7 ± 1.9	16.5 ± 3.1

Adapted from de Jong (1981*c*).

SCFA play a role in short-term feeding in the non-lactating goat, the feedback is not generated from portal or peripheral blood.

Baile (1971) found that infusions of 4 M sodium propionate or acetate during spontaneous meals reduced the daily intake of grain (meal length and number of meals remained unaffected) in goats and sheep when infused into the ruminal vein, but not into a mesenteric vein, the portal vein or the carotid artery. Therefore, it seems that portal infusion of SCFA, even at very high rates as used by Baile, will not affect feeding. Baile proposed that the function of propionate receptors in the ruminal veins is to control feeding. Infusion into a small ruminal vein – upstream from the portal site – may be effective. However, Baile's work can be criticized on some points: high doses without appropriate controls were used and the infusions were given during meals only, whereas the absorption of SCFA produced after a meal takes place over a period of hours and spontaneous meals are not related to blood SCFA. SCFA were not measured to ascertain the physiological significance of the infused SCFA. As far as I know, the above ruminal vein findings have not been confirmed in additional studies and the postulated propionate receptors in the ruminal vein wall have not been demonstrated by electrophysiological techniques.

In contrast to the results of Baile and our group, Anil & Forbes (1980) and Elliot, Symonds & Pike (1985) observed that the infusion of propionate into the hepatic portal region reduced feeding in sheep and steers. Acetate had no effect. In the steers, at least a three-fold increase in systemic propionate levels was achieved. In the latter study, in which the animals were not fed *ad libitum*, the feeding responses to propionate were less consistent than in the former study, despite the clear increase in systemic propionate. Part of the conflicting results might be explained by the fact that osmotic controls were not used in either study. On the other hand, it remains unexplained that sodium propionate proved effective and sodium acetate at a higher dose did not (Anil & Forbes, 1980). Differences in the energy status of the animals may account for part of the conflicting results (Elliot *et al.*, 1985). This may be true, as infusions of propionate into the visceral circulation in sheep fed restricted amounts of food at a rate 20% lower than that used by Anil & Forbes (1980) resulted in triple propionate levels in systemic and portal blood, but did not reduce intake (Peters, Bergman & Elliot, 1983).

The liver contains receptors sensitive to propionate, and nervous pathways are important links between liver and brain, conveying the rate of utilization of propionate (Anil & Forbes, 1980). These findings fit in with the fact that propionate – a ruminant's main substrate for gluconeogenesis – is extensively metabolized by the liver. It is not known how propionate stimulates these receptors. However, this does not imply that these receptors control food intake under physiological conditions, though they may act as a safety mechanism.

To summarize the influence of blood SCFA on meal patterning, intrajugular infusions of SCFA did not affect food intake in the majority of the trials and, if a decrease was observed, non-physiological conditions may have been responsible. Whilst our results suggest that SCFA in hepatic portal blood do not govern meal size or frequency, some other studies showed reduced intake after propionate infusions. Differences in the energy status of the animals, in hypertonicity and rates of infusion may explain only some of the inconsistencies.

Rumen fluid

Considerable research on intraruminal infusions of SCFA was carried out in the 1960s in schedule-fed sheep and cattle (for reviews, see Baile & Forbes, 1974; Papas & Hatfield, 1978). Acetate was usually a potent inhibitor of feed intake, whereas propionate and *n*-butyrate had varying effects. However, experimental conditions were often non-physiological and SCFA in rumen fluid or blood were not measured, even though large doses of chemicals were given.

Intraruminal lactate did not show a convincing influence either (see e.g. Baile & Pfander, 1966). On the other hand, intraduodenal infusions of DL-lactate, at pharmacological doses and without measurement of duodenal or circulating lactate, effectively depressed feeding (Buéno, 1975). Moreover, it is unknown whether duodenal lactate is related to a meal. Therefore, the role of duodenal lactate as a major regulator of normal ruminant feeding seems doubtful.

In the subsequent years work was done on free-feeding ruminants. In freely fed goats, intraruminal infusions of SCFA decreased meal size (Baile & Mayer, 1969; Focant, Gallouin & Leclercq, 1979). Baile and McLaughlin (1970) believed that, in the case of acetate, this effect was mediated by receptors in the wall of the dorsal sac of the reticulorumen. However, Leek (1986) questioned this hypothesis, because very high concentrations were required to activate these ruminal receptors and they are similarly sensitive to acids other than acetic acid. Some points in the investigations of Baile and co-workers are open to criticism (for details see de Jong, 1981*c*; Grovum, 1987). In most studies a control for the sodium content of the SCFA infusions was absent; consequently there were no proper controls for the tonicity of the SCFA solutions. Very large water consumption in these studies confirmed the osmotic load (Baile & Mayer, 1968; Baile & McLaughlin, 1970). The increased tonicity rather than the SCFA themselves could account for the observed decreases in intake (see below). Baile & Mayer (1969), however, demonstrated in a trial of limited value that sodium did not contribute to satiety because sodium propionate and propionic acid caused similar anorexic effects. Furthermore, the infusion rates – during meals only – greatly exceeded that of ruminal SCFA production (see e.g. Baile & Pfander, 1966). The changes in the rumen fluid during and immediately after the infusions are unknown (Baile & Mayer, 1969). It should also be stressed that infusions may cause extreme local changes in the rumen before mixing takes place.

Virtually all studies on the role of SCFA in the control of feeding in ruminants have been conducted on non-lactating animals. In ruminants consuming high amounts of feed, such as high-producing dairy cattle, however, control mechanisms may differ from those in dry animals. Interestingly, Faverdin, Richou & Peyraud (1992) reported that intraruminal infusions of SCFA mixtures suppressed intake in lactating cows but had no significant effects in dry cows. The inhibitory effects on food intake could not be attributed to osmolality changes. These results support the view that the sensitivity of the animal to SCFA depends on its physiological status (Elliot *et al.*, 1985). On the other hand, in lactating cows in late lactation a clear-cut effect on intake was seen after intraruminal infusions of sodium acetate

(Mbanya, Anil & Forbes, 1988). This intake reduction, however, became obvious only at rates that elevated ruminal acetate to at least twice the normal level (Forbes & Barrio, 1992; Anil *et al.*, 1993). In the light of these findings, more research on highly productive cows is needed. In particular, the requirement for a satiety cue (i.e. eating must change the concentration during the meal) should be addressed.

Negative results on the other hand may also be of interest. For instance, in sheep fed a hay ration, satiation was not affected by large increases in ruminal and (presumably) blood SCFA levels induced by the prefeeding of concentrates (Duranton & Buéno, 1985). Furthermore, Phillip, Buchanan-Smith & Grovum (1981) showed that intraruminal infusions of large amounts of acetic acid had no effect on the food intake of sheep. These workers pointed out that changes in ruminal osmolality may play a role in short-term control of feeding. This does not apply to pH and rumen motility. Indeed, intraruminal loads of sodium acetate and sodium propionate were as effective in depressing the intake of hungry sheep as were equimolar loads of sodium chloride (Ternouth & Beattie, 1971; Grovum & Bignell, 1989). The wall of the reticulorumen was the site mediating the anorexic effects of ruminal hypertonicity (Carter & Grovum, 1990). Grovum, one of the first to recognize the possible impact of rumen osmolality in feeding control, suggested that rumen tonicity was a major factor in intake control and refuted SCFA per se as satiety signals. On the other hand, this hypothesis cannot explain the fact that sometimes one sodium SCFA proved more effective in depressing intake than equimolar doses of sodium salts of other SCFA or NaCl. For example, Engku Azahan & Forbes (1992) found in sheep having continuous as well as brief access to food that both sodium chloride and sodium acetate depressed the intake of concentrates (but not of hay). Acetate tended to have a greater and more prolonged anorexic effect. However, the elicited rumen acetate levels were outside the physiological range. In goats receiving partially neutralized SCFA solutions to minimize hypernatraemia, we also observed a marked reduction of intake after intraruminal acetate infusions. These were characterized by long latencies and intermeal intervals as well as a tendency towards a prolonged effect lasting for some hours after the infusion period. Despite precautions, rumen sodium levels rose markedly. Since high ruminal and blood acetate concentrations were required to provoke satiety (de Jong, 1981*c*), a physiological role for ruminal acetate in the regulation of food intake is highly doubtful.

We should note that drinking water was withheld in Grovum's experiments, which could have overemphasized the role of osmolality as a physiological controller of food intake. Furthermore, although rumen osmolality increases during and after large meals, it is unknown whether the tonicity of ruminal fluid is related to eating; are spontaneous meals initiated when tonicity is low and do meals cease when tonicity increases? Finally, osmoreceptors have not been identified so far in the rumen wall.

In conclusion, whilst some researchers suggest that ruminal acetate acts on intake via more than just an osmotic mechanism (Forbes & Barrio, 1992), others hold that the anorexic effects of salts of SCFA are the result of only their osmotic properties (Grovum & Bignell, 1989). More experiments are required to solve this controversy, but – irrespective of the outcome – it should be noted that, in all studies, non-physiological increments in ruminal acetate levels were required, to elicit intake depressions.

Pancreactic hormones

Hormones may act as essential links in satiety. Below, we shall consider briefly the possible involvement of insulin and glucagon in relation to SCFA metabolism in the regulation of food intake (for fuller details of SCFA metabolism and pancreatic hormones, see Chapter 14). Pancreatic hormones are at the centre of metabolic regulation and may thus be important for the regulation of energy balance (Bassett, 1975; Brockman, 1986). The hypothalamus is not only involved in the regulation of food intake and body weight, but also implicated in the regulation of the endocrine pancreas (Woods *et al.*, 1986; Steffens *et al.*, 1990). This emphasizes the significance of insulin and glucagon. There is little evidence that somatostatin and pancreatic polypeptide are normally involved in appetite control (de Jong, 1986).

Insulin

Both in schedule-fed (Bassett, 1972; Mineo *et al.*, 1990*c*) and free-fed (Chase *et al.*, 1977*b*; de Jong, 1981*b*) ruminants, eating induces a small but significant increase in the plasma insulin level. With spontaneous meals this increase frequently occurs as rapidly as that seen in monogastric animals and humans (Fig. 17.1). With schedule-fed ruminants the increase in insulin may be due to meal-induced increases in SCFA (Evans *et al.*, 1975), because peripheral insulinogenic SCFA and insulin levels increase concomitantly. However, acetate can be excluded as a physiological regulator, as an injection of acetate elicits a small response, if any, after only very high doses (Ambo, Takahashi & Tsuda, 1973; Mineo *et al.*, 1990*b*). Furthermore, *n*-valerate and branched-chain fatty acids – though very potent insulinogenic stimuli, even more so than propionate or butyrate (Ambo *et al.*, 1973; Mineo *et al.*, 1990*a*) – are

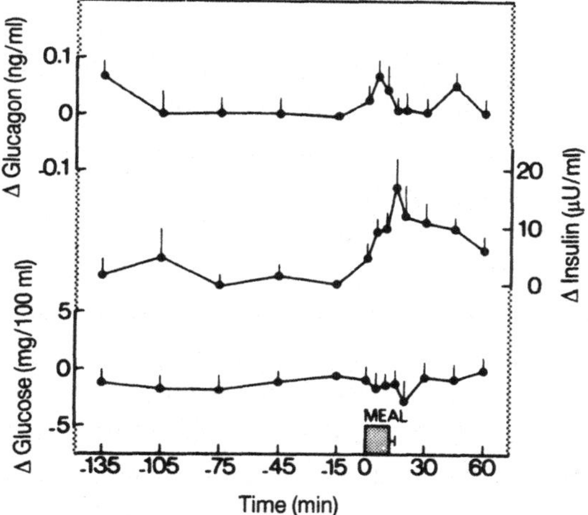

Fig. 17.1. Effect of spontaneous meals on changes in blood glucose, plasma insulin and glucagon concentrations in goats. Mean ± SEM ($n = 5$). Adapted from de Jong (1981*c*).

unlikely to control insulin, because of their extremely low and relatively constant peripheral levels (de Jong, 1982).

While clear-cut effects of large quantities of propionate and butyrate were observed, assessment of physiological relevance remains difficult (Stern, Baile & Mayer, 1970; de Jong, 1982; Bines & Hart, 1984). De Jong (1982) suggested that relative changes in, rather than absolute levels of, peripheral SCFA may be important. This hypothesis was studied in cows maintained on intragastric infusion of SCFA and casein (Istasse *et al.*, 1987). Propionic acid was either infused continuously (to simulate *ad libitum* feeding) or part of it was infused in two 3-h pulses at 12-h intervals (to mimic twice daily feeding). While the intraruminal pulses of propionate – causing six-fold increases in peripheral propionate levels – coincided with sharp peaks in insulin levels, during the continuous infusions plasma insulin was relatively constant. Similarly, in lactating cows clear fluctuations in the levels of ruminal and blood SCFA were prevented by increasing the feeding frequency, which in turn eliminated insulin peaks and, in general, decreased insulin levels (Sutton *et al.*, 1986). Diets favouring greater ruminal propionate production are usually associated with greater insulin concentrations, which supports the view that propionate may, at least to some extent, control insulin secretion. A physiological role of butyrate is questionable, due to its very low peripheral concentrations (Bines & Hart, 1984), although marked fluctuations in peripheral butyrate levels may occur, the insulinogenic properties of pharmacological doses of butyrate are higher than those of propionate (Bassett, 1972; Ambo *et al.*, 1973) and absolute levels rather than the rate of butyrate changes were examined. Chronic intramesenteric (Reynolds, Tyrrell & Armentano, 1992) or intraruminal (Krehbiel, Harmon & Schnieder, 1992) infusions of butyrate in steers failed to affect portal insulin release, despite an approximately four-fold increment in arterial butyrate levels in the latter study.

The above work suggests that the rate of increase in insulinogenic SCFA influences insulin secretion, so that at least in schedule-fed ruminants, these SCFA may stimulate insulin secretion. Of the SCFA, propionate may be the major regulator, although an additive role of the butyrate cannot be excluded. It is surely not the only way in which the insulin release is governed. For instance, the limited role of SCFA becomes clear from work on fattening ruminants. The increase in insulin levels in obese sheep (see below) is unlikely to be caused by insulinogenic SCFA or other insulin-releasing nutrients, because several weeks of excessive food intake, resulting in very high ruminal SCFA production, preceded insulin increments (van der Meerschen-Doizé *et al.*, 1983; McCann, Bergman & Beermann, 1992). Similarly, van der Meerschen-Doizé *et al.* (1984) showed that plasma insulin levels in obese sheep were 25 times those in pair-fed lean sheep. The effect on insulin upon meal initiation in ruminants as well as in monogastrics also appears to be due to a vagal reflex triggered by oral stimulation during eating (de Jong, Strubbe & Steffens, 1977; Faverdin, 1986*a*), as insulin is released – especially during spontaneous meals – almost as soon as eating starts, i.e. before blood SCFA levels are affected (Chase *et al.*, 1977*b*; de Jong, 1981*b*). This was also seen in a sham-fed sheep (Bassett, 1975).

An increase in insulin in response to a meal does not simply imply involvement in the control of feeding; the cause-and-effect relationships must be established. Indeed, insulin may function as part of a feedback mechanism for meal termination. Intrajugular (Deetz & Wangsness, 1981) or intraportal (Deetz *et al.*, 1980) administration of physiological doses of insulin to sheep fed various diets slightly decreased food intake, even though plasma insulin levels were increased for half an hour at most and blood glucose remained unaffected. This also applied to pigs (Anika, Houpt & Houpt, 1980). Insulin depressed the rate of eating in lactating cows fasted overnight (Faverdin, 1986*b*). The reduced intake may be mediated by insulin receptors in brain areas devoid of the blood–brain barrier, e.g. in cerebral microvessels, or be due to an increased rate of peripheral nutrient utilization, e.g. hepatic glucose utilization.

On the other hand, insulin seems to have a function in long-term regulation of intake. In ruminants voluntary food intake begins to decline with fatness

(Graham, 1969; van der Meerschen-Doizé *et al.*, 1982; McCann *et al.*, 1992). As in non-ruminants and humans (Steffens *et al.*, 1990), plasma insulin is strongly correlated with the degree of adiposity and body weight (de Jong, 1981*b*; van der Meerschen-Doizé *et al.*, 1983). In fact, in fattening ruminants the plasma insulin rose and intake declined coincidentally. Changes in other blood parameters were much less marked (van der Meerschen-Doizé *et al.*, 1983; McCann *et al.*, 1992). Woods *et al.* (1986) found that the concentration of insulin in the cerebrospinal fluid reflected blood insulin levels over time. Specific insulin receptors exist in the brain. Moreover, chronic elevation of insulin in the cerebrospinal fluid by intraventricular or peripheral application of small doses of insulin resulted in a depressed intake in monogastrics (Plata-Salaman & Oomura, 1986; Woods *et al.*, 1986), and in some cases in sheep (Rivière & Buéno, 1987). So far we can conclude that insulin is a clear candidate to mediate intake reduction in fat animals. Ruminal and circulating SCFA can probably be excluded as direct regulators of body weight.

Glucagon

Plasma glucagon levels increase in response to feeding in schedule-fed sheep (Bassett, 1972; Mineo *et al.*, 1990*c*), but not in lactating cows (de Boer, Trenkle & Young, 1985; Sutton *et al.*, 1986). Only moderate effects of spontaneous meals on glucagon levels were observed in goats (Fig. 17.1; de Jong, 1981*b*). Although secretion of glucagon, like that of insulin, can be stimulated by manipulating the gut hormones, the autonomic nervous system and nutrients such as SCFA with 3–5 carbon atoms (Bassett, 1975; Brockman, 1982; Mineo *et al.*, 1990*a*), it is still not clear to what extent these factors underlie the meal-induced release of glucagon.

The physiological role of the glucagonogenic SCFA for the regulation of glucagon secretion is difficult to determine, even considering studies that include the determination of peripheral SCFA (Bassett, 1972; de Jong, 1982; Peters *et al.*, 1983; Sano *et al.*, 1993). From many studies it is evident, however, that a regulating function for SCFA is much less likely than in the case of insulin control (Bloom & Edwards, 1985). A role for branched-chain fatty acids in the release of glucagon can be excluded, if only because supraphysiological doses of these SCFA are required to enhance glucagon secretion.

Whilst in monogastric animals and humans pancreatic glucagon may act as a short-term satiety signal (Langhans & Scharrer, 1992), such evidence is very scanty in ruminants. In sheep, intravenous injections of glucagon during spontaneous meals reduced daily food intake (Deetz & Wangsness, 1981). Although blood glucagon immediately after administration was not measured, it should have been within the physiological range. Simultaneous injection of the gluconeogenesis substrate propionate did not enhance this reduction.

Summary

Feeding is a complex behaviour that is finally controlled by the central nervous system, which is responsive to gastrointestinal, metabolic and sensory signals. Teleologically the existence of multiple feedback systems makes sense. Therefore, the decision to start or stop eating depends on the balance of several cues (for review, see Forbes & Barrio, 1992). In the search for such feedback mechanisms it is essential to correlate metabolic and hormonal changes with hunger and satiety.

SCFA presumably play a minor role in controlling short-term food intake in ruminants under normal conditions. Generally, spontaneous meals and changes in plasma or ruminal SCFA do not go hand-in-hand, and there is little evidence that manipulation of blood or ruminal SCFA concentrations influences the initiation or termination of a meal. They may, however, operate as an emergency mechanism, e.g. under certain conditions in high-producing dairy cows or in schedule-fed ruminants eating very large meals. On the other hand, compelling evidence was found that tonicity of ruminal fluid is involved in satiety. Much of the observed anorexic effects of rumen SCFA can be attributed to an increase in rumen tonicity.

Pancreatic hormones may mediate SCFA-elicited satiety. Whilst insulin may function as a short-term satiety signal, for glucagon such evidence is very scanty in herbivores. As regards insulin secretion, the rate of increase of propionate and perhaps butyrate levels may act as a physiological control. A physiological role for glucagonogenic SCFA is less likely, in spite of clear-cut pharmacological effects. In the case of large meals, SCFA may evoke satiety via insulin. In long-term regulation, insulin may act as an adiposity signal, causing ruminants to eat less when fat than when thin.

References

Adams, G. B. & Forbes, J. M. (1982). Metabolite levels in hepatic portal blood of sheep during *ad libitum* feeding. *Journal of Physiology*, **330**, 47P–48P.

Ambo, K., Takahashi, H. & Tsuda, T. (1973). Effects of feeding and infusion of short-chain volatile fatty acids and glucose on plasma insulin and blood glucose levels in sheep. *Tohoku Journal of Agricultural Research*, **24**, 54–62.

Anika, S. M., Houpt, T. R. & Houpt, K. A. (1980). Insulin as a satiety hormone. *Physiology and Behavior*, **25**, 21–3.

Anil, M. H. & Forbes, J. M. (1980). Feeding in sheep during intraportal infusions of short-chain fatty acids and the effect of liver denervation. *Journal of Physiology*, **298**, 407–14.

Anil, M. H., Mbanya, J. N., Symonds, H. W. & Forbes, J. M. (1993). Responses in the voluntary intake of hay or silage by lactating cows to intraruminal infusions of sodium acetate or sodium propionate, the tonicity of rumen fluid or rumen distension. *British Journal of Nutrition*, **69**, 699–712.

Baile, C. A. (1971). Metabolites as feedbacks for control of feed intake and receptor sites in goats and sheep. *Physiology and Behavior*, **7**, 819–26.

Baile, C. A. & Forbes, J. M. (1974). Control of feed intake and regulation of energy balance in ruminants. *Physiological Reviews*, **54**, 160–214.

Baile, C. A. & Mayer, J. (1968). Effects of intravenous versus intraruminal injections of acetate on feed intake of goats. *Journal of Dairy Science*, **51**, 1490–4.

Baile, C. A. & Mayer, J. (1969). Depression of feed intake of goats by metabolites injected during meals. *American Journal of Physiology*, **217**, 1830–6.

Baile, C. A. & McLaughlin, C. L. (1970). Feed intake of goats during volatile fatty acid injections into four gastric areas. *Journal of Dairy Science*, **53**, 1058–63.

Baile, C. A. & Pfander, W. H. (1966). A possible chemosensitive regulatory mechanism of ovine feed intake. *American Journal of Physiology*, **210**, 1243–8.

Baldwin, B. A. (1985). Neural and hormonal mechanisms regulating food intake. *Proceedings of the Nutrition Society*, **44**, 303–11.

Barnes, R. J., Comline, R. S. & Dobson, A. (1986). The control of splanchnic blood flow. In *Control of Digestion and Metabolism in Ruminants*, ed. L. P. Milligan, W. L. Grovum & A. Dobson, pp. 41–59. Englewood Cliffs, NJ: Prentice-Hall.

Bassett, J. M. (1972). Plasma glucagon concentrations in sheep; their regulation and relation to concentrations of insulin and growth hormone. *Australian Journal of Biological Sciences*, **25**, 1277–87.

Bassett, J. M. (1975). Dietary and gastro-intestinal control of hormones regulating carbohydrate metabolism in ruminants. In *Digestion and Metabolism in the Ruminant*, ed. I. W. McDonald & A. C. I. Warner, pp. 383–98. Armidale: The University of New England Publishing Unit.

Bines, J. A. & Hart, I. C. (1984). The response of plasma insulin and other hormones to intraruminal infusion of VFA mixtures in cattle. *Canadian Journal of Animal Science*, **64** (Suppl.), 304–5.

Bloom, S. R. & Edwards, A. V. (1985). Pancreatic neuroendocrine responses to butyrate in conscious sheep. *Journal of Physiology*, **364**, 281–8.

Bragg, D. St A., Murphy, M. R. & Davis, C. L. (1986). Effect of source of carbohydrate and frequency of feeding on rumen parameters in dairy steers. *Journal of Dairy Science*, **69**, 392–402.

Brockman, R. P. (1982). Insulin and glucagon responses in plasma to intraportal infusions of propionate and butyrate in sheep (*Ovis aries*). *Comparative Biochemistry and Physiology*, **73A**, 237–8.

Brockman, R. P. (1986). Pancreatic and adrenal hormonal regulation of metabolism. In *Control of Digestion and Metabolism in Ruminants*, ed. L. P. Milligan, W. L. Grovum & A. Dobson, pp. 405–19. Englewood Cliffs, NJ: Prentice-Hall.

Buéno, L. (1975). Rôle de l'acide DL-lactique dans le contrôle de l'ingestion alimentaire chez le mouton. *Annales de Recherches vétérinaires*, **6**, 325–36.

Carter, R. R. & Grovum, W. L. (1990). Factors affecting the voluntary intake of food by sheep. 5. The inhibitory effect of hypertonicity in the rumen. *British Journal of Nutrition*, **64**, 285–99.

Chase, L. E., Wangsness, P. J., Kavanaugh, J. F., Griel, L. C. Jr. & Gahagan, J. H. (1977*a*). Changes in portal blood metabolites and insulin with feeding steers twice daily. *Journal of Dairy Science*, **60**, 403–9.

Chase, L. E., Wangsness, P. J. & Martin, R. J. (1977*b*). Portal blood insulin and metabolite changes with spontaneous feeding in steers. *Journal of Dairy Science*, **60**, 410–15.

Conrad, H. R. (1966). Symposium on factors influencing the voluntary intake of herbage by ruminants: physiological and physical factors limiting feed intake. *Journal of Animal Science*, **25**, 227–35.

de Boer, G., Trenkle, A. & Young, J. W. (1985). Glucagon, insulin, growth hormone, and some metabolites during energy restriction ketonemia of lactating cows. *Journal of Dairy Science*, **68**, 326–37.

Deetz, L. E. & Wangsness, P. J. (1981). Influence of intrajugular administration of insulin, glucagon and propionate on voluntary feed intake of sheep. *Journal of Animal Science*, **53**, 427–33.

Deetz, L. E., Wangsness, P. J., Kavanaugh, J. F. & Griel, L. C. Jr (1980). Effect of intraportal and continuous intrajugular administration of insulin on feeding in sheep. *Journal of Nutrition*, **110**, 1983–91.

de Jong, A. (1981*a*). The effect of feed intake on nutrient and hormone levels in jugular and portal blood in goats. *Journal of Agricultural Science, Cambridge*, **96**, 643–57.

de Jong, A. (1981*b*). Short- and long-term effects of eating on blood composition in free-feeding goats. *Journal of Agricultural Science, Cambridge*, **96**, 659–68.

de Jong, A. (1981*c*). Regulation of food intake in the goat: circulating metabolites and hormones in relation to eating. PhD thesis, State University of Groningen, Groningen.

de Jong, A. (1982). Patterns of plasma concentrations of insulin and glucagon after intravascular and intraruminal administration of volatile fatty acids in the goat. *Journal of Endocrinology*, **92**, 357–70.

de Jong, A. (1986). The role of metabolites and hormones as feedbacks in the control of food intake in ruminants. In *Control of Digestion and Metabolism in Ruminants*, ed. L. P. Milligan, W. L. Grovum & A. Dobson, pp. 459–78. Englewood Cliffs, NJ: Prentice-Hall.

de Jong, A. (1987). Metabolic and endocrine controls of food intake in ruminants. In *Physiological and Pharmacological Aspects of the Reticulo-Rumen*, ed. L. A. A. Ooms, A. D. Degryse & A. S. J. P. A. M. van Miert, pp. 171–97. Dordrecht: Martinus Nijhoff.

de Jong, A., Steffens, A. B. & de Ruiter, L. (1981). Effects of portal volatile fatty acid infusions on meal patterns and blood composition in goats. *Physiology and Behavior*, **27**, 683–9.

de Jong, A., Strubbe, J. H. & Steffens, A. B. (1977). Hypothalamic influence on insulin and glucagon release in the rat. *American Journal of Physiology*, **233**, E380–E388.

Duranton, A. & Buéno, L. (1985). Influence of regimen (roughage vs. concentrates) on satiety and forestomach motility in sheep. *Physiology and Behavior*, **35**, 105–8.

Elliot, J. M., Symonds, H. W. & Pike, B. (1985). Effect on feed intake of infusing sodium propionate or sodium acetate into a mesenteric vein of cattle. *Journal of Dairy Science*, **68**, 1165–70.

Engku Azahan, E. A. & Forbes, J. M. (1992). Effects of intraruminal infusions of sodium salts on selection of hay and concentrate foods by sheep. *Appetite*, **18**, 143–54.

Evans, E., Buchanan-Smith, J. G. & MacLeod, G. K. (1975). Postprandial patterns of plasma glucose, insulin and volatile fatty acids in ruminants fed low- and high-roughage diets. *Journal of Animal Science*, **41**, 1474–9.

Faverdin, P. (1986*a*). Variations de l'insulinémie en début de repas chez la vache en lactation. *Reproduction, Nutrition, Development*, **26**, 381–2.

Faverdin, P. (1986*b*). Injections de doses physiologiques d'insuline chez la vache en lactation: effets sur les quantités ingérées et les métabolites sanguins. *Reproduction, Nutrition, Development*, **26**, 383–4.

Faverdin, P., Richou, B. & Peyraud, J. L. (1992). Effects of digestive infusions of volatile fatty acids or glucose on food intake in lactating or dry cows. *Annales de Zootechnie*, **41**, 93.

Focant, M., Gallouin, F. & Leclercq, M. (1979). Volatile fatty acids and rumination in the goat. *Annales de Recherches vétérinaires*, **10**, 226–8.

Forbes, J. M. (1992). Metabolic aspects of satiety. *Proceedings of the Nutrition Society*, **51**, 13–19.

Forbes, J. M. & Barrio, J. P. (1992). Abdominal chemo- and mechanosensitivity in ruminants and its role in the control of food intake. *Experimental Physiology*, **77**, 27–50.

Graham, N. C. Mc. (1969). The influence of body weight (fatness) on the energetic efficiency of adult sheep. *Australian Journal of Agricultural Research*, **20**, 375–85.

Grovum, W. L. (1987). A new look at what is controlling food intake. In *Feed Intake by Beef Cattle*, ed. F. N. Owens, pp. 1–40. Stillwater: Oklahoma State University.

Grovum, W. L. & Bignell, W. W. (1989). Results refuting volatile fatty acids per se as signals of satiety in ruminants. *Proceedings of the Nutrition Society*, **48**, 3A.

Istasse, L. Hovell, F. D. DeB., MacLeod, N. A. & Ørskov, E. R. (1987). The effects of continuous or intermittent infusion of propionic acid on plasma insulin and milk yield in dairy cows nourished by intragastric infusion of nutrients. *Livestock Production Science*, **16**, 201–14.

Ketelaars, J. & Tolkamp, B. (1991). Toward a new theory of feed intake regulation in ruminants. PhD thesis, Agricultural University Wageningen, Wageningen.

Krehbiel, C. R., Harmon, D. L. & Schnieder, J. E. (1992). Effect of increasing ruminal butyrate on portal and hepatic nutrient flux in steers. *Journal of Animal Science*, **70**, 904–14.

Langhans, W. & Scharrer, E. (1992). Metabolic control of eating. *World Review of Nutrition and Dietetics*, **70**, 1–67.

Leek, B. F. (1986). Sensory receptors in the ruminant alimentary tract. In *Control of Digestion and Metabolism in Ruminants*, ed. L. P. Milligan, W. L. Grovum & A. Dobson, pp. 3–17. Englewood Cliffs, NJ: Prentice-Hall.

Mbanya, J. N., Anil, M. H. & Forbes, J. M. (1988). Effects of intraruminal infusions of sodium acetate on silage intake by dairy cows. *Proceedings of the Nutrition Society*, **47**, 177A.

McCann, J. P., Bergman, E. N. & Beermann, D. H. (1992). Dynamic and static phases of severe dietary obesity in sheep: food intakes, endocrinology and carcass and organ chemical composition. *Journal of Nutrition*, **122**, 496–505.

Mineo, H., Kanai, M., Kato, S. & Ushijima, J.-I. (1990*a*). Effects of intravenous injection of butyrate, valerate and their isomers on endocrine pancreatic responses in conscious sheep (*Ovis aries*). *Comparative Biochemistry and Physiology*, **95A**, 411–16.

Mineo, H., Kitade, A., Kawakami, S., Kato, S. & Ushijima, J. (1990*b*). Effect of intravenous injection of acetate on the pancreas of sheep. *Research in Veterinary Science*, **48**, 310–13.

Mineo, H., Oyamada, T., Yasuda, T., Akiyama, M., Kato, S. & Ushijima, J.-I. (1990*c*). Effect of feeding frequency on plasma glucose, insulin and glucagon concentrations in sheep. *Japanese Journal of Zootechnical Science*, **61**, 411–16.

Papas, A. & Hatfield, E. E. (1978). Effect of oral and abomasal administration of volatile fatty acids on voluntary feed intake of growing lambs. *Journal of Animal Science*, **46**, 288–96.

Peters, J. P., Bergman, E. N. & Elliot, J. M. (1983). Changes of glucose, insulin and glucagon associated with propionate infusion and vitamin B-12 status in sheep. *Journal of Nutrition*, **113**, 1229–40.

Phillip, L. E., Buchanan-Smith, J. G. & Grovum, W. L. (1981). Effects of infusing the rumen with acetic acid and nitrogenous constituents in maize silage extracts on food intake, ruminal osmolality and blood acid-base balance in sheep. *Journal of Agricultural Science, Cambridge*, **96**, 429–38.

Plata-Salaman, C. R. & Oomura, Y. (1986). Effect of intra-third ventricular administration of insulin on food intake after food deprivation. *Physiology and Behavior*, **37**, 735–40.

Rayner, D. V. (1992). Gastrointestinal satiety in animals other than man. *Proceedings of the Nutrition Society*, **51**, 1–6.

Reynolds, C. K., Tyrrell, H. F. & Armentano, L. E. (1992). Effects of mesenteric vein *n*-butyrate infusion on liver metabolism by beef steers. *Journal of Animal Science*, **70**, 2250–61.

Rivière, P. & Buéno, L. (1987). Influence of regimen and insulinemia on orexigenic effects of GRF 1-44 in sheep. *Physiology and Behavior*, **39**, 347–50.

Robinson, P. H., Tamminga, S. & van Vuuren, A. M. (1986). Influence of declining level of feed intake and varying the proportion of starch in the concentrate on rumen fermentation in dairy cows. *Livestock Production Science*, **15**, 173–89.

Sano, H., Hattori, N., Todome, Y., Tsuruoka, F., Takahashi, H. & Terashima, Y. (1993). Plasma insulin and glucagon responses to intravenous infusion of propionate and their autonomic control in sheep. *Journal of Animal Science*, **71**, 3414–22.

Silver, A. J. & Morley, J. E. (1991). Role of CCK in regulation of food intake. *Progress in Neurobiology*, **36**, 23–34.

Simkins, K. L. Jr, Suttie, J. W. & Baumgardt, B. R. (1965). Regulation of food intake in ruminants. 3. Variation in blood and rumen metabolites in relation to food intake. *Journal of Dairy Science*, **48**, 1629–34.

Steffens, A. B., Strubbe, J. H., Balkan, B. & Scheurink, A. J. W. (1990). Neuroendocrine mechanisms involved in the regulation of body weight, food intake and metabolism. *Neuroscience & Biobehavioural Reviews*, **14**, 305–19.

Stern, J. S., Baile, C. A. & Mayer, J. (1970). Are propionate and butyrate physiological regulators of plasma insulin in ruminants? *American Journal of Physiology*, **219**, 84–91.

Sutton, J. D., Hart, I. C., Broster, W. H., Elliot, R. J. & Schuller, E. (1986). Feeding frequency for lactating cows: effects on rumen fermentation and blood metabolites and hormones. *British Journal of Nutrition*, **56**, 181–92.

Ternouth, J. H. & Beattie, A. W. (1971). Studies of the food intake of sheep at a single meal. *British Journal of Nutrition*, **25**, 153–65.

Theurer, C. B. & Wanderley, R. C. (1987). Role of absorbed nutrients in feed intake control. In *Feed Intake by Beef Cattle*, ed. F. N. Owens, pp. 275–89. Stillwater: Oklahoma State University.

van der Meerschen-Doizé, F., Bouchat, J.-C., Bouckoms-van der Meir, M.-A. & Paquay, R. (1983). Effects of long-term *ad libitum* feeding on plasma lipid components and blood glucose, β-hydroxybutyrate and insulin concentrations in lean adult sheep. *Reproduction, Nutrition, Development*, **23**, 51–63.

van der Meerschen-Doizé, F., Bouchat, J. C., Bouckoms-van der Meir, M.-A. & Paquay, R. (1984). Influence of the state of fatness on body composition and blood constituents (lipids, glucose, ketone bodies and insulin) in adult sheep. *Journal of Animal Physiology and Nutrition*, **52**, 105–12.

van der Meerschen-Doizé, F., Bouckoms-van der Meir, M.-A. & Paquay, R. (1982). Effects of long-term *ad libitum* feeding on the voluntary food intake, body weight, body composition and adipose tissue morphology of lean adult sheep. *Reproduction, Nutrition, Development*, **22**, 1049–60.

Woods, S. C., Taborsky, G. J. Jr & Porte, D. Jr (1986). CNS control of nutrient homeostasis. In *Handbook of Physiology, Section 1: The Nervous System*, vol. IV, ed. F. Bloom, pp. 365–411. Bethesda, MD: American Physiological Society.

18

Effects of butyrate on cell proliferation and gene expression

J. KRUH, N. DEFER AND L. TICHONICKY

Introduction

Butyrate presents several unexpected properties when added to cells in culture and also *in vivo*. The main effects can be summarized as follows:

Arrest of cell proliferation;
Alteration of cell morphology and ultrastructure;
Alteration of gene expression.

It is important to note that all the effects of butyrate are reversible. Shortly after the removal of butyrate from the medium, the cells recover their initial molecular and cellular characteristics. Furthermore, the other short-chain fatty acids (SCFA) are much less effective or not effective at all in cell growth and gene expression.

Butyrate strongly inhibits histone deacetylases, which results in hyper-acetylation of histones. It has been postulated that this is the mechanism of action of butyrate (Kruh, 1982). In this chapter we emphasize the more recent studies.

Effect on cell proliferation

Butyrate reduces the cell growth rate of Chinese hamster ovary (CHO) cells (Wright, 1972), of chick fibroblasts and HeLa cells (Hagopian *et al.*, 1977) and of myoblasts (Leibovitch & Kruh, 1979). The addition of butyrate to cell cultures leads to an arrest of cell growth at the G_1 phase of the cell cycle (d'Anna *et al.*, 1980*a*). This observation was confirmed by us on HTC cells. A time-lapse cinematography study showed that the arrest of the cells in cell cycle occurred at a specific step, immediately after mitosis, at early G_1. In addition, butyrate did not alter the interphase duration after removal of the compound, indicating that butyrate could be used for cell growth synchronization (van Wijk, Tichonicky & Kruh, 1981). Human breast cancer cells accumulated at the G_0/G_1 phase when treated with butyrate (Guilbaud *et al.*, 1990; Planchon *et al.*, 1991).

The butyrate-induced arrest of cell growth could at least partly result from an effect of this compound on gene expression. In Swiss 3T3 cells, butyrate reduced the expression of c-*myc*, of p53 and of thymidine kinase, and increased the expression of c-*fos* (Toscani, Soprano & Soprano, 1988). Butyrate inhibited the expression of CDC2, a gene involved in the control of cell proliferation (Charollais, Bucket & Mester, 1990).

Butyrate is able to induce proteins specific to non-dividing cells. It induces histone $H1^0$ in neuroblastoma cells (Hall & Cole, 1986). Histone H1 is usually phosphorylated in proliferating cells. Butyrate treatment of CHO cells produced a dephosphorylation of H1 (d'Anna, Tobey & Gurley, 1980*b*).

Effect of gene expression

Butyrate is able to alter the expression of many genes.

Haemoglobin

Butyrate induced the synthesis of haemoglobin in murine erythroleukaemia cells infected with Friend virus (Leder & Leder, 1975). Butyrate was able to enhance the transcription of human globin gene cluster injected into *Xenopus* (Partington, Yarwood & Rutherford, 1984). In general, butyrate induces the synthesis of fetal and embryonic haemoglobins and has no effect on, or even inhibits, the synthesis of adult haemoglobin. In human cord blood erythroid progenitors treated with α-aminobutyric acid, the synthesis of γ-globin was stimulated whereas the synthesis of β-globin was inhibited (Perrine *et al.*, 1987). Injection of butyrate increased 5–10-fold the expression of the embryonic globin gene in the Leghorn chicken (Ginder, Whitters & Pohlman, 1984). When injected into fetal lambs *in utero*, butyrate delayed or even suppressed the switch from fetal to adult haemoglobin (Perrine *et al.*, 1988).

Butyrate or α-aminobutyrate, when administered for 5 days to normal or anaemic baboons, increased the level of fetal haemoglobin 5 times. The same effect was observed in baboon erythroid progenitor cell cultures (Constantoulakis, Papayannopoulou & Stomatoyannopoulos, 1988). Butyrate stimulated the expression of the human γ-globin gene transfected into mouse erythroleukaemia cells, as well as that of the endogenous embryonic haemoglobin gene (Zhang *et al.*, 1990). The embryonic globin gene was induced with butyrate in erythroleukaemia cells transfected with chicken globin genes.

This induction required the presence of a 5′-flanking sequence extending from −569 to −725 base pairs upstream from the gene CAP site (Glauber *et al.*, 1991).

The importance of these observations relies on the possible use of butyrate or an analogue in human therapeutics, more precisely in β-thalassaemia and in sickle cell anaemia, since an elevated production of fetal haemoglobin could strongly improve the clinical symptoms of these diseases. Butyrate and α-aminobutyrate, when added to erythroid progenitors of patients, increased the fetal haemoglobin expression from 7 to 30%, which is sufficient for ameliorating clinical symptoms (Perrine *et al.*, 1989). Recently, humans with sickle cell anaemia or β-thalassaemia were perfused for one week with butyrate. A strong rise in γ-globin was observed without any toxic symptoms (Olivieri *et al.*, 1991).

Other proteins

Butyrate is able to induce the synthesis of a number of proteins, including peptidic and glycoprotein hormones and hormone receptors. An ectopic synthesis has often been observed. In contrast, butyrate inhibits the expression of proteins in cells in which its level is high. In general, butyrate acts at the level of specific mRNAs, mainly by altering gene transcription (Table 18.1).

Hormone-induced protein synthesis

Several hormones are able to induce protein synthesis by acting in most cases at a pre-translational level. In general, butyrate inhibits the induction without altering the number of hormone receptors and the hormone-binding characteristics (Table 18.2).

Effect on cell morphology and ultrastructure

Butyrate induces morphological modifications in cells. The nature of the modifications varies from one cell type to another; however, they have several common features. These modifications are at least partly related to the effects of butyrate on the cytoskeleton and on the external matrix. When added to cancer cells, butyrate often induces cell differentiation and the reappearance of a differential structure. These modifications are prevented by cycloheximide and actinomycin which is consistent with an effect of butyrate on transcription and protein synthesis.

In many cell types butyrate treatment results in the appearance of

Table 18.1. *Effect of butyrate on gene expression. Butyrate induces synthesis (↗) of several specific proteins in cells in which synthesis is low, and inhibits synthesis (↘) in cells in which it is high*

Protein	Cell type	Reference
Pituitary glycoprotein hormones		
↗ FSH, hCG	HeLa cells	Ghosh & Cox (1977); Ghosh *et al.* (1977)
↗ hCG	Chago cells	Chou *et al.* (1977)
↘ hCG	Trophoblastic cells	Chou *et al.* (1977)
Other hormones		
↗ Insulin, glucagon	Insulinoma cells	Philipe *et al.* (1987)
↗ Calcitonin	Thyroid carcinoma cells	Nakagawa *et al.* (1988)
↘ Calcitonin-related protein	Thyroid carcinoma cells	Nakagawa *et al.* (1988)
Hormone receptors		
↘ Thyroid hormone receptor	Rat pituitary cells	Samuels *et al.* (1980); Lazar (1990)
↗ Thyroid hormone receptor	Hepatocytes, hepatomas, fibroblasts	Matsuhashi *et al.* (1987)
↘ Insulin receptors	Glial cells	Montiel *et al.* (1989)
↗ Insulin receptors	Lymphoma cells	Newman *et al.* (1989)
↗ β-Adrenergic receptors	HeLa cells	Tallman *et al.* (1977); Kassis (1985)
↘ Oestrogen receptor	Human mammary cancer cells	Stevens *et al.* (1984); Planchon *et al.* (1991)
Alkaline phosphatase		
↗ (Intestinal form)	Human colon cells	Herz *et al.* (1981)
↗ (Placental form)	Human rectal cancer cells	Morita *et al.* (1982)
	Choriocarcinoma cells	Ito & Chou (1984)
Metallothionein		
↗	Rat hepatoma cells	Birren & Herschman (1986)
↗	Teratocarcinoma cells	Andrews & Adamson (1987)

FSH, follicle stimulating hormone; hCG, human chorionic gonadotrophin.

fibroblastic-type cells, which display long membranous processes (Henneberry & Fishman, 1976). In HTC cells, which display a polygonal shape, we observed a loss of contiguity, elongation and formation of protrusions. As early as 1 h after the addition of butyrate, the nucleoli became larger, with more diffuse granules. Later, irregular-shaped nuclei were observed (Guillouzo *et al.*, 1980). When treated with butyrate, F9 embryonal carcinoma cells changed from a typical stem-cell morphology to a flat polygonal shape with processes at each angle, simultaneously with the production of plasminogen activator and other differentiation markers (Kosaka *et al.*, 1991). In pancreatic adenocarcinoma cells, addition of butyrate induced a secretory differentiation with increase in the rough endoplasmic reticulum and Golgi apparatus and

Table 18.2. *Hormone-induced protein synthesis*

Protein	Hormone	Cell type	Reference
Ovalbumin, transferrin	Oestradiol	Chick embryo oviduct cells	McKnight *et al.* (1980)
Tyrosine amino transferase	Glucocorticoid	HTC cells	Tichonicky *et al.* (1981)
Glycerol phosphate dehydrogenase	Glucocorticoid	Glial cells	Kumar *et al.* (1985)
Growth hormone	Thyroid hormone	Pituitary cells	Cattini *et al.* (1988)
Casein	Prolactin	Mammary explants	Martel *et al.* (1983)

progressive appearance of an intracellular lumen (Mullins, Kern & Metzgar, 1991). Restoration of the cytoskeleton and external matrix was observed in many cell types: kidney cells transformed by sarcoma virus (Altenburg, Via & Steiner, 1976), hepatoma cells (Borenfreund *et al.*, 1980), rat kidney cells (Hayman, Engvall & Ruoslahti, 1980) and human pancreatic carcinoma cells (Bryant *et al*, 1986).

Butyrate has a strong effect on cell surface mucopolysaccharides, glycolipids and glycoconjugates, which correlates with the loss of malignant characteristics, as observed in cultured chondrocytes (Bretton & Pennypacker, 1989), murine sarcoma virus (MSV)-transformed kidney cells (Via *et al.*, 1980) and pancreatic tumour cells (Bloom *et al.*, 1989).

Many of the effects of butyrate – arrest of cell growth, induction of molecular and cellular differentiation of the cytoskeleton and external matrix, decrease in tumorigenicity – result in a loss of most of the malignant characteristics of the cancerous cell. Butyrate is therefore a potential drug for cancer therapy.

Effect on the oncogene expression

Butyrate modulates the expression of several oncogenes. It inhibits the expression of c-*myc* in 3T3 cells (Toscani *et al.*, 1988), in Burkitt lymphoma cells (Polack *et al.*, 1987) and in rectal carcinoma cells (Herold & Rothberg, 1988). It acts at the mRNA level. This effect of butyrate is independent of its effect on cell growth (Tichonicky, Kruh & Defer, 1990).

Butyrate induces c-*fos* expression in a variety of cells: Swiss 3T3 cells (Toscani *et al.*, 1988), pheochromocytoma cells (Naranjo *et al.*, 1990) and HTC cells, in which this induction is independent of the cell-cycle phase (Tichonicky *et al.*, 1990). Butyrate increases c-*erb* A oncogene expression in human colon fibroblasts (Bahn, Zeller & Smith, 1988).

In colon carcinoma cells, butyrate reduces the level of $pp60^{c\text{-}src}$ and $p56^{lck}$; this diminution is associated with the induced cell differentiation (Foss *et al.*, 1989). Butyrate suppresses the transforming activity of an activated N-*ras* oncogene in human colon carcinoma cells (Stoddart, Lane & Niles, 1989).

Mechanism of action

Chromatin protein acetylation

Butyrate causes a hyperacetylation of histones (Riggs *et al.*, 1977; Vidali *et al.*, 1978), due to a strong inhibition of histone deacetylases (Sealy & Chalkley, 1978*a*). These observations were confirmed in a great variety of cell types. It is usually admitted that histone acetylation results in gene activation (Csordas, 1990). Chromatin containing highly acetylated histones, when transcribed by *Escherichia coli* or HeLa cell RNA polymerases, presents an increase in template activity (Dobson & Ingram, 1980).

Chromatin protein phosphorylation

Butyrate inhibits phosphorylation of histone H1 and H2A in HeLa cells (Boffa, Gruss & Allfrey, 1981). In these cells, butyrate enhances the phosphorylation of two other chromatin proteins: HMG14 and 17 (Levy-Wilson, 1981).

DNA methylation

A small fraction of cytosine is methylated in DNA. In a human embryonic lung fibroblast culture, butyrate caused a hypermethylation of cytosine: 6% instead of 3% cytosine became methylated (de Haan, Gevers & Parker, 1986). Azacytidine inhibits DNA methylation. In Leghorn chickens, azacytidine increased 5–10-fold the level of embryonic globin mRNA (Ginder *et al.*, 1984). The combination of azacytidine and α-aminobutyrate resulted in synergistic induction of fetal haemoglobin in the adult baboon (Constantoulakis *et al.*, 1988).

Chromatin structure and expression

Butyrate alters chromatin structure in such a way that it increases the sensitivity to DNase I and micrococcal nuclease, as shown in HeLa cells (Mathis *et al.*, 1978) and in HTC cells (Sealy & Chalkley, 1978*b*; Kitzis *et al.*, 1980). This alteration was confirmed by calorimetric study of the thermal transition (Touchette, Anton & Cole, 1986).

Butyrate induces alterations of the mRNA population in myoblasts (Leibovitch *et al.*, 1982) and in HTC cells (Raymondjean, Tichonicky & Kruh, 1985). We found in both cases a strong modification of the hybridization kinetics of the RNA in butyrate-treated cells as compared to untreated cells.

Since butyrate acts on a limited number of genes and since butyrate is able to inhibit the expression of several genes, mechanisms involving global modifications of chromatin proteins and changes in chromatin structure cannot explain the discrete alteration of gene expression induced by butyrate. Other mechanisms have to be involved to explain the butyrate effects.

Relation between butyrate and other morphogenic and anti-tumour compounds

Butyrate could modulate the effect of such compounds.

Retinoic acid

Butyrate and retinoic acid both inhibit the proliferation of human retinoblastoma in a synergistic fashion and could be used in therapeutics (Kyristis, Joseph & Chader, 1984). Butyrate and retinoic acid produce a partial remission of acute myelogenous leukaemia (Novogrodsky, Dvir & Ravid, 1983). Both butyrate and retinoic acid act synergistically on the differentiation of myeloid leukaemia cells (Breitman & He, 1990).

Hormone D_3

This derivative of vitamin D_3 suppresses colony formation in soft agar and increases the alkaline phosphate activity in rat osteosarcoma cells. These effects are enhanced by butyrate (Yoneda, Aya & Sakuda, 1984). Hormone D_3 greatly enhances the butyrate-induced enterocyte differentiation of human colonic carcinoma cells (Tanaka *et al.* 1990).

Interferons

Interferons have an anti-tumour effect on mice inoculated with sarcoma cells. The survival of these mice is strongly prolonged when both interferon and butyrate are used (Bourgeade, Cerruti & Chany, 1979). Butyrate enhances the antiviral effect of interferon on MSV-transformed hamster cells (Bourgeade & Chany, 1979).

Effect of butyrate on gene promoters and regulators

DNA sequences flanking the genes induced by butyrate could be required for butyrate action. In K562 cells, the CAT box is involved in γ-globin induction. After transfection of DNA in murine erythroleukaemia cells, the induction of chicken embryonic globin requires a DNA sequence from -569 to -725 base pairs (Glauber *et al.*, 1991). The activation of the human immunodeficiency virus requires the presence of the LTR sequence (Bohan, York & Srinavasan, 1987) and of the TATA box (Golub, Li & Volski, 1991).

These observations strongly suggest that butyrate could be a cofactor of transacting proteins that regulate the expression of genes. Such a mechanism of action would explain the specific effects of butyrate on the expression of a limited number of genes. However, more experiments are required to assess the importance of this mechanism.

Therapeutic use of butyrate

Sodium butyrate has been considered for therapeutic use in two types of diseases: haematological diseases and cancer.

In the haematological diseases β-thalassaemia and sickle-cell anaemia, clinical trials have been initiated to take advantage of the induction by butyrate of fetal haemoglobin. High doses are required (infusion of 500–1500 mg/kg per day); toxicity is low; however, very high doses are associated with a neuropathological picture.

In cancer and more precisely leukaemia, advantage is taken of the specific properties of butyrate on cell proliferation and differentiation. The need for high doses of butyrate results from its rapid degradation. Butyrate derivatives that are more stable and possibly more active would be highly welcome. Several such derivatives have been described and stable butyrate derivatives have been synthesized. The most active are the monoacetone glucose 3-butyrate and monoacetone glucose 6-butyrate. These compounds presented a low-level toxicity and high anti-tumour activity in mice inoculated with Crocker tumour cells (Pouillart *et al.*, 1990; Planchon *et al.*, 1991). With the same mice, 1-octylbutyrate and poly(ethylene glycol) dibutyrate gave anti-tumour protection (Wakselman, Cerruti & Chany, 1990).

Pivalyloxymethyl butyrate inhibited the proliferation of leukaemia cells and increased the survival of mice with lung carcinoma primary cancer (Rephaeli *et al.*, 1991).

It is clear that the study of butyrate, initiated some 15 years ago, is far from being terminated.

References

Altenburg, B. C., Via, D. P. & Steiner, S. H. (1976). Modification of the phenotype of murine sarcoma virus-transformed cells by sodium butyrate. *Experimental Cell Research*, **102**, 223–31.

Andrews, G. K. & Adamson, E. D. (1987). Butyrate selectively activates the metallothionein gene in teratocarcinoma cells and influences hypersensitivity to metal induction. *Nucleic Acids Research*, **15**, 5461–75.

Bahn, R. S., Zeller, J. C. & Smith, T. J. (1988). Butyrate increases c-*erb* A oncogene expression in human colon fibroblasts. *Biochemical and Biophysical Research Communications*, **150**, 259–62.

Birren, B. W. & Herschman, H. R. (1986). Regulation of the rat metallothionein I gene by sodium butyrate. *Nucleic Acids Research*, **14**, 853–67.

Bloom, E. J., Siddiqui, B., Hicks, J. W. & Kim, Y. S. (1989). Effect of sodium butyrate, a differentiating agent, on cell surface glycoconjugates of a human pancreatic cell line. *Pancreas*, **4**, 59–64.

Boffa, L. C., Gruss, R. J. & Allfrey, V. G. (1981). Manifold effects of sodium butyrate on nuclear function. *Journal of Biological Chemistry*, **256**, 9612–21.

Bohan, C., York, D. & Srinavasan, A. (1987). Sodium butyrate activates human immunodeficiency virus long terminal repeat-directed expression. *Biochemical and Biophysical Research Communications*, **148**, 899–905.

Borenfreund, E., Schmid, E., Bendich, A. & Franke, W. W. (1980). Constitutive aggregates of intermediate-sized filaments of the vimentin and cytokeratin type in cultured hepatoma cells and their dispersal by butyrate. *Experimental Cell Research*, **127**, 215–35.

Bourgeade, M. F., Cerruti, I. & Chany, C. (1979). Enhancement of interferon antitumor action by sodium butyrate. *Cancer Research*, **39**, 4720–3.

Bourgeade, M. F. & Chany, C. (1979). Effect of sodium butyrate on the antiviral and anticellular action of interferon in normal and MSV-transformed cells. *International Journal of Cancer*, **24**, 314–18.

Breitman, T. R. & He, R. (1990). Combination of retinoic acid with either sodium butyrate, dimethylsulfoxide or hexamethylene bisacetamide synergistically induce differentiation of the human myeloid leukemia cell line HL60. *Cancer Research*, **50**, 6268–73.

Bretton, R. H. & Pennypacker, J. P. (1989). Butyric acid causes morphological changes in cultured chondrocytes through alterations in the extracellular matrix. *Journal of Cellular Physiology*, **138**, 197–204.

Bryant, G., Haberem, C., Rao, C. N. & Liotta, L. A. (1986). Butyrate induced reduction of tumor cell laminin receptors. *Cancer Research*, **46**, 807–11.

Cattini, P. A., Kardami, E. & Eberhardt, N. L. (1988) Effect of butyrate on thyroid hormone-mediated gene expression in rat pituitary tumor cells. *Molecular and Cellular Endrocrinology*, **56**, 263–70.

Charollais, R. H., Bucket, C. & Mester, J. (1990). Butyrate blocks the accumulation of CDC2 mRNA in late G_1 phase but inhibits both the early and the late G_1 progression in chemically transformed mouse fibroblasts BP-A31. *Journal of Cellular Physiology*, **145**, 46–52.

Chou, J. Y., Robinson, J. C. & Wang, S. S. (1977). Effects of sodium butyrate on human chorionic gonadotrophin in trophoblastic and non-trophoblastic tumors. *Nature*, **268**, 543–4.

Constantoulakis, P., Papayannopoulou, T. & Stomatoyannopoulos, G. (1988). α-Amino *N*-butyric acid stimulates fetal hemoglobin in the adult. *Blood*, **72**, 1961–7.

Csordas, A. (1990). On the biological role of histone acetylation. *Biochemical Journal*, **265**, 23–38.

d'Anna, J. A., Gurley, L. R., Becker, R. R., Barham, S. S., Tobey, R. A. & Walters, R. A. (1980*a*). Amino acid analysis and cell cycle dependent phosphorylation of an H1-like, butyrate enhanced protein from Chinese hamster cells. *Biochemistry*, **19**, 4331–41.

d'Anna, J. A., Tobey, R. A. & Gurley, L. R. (1980*b*). Concentration-dependent effects of sodium butyrate in Chinese hamster cells: cell-cycle progression, inner histone acetylation, histone H1 dephosphorylation and induction of an H1-like protein. *Biochemistry*, **19**, 2656–71.

de Haan, J. B., Gevers, W. & Parker, M. I. (1986). Effects of sodium butyrate on the synthesis and methylation of DNA in normal cells and their transformed counterpart. *Cancer Research*, **46**, 713–16.

Dobson, M. E. & Ingram, V. M. (1980), *In vitro* transcription of chromatin containing histones hyperacetylated *in vivo*. *Nucleic Acids Research*, **8**, 4201–19.

Foss, F. M., Veillette, A., Sartor, O., Rosen, N. & Bolen, J B. (1989). Alteration of the expression of $pp60^{c\text{-}src}$ and $p56^{lck}$ associated with butyrate-induced differentiation of human colon carcinoma cells. *Oncogene Research*, **5**, 13–23.

Ghosh, N. K. & Cox, R. P. (1977). Induction of human follicle-stimulating hormone in HeLa cells by sodium butyrate. *Nature*. **267**, 435–7.

Ghosh, N. K., Ruckenstein, A. & Cox, R. P. (1977). Induction of human choriogonadotrophin in HeLa cell culture by aliphatic monocarboxylates and inhibitors of deoxyribonucleic acid synthesis. *Biochemical Journal*, **166**, 265–74.

Ginder, G. D., Whitters, M. J. & Pohlman, J. K. (1984). Activation of a chicken embryonic globin gene in adult erythroid cells by 5-azacytidine and sodium butyrate. *Proceedings of the National Academy of Sciences, USA*, **81**, 3954–8.

Glauber, J. G., Wandersee, N. J., Little J. A. & Glinder, G. D. (1991). 5′ flanking sequences mediate butyrate stimulation of embryonic globin gene expression in adult erythroid cells. *Molecular and Cellular Biology*, **11**, 4690–7.

Golub, E. I., Li, G. & Volski, D. J. (1991). Induction of dormant HIV-1 by sodium butyrate: involvement of the TATA box on the activation of the HIV-1 promoter. *AIDS*, **5**, 663–8.

Guilbaud, N. F., Gas, N., Dupont, M. A. & Valette, A. (1990). Effects of differentiation-inducing agents on maturation of human MCF-7 breast cancer cells. *Journal of Cellular Physiology*, **145**, 162–72.

Guillouzo, A., Tichonicky, L., Boisnard-Rissel, M. & Kruh, J. (1980). Early reversible nuclear alterations induced by sodium butyrate in cultured hepatoma cells. *Cell Biology International Reports*, **4**, 961–8.

Hagopian, H. K., Riggs, M. G., Swartz, L. A. & Ingram, V. M. (1977). Effects of *n*-butyrate on DNA synthesis in chick fibroblasts and HeLa cells. *Cell*, **12**, 855–60.

Hall, J. M. & Cole, R. D. (1986). Mechanisms of $H1^0$ accumulation in mouse neuroblastoma cells differ with different treatments. *Journal of Biological Chemistry*, **261**, 5168–74.

Hayman, E. G., Engvall, E. & Ruoslahti, E. (1980). Butyrate restores fibronectin at cell surface of transformed cells. *Experimental Cell Research*, **127**, 478–81.

Henneberry, R. C. & Fishman, P. H. (1976). Morphological and biochemical differentiation in HeLa cells. *Experimental Cell Research*, **103**, 55–62.

Herold, K. M. & Rothberg, P. G. (1988). Evidence for a labile intermediate in the butyrate induced reduction of the level of c-*myc* RNA in SW837 rectal carcinoma cells. *Oncogene*, **3**, 423–8,

Herz, F., Schermer, A., Halwer, M. & Bogart, L. M. (1981). Alkaline phosphatase in HT-29, a human colon cancer cell line. Influence of sodium butyrate and hyperosmolality. *Archives of Biochemistry and Biophysics*, **216**, 581–91.

Ito, F. & Chou, J. Y. (1984). Induction of placental alkaline phosphatase biosynthesis by sodium butyrate. *Journal of Biological Chemistry*, **259**, 2526–30.

Kassis, S. (1985). Modulation of the receptor-coupled adenyl-cyclase system in HeLa cells by sodium butyrate. *Biochemistry*, **24**, 5666–72.

Kitzis, A., Tichonicky, L., Defer, N. & Kruh, J. (1980). Effect of sodium butyrate on chromatin structure. *Biochemical and Biophysical Research Communications*, **93**, 833–41.

Kosaka, M., Nishina, Y., Takeda, M., Matsumoto, K. & Nishiyune, Y. (1991). Reversible effects of sodium butyrate on the differentiation of F9 embryonal carcinoma cells. *Experimental Cell Research*, **192**, 46–51.

Kruh, J. (1982). Effects of sodium butyrate, a new pharmacological agent, on cells in culture. *Molecular and Cellular Biochemistry*, **42**, 65–82.

Kumar, S., Sachar, K., Huber, J., Weingarten, D. P. & de Vellis, J. (1985). Glucocorticoids regulate the transcription of glycerol phosphate dehydrogenase in cultured glial cells. *Journal of Biological Chemistry*, **260**, 14743–7.

Kyristis, A., Joseph, G. & Chader, G. J. (1984). Effect of butyrate, retinol and retinoic acid on human Y-79 retinoblastoma cells growing in monolayer cultures. *Journal of National Cancer Institute*, **73**, 649–54.

Lazar, M. A. (1990). Sodium butyrate selectively alters thyroid hormone receptor gene expression in GH3 cells. *Journal of Biological Chemistry*, **265**, 17474–7.

Leder, A. & Leder, P. (1975). Butyric acid, a potent inducer of erythroid differentiation in cultured erythroleukemia cells. *Cell*, **5**, 319–22.

Leibovitch, M. P. & Kruh, J. (1979). Effect of sodium butyrate on myoblast growth and differentiation. *Biochemical and Biophysical Research Communications*, **87**, 896–903.

Leibovitch, M. P., Leibovitch, S. A., Harel, J. & Kruh, J. (1982). Effect of sodium butyrate on messenger RNA populations in myogenic cells in culture. *Differentiation*, **22**, 106–12.

Levy-Wilson, B. (1981). Enhanced phosphorylation of high mobility group proteins in nuclease sensitive mononucleosomes from butyrate-treated HeLa cells. *Proceedings of the National Academy of Sciences, USA*, **78**, 2189–93.

Martel, P., Houdebine, L. M. & Teyssot, B. (1983). Effect of sodium butyrate on the stimulation of casein gene expression by prolactin. *FEBS Letters*, **154**, 55–9.

Mathis, D. J., Oudet, P., Wasylyk, B. & Chambon, P. (1978). Effect of histone acetylation on structure and *in vitro* transcription of chromatin. *Nucleic Acids Research*, **5**, 3523–47.

Matsuhashi, T., Uchimura, H. & Takaku, F. (1987). *n*-Butyrate increases the level of thyroid hormone nuclear receptor in non-pituitary cultured cells. *Journal of Biological Chemistry*, **262**, 3993–9.

McKnight, G. S., Hager, L. & Palmiter, R. D. (1980). Butyrate and related inhibitors of histone deacetylation block the induction of egg white genes by steroid hormones. *Cell*, **22**, 469–77.

Montiel, F., Ortiz-Caro, J., Villa, A., Pascual, A. & Aranda, A. (1989). Presence of insulin receptors in cultured glial C6 cells. Regulation by butyrate. *Biochemical Journal*, **258**, 147–55.

Morita, A., Tsao, D. & Kim, Y. S. (1982). Effect of sodium butyrate on alkaline phosphatase in HRT-18, a human rectal cancer cell line. *Cancer Research*, **42**, 4540–5.

Mullins, T. D., Kern, H. F. & Metzgar, R. S. (1991). Ultrastructural differentiation of sodium butyrate-treated human pancreatic adenocarcinoma cell lines. *Pancreas*, **6**, 578–87.

Nakagawa, T., Nelkin, B. D., Baylin, S. B. & de Bustros, A. (1988). Transcriptional and post-transcriptional modulation of calcitonin gene expression by sodium butyrate in cultured human medullary thyroid carcinoma. *Cancer Research*, **48**, 2096–100.

Naranjo, J. R., Mellstrom, B., Auwerx, J., Mollinedo, F. & Sassone-Corsi, P. (1990). Unusual c-*fos* induction upon chromaffin PC12 differentiation by sodium butyrate: loss of *fos* autoregulatory functions. *Nucleic Acids Research*, **18**, 3605–10.

Newman, J. D., Eckardt, G. S., Boyd, A. & Harrison, L. C. (1989). Induction of the insulin receptor and other differentiation markers by sodium butyrate in the Burkitt lymphoma cell RAJI. *Biochemical and Biophysical Research Communications*, **161**, 101–6.

Novogrodsky, A., Dvir, A. & Ravid, A. (1983). Effect of polar organic compounds in leukemia cells. Butyrate-induced partial remission of acute myelogenous leukemia in a child. *Cancer*, **51**, 9–14.

Olivieri, N., Dover, G., Ginder, G., Papayannopoulou, T., Miller, B., Lee, S., Li, S. T., Shafer, F., Vichinsky, E. & Perrine, S. (1991). Butyrate stimulates α globin synthesis in patients with β globin gene disorders. *Blood*, **78** (Suppl. 1), 368a.

Partington, G. A., Yarwood, N. J. & Rutherford, T. R. (1984). Human globin gene transcription in injected xenopus oocytes: enhancement by sodium butyrate. *EMBO Journal*, **3**, 2787–92.

Perrine, S. P., Miller, B. A., Faller, D. V., Cohen, R. A., Vichinsky, E. P., Hurst, D., Lubin, B. H. & Papayannopoulou, T. (1989). Sodium butyrate enhances fetal globin gene expression in erythroid progenitors of patients with Hb SS and β thalassemia. *Blood*, **74**, 454–9.

Perrine, S. P., Miller, B. A., Green, M. F., Cohen, R. A., Cook, N., Shackleton, C. & Faller, D. V. (1987). Butyric acid analogues augment γ globin gene expression in neonatal erythroid progenitors. *Biochemical and Biophysical Research Communications*, **148**, 694–700.

Perrine, S. P., Rudolph, A., Faller, D. V., Roman, C., Cohen, R. A., Chen, S. J. & Kan, Y. W. (1988). Butyrate infusions in the ovine fetus delay the biological clock for globin gene switching. *Proceedings of the National Academy of Sciences, USA*, **85**, 8540–2.

Philipe, J., Drucker, D. J., Chick, W. L. & Habener, J. F. (1987). Transcriptional regulation of genes encoding insulin, glucagon and angiotensinogen by sodium butyrate in a rat islet cell line. *Molecular and Cellular Biology*, **7**, 560–3.

Planchon, P. Raux, H., Magnien, V., Ronco, G., Villa, P., Crepin, M. & Brouty-Boye, D. (1991). New stable butyrate derivatives alter proliferation and differentiation in human mammary cells. *International Journal of Cancer*, **48**, 443–9.

Polack, A., Eick, D., Koch, E. & Bornkamm, G. W. (1987). Truncation does not abrogate transcriptional down regulation of the c-*myc* gene by sodium butyrate in Burkitt's lymphoma cells. *EMBO Journal*, **6**, 2959–64.

Pouillart, P., Ronco, G., Cerruti, I., Chany, C. & Villa, P. (1990). Low level toxicity and antitumor activity of butyric mono- and polyester monosaccharide derivatives in mice. *Journal of Biological Regulatory and Homeostatic Agents*, **4**, 135–41.

Raymondjean, M., Tichonicky, L. & Kruh, J. (1985). Effect of sodium butyrate on the complexity and the translation activity in HTC cell RNAs. *Biology of the Cell*, **54**, 39–48.

Rephaeli, A., Rabizadeh, E. Aviram, E., Shaklai, M., Ruse, M. & Nudelman, A. (1991). Derivatives of butyric acid as potential anti-neophasic agents. *International Journal of Cancer*, **49**, 66–72.

Riggs, M. G., Whittaker, R. G., Neumann, J. R. & Ingram, V. M. (1977). *n*-Butyrate causes histone modification in HeLa and Friend erythroleukemia cells. *Nature*, **268**, 462–4.

Samuels, H. H., Stanley, F., Casanova, J. & Shao, T. C. (1980). Thyroid hormone nuclear receptor levels are influenced by the acetylation of chromatin-associated proteins. *Journal of Biological Chemistry*, **255**, 2499–508.

Sealy, L. & Chalkley, R. (1978*a*). The effect of sodium butyrate on histone modification. *Cell*, **14**, 115–21.

Sealy, L. & Chalkley, R. (1978*b*). DNA associated with hyperacetylated histone is preferentially digested by DNase 1. *Nucleic Acids Research*, **5**, 1863–76.

Stevens, M. S., Aliabadi, Z. & Moore, M. R. (1984). Associated effects of sodium butyrate on histone acetylation and estrogen receptor in the human breast cancer cell line MCF-7. *Biochemical and Biophysical Research Communications*, **119**, 132–8.

Stoddart, J. H., Lane, M. A. & Niles, R. M. (1989). Sodium butyrate suppresses the transforming activity of an activated N-*ras* oncogene in human colon carcinoma cells. *Experimental Cell Research*, **184**, 16–27.

Tallman, J. F., Smith, C. C. & Henneberry, R. C. (1977). Induction of functional β adrenergic receptors in HeLa cells. *Proceedings of the National Academy of Sciences, USA*, **74**, 873–7.

Tanaka, Y., Bush, K. K., Eguchi, T. Ikekawa, N., Taguchi, T., Kobayashi, Y. & Higgins, P. J. (1990). Effects of 1,25 hydroxyvitamin D_3 and its analogs on butyrate-induced differentiation of HT-29 human colonic carcinoma cells and on reversal of the differentiated phenotype. *Archives of Biochemistry and Biophysics*, **276**, 415–23.

Tichonicky, L., Kruh, J. & Defer, N. (1990). Sodium butyrate inhibits c-*myc* and stimulates c-*fos* expression in all the steps of the cell-cycle in hepatoma tissue cultured cells. *Biology of the Cell*, **69**, 63–7.

Tichonicky, L., Santana Calderon, M. A., Defer, N., Giesen, E. M., Beck, G. & Kruh, J. (1981). Selective inhibitors by sodium butyrate of glucocorticoid-induced tyrosine amino-transferase synthesis in hepatoma tissue cultured cells. *European Journal of Biochemistry*, **130**, 427–33.

Toscani, A., Soprano, D. R. & Soprano, K. J. (1988). Molecular analysis of sodium butyrate induced growth arrest. *Oncogene Research*, **3**, 223–38.

Touchette, N. A., Anton, E. & Cole, R. D. (1986). A higher order chromatin structure that is lost during differentiation of mouse neuroblastoma cells. *Journal of Biological Chemistry*, **261**, 2185–8.

van Wijk, R., Tichonicky, L. & Kruh, J. (1981). Effect of sodium butyrate on the hepatoma cell cycle: possible use for cell synchronization. *In vitro*, **17**, 859–62.

Via, D. P., Sramer, S., Larriba, G. & Steiner, S. (1980). Effects of sodium butyrate on the membrane glycoconjugates of murine sarcoma virus transformed rat cells. *Journal of Cell Biology*, **84**, 225–34.

Vidali, G., Boffa, L. C., Mann, R. S. & Allfrey, V. G. (1978). Reversible effects of Na-butyrate on histone acetylation. *Biochemical and Biophysical Research Communications*, **62**, 223–7.

Wakselman, M., Cerruti, I. & Chany, C. (1990), Anti-tumor protection induced in mice by fatty acid conjugates: alkyl butyrate and poly(ethylene glycol) dibutyrates. *International Journal of Cancer*, **46**, 462–7.

Wright, J. A. (1972). Morphology and growth rate changes in Chinese hamster cells cultured in presence of sodium butyrate. *Experimental Cell Research*, **78**, 456–60.

Yoneda, T., Aya, S. & Sakuda, M. (1984). Sodium butyrate augments the effects of 1,25-dihydroxyvitamin D_3 on neoplastic and osteoblastic phenotype in clonal rat osteosarcoma cells. *Biochemical and Biophysical Research Communications*, **121**, 796–801.

Zhang, J., Raich, N., Enver, T., Anagnou, N. P. & Stamatoyannopoulos, G. (1990). Butyrate induces expression of transfected human fetal and endogenous mouse embryonic globin gene in GM979 erythroleukemia cells. *Developmental Genetics*, **11**, 168–74.

19

Effects of short-chain fatty acids on the proliferation of gut epithelial cells *in vivo*[1]

T. SAKATA

Introduction

Many vertebrate species depend on microbial activities in their digestive tracts for metabolic energy (Parra, 1978). Short-chain fatty acids (SCFA) such as acetic, propionic, butyric and valeric acids represent energy-carrying nutrients produced by gut fermentation (Bugaut, 1987). The contribution of these acids to the host's energy economy varies among animals of different food habits. However, all reptiles, birds and mammals employ gut fermentation (Stevens, 1988). SCFA and their major fermentation products with gases (carbon dioxide, methane and hydrogen) are always found in significant concentrations in the fermentation chambers of the forestomach and hindgut. Gut fermentation and the production of SCFA are basic functions of land vertebrates. It is therefore reasonable to expect SCFA to act as the signal that tells the host animal to react to changes in microbial activity in the digestive system.

Functions of the digestive tract, such as digestion, absorption, secretion and metabolism, depend on the number and functional status of gut epithelial cells. Epithelial cell number is the result of a dynamic equilibrium between cell proliferation and cell loss (desquamation plus apoptosis). This chapter reviews the *in vivo* effect of SCFA on epithelial cell proliferation both of ruminant and non-ruminant animals. The effects of SCFA on motility, absorption and secretion in the digestive tract are discussed by other authors in this book.

[1] To the memory of the late Professor emeritus Hideo Tamate, who was one of the initiators of physiological studies on SCFA in the late 1950s. Professor emeritus Hideo Tamate, Sendai, born August 9, 1922, deceased October 17, 1988.

Stimulatory effect of SCFA on proliferation of rumen epithelial cells

Effects on rumen development during weaning

The development of the forestomach is a prerequisite for a ruminant to be a successful herbivore. In ruminant species, a very large part of the forestomach (rumen plus reticulum) functions as a fermentation chamber, with volumes greater than 100 l in modern domestic cattle. Abundant rumen papillae increase the inner surface area approximately sevenfold in adult domestic ruminants. However, their stomach at birth is amost as small as that of the human with a relatively flat mucosal surface and poorly developed rumen papillae. Weaning promotes dramatic growth of the forestomach; prolonged suckling retards its growth (Tamate, 1957; Fig. 19.1).

SCFA as the chemical lumen trophic factor for rumen mucosa in weaning ruminants

Weaning has two functions for the ruminant: introduction of physical stimuli such as abrasion that do not exist in a liquid diet and stimulation of microbial activities in the rumen. Fluid bypasses the rumen and reticulum to enter the abomasum in suckling ruminants (Tamate *et al.*, 1962). Tamate *et al.* (1962, 1964) tried to stimulate weaning by introducing either SCFA, the main

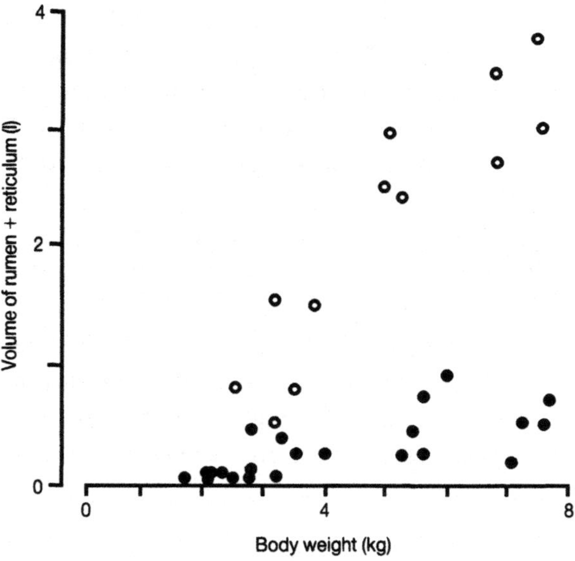

Fig. 19.1. Growth of the volume of the rumen plus reticulum of milk-fed (filled circles) and solid-fed (open circles) goats. Data from Tamate (1957).

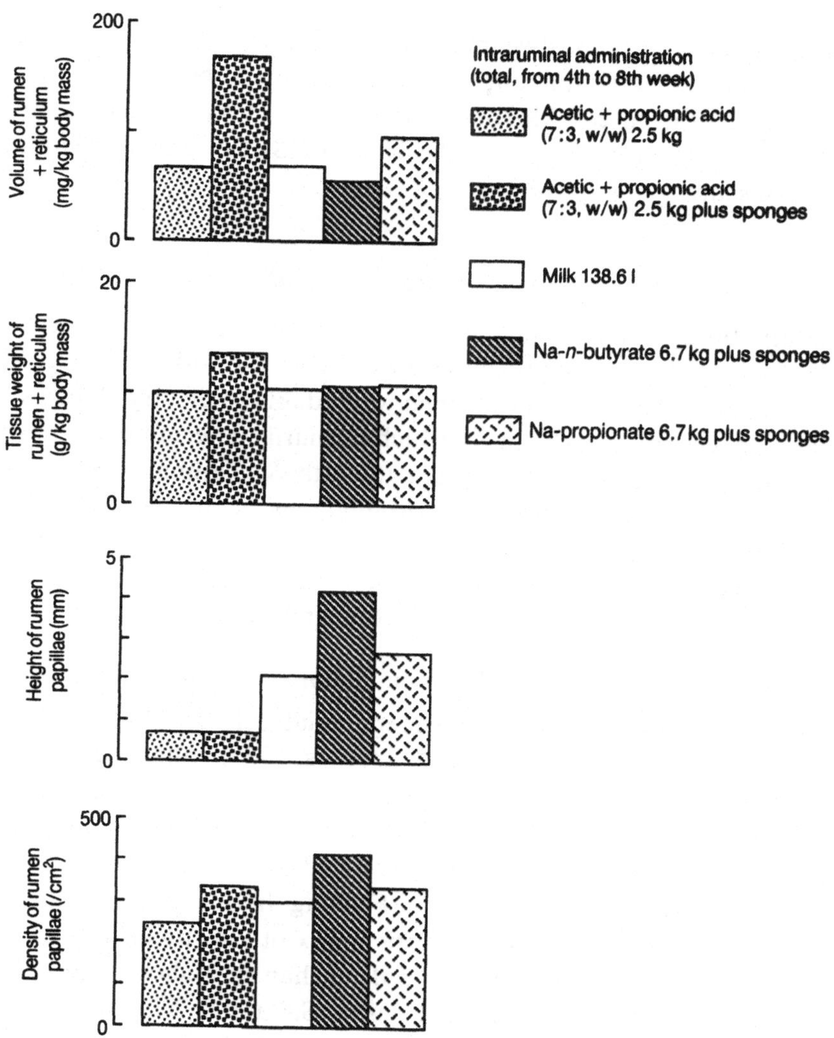

Fig. 19.2. Effects of SCFA and physical stimuli (sponges) on the growth of rumen plus reticulum and on the development of rumen papillae. Data from Tamate *et al.* (1962).

products of rumen fermentation, or sponges into the rumen of a 4-week-old goat. They found that physical stimuli (sponges) were responsible for an increase in the capacity of the rumen plus reticulum, whilst the development of rumen papillae depended on SCFA (Fig. 19.2). To my knowledge, this was the first demonstration of a chemically defined lumen trophic factor for gut epithelial cells.

However, SCFA are not responsible for muscle growth in the ruminant forestomach during the postweaning period (Tamate *et al.*, 1962, 1964). This is also the case in non-ruminant species, as discussed below.

Thus far, epithelial cell kinetics in the rumen at weaning have not been investigated. The mechanism for the effect of SCFA during weaning also remains obscure.

Effects of SCFA on adult rumen epithelial cell proliferation

The adaptational capacity of the ruminant digestive system, especially the rumen, is one of the key features that have led to the wide and successful use of ruminants in agriculture. The rumen wall adapts to dietary changes mainly by changing its epithelial cell mass, which primarily determines the absorptive and metabolic capacity of the organ (Sakata & Yajima, 1984). However, ruminants sometimes fail to adapt to high levels of feed intake or high proportions of easily fermentable feed, especially finely ground grains, mainly due to failure in mucosal adaptation such as hyper- and parakeratosis, which may lead to liver abscess (Fell *et al.*, 1968; Ørskov, 1973).

Influence of feeding condition on rumen epithelial cell kinetics

The influence of feeding on rumen epithelial cell proliferation has been studied. Increased feed intake (Fell & Weekes, 1975) enhanced the epithelial cell number in lactating sheep and increased the mitotic index (number of mitotic figures/1000 basal layer cells) of the rumen epithelium (Sakata & Tamate, 1978*c*). Fasting decreased and re-feeding increased the mitotic index (Tamate, Kikuchi & Sakata, 1974). Feeding frequency also affected the mitotic index of the rumen. The mitotic index of the rumen was higher in a sheep fed a certain amount once in 3 days than in a sheep pair fed once a day (i.e. fed one-third of the amount daily) (Sakata & Tamate, 1974). Grain feeding increased and hay feeding decreased the epithelial mitotic index of the rumen (Goodlad & Fell, 1981). These results indicate that conditions that increase the rate or amount of SCFA production in the rumen stimulate epithelial cell mitosis.

Effects of intraruminal infusion of SCFA on rumen epithelial cell mitosis

Intraruminal administration of sodium *n*-butyrate, sodium propionate or sodium acetate (18 mmol/kg body mass per day) increased rumen epithelial cell mitosis even in fasted (i.e. energy-deficient) adult sheep (Sakata & Tamate, 1978*b*, 1979). Butyrate had a stronger effect than had acetate or propionate. The effect of SCFA was transitional in spite of continued daily administration in fasted sheep (Fig. 19.3). The stimulatory effect of sodium

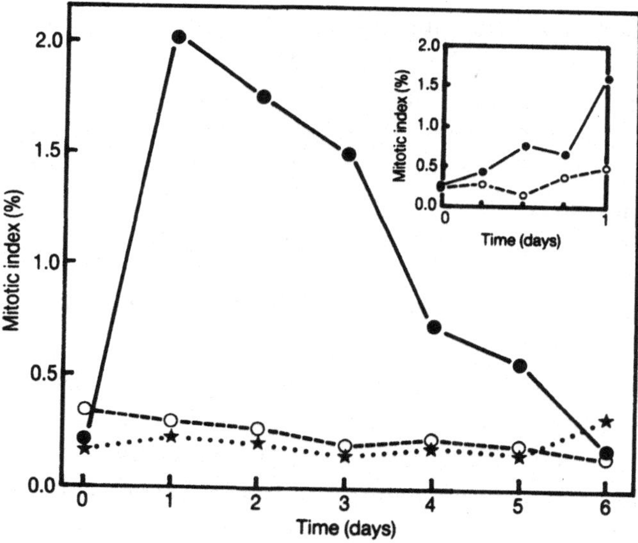

Fig. 19.3. Effects of rapid (within 10 s, once a day; filled circles) or continuous (over 20–24 h daily; open circles) infusion into the rumen of sodium *n*-butyrate, compared with saline solution (stars) on the epithelial cell mitotic index in fasted adult sheep. Data from Sakata & Tamate (1978*b*).

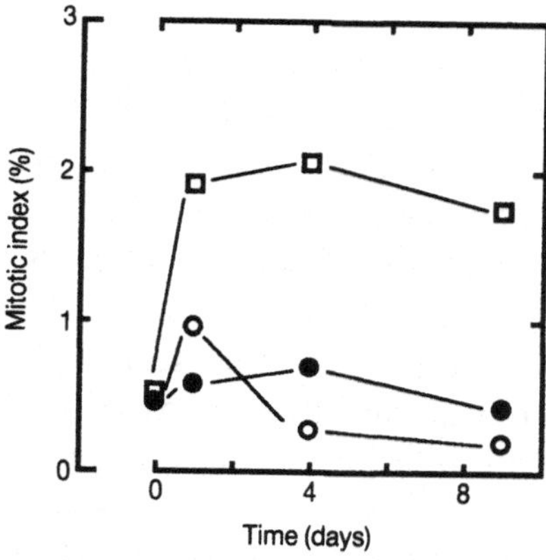

Fig. 19.4. Effects of rapid (open squares) or continuous (open circles) infusion into the rumen of sodium *n*-butyrate, compared with saline solution (filled circles) on the epithelial cell mitotic index in fed adult sheep. Data from Galfi *et al.* (1986).

n-butyrate persisted at least for 1 week with daily administration into the rumen of fed sheep (Galfi *et al.*, 1986; Fig. 19.4).

The stimulatory effect of butyrate on the rumen epithelium depended on the administration rate (Sakata & Tamate, 1978*b*; Galfi, Neogrady & Kutas,

1986); rapid administration of sodium *n*-butyrate, within 10 s resulted in a marked increase in the mitotic index within a day, but the same dose had no effect when infused intraruminally over 20 h. These results suggest that ruminants sense either the increment of SCFA concentrations or the oscillation in the SCFA concentrations in the rumen. In other words, it is not the amount of SCFA produced in the rumen but either the rate or the change in rate of SCFA production that influences epithelial cell proliferation.

Mechanism for the trophic effect of SCFA in adult ruminants: involvement of insulin

It is not likely that low pH alone can stimulate the epithelial cell mitosis of the rumen, as is often suggested (Fell *et al.*, 1968; Ørskov, 1973). The above studies used sodium salts of SCFA and no rumen acidification was detected, but an increase in the rumen mitotic index occurred (Sakata & Tamate, 1978*b*; Galfi *et al.*, 1986). However, this does not necessarily rule out the possible enhancement of mitotic stimulation of SCFA by low pH.

Since the SCFA inhibit rumen epithelial cell proliferation *in vitro* (Galfi *et al.*, 1981), the stimulatory effect of SCFA on rumen epithelial cells *in vivo* must be indirect and overcomes the direct inhibitory effect (Sakata *et al.*, 1980*b*). Therefore, humoral mediation of indirect stimulation was proposed. Insulin was the first possible humoral mediator to be tested, since butyrate and propionate (but not acetate) stimulate insulin release from sheep pancreatic islets (Manns, Boda & Willes, 1967; Manns & Boda, 1967).

Intravenous infusion of insulin (0.125 IU/kg per h plus glucose 300 mg/kg per h for 6 h; the latter to prevent hypoglycaemia) increased the epithelial mitotic index of fasted adult sheep within 3 h of the start of the infusion, and returned to initial levels within 42 h of the end (Sakata *et al.*, 1980*b*; Fig. 19.5). This increase in mitotic index was larger than that seen with glucose infusion alone (300 mg/kg per h for 6 h) in the same study. Furthermore, blood insulin levels in sheep given an infusion of insulin plus glucose resembled those after butyrate infusion in previous studies (Sakata *et al.*, 1980*a*). The stimulatory effect of SCFA on rumen epithelial cell mitosis is therefore at least partly mediated by insulin.

Such mediation by insulin was confirmed by *in vitro* experiments (Galfi, Neogrady & Sakata, 1991; Fig. 19.6). Insulin (1.6×10^{-6} or 1.6×10^{-7} mmol/l) stimulated the proliferation of a primary culture of rumen epithelial cells independently of the inhibitory action of co-existing butyric acid (2 or 10 mmol/l). Both the stimulatory effect of insulin and the inhibitory effect of butyrate were dose-dependent.

Glucagon, which is also released by SCFA (Mineo *et al.*, 1990), stimulates

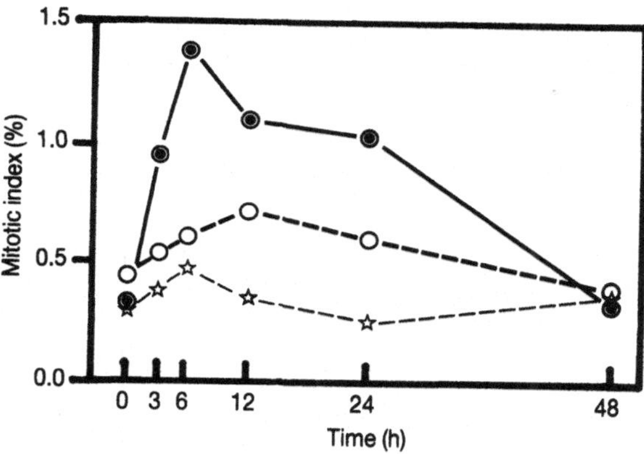

Fig. 19.5. Mitotic index of the rumen epithelium of sheep following infusion for 6 h of 300 mg/glucose/kg per h, with (ringed circles) or without (open circles) simultaneous infusion of 0.125 U insulin/kg per g. Results are compared to those for 6-h infusion of 0.9% (w/v) saline solution (stars) (Sakata *et al.*, 1980*b*).

the proliferation of primary cultures of rumen epithelial cells, but only in the absence of butyrate (Galfi *et al.*, 1991). Therefore, glucagon cannot be a physiological mediator for the trophic action of SCFA *in vivo*.

Implications of the tropic effect of SCFA in adult ruminants

The stimulatory effect of SCFA *in vivo* may facilitate adaptation of the rumen mucosa to an increased intake of readily fermentable feed such as grains or fruits for the forestomach fermenter. Readily fermentable substrates can be degraded rapidly in the forestomach to produce SCFA, resulting in an increase in epithelial cell mass, as observed after the rapid intraruminal administration of sodium *n*-butyrate (Sakata & Tamate, 1978*a*). This should facilitate the absorption and metabolism of SCFA, rapidly produced in the forestomach, by increasing the number of functional epithelial cells. However, whether the rapid infusion of SCFA really increases the number of rumen epithelial cells and thereby absorptive and metabolic capacity of the rumen is yet to be studied. In this regard, Gäbel *et al.* (1987) found that increasing the proportion of grains against hay, which should have accelerated the rate of SCFA production (especially of propionic and *n*-butyric acids) and the rate of rumen epithelial cell proliferation, increased the surface area of rumen papillae and the absorption of sodium, chloride and magnesium.

In spite of possible adaptational advantages, the increase in cell proliferation rate is usually accompanied by an increase in cell loss rate in non-cancerous regenerating tissues, leading to an increase in endogenous nitrogen loss via

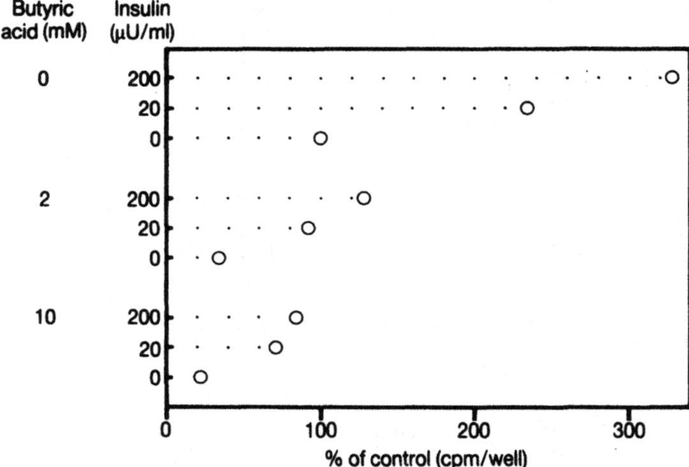

Fig. 19.6. Effects of insulin and butyric acid on the proliferation measured as ^{3}H-thymidine uptake in counts per min (cpm) of a primary culture of rumen epithelial cells. Data from Galfi *et al.* (1991).

sloughed epithelial cells. This can be problematic when the forestomach fermenters eat readily fermentable but nitrogen-poor feed. In this regard, it would be worthwhile to study the influence of SCFA on rumen epithelial cell production under conditions of different nitrogen intake. It also remains unclear whether ruminal SCFA stimulate the epithelial mitotic activity of other gut segments and whether the SCFA produced in the hindgut of ruminants, especially before weaning, stimulate epithelial cell proliferation in the rumen.

Influence of SCFA on epithelial cell division in the digestive tract of non-ruminant animals *in vivo*

Conditions that reduce the production of SCFA depress epithelial cell proliferation not only of the large intestine but also of the small intestine. Caecocolonic bypass surgery (Sakata, 1988), parenteral nutrition (Jane, Carpentier & Willems, 1977), feeding of a substrate-free diet (Goodlad & Wright, 1983) and germ-free conditions (Komai, Takehisa & Kimura, 1982) depress the mitotic activity of intestinal epithelia. These results clearly indicate the importance of hindgut fermentation in maintaining the level of epithelial cell proliferation of the small and large intestine.

The stimulatory effect of SCFA on intestinal epithelial cell proliferation was studied using rats with Roux-en-Y ileostomy for the administration of

SCFA (Sakata, 1986, 1987). In these studies, SCFA were injected into the hindgut of rats in which the production of SCFA was depressed (either rats which had been fed a fibre-free elemental diet or germ-free rats) (Sakata, 1986, 1987). In other words, these studies were intended to stimulate the depressed epithelial cell proliferation due to lowered SCFA production by injecting SCFA into the hindgut lumen.

Mode of the trophic effect of SCFA on intestinal epithelium in rats

The stimulatory effect of SCFA on intestinal epithelial cell proliferation appeared within a few days of daily administration and lasted for at least 2 weeks (Sakata, 1987). Daily administration of approximately 10% of the daily production of SCFA (acetic, propionic and *n*-butyric acids, 100, 20 and 60 mM, respectively, pH 6.1, 3 ml twice daily) into the caecum via the ileostomy at the terminal ileum increased the crypt production rate in the caecum and distal colon within 1–2 days (Sakata, 1987; Fig. 19.7). SCFA increased the crypt cell production rate in the jejunum and distal colon 3–4-fold without changing the pattern of circadian fluctuation (Sakata, 1987; Fig. 19.8). The stimulatory effect of SCFA is independent of the physical effect of non-fermentable dietary bulk, which stimulates the growth of non-mucosal tissue of the intestine (Sakata, 1986). These results suggest that mechanisms for the trophic effects of fermentable and non-fermentable dietary fibres are different.

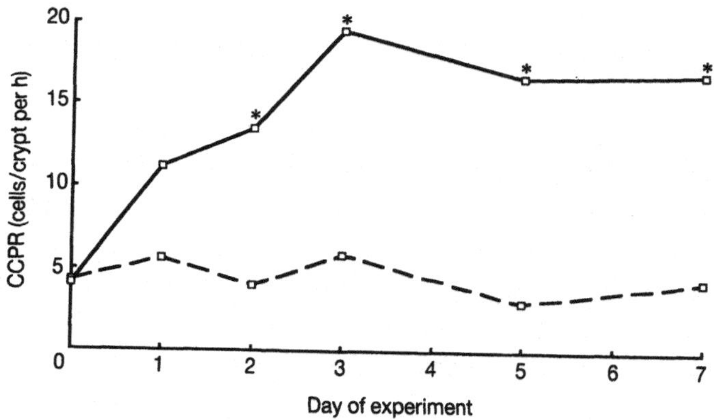

Fig. 19.7. Time-course of the trophic effect (crypt cell production rate; CCPR) of short-chain fatty acids (acetic, 100 mM, propionic, 20 mM, *n*-butyric, 60 mM, pH 6.1, 3 ml twice faily per ileostomy; unbroken line) on the distal colon of rats fed on an elemental diet. Control (dashed line): sodium chloride solution, 180 mM, pH 6.1. Asterisk, $p < 0.05$ (12 degrees of freedom). Data from Sakata (1987).

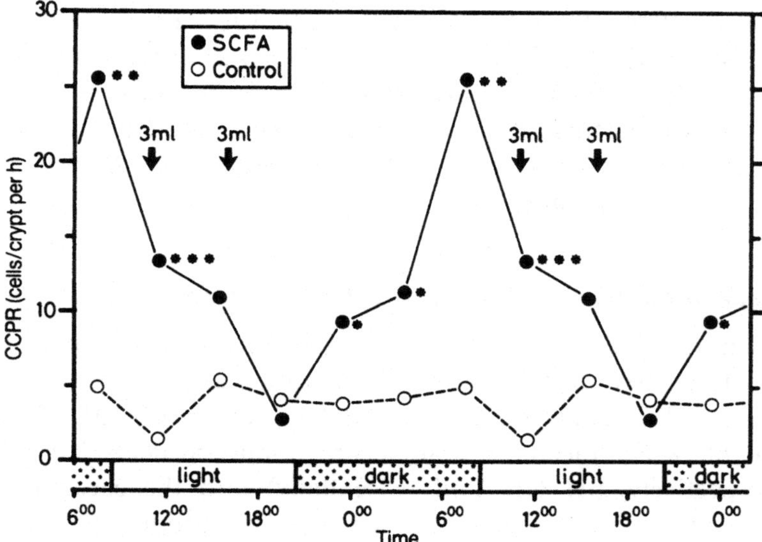

Fig. 19.8. Circadian fluctuation of epithelial cell proliferation (crypt cell production rate, CCPR) in the jejunum of rats given short-chain fatty acids (SCFA: acetic 100 mM, propionic 20 mM, *n*-butyric 60 mM), pH 6.1, 3 ml twice daily per ileostomy) and fed on an elemental diet. ***, ** and *: $p < 0.001$, $p < 0.01$ and $p < 0.05$, respectively (12 degrees of freedom). Data from Sakata (1987).

Acetic, propionic and *n*-butyric acids (except acetic acid in the jejunum) showed a dose-dependent stimulatory effect on epithelial cell production rates in the jejunum and distal colon (Sakata, 1987; Fig. 19.9). The effectiveness was in the order: *n*-butyric > propionic > acetic acid.

Rombeau's group (Kripke *et al.*, 1989) found that continuous infusions of either butyric acid (20–150 mM) or a mixture of SCFA (acetic, propionic and *n*-butyric acids; 70, 35 and 20 mM, respectively; pH 6.1) into the colon increased the mucosal DNA content of the jejunum and proximal colon of caecectomized rats. Their findings suggest that SCFA at physiological rates of administration can stimulate epithelial cell proliferation in the intestine (Sakata, 1991). This is different from the results in ruminants discussed above.

Mechanism of the trophic effect of SCFA in rats

The trophic effect of SCFA does not need bacterial metabolism; SCFA induced trophism in germ-free rats (Sakata, 1987). It is not hydrogen ions, but protonated SCFA or SCFA anions that have the stimulatory effect; the

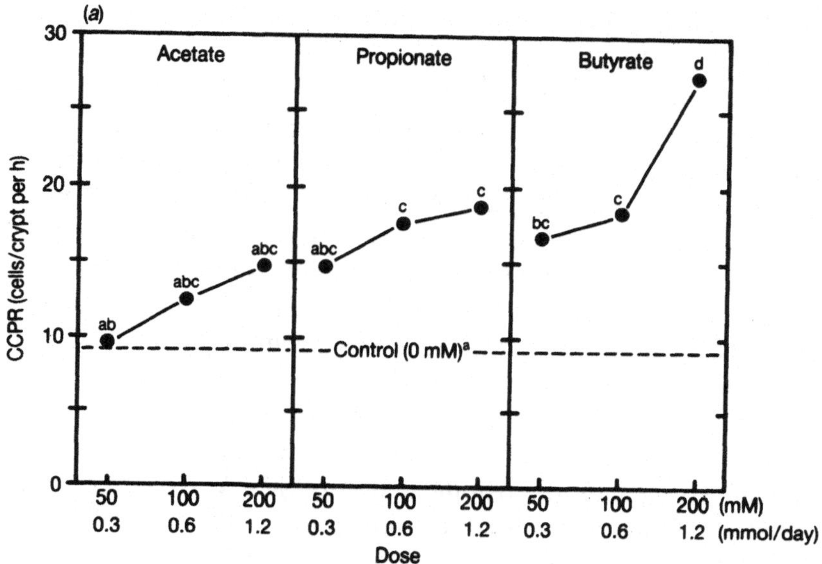

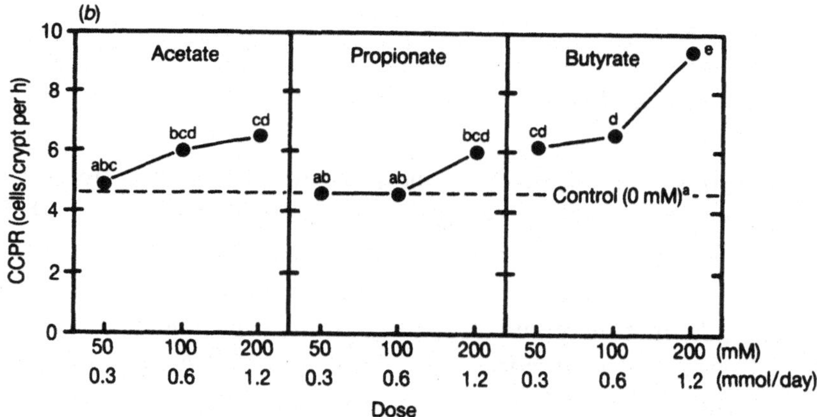

Fig. 19.9. Comparison of dose-response relation to three short-chain fatty acids (pH 6.1) on epithelial cell proliferation (crypt cell production rate, CCPR) in the jejunum (*a*) and distal colon (*b*) of rats fed an elemental diet, a, b, c: Means in each segment not sharing a common letter differed significantly, $p < 0.05$ (20 degrees of freedom). Control: sodium chloride solution, 200 mM, pH 6.1. Data from Sakata (1987).

pH of test solutions and control solutions was adjusted to 6.1 in the experiments of Sakata 1967) and Kripke *et al.* (1989). However, this does not necessarily exclude the possibility of mitotic stimulation by low lumenal pH. It is possible that low lumenal pH, caused by the accumulation of succinic or lactic acid, enhances the stimulatory effect of SCFA on intestinal epithelial cells (Hoshi *et al.*, 1994).

It is unlikely that SCFA directly stimulate intestinal epithelial proliferation. Firstly, it is hard to explain the effect of SCFA infused into the large intestine on jejunal epithelium (about 70 cm orad to the site of administration in rats) by a direct mechanism (Sakata, 1987), suggesting that the trophic action of SCFA on intestinal epithelial cells can be transmitted via a systemic mediatory mechanism. Secondly, SCFA generally inhibit the proliferation of cell cultures (Ginsburg *et al.*, 1973; see also Chapter 18, this volume) including epithelial cells of short-term cultures of rat caecum (Sakata, 1987), although the caecal preparations included histologically identifiable intestinal nerve-system and enteroendocrine cells. The latter finding indicates that local mechanisms such as the enteric nerve system or enteroendocrine system are not sufficient to mediate the trophic action of SCFA. However, it should be noted that the function of these local mediatory systems was not tested in the short-term culture of Sakata (1987), leaving the possibility of local and indirect mediation of the trophic effect of SCFA on hindgut epithelial cells.

Reception and systemic transmission of the trophic effect of SCFA in rats

The receptors for SCFA probably lie in or just below the hindgut mucosa (Sakata, 1991). This location is suggested because epithelial cells of the large intestine consume most of the *n*-butyric acid absorbed from the lumen, making its concentration in portal blood very low (Chapter 22). It is, therefore, difficult to explain the strong stimulatory effect of *n*-butyric acid on proliferation by post portal reception. The SCFA receptor studied by Yajima (Chapter 13) may also be responsible for the trophic effect of hindgut SCFA.

The efferent transmission of the trophic effect of SCFA is non-neural and very likely to be vascularly mediated (Sakata, 1989). In a study in which a small segment of jejunum was autografted under the skin, with or without its mesenteric innervation, disruption of the mesenteric innervation did not abolish the stimulatory effect of caecally administered SCFA on epithelial cell proliferation of the grafted segment (Fig. 19.10).

Enteroglucagon or intestinal peptide PYY may be the mediator(s) for the trophic action of SCFA. Feeding of pectin or guar gum increases blood levels of these gut peptides in rats. These peptides stimulate proliferation of intestinal epithelial cells both *in vivo* and *in vitro* (Goodlad *et al.*, 1987). Insulin

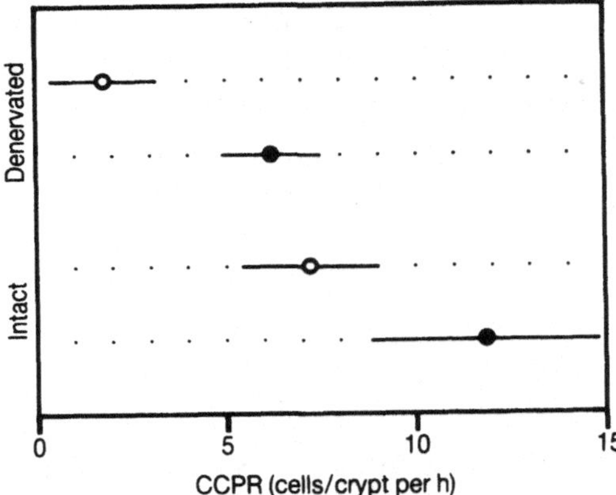

Fig. 19.10. Effect of short-chain fatty acids (acetic 100 mM, propionic 20 mM and *n*-butyric 60 mM, pH 6.1, 3 ml twice daily per ileostomy: filled circles) on epithelial cell proliferation (crypt cell production rate, CCPR) between 11.30 and 12.30 in rats fed an elemental diet and with their mesenteric connection to the subcutaneous jejunal graft either disconnected or maintained. Means with SD ($n = 4$ or 5). Control (open circles): sodium chloride solution, 180 mM, pH 6.1. Effects of denervation on CCPR, $p < 0.001$; effects of SCFA administration on CCPR, $p < 0.001$; effects of two-way interaction (denervation × SCFA) on CCPR, $p > 0.9$. Data from Sakata (1989).

does not appear to be the efferent mediator in those non-ruminant species in which SCFA do not stimulate insulin release (Horino *et al.*, 1968).

Recent studies with the use of rats with microsurgical denervation of the caecum showed that the afferent transmission for the trophic effect of SCFA requires an autonomic nerve mechanism (Frankel *et al.*, 1992). These studies also suggested that a part of the trophic effect of SCFA on colonic epithelium is locally mediated. This does not agree with the earlier study using short-term culture of caecal tissue (Sakata, 1987; Fig. 19.10). The effect of SCFA on epithelial cell proliferation in the primary culture of intestinal segments having a functionally intact intestinal nervous system and enteroendocrine system remains to be tested. Involvement of the autonomic nervous system for transmission of the trophic effect of SCFA may at least partly explain why normal function of the autonomic nervous system is necessary to maintain the normal level of epithelial cell proliferation in the intestine (Klein, 1980; Sakata, 1989).

There are suggestions that increased blood flow (Kvietys & Granger, 1967; Chapter 26) or energy supply to hindgut epithelial cells (Roediger, Chapter 22) by SCFA are responsible for their trophic effect. However, the principal mechanism may be neither of these processes, because SCFA in the hindgut exert their enterotrophic effects proximally, while their effects on blood flow and cell metabolism are local. Nevertheless, investigations of the effects of SCFA on blood flow and fuel supply to sustain higher levels of epithelial cell proliferation appear warranted.

Conclusions

The gastrointestinal segments in which fermentation occurs (forestomach and large intestine) seem to adapt to changes in feeding and microbial conditions through a response to the production of SCFA. Thus, recognized signals are proposed that stimulate epithelial cell proliferation and enhance gut motility (Chapter 12), chloride secretion from the colon (Chapter 13), salivary flow (Chapter 15) and pancreatic secretions (Chapter 14).

Animals probably do not respond to increased mass and abrasion in the gut lumen by increasing epithelial cell production (Tamate *et al.*, 1962, 1964; Sakata, 1986). The trophic effect of SCFA might be an alternative mechanism by which to respond to the increase in the functional load on the hindgut and forestomach, due to eating a larger amount of fibrous materials. However, this mechanism may not be beneficial when the diet contains high amounts of indigestible and fermentable materials with low nitrogen content. Humans and animals cannot compensate for the increased epithelial cell loss (i.e. increased endogenous nitrogen excretion) due to the stimulatory effect of SCFA on epithelial cell proliferation.

It is interesting that most of the physiological effects of SCFA are dose-dependent and vary anong acids. Responses of the digestive organs to substrate can be influenced by the mode of fermentation, i.e. the rate of fermentation and molar proportion of SCFA. Accordingly, the chemical composition of the diet per se is not a good predictor of the postprandial responses of these organs. Other factors, such as particle size of the food, or entry rate of substrate into the fermentation chamber, have considerable influences on both production rate and molar proportions of microbially produced SCFA.

Therefore, investigation of foods or food components as physiological stimuli cannot be made from simple chemical analysis alone. Instead, it is very important to assess the production rate of each SCFA from the food (components) in the fermentation chamber, perhaps using an *in vitro* approach (Kikuchi & Sakata, 1992; Kiriyama, Hariu & Sakata, 1992).

References

Bugaut, M. (1987). Occurrence, absorption and metabolism of short chain fatty acids in the digestive tract of mammals. *Comparative Biochemistry and Physiology*, **86B**, 439–72.

Fell, B. F., Kay, M., Whitelaw, F. G. & Boyne, R. (1968). Observations on the development of ruminal lesions in calves fed on barley. *Research in Veterinary Sciences*, **9**, 458–66.

Fell, B. F. & Weekes, T. E. C. (1975). Food intake as a mediator of adaptation in the ruminal epithelium. In *Digestion and Metabolism in the Ruminant*, ed. I. W. McDonald & A. C. I. Warner, pp. 101–18. Armidale: The University of New England Publishing Unit.

Frankel, W., Zhang, W., Singh, A., Klurfeld, D., Sakata, T., Modlin, I. & Rombeau, J. (1992). Stimulation of the autonomic nervous system (ANS) mediates short-chain fatty acid (SCFA)-induced jejunal trophism. *Surgical Forum*, **43**, 24–5.

Gäbel, G., Martens, H., Suendermann, M. & Galfi, P. (1987). The effect of diet, intraruminal pH and osmolarity on sodium, chloride and magnesium absorption from the temporarily isolated and washed reticulo-rumen of sheep. *Quarterly Journal of Experimental Physiology*, **72**, 501–11.

Galfi, P., Neogrady, S. & Kutas, F. (1986). Dissimilar ruminal epithelial response to short-term and continuous intraruminal infusion of sodium *n*-butyrate. *Journal of Veterinary Medicine*, **A33**, 47–52.

Galfi, P., Neogrady, S. & Sakata, T. (1991). Effects of volatile fatty acids on the epithelial cell proliferation of the digestive tract and its hormonal mediation. In *Physiological Aspects of Digestion and Metabolism in Ruminants*, ed. T. Tsuda, Y. Sasaki & R. Kawashima, pp. 50–9. San Diego: Academic Press.

Galfi, P., Veresegyhazy, T., Neogrady, S. & Kutas, F. (1981). Effect of sodium *n*-butyrate on primary ruminal epithelial cell culture. *Zentralblatt für Veterinär Medizin*, **A28**, 259–61.

Ginsburg, E. Salamon, D., Sreevalsan, T. & Freese, E. (1973). Growth inhibition and morphological changes caused by lipophilic acids in mammalian cells. *Proceedings of the National Academy of Sciences of the USA*, **70**, 2457–61.

Goodlad, R. A. & Fell, B. F. (1981). Some effects of diet on the mitotic index and the cell cycle of the ruminal epithelium of sheep. *Quarterly Journal of Experimental Physiology*, **66**, 487–99.

Goodlad, R. A., Lenton, W., Ghatei, M. A., Adrian, T. E., Bloom, S. R. & Wright, N. A. (1987). Proliferative effects of 'fibre' on the intestinal epithelium: relationship to gastrin, enteroglucagon and PYY. *Gut*, **28** (S1), 221–6.

Goodlad, R. A. & Wright, N. A. (1983). Effects of addition of kaolin or cellulose to an elemental diet on intestinal cell proliferation in the rat. *British Journal of Nutrition*, **50**, 91–8.

Horino, M. L., Machlin, J., Hertelendy, F. & Kipnis, D. M. (1968). Effects of short-chain fatty acids on plasma insulin in ruminant and nonruminant species. *Endocrinology*, **83**, 118–28.

Hoshi, H., Sakata, T., Mikuni, K., Hashimoto, H. & Kimura, S. (1994). Galactosylsucrose and xylosylfructoside alter digestive tract size and concentrations of cecal organic acids in rat fed diets containing cholesterol and cholic acid. *Journal of Nutrition*, **124**, 52–60.

Jane, P., Carpentier, Y. & Willems, G. (1977). Colonic mucosal atrophy induced by a liquid elemental diet in rats. *American Journal of Digestive Diseases*, **22**, 808–12.

Kikuchi, H. & Sakata, T. (1992). Qualitative and quantitative estimation of soluble indigestible polysaccharides as substrate for hindgut fermentation by mini-scale batch culture. *Journal of Nutritional Sciences and Vitaminology*, **38**, 287–96.

Kiriyama, H., Hariu, Y. & Sakata, T. (1992). Comparison of *in vitro* productivities of short-chain fatty acids and gases from aldoses and the corresponding alcohols by pig cecal bacteria. *Journal of Nutritional Biochemistry*, **3**, 447–51.

Klein, R. M. (1980). Influence of guanethidine-induced sympathectomy on crypt cell proliferation in the pre- and post-closure ileum of the neonatal rat. In *Cell Proliferation in the Gastrointestinal Tract*, ed. D. R. Appleton, J. P. Sunter & A. J. Watson, pp. 109–22. Tunbridge Wells: Pitman Medical.

Komai, M., Takehisa, F. & Kimura, S. (1982). Effect of dietary fiber on intestinal epithelial cell kinetics of germ-free and conventional mice. *Nutritional Report International*, **26**, 255–61.

Kripke, S. A., Fox, A. D., Berman, J. M., Settle, R. G. & Rombeau, J. L. (1989). Stimulation of intestinal mucosal growth with intracolonic infusion of short-chain fatty acids. *Journal of Parenteral and Enteral Nutrition*, **13**, 109.

Kvietys, P. R. & Granger, D. N. (1967). Effects of volatile fatty acids on blood flow and oxygen uptake by the dog colon. *Gastroenterology*, **80**, 962–9.

Manns, J. G. & Boda, J. M. (1967). Insulin release by acetate, propionate, butyrate and glucose in lambs and adult sheep. *American Journal of Physiology*, **212**, 745–55.

Manns, J. G., Boda, J. M. & Willes, R. F. (1967). Probable role of propionate and butyrate in control of insulin secretion in sheep. *American Journal of Physiology*, **212**, 756–64.

Mineo, H., Kanai, M., Kato, S. & Ushijima, J. (1990). Effects of intravenous injection of butyrate, valerate and their isomers on endocrine pancreatic responses in conscious sheep (*Ovis aries*). *Comparative Biochemistry and Physiology*, **95A**, 411–16.

Ørskov, E. R. (1973). The effect of not processing barley on rumenitis in sheep. *Research in Veterinary Sciences*, **14**, 110–12.

Parra, R. (1978). Comparison of foregut and hindgut fermentation in herbivores. In *The Ecology of Arboreal Folivores*, ed. G. G. Montgomery, pp. 205–29. Washington, DC: Smithsonian Institution Press.

Sakata, T. (1986). Effects of indigestible dietary bulk and short chain fatty acids on the tissue weight and epithelial cell proliferation rate of the digestive system. *Journal of Nutritional Sciences and Vitaminology*, **32**, 355–62.

Sakata, T. (1987). Stimulatory effect of short-chain fatty acids on epithelial cell proliferation in the rat intestine: a possible explanation for trophic effects of fermentable fibre, gut microbes and luminal trophic factors. *British Journal of Nutrition*, **58**, 95–103.

Sakata, T. (1988). Depression of intestinal epithelial cell production rate by hindgut bypass in rats. *Scandinavian Journal of Gastroenterology*, **23**, 1200–2.

Sakata, T. (1989). Stimulatory effect of short-chain fatty acids on epithelial cell proliferation of isolated and denervated jejunal segment of the rat. *Scandinavian Journal of Gastroenterology*, **24**, 886–90.

Sakata, T. (1991). Effects of short-chain fatty acids on epithelial cell proliferation and mucus release in the intestine. In *Short-Chain Fatty Acids: Metabolism, and Clinical Importance*, ed. J. H. Cummings, J. L. Rombeau & T. Sakata, pp. 63–7. Columbus, OH: Ross Laboratories.

Sakata, T., Hikosaka, K., Shimomura, Y. & Tamate, H. (1980*a*). Stimulatory effect of insulin on ruminal epithelium cell mitosis in adult sheep. *British Journal of Nutrition*, **44**, 325–31.

Sakata, T., Hikosaka, K., Shiomura, T. & Tamate, H. (1980*b*). The stimulatory effect of butyrate on epithelial cell proliferation in the rumen of the sheep, and its mediation by insulin; differences between *in-vivo* and *in-vitro* studies. In *Cell Proliferation in the Gastrointestinal Tract*, ed. D. R. Appleton, J. P. Sunter & A. J. Watson, pp. 123–37. Tunbridge Wells: Pitman Medical.

Sakata, T. & Tamate, H. (1974). Effect of the intermittent feeding on the mitotic index and the ultrastructure of basal cells of the ruminal epithelium in the sheep. *Tohoku Journal of Agricultural Research*, **25**, 156–63.

Sakata, T. & Tamate, H. (1978*a*). Influence of butyrate on microscopic structure of ruminal mucosa in adult sheep. *Japanese Journal of Zootechnical Sciences*, **49**, 687–96.

Sakata, T. & Tamate, H. (1978*b*). Rumen epithelial cell proliferation accelerated by rapid increase in intraruminal butyrate. *Journal of Dairy Science*, **61**, 1109–13.

Sakata, T. & Tamate, H. (1978*c*). Presence of circadian rhythm in the mitotic index of the ruminal epithelium in sheep. *Research in Veterinary Sciences*, **24**, 1–3.

Sakata, T. & Tamate, H. (1979). Rumen epithelial cell proliferation accelerated by propionate and acetate. *Journal of Dairy Science*, **62**, 49–52.

Sakata, T. & Yajima, T. (1984). Influence of short chain fatty acids on the epithelial cell division of digestive tract. *Quarterly Journal of Experimental Physiology*, **69**, 639–48.

Stevens, C. E. (1988). *Comparative Physiology of the Vertebrate Digestive System.* Cambridge: Cambridge University Press.

Tamate, H. (1957). The anatomical studies on the stomach of the goat. II. The post-natal changes in the capacities and the relative sizes of the four divisions of the stomach. *Tohoku Journal of Agricultural Research*, **7**, 209.

Tamate, H. Kikuchi, T. & Sakata, T. (1974). Ultrastructural changes in the ruminal epithelium after fasting and refeeding. *Tohoku Journal of Agricultural Research*, **25**, 142–55.

Tamate, H., McGilliard, A. D., Jacobson, N. L. & Getty, R. (1962). Effect of various diets on the anatomical development of the stomach in the calf. *Journal of Dairy Science*, **45**, 408–20.

Tamate, H. McGilliard, A. D., Jacobson, N. L. & Getty, R. (1964). The effect of various diets on the histological development of the stomach in the calf. *Tohoku Journal of Agricultural Research*, **14**, 171–93.

20

Short-chain fatty acids and colon tumorigenesis: animal models

J. R. LUPTON

It is crucial to understand the relationship between short-chain fatty acids (SCFA) (the major anions in colonic contents) and colon tumour development in the intact animal, since it is clear that information obtained from studies with cell lines is not always in agreement with data *in vivo*. As important as the task is, however, there are major problems in accomplishing it. A direct assessment of the effect of specific SCFA on colon tumour development in the whole animal system is not possible. Colonic epithelial cells are exposed to a heterogeneous mixture of substances in addition to SCFA, including undigested dietary residues, bacterial metabolites and sloughed cells. Diet affects all of these factors in an interactive, site-specific manner (Chapkin *et al.*, 1993), making it difficult to attribute a particular effect to SCFA production alone. Feeding individual SCFA does not help clarify their role in colon carcinogenesis, since most SCFA are absorbed in the upper gastrointestinal tract and therefore never reach the colon. Intrarectal instillation of SCFA is impractical for long-term tumour studies and also fails to mimic the way in which SCFA are actually produced in the colon.

Despite these very real limitations, this chapter will attempt to provide an overall assessment of the relationship of SCFA to colon cancer by approaching the problem in an indirect manner. Three types of study are reviewed: (1) fibre/experimental carcinogen studies; (2) fibre/SCFA colonic cell proliferation studies; and (3) SCFA/experimental carcinogen studies, including the role of butyrate as a potential antineoplastic agent. From a review of these studies, hypotheses are made as to the mechanisms by which SCFA may promote and/or protect against colon carcinogenesis.

Dietary fibre and experimental colon carcinogenesis studies

Since dietary fibre is the usual substrate for SCFA production, a review of the fibres that are protective and those that fail to protect against colon cancer, combined with data on the fermentability of the fibre, should provide indirect evidence of the role of SCFA in tumorigenesis. Although the majority of epidemiological studies support a protective role of dietary fibres against colon carcinogenesis (Heilbrun *et al.*, 1989; Trock, Lanza & Greenwald, 1990), experiments in the murine model using a variety of fibres and carcinogens have produced conflicting results (Rogers & Nauss, 1984; Jacobs & Lupton, 1986). This is not surprising, since fibres are a heterogeneous group of compounds with different physicochemical properties. A review of all of the fibre/experimental carcinogen studies reveals a relatively consistent pattern: the less fermentable the fibre, the more protective it is against colon carcinogenesis. Although there are exceptions (Heitman, Hardman & Cameron, 1992), the poorly fermented wheat bran and cellulose generally protect against experimentally-induced colon cancer (Wilson, Hutcheson & Wideman, 1977; Barbolt & Abraham, 1978; Watanabe *et al.*, 1979; Cameron *et al.*, 1989; Heitman *et al.*, 1989) whereas the highly fermentable pectin, guar gum, oat bran, agar and carrageenan fail to protect and may actually enhance tumorigenesis (Watanabe *et al.*, 1979; Bauer *et al.*, 1981; Jacobs & Lupton, 1986). Most of the dietary fibre colon carcinogenesis studies are summarized in a review (Cameron *et al.*, 1990) and in a recent publication (Heitman *et al.*, 1992). These data indirectly support a promotive role for SCFA with respect to colon carcinogenesis.

It should be noted that SCFA production is not the only consequence of fibre fermentation (see Fig. 20.1). As fibre is fermented, it loses its dilution potential. We have previously shown that wheat bran and cellulose are far better *in vivo* dilutors of a non-absorbable marker than are the more fermentable fibres pectin, guar or oat bran (Gazzaniga & Lupton, 1987). This is important, because carcinogens and promoters (such as bile acids and ammonia) may be diluted in a bulky stool, but not if the fibre has been fermented to SCFA. Thus the fermentability of a fibre may be positively correlated with experimental tumorigenesis because of the loss of dilution potential rather than the production of SCFA.

Fibre/SCFA/colonic cell proliferation studies

A large number of reports support the hypothesis that early changes in cell division patterns are characteristic of and predictive for neoplasia (Farber, 1984; Romagnoli *et al.*, 1984; Williamson & Rainey, 1984). For this reason, measurements of cell proliferation are often considered the 'gold standard'

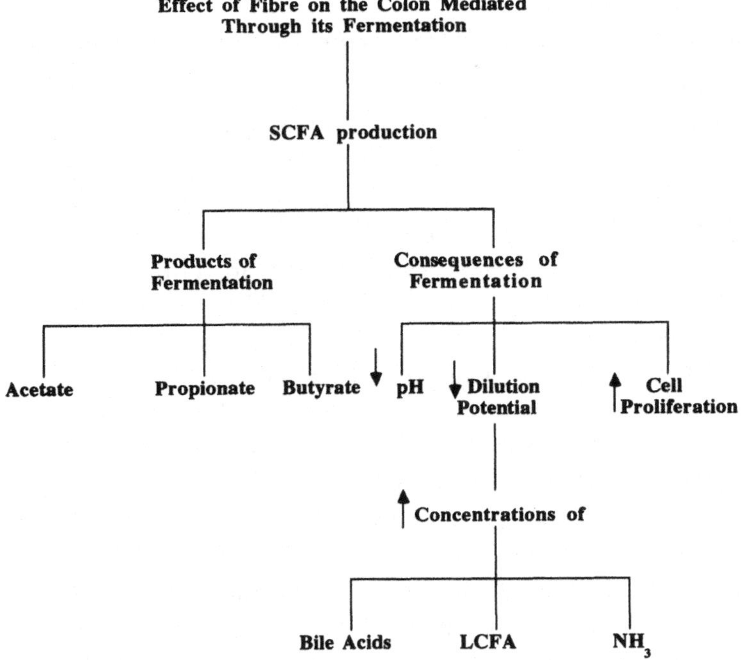

Fig. 20.1. The effect of fibre on the colon is mediated through its fermentation. As fibre is fermented, short-chain fatty acids (SCFA) are produced, primarily acetate, propionate and butyrate. As a consequence of the fermentation of fibre, the pH decreases, as does the dilution potential of the fibre. Luminal concentrations of bile acids, long-chain fatty acids (LCFA) and ammonia increase. There is a corresponding increase in cell proliferation.

of intermediate markers for colon carcinogenesis. Studies on the effect of fibres and SCFA on colonic cell proliferation should therefore provide important indirect information on their effect on tumorigenesis. The fermentability of different fibres to SCFA and their effect on cell proliferation are reviewed by Newmark & Lupton (1990). Studies indicate that fibre fermentability is important in determining mucosal cell proliferation (Jacobs & Lupton, 1984, 1986; Lupton, Coder & Jacobs, 1988), with the most fermentable fibres resulting in the greatest increases in cell proliferation. Sakata and co-workers (Sakata & von Engelhardt, 1983; Sakata & Yajima, 1984; Sakata, 1987) have conducted a series of carefully designed studies to determine the effects of SCFA on gastrointestinal epithelial cell proliferation. These studies, which are reviewed in detail elsewhere in this book (Chapter 19) clearly show that SCFA are mitogenic to the colonic mucosa.

SCFA/experimental carcinogen studies and the role of butyrate

Only two studies have reported both SCFA concentrations and tumour incidence, and both have involved the *in vivo* manipulation of butyrate levels. A number of studies have shown butyrate to be a differentiating agent and inhibitor of cell proliferation in various human colon cancer cell lines (Kim, Tsao & Siddiqui, 1980; Prasad, 1980; Kruh, 1982; Augeron & Laboisse, 1984; Siddiqui & Kim, 1984; Chung *et al.*, 1985; Whitehead, Young & Bhatal, 1986; Gum *et al.*, 1987). In large part due to these studies, butyrate is considered antineoplastic. There is therefore great interest in this SCFA as a chemotherapeutic and chemopreventive agent (Rephaeli *et al.*, 1991).

In the first *in vivo* butyrate study, Freeman (1986) provided 1% or 2% sodium butyrate in the drinking water of rats treated with the experimental colon carcinogen 1,2-dimethylhydrazine (DMH). More butyrate-treated animals at both the 1% and the 2% levels had bowel tumours (85% and 70%, respectively) than control rats (50%). In the second study, Deschner *et al.* (1990) hypothesized that the promotive effect of butyrate on DMH-induced colonic tumours in the Freeman study may have been due to the high amount of sodium consumed by the animals. They therefore provided butyrate as tributyrin to female CF1 mice using azoxymethane (AOM) as the experimental carcinogen. Although feeding of tributyrin resulted in a tenfold increase in faecal butyric acid levels, there were no differences in tumour incidence between tributyrin-fed and control mice. Thus, of the two studies, one showed a promotive effect of butyrate and the other showed no effect.

Almost all of the work on butyrate and cancer has been done *in vitro*, with the use of transformed cells. There is good evidence that the effect of SCFA on colonocytes is different in normal cells v. transformed cells (Prasad, 1980; Scheppach *et al.*, 1992). Butyrate appears to inhibit growth in transformed cells, while enhancing proliferation in normal human (Scheppach *et al.*, 1992) and rat (Sakata, 1987) mucosa. The apparent dichotomy between the *in vivo* and *in vitro* data has not been satisfactorily resolved. Boffa *et al.* (1992) addressed the issue of *in vivo/in vitro* discrepancies in the butyrate literature by replicating some of their *in vitro* work *in vivo*. Differing molarities of butyrate were created in the colonic lumen of rats by feeding different amounts of wheat bran, and their effect on epithelial cell histone acetylation and cytokinetics was evaluated. There was a significant inverse correlation between luminal butyrate levels and colonic cell proliferation, but no induction of terminal differentiation was detectable. There was a positive linear correlation between luminal butyric acid levels and colon epithelial cell histone acetylation. The histone acetylation data were similar to what has been observed *in vitro*, that the DNA strand is in a more open position in cells treated with butyrate (Ausio & van Holde, 1986). This makes the DNA more prone to carcinogen damage and to damage repair (Bohr, Phillips & Hanawalt, 1987). The lack of terminal differentiation was contrary to what has been observed for transformed cells in culture.

One possible conclusion from this study is that butyrate-induced hyperacetylation of histones may be protective against tumours at certain times (during DNA damage repair) and promotive at other times (during carcinogen administration). One other study lends support to this hypothesis. Jacobs (1983) supplemented rats with wheat bran during carcinogen administration, during promotion, or both. Wheat bran (which produces butyrate, particularly in the distal colon) was promotive if provided during carcinogen administration, but protective if provided during the promotion phase. A definitive resolution of these seeming inconsistencies awaits further research. In the meantime, however, the available data suggest that caution should be exercised in extrapolating from *in vitro* data to *in vivo* models, and from healthy colonic epithelial cells to their transformed counterparts.

Mechanisms by which SCFA may promote and/or protect against colon carcinogenesis

The process by which a luminal metabolite, such as SCFA, may initiate a signal for cell division is complex. A direct effect of SCFA on colonocytes has been proposed, as has a variety of indirect effects (Sakata & von Engelhardt, 1983). This subject is discussed in detail in Chapter 19. A few potentially pertinent observations are added here.

Effects of SCFA are mediated through changes in intracellular pH

It is well known that SCFA are rapidly absorbed by colonocytes (see Chapters 9 and 10), but their postabsorptive fate is less clear. In fact, the mechanism of absorption has not been clearly delineated, nor has the effect of SCFA absorption on intracellular pH. A certain proportion of SCFA may be absorbed by non-ionic diffusion (Mascolo, Rajendran & Binder, 1991), resulting in a rapid dissociation within the cell and a drop in intracellular pH. Non-ionic diffusion is not the only route of absorption, however, since SCFA are 99% ionized in the colonic lumen at a pH of 7.0 (pK_a 4.8) (Newmark & Lupton, 1990). Several anion exchange pathways have been proposed, although universal agreement has not been reached (Binder & Mehta, 1989; Sellin & DeSoignie, 1990; Harig *et al.*, 1991; Mascolo *et al.*, 1991). Again, although this is not yet reported, intracellular pH changes should result from the absorption of SCFA by an anion exchange system. This information is important because of the known relationship between changes in intracellular pH and cell division (Epel & Dube, 1987). Differences have been observed between pH values in many human tumours as compared to their respective normal tissues (Oberhaensli *et al.*, 1986; Vaupel, Kallinowski & Okunieff, 1989). An understanding of this phenomenon may make it possible to exploit differences in intracellular pH between tumours and normal tissues to develop new approaches to cancer therapy (Anon., 1992).

Effects of SCFA are mediated through changes in cellular metabolic events

SCFA have a profound effect on the metabolism of colonocytes, as shown by the atrophy of colonocytes deprived of SCFA (Glotzer, Glick & Goldman, 1981; Agarwal & Schimmel, 1989) and their recovery when SCFA were reintroduced (Harig *et al.*, 1989). The metabolism of butyrate by colonocytes with production of ketone bodies is a major difference between the large- and small-intestinal mucosae (Henning & Hird, 1972; Watford, Lund & Krebs, 1979) and may help explain diseases that are limited to the small- or large-bowel mucosae (Roediger, 1982). One consequence of the metabolism of SCFA such as butyrate is an increase in energy available to the cell. The energy, in theory, can be used for ATP-requiring reactions. Roediger & Moore (1981) showed that butyrate enhanced ATP-dependent sodium absorption twofold in freshly defunctioned human colonic loops. They suggested that this increased absorption of sodium in the presence of butyrate could have clinical implications in the genesis of postoperative diarrhoea.

Effects of SCFA are mediated through signalling events originating in changes in membrane lipids

Recent results from our laboratory show that the effects of fibre on cell proliferation are dependent on the source of fat in the diet (Chapkin *et al.*, 1993). How fat and fibre interact is not known, but data from Awad, Horvath & Andersen (1991) suggest that butyrate selectively affects the incorporation of dietary long-chain fatty acids (LCFA) into colonic cell membranes of certain tumour cells. In addition, butyrate enhanced differentiation in cells supplemented with certain LCFA but not with others. Changes in membrane lipids can, in turn, affect the activity of protein kinase C (PKC), which may play a crucial role in cellular growth regulation, differentiation and malignant transformation (Sakanoue *et al.*, 1991). Our data (Chapkin *et al.*, 1993) show an effect of fibre on PKC activity, and a significant correlation between this activity and cell proliferation.

Effects of SCFA are mediated through release of peptides

Peptide tyrosine (PYY) is a peptide of 36 amino acid residues that has been localized to endocrine cells of the intestinal mucosa (El-Salhy & Grimelius, 1983). Clinically, plasma levels of PYY are elevated in patients with malabsorption syndromes, inflammatory bowel disease or dumping syndrome, and after intestinal resection (Adrian *et al.*, 1986). In a recent study in isolated perfused rabbit colon, Longo *et al.* demonstrated that SCFA stimulated the release of PYY (Longo *et al.*, 1991), suggesting that SCFA act directly on the distal colonic mucosa in stimulating the release of PYY.

Therapeutic implications for humans

Few studies have been performed in humans in which SCFA are related to tumour incidence or cell proliferation. The one wheat-bran study that provided some evidence for a protective effect against benign large-bowel neoplasia (DeCosse, Miller & Lesser, 1989) was conducted in patients with familial adenomatous polyposis with total colectomies. Although SCFA were not measured in this study, it is unlikely that much fibre fermentation would have occurred in these individuals. In fact, Mitchell *et al.* (1985) found no relationship between fibre intake and either total or individual SCFA concentrations in digesta taken from the stomata of patients who had undergone large-bowel surgery.

In a recent study (Kashtan *et al.*, 1992) the effect of soluble fibre on indexes of colon-cancer risk in postpolypectomy and non-polyp patients was evaluated. Half the group received oat-bran supplements and the other half took wheat-bran supplements. Colonic biopsies taken before and after the intervention showed no difference in the index of thymidine colonic crypt cell labelling, despite increased fermentation by oat bran as evaluated by a drop in faecal pH with oat bran as compared to wheat bran.

Weaver *et al.* (1988) investigated the distribution of SCFA in enema samples taken from subjects before sigmoidoscopy as an indicator of possible microbial differences between subjects subsequently diagnosed as normal or those having colonic disorders. A significantly higher ratio of acetate to total SCFA and lower ratio of butyrate to total SCFA was found for polyp–colon cancer subjects than for normal subjects. The authors concluded that polyp–cancer patients have an increased capacity to produce acetate and a decreased capacity to form butyrate. An alternative hypothesis which they noted, but discarded, was that there was decreased utilization of butyrate by polyp–colon cancer subjects. A third explanation is that the habitual diets of individuals in these two groups were different, providing differing substrates for the microflora. It is of interest that a separate study found that subjects with polyps malabsorb less starch than do normal subjects (Thornton *et al.*, 1987) and resistant starch is known to produce fermentations high in butyrate (Englyst, Hay & Macfarlane, 1987).

In conclusion, data are lacking that directly relate colonic SCFA to tumour incidence. Although epidemiological data support a protective role for dietary fibre against colon cancer, experimental studies suggest that it is the less fermentable fibres that produce the beneficial effects. Studies on SCFA infused into the colon or produced from bacterial fermentation show that SCFA are mitogenic to the colonic mucosa. In general, agents that stimulate colonic cell proliferation enhance tumorigenesis. Butyrate is receiving intense scrutiny as an antineoplastic agent because of its differentiating and anti-proliferative effects in a variety of cancer cell lines. However, *in vivo* data on a protective effect of butyrate against colon carcinogenesis are lacking. Because of the very positive benefits of SCFA on maintaining a healthy mucosa, and on returning an atrophic mucosa to a normal proliferative state, it may well be that the timing and degree of SCFA-induced colonic proliferation is the key to understanding putative discrepancies in normal v. cancer cells and *in vivo* v. *in vitro* studies.

References

Adrian, T. E., Savage, T. E., Bacarese-Hamilton, A. J. *et al.* (1986). Peptide YY abnormalities in gastrointestinal disease. *Gastroenterology*, **90**, 379–84.

Agarwal, V. P. & Schimmel, E. M. (1989). Diversion colitis: a nutritional deficiency syndrome? *Nutrition Review*, **47**, 257–61.

Anon. (1992). Tumor pH. *Lancet*, **340**, 342–3.

Augeron, C. & Laboisse, C. L. (1984). Emergence of permanently differentiated cell clones in a human colonic cancer cell line in culture after treatment with sodium butyrate. *Cancer Research*, **44**, 3961–9.

Ausio, J. & van Holde, K. E. (1986). Histone hyperacetylation: its effects on nucleosome conformation and stability. *Biochemistry*, **25**, 1421–8.

Awad, A. B., Horvath, P. J. & Andersen, M. S. (1991). Influence of butyrate on lipid metabolism, survival and differentiation of colon cancer cells. *Nutrition and Cancer*, **16**, 125–33.

Barbolt, T. A. & Abraham, R. (1978). The effect of bran in dimethylhydrazine-induced colon carcinogenesis of the rat. *Proceedings of the Society of Experimental Biology and Medicine*, **157**, 656–9.

Bauer, H. G., Asp. N.-G., Dahlqvist, A., Fredlung, P. E., Nyman, M. & Oste, R. (1981). Effect of two kinds of pectin and guar gum on 1,2-dimethylhydrazine initiation of colon tumors and on fecal β-glucuronidase activity in the rat. *Cancer Research*, **41**, 2518–23.

Binder, H. J. & Mehta, P. (1989). Short-chain fatty acids stimulate active sodium and chloride absorption *in vitro* in the rat distal colon. *Gastroenterology*, **96**, 989–96.

Boffa, L. C., Lupton, J. R., Mariani, M. R., Ceppi, M., Newmark, H. L., Scalmati, A. & Lipkin, M. (1992). Modulation of colonic epithelial cell proliferation, histone acetylation, and luminal short chain fatty acids by variation of dietary fiber (wheat bran) in rats. *Cancer Research*, **52**, 5906–12.

Bohr, V. A., Phillips, D. H. & Hanawalt, P. C. (1987). Heterogeneous DNA damage and repair in the mammalian genome. *Cancer Research*, **47**, 6426–36.

Cameron, I. L., Ord, V. A., Hunter, K. E. & Heitman, D. W. (1990). Colon carcinogenesis: modulation of progression. In *Colon Cancer Cells*, ed. M. P. Moyer and G. H. Poste, pp. 63–84. Academic Press.

Cameron, I. L., Ord, V. A., Hunter, K. E., Padilla, G. M. & Heitman, D. W. (1989). Suppression of a carcinogen (1,2-dimethylhydrazine dihydrochloride)-induced increase in mitotic activity in the colonic crypts of rats by addition of dietary cellulose. *Cancer Research*, **49**, 991–5.

Chapkin, R. S., Gao, J., Lee, D.-Y. K. & Lupton, J. R. (1993). Dietary fibers and fats alter rat colon protein kinase C activity: correlation to cell proliferation. *Journal of Nutrition*, **123**, 649–55.

Chung, Y. S., Song, I. S., Erickson, R. H., Sleisenger, M. H. & Kim, Y. S. (1985). Effect of growth and sodium butyrate on brush border membrane-associated hydrolases in human colorectal cancer cell lines. *Cancer Research*, **45**, 2976–82.

DeCosse, J. J., Miller, H. H. & Lesser, M. L. (1989). Effect of wheat fiber and vitamins C and E on rectal polyps in patients with familial adenomatous polyposis. *Journal of the National Cancer Institute*, **81**, 1290–7.

Deschner, E. E., Ruperto, J. F., Lupton, J. R. & Newmark, H. L. (1990). Dietary butyrate (tributyrin) does not enhance AOM-induced colon tumorigenesis. *Cancer Letters*, **52**, 79–82.

El-Salhy, T. & Grimelius, L. (1983). Immunocytochemical demonstration of poly-peptide YY (PYY) in the gastrointestinal tract of the monkey, *Macaca rhesus*: a light and electron microscopic study. *Biomedically Research*, **4**, 289–94.

Englyst, H. N., Hay, S. & Macfarlane, G. T. (1987). Polysaccharide breakdown by mixed populations of human fecal bacteria. *FEMS Microbiology Ecology*, **95**, 163–71.

Epel, D. & Dube, F. (1987). Intracellular pH and cell proliferation. In *Control of Animal Cell Proliferation II*, ed. A. L. Boynton & H. L. Leffert, pp. 364–93. Academic Press.

Farber, E. (1984). Cellular biochemistry of the stepwise development of cancer with chemicals. G. H. A. Clowes memorial lecture. *Cancer Research*, **44**, 5463–74.

Freeman, H. J. (1986). Effects of differing concentrations of sodium butyrate on 1,2-dimethylhydrazine-induced rat intestinal neoplasia. *Gastroenterology*, **91**, 596–602.

Gazzaniga, J. M. & Lupton, J. R. (1987). Dilution effect of dietary fiber sources: an *in vivo* study in the rat. *Nutrition Research*, **7**, 1261–8.

Glotzer, D. J., Glick, M. E. & Goldman, H. (1981). Proctitis and colitis following diversion of the fecal stream. *Gastroenterology*, **80**, 438–41.

Gum, J. R., Kam, W. K., Byrd, J. C., Hicks, J. W., Sleisenger, M. H. & Kim, Y. S. (1987). Effects of sodium butyrate on human colonic adenocarcinoma cells: induction of placental-like alkaline phosphatase. *Journal of Biological Chemistry*, **262**, 1092–7.

Harig, J. M., Soergel, K. H., Barry, J. A. & Ramaswamy, K. (1991). Transport of propionate by human ileal brush-border membrane vesicles. *American Journal of Physiology*, **260**, G776–G782.

Harig, J. M., Soergel, K. H., Komorowski, R. A. & Wood, C. M. (1989). Treatment of diversion colitis with short-chain fatty acid irrigation. *New England Journal of Medicine*, **320**, 23–8.

Heilbrun, L. K., Nomura, A., Hankin, J. H. & Stemmermann, G. N. (1989). Diet and colorectal cancer with special reference to fiber intake. *International Journal of Cancer*, **44**, 1–6.

Heitman, D. W., Hardman, W. E. & Cameron, I. L. (1992). Dietary supplementation with pectin and guar gum on 1,2-dimethylhydrazine-induced colon carcinogenesis in rats. *Carcinogenesis*, **13**, 815–18.

Heitman, D. W., Ord, V. A., Hunter, K. E. & Cameron, I. L. (1989). Effect of dietary cellulose on cell proliferation and progression of 1,2-dimethylhydrazine-induced colon carcinogenesis in rats. *Cancer Research*, **49**, 5581–5.

Henning, S. J. & Hird, F. J. R. (1972). Ketogenesis from butyrate and acetate by the caecum and the colon of rabbits. *Biochemical Journal*, **130**, 785–90.

Jacobs, L. R. (1983). Enhancement of rat colon carcinogenesis by wheat bran consumption during the stage of 1,2-dimethylhydrazine administration. *Cancer Research*, **43**, 4057–61.

Jacobs, L. R. & Lupton, J. R. (1984). Effect of dietary fibers on rat large bowel mucosal growth and cell proliferation. *American Journal of Physiology*, **246**, G367–G385.

Jacobs, L. R. & Lupton, J. R. (1986). Relationship between colonic luminal pH, cell proliferation, and colon carcinogenesis in 1,2-dimethylhydrazine-treated rats fed high fiber diets. *Cancer Research*, **46**, 1727–34.

Kashtan, H., Stern, H. S., Jenkins, D. J., Jenkins, A. L., Thompson, L. U., Hay, K., Marcon, N., Minkin, S. & Bruce, W. R. (1992). Colonic fermentation and markers of colorectal-cancer risk. *American Journal of Clinical Nutrition*, **55**, 723–8.

Kim, Y. S., Tsao, D. & Siddiqui, B. (1980). Effects of sodium butyrate and dimethylsulfoxide on biochemical properties of human colon cancer cells. *Cancer*, **45**, 1185–92.

Kruh, J. (1982). Effects of sodium butyrate, a new pharmacological agent, on cells in culture. *Molecular Cell Biochemistry*, **42**, 65–82.

Longo, W. E., Ballantyne, G. H., Savoca, P. E., Adrian, T. E., Bilchik, A. J. & Modlin, I. M. (1991). Short-chain fatty acid release of peptide YY in the isolated rabbit distal colon. *Scandinavian Journal of Gastoenterology*, **26**, 442–8.

Lupton, J. R., Coder, D. M. & Jacobs, L. R. (1988). Long term effects of fermentable fibers on rat colonic pH and epithelial cell cycle. *Journal of Nutrition*, **188**, 840–5.

Mascolo, N., Rajendran, V. M. & Binder, H. J. (1991). Mechanism of short-chain fatty acid uptake by apical membrane vesicles of rat distal colon. *Gastroenterology*, **101**, 331–8.

Mitchell, B. L., Lawson, M. J., Davis, M., Grant, A. K., Roediger, W. E. W.,

Illman, R. J. & Topping, D. L. (1985). Volatile fatty acids in the human intestine: studies in surgical patients. *Nutrition Research*, **5**, 1089–92.

Newmark, H. L. & Lupton, J. R. (1990). Determinants and consequences of colonic luminal pH: implications for colon cancer. *Nutrition and Cancer*, **14**, 161–73.

Oberhaensli, R. D., Hilton-Jones, D., Bore, P. J., Hands, L. J., Rampling, R. P. & Radda, G. K. (1986). Biochemical investigation of human tumours *in vivo* with phosphorus-31 magnetic resonance spectroscopy. *Lancet*, **2**, 8–11.

Prasad, K. N. (1980). Butyric acid: a small fatty acid with diverse functions. *Life Science*, **27**, 1351–8.

Rephaeli, A., Rabizadeh, E., Aviram, A., Shaklai, M., Ruse, M. & Nudelman, A. (1991). Derivatives of butyric acid as potential anti-neoplastic agents. *International Journal of Cancer*, **49**, 66–72.

Roediger, W. E. W. (1982), Utilization of nutrients by isolated epithelial cells of the rat colon. *Gastroenterology*, **83**, 424–9.

Roediger, W. E. W. & Moore, A. (1981). Effect of short-chain fatty acid on sodium absorption in isolated human colon perfused through the vascular bed. *Digestive Diseases and Sciences*, **26**, 100–6.

Rogers, A. E. & Nauss, K. M. (1984). Contributions of laboratory animal studies of colon carcinogenesis. In *Large Bowel Cancer*, ed. A. J. Mastromarino & M. G. Brattain, pp. 1–45. New York: Praeger.

Romagnoli, P. Filipponi, F. Bandettini, L. & Bregnola, D. (1984). Increase of mitotic activity in the colonic mucosa of patients with colorectal cancer. *Diseases of the Colon and Rectum*, **27**, 305–8.

Sakanoue, Y., Hatada, T., Kusunoki, M., Yanagi, H., Yamamura, T. & Utsunomiya, J. (1991). Protein kinase C activity as marker for colorectal cancer. *International Journal of Cancer*, **48**, 803–6.

Sakata, T. (1987). Stimulatory effect of short-chain fatty acids on epithelial cell proliferation in the rat intestine: a possible explanation for trophic effect of fermentable fibre, gut microbes and luminal trophic factors. *British Journal of Nutrition*, **58**, 95–103.

Sakata, T. & von Engelhardt, W. (1983). Stimulatory effect of short chain fatty acids on the epithelial cell proliferation in rat large intestine. *Comparative Biochemistry Physiology*, **74A**, 459–62.

Sakata, T. & Yajima, T. (1984). Influence of short chain fatty acids on the epithelial cell division of digestive tract. *Quarterly Journal of Experimental Physiology*, **69**, 639–48.

Scheppach, W., Bartram, P., Richter, F., Liepold, H. Dusel, G., Hofstetter, G., Ruthlein, J. & Kasper, H. (1992). The effect of short-chain fatty acids on the human colonic mucosa *in vitro*. *Journal of Parenteral and Enteral Nutrition*, **16**, 43–8.

Sellin, J. H. & DeSoignie, R. (1990). Short-chain fatty acid absorption in rabbit colon *in vitro*. *Gastroenterology*, **99**, 676–83.

Siddiqui, B. & Kim, J. S. (1984). Effects of sodium butyrate, dimethyl sulfoxide, and retinoic acid on glycolipids of human rectal adenocarcinoma cells. *Cancer Research*, **44**, 1648–52.

Thornton, J. R., Dryden, A., Kelleher, J. & Losowsky, M. S. (1987). Super-efficient starch absorption. A risk factor for colonic neoplasia. *Digestive Diseases and Sciences*, **32**, 1088–81.

Trock, B., Lanza, E. & Greenwald, P. (1990). Dietary fiber, vegetables, and colon cancer: a critical review and meta-analysis of the epidemiologic evidence. *Journal of the National Cancer Institute*, **82**, 650–61.

Vaupel, P., Kallinowski, F. & Okunieff, P. (1989). Blood flow, oxygen and nutrient supply, and metabolic microenvironment of human tumours: a review. *Cancer Research*, **49**, 6449–65.

Watanabe, K., Reddy, B. S., Weisburger, J. H. & Kritchevsky, D. (1979). Effect of dietary alfalfa, pectin and wheat bran on azoxymethane- or methylnitrosourea-induced colon carcinogenesis in F344 rats. *Journal of the National Cancer Institute*, **63**, 141–5.

Watford, M., Lund, P. & Krebs, H. A. (1979). Isolation and metabolic characteristics of rat or chicken enterocytes. *Biochemical Journal*, **178**, 589–96.

Weaver, G. A., Krause, J. A., Miller, T. L. & Wolin, M. J. (1988). Short chain fatty acid distributions of enema samples from a sigmoidoscopy population: an association of high acetate and low butyrate ratios with adenomatous polyps and colon cancer. *Gut*, **29**, 1539–43.

Whitehead, R. H., Young, G. P. & Bhatal, P. S. (1986). Effects of short chain fatty acids on a new human colon carcinoma cell line (LIM1215). *Gut*, **27**, 1457–63.

Williamson, R. C. N. & Rainey, J. R. (1984). The relationship between intestinal hyperplasia and carcinogenesis. *Scandinavian Journal of Gastroenterology*, **9** (Suppl. 104), 57–76.

Wilson, R. B., Hutcheson, D. P. & Wideman, L. (1977). Dimethylhydrazine-induced colon tumors in rats fed diets containing beef fat and corn oil with and without wheat bran. *American Journal of Clinical Nutrition*, **30**, 176–81.

21

Butyrate and the human cancer cell

G. P. YOUNG AND P. R. GIBSON

Introduction

In normal colonic epithelium, the dividing cells are located in the mid to lower portion of the crypt. Daughter cells migrate towards the luminal surface and mature (Colony, 1989). The mature colonocyte is highly polarized, with an apical brush border linked to adjacent cells by tight junctions at the level of the terminal web (Colony, 1989). Cell-to-cell interactions maintain the polarized state. Membrane biogenesis must proceed normally for differentiation to occur, i.e. membrane components such as vasoactive intestinal peptide (VIP) receptors and Na/K-ATPase must be present.

In cancers, the normal crypt structure is disrupted as cells proliferate and invade the basement membrane. Cells also fail to show the usual characteristics of differentiation; as aplasia increases there is increasing disorganization of subcellular architecture and loss of polarity (Higgins, 1989). Levels of the brush border membrane enzyme alkaline phosphatase, a marker of differentiation, are lower in tumours compared to normal epithelium (Bell & Williams, 1979). Expression of the brush border hydrolases aminopeptidase-N and diaminopeptidylpeptidase-IV, also markers of differentiation, are perturbed in the neoplastic process in the colon (Young *et al.*, 1992).

Of the principal short-chain fatty acids (SCFA) produced in the colon as an energy source for the normal epithelium, butyrate is especially important (Roediger, 1982; Butler *et al.*, 1990). It also has interesting and unique effects on tumour cells. Addition of butyrate to cultured tumour cell lines has revealed two major effects of special relevance to colorectal tumorigenesis.

(1) Butyrate inhibits DNA synthesis and arrests cultured tumour cells in the G_1 phase of the cell cycle (see Toscani, Soprano & Soprano, 1988). In concentrations that have this effect, it is not toxic to cells; it only marginally inhibits RNA and protein synthesis and the cells remain viable and functional.

(2) Butyrate is a potent inducer of differentiation of tumour cells, producing a phenotype typically associated with the normal mature cell (Whitehead, Young & Bhathal, 1989).

As butyrate is produced during fermentation of dietary fibre, it might account for the protective effect of certain types of fibre for colonic tumorigenesis.

In this chapter, we discuss aspects of epithelial cell biology and molecular biology in normal and neoplastic human cells that are likely to be influenced by butyrate.

Butyrate and the cancer cell

Effects on in vitro *cell proliferation*

The LIM1215 cell line is a moderately differentiated line with morphological features of colonocytes, derived from a 35-year-old patient belonging to a hereditary non-polyposis colorectal cancer kindred. We have shown that addition of butyrate at concentrations of 1–10 mM markedly slowed proliferation in the cell line (Fig. 21.1); the cell doubling time in monolayer culture increased from 26 h to 72 h and cloning efficiency fell from 1.1 to 0.05% (Whitehead *et al.*, 1986).

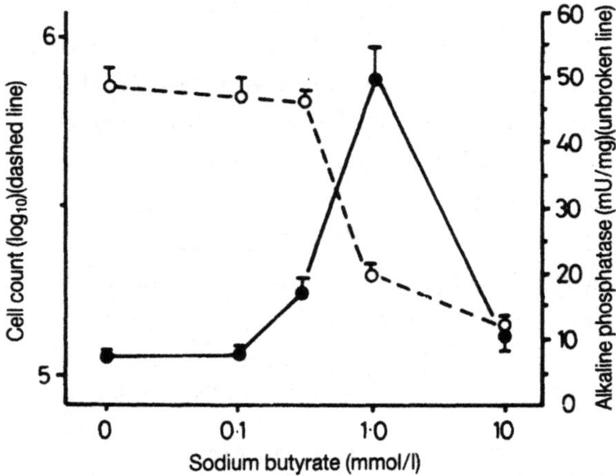

Fig. 21.1. Effect of various concentrations of butyrate on cell growth and alkaline phosphatase activity of LIM1215 colon cancer cells in monolayer culture as reported by Whitehead *et al.* (1986). Reproduced with permission of the publisher.

Butyrate slowed cell proliferation and/or blocked DNA synthesis *in vitro* in a range of other colorectal cancer cell lines as well, including SW480, SW620, HRT-18, HE-29, CaCo-2 and LS180 (Kim *et al.*, 1980; Tsao *et al.*, 1982; Whitehead *et al.*, 1986; Czerniak, *et al.*, 1987; Colony, 1989; Barnard & Warwick, 1992; Souleimani & Asselin, 1992). In the HRT-18 cell line it blocked anchor-independent growth (Tsao *et al.*, 1982). At 2 mM, this effect occurred without loss of cell viability. At 5 mM, there was complete inhibition of growth but viability was also lost due to toxicity. Slowing of proliferation was not permanent, however, and on withdrawal of butyrate the growth rate rapidly increased. Butyrate also caused HRT-18 cells to become larger and arranged in a polygonal epithelioid fashion.

These effects probably occurred because butyrate arrests cells in the G_1 phase of the cell cycle (Toscani *et al.*, 1988; Barnard & Warwick, 1992). The specific mechanism by which this might be achieved is discussed below.

Effect on differentiation markers

The effect of the principal SCFA on expression of various markers of differentiation has been examined in the LIM1215 cancer cell line (Whitehead *et al.*, 1986). Acetate, propionate and butyrate are all produced as a result of fermentation of fibre, but butyrate had the most marked effects. At 1 mM, it increased alkaline phosphatase activity by 600% (Fig. 21.1); acetate and propionate increased activity by only 50–100%. Butyrate also increased diaminopeptidylpeptidase-IV activity (by 35%) and the number of cells expressing the enzyme (from 3% to 60%). Suppression of proliferation and induction of alkaline phosphatase activity occurred at the same time-point in culture, suggesting a close link between the differentiating and anti-proliferative effects.

Other studies have not examined the range of fermentation products but have shown similar effects for butyrate. Chung *et al.* (1985) tested the effect of butyrate on four brush-border membrane hydrolases in 14 cell lines. Responses varied:

(1) Alkaline phosphatase: butyrate increased activity in 10 of the 14 lines, with increases ranging from two- to 123-fold! Increased activity was blocked by cycloheximide in the HRT-18 line, indicating that the increase was due to new protein synthesis and not to slowed degradation (Tsao *et al.*, 1982).
(2) Diaminopeptidylpeptidase: butyrate caused either a slight rise or no effect.
(3) Aminopeptidase: butyrate decreased activity in 12 of 14 cell lines.
(4) Sucrase: butyrate increased activity in seven of 14 cell lines.

There was no correlation between alkaline phosphatase induction and effects on the other enzymes, but there was a relationship between alkaline phosphatase inducibility and degree of differentiation (i.e. by morphology).

Barnard & Warwick (1992) have demonstrated that butyrate induces 'enterocytic' differentiation in HT-29 cells and alkaline phosphatase mRNA.

On the basis of these findings, we can conclude that butyrate can induce some cancer cells to acquire a phenotype more consistent with the normal differentiated cell, but this effect does not occur in all cell lines, suggesting that some are resistant to this 'antitumour' effect.

Differentiation as a key factor in cell behaviour

In normal colonic epithelium, differentiation is causally linked with loss of ability to undergo cell division. Differentiation may be defined as a cell locked in the G_1 phase of the cell cycle with the necessary components for cell function being properly integrated (Higgins, 1989). One hypothesis concerning the genesis of neoplasia is that it results from a disorder that allows cells to escape this state of terminal differentiation (Kim *et al.*, 1980). This has generated great interest in the ability of so-called 'differentiating agents' to suppress the rate of growth of cancer cells by returning cells to G_1 and inducing expression of a differentiated phenotype.

Significance of butyrate production in vivo *for tumorigenesis*

The importance of these *in vitro* effects on proliferation and differentiation for the whole animal are not clear, for a number of reasons. The 'antitumour' effects occur *in vitro* at low concentrations of butyrate (1–5 mM), yet luminal concentrations reach as high as 30 mM (McIntyre *et al.*, 1991) without apparent detrimental effect. Perhaps mucus at the luminal surface of the epithelium creates a microenvironment that effectively reduces the concentration of butyrate to which the colonocyte is exposed.

There is no simple way to deliver butyrate to the colon. Orally administered butyrate is absorbed before it reaches the colon (Freeman, 1986). Butyrate esters and tributyrin influence proximal colonic butyrate levels in animals, but have not been tried in humans. The predominance of cancers in the distal colon suggests that it is important that distal colonic and faecal levels of butyrate are increased, before its effect can adequately be evaluated *in vivo*.

A recent study has shown that faecal levels of butyrate vary considerably when animals are fed different fibres (McIntyre *et al.*, 1991). In the rat (McIntyre *et al.*, 1991) and humans (Kashtan *et al.*, 1992) the slowly fermentable fibre wheat bran was more effective than more completely fermentable and soluble fibres at maintaining high butyrate levels along the length of the large bowel. Therefore feeding wheat bran is the best way known to deliver butyrate to the distal colon.

In animal models of bowel cancer, when wheat bran is given throughout the period of study, it commonly protects against tumours (Young, 1990). This is not the case for soluble fibres such as guar gum or pectin, which do not elevate distal colonic and faecal butyrate. Furthermore, there is a significant inverse relationship between tumour mass and faecal butyrate levels in the rat model (McIntyre, Gibson & Young. 1993). Direct interventional studies in humans have shown that administration of wheat bran (as bran cereal flakes) to patients with familial adenomatous polyposis and rectum remaining intact resulted in a reduction of adenoma formation within 9 months (De Cosse, Miller & Lesser, 1989).

Such findings give indirect evidence for a tumour protective effect of butyrate, but a contrary view has been expressed. Paraskeva *et al.* (1990), suggested that butyrate actually selects out butyrate-resistant cells by killing off these that are sensitive; they propose that the resistant cells have a greater than usual malignant potential. It is difficult to test such a possibility *in vivo*. This raises the question of whether butyrate-sensitivity or resistance is dependent on the stage a cell has reached in the process of tumorigenesis. To address this, we need to compare the effects of butyrate on normal and neoplastic cells.

Butyrate and normal colonic epithelium

Butyrate plays roles in several key areas of the biology of colonic epithelium.

Energy supply

Consumption of energy by colonic epithelium is likely to be high as a result of high cell turnover in the epithelium and the transport and barrier functions it carries out. Studies of utilization of potential metabolic substrates have demonstrated that butyrate is the major fuel; it seems to be the preferred energy source, as it has a sparing effect on oxidation of the alternative substrates, glucose and glutamine (Roediger, 1980; Roediger, 1982; Ardawi & Newsholme, 1985; Butler *et al.*, 1990).

Faecal desiccation

One of the major functions of colonic epithelium is to desiccate luminal contents. Luminal SCFA stimulate epithelial absorption of sodium (Ruppin, Bar-Meir & Soergel, 1980; Roediger & Moore, 1981). This process appears at least in part to be dependent on the generation of carbon dioxide from the oxidation of butyrate (Roediger, 1989). Additional mechanisms might include upregulation of Na^+/H^+ transport by inducing transcription of mRNA for the Na^+/H^+ exchanger, as recently described in CaCo-2 cells (Bishop *et al.*, 1992). This effect is also of relevance to the control of intracellular pH, since SCFA acidify the intracellular environment and regulation of such acidification involves Na^+/H exchange (Sellin & DeSoignie, 1992).

Cell adhesion

Another major function of colonic epithelium is to provide a tight and efficient barrier between the internal milieu and the chemically complex luminal environment. The efficiency of the barrier depends upon cell–cell and cell–substratum adhesion as well as on the tight junctions. Colonic epithelial cells must also be able to break such cell adhesions in order to migrate up the crypt and to be shed from the surface into the lumen. Factors controlling adhesion and migration are poorly understood. One mechanism of importance in migration of keratinocytes, monocytes and fibroblasts (Kirchheimer & Binder, 1991; Lazarus & Jensen, 1991) is the activity of cell-surface, receptor-bound urokinase, a neutral protease that activates plasminogen. The wide range of substrates for plasmin includes basement-membrane components such as laminin, proteoglycan and fibronectin, which have specific binding sites on cell-surface proteins such as integrins. Urokinase receptors appear to reside in clusters around cell–cell and cell–substratum contact points (Pollanen *et al.*, 1987; Takahashi *et al.*, 1990; Schmitt *et al.*, 1991). If such receptor localization occurs in colonic epithelium, a role for urokinase in the control of colonic epithelial cell adhesion and migration would seem reasonable.

We have recently demonstrated that colonic epithelial cells have urokinase associated with their plasma membrane (Gibson, van de Pol & Doe, 1991*b*) and that *in vitro* they constitutively secrete urokinase and at least one of its specific inhibitors, plasminogen activator inhibitor-1 (PAI-1) (P. R. Gibson, O. Rosella, G. Rosella & G. P. Young, unpublished data). Butyrate at non-toxic concentrations (1–4 mM) markedly inhibits the secretion of urokinase (but not PAI-1) to a degree similar to that exhibited by pharmacological concentrations of dexamethasone, a potent inhibitor of urokinase production in many other cell types (Gibson *et al.*, 1993*b*). Butyrate acts at least in part by inhibiting transcription of u-PA mRNA (Gibson *et al.*, 1993*b*). Dietary elevation of luminal butyrate concentrations in the distal colon and rectum of rats is associated with significantly lower mucosal urokinase activity (Gibson *et al.*, 1993*a*), suggesting that butyrate also reduces urokinase secretion *in vivo*. The relationship, however, between butyrate's effect on the urokinase system and functional aspects of colonic epithelium (such as barrier function or epithelial repair) remains speculative at present.

Proliferation and differentiation

Evidence is now compelling that luminal butyrate plays a key role in colonic mucosal growth and epithelial proliferation. When luminal butyrate production is markedly suppressed by a reduction in the delivery of fermentable substrates to the colon, e.g. by an elemental diet (Janne, Carpenter & Willems, 1977; Goodlad & Wright, 1983) or by diversion of the faecal stream (Sakata, 1988), mucosal atrophy occurs. Subsequent instillation of SCFA into the lumen results in mucosal regeneration characterized by increased mucosal weight and DNA content, crypt length and mitotic index (Sakata 1984; Kripke *et al.*, 1989). These effects are mainly due to butyrate (Kripke *et al.*, 1989; Sakata, 1987).

Whether butyrate modulates cell differentiation as well as proliferation *in vivo* is uncertain, but elevation of luminal butyrate concentrations in rats by ingestion of wheat bran does not change the mucosal expression of the brush-border hydrolases, alkaline phosphatase and dipeptidyl peptidase IV (Young & Gibson, 1991).

The mechanisms by which butyrate promotes intestinal growth are far from elucidated. Considerable evidence supports an *indirect* systemic effect, especially since SCFA mixtures stimulate the mitotic index not only in colonic epithelium exposed to luminal SCFA but also in unexposed adjacent colonic epithelium, ileum and jejunum (Sakata & von Engelhardt, 1983; Sakata, 1987; Kripke *et al.*, 1989). Colonic perfusion of SCFA stimulates mucosal growth in unperfused, isolated, denervated loops of jejunum (Sakata, 1989). However, a *direct* action cannot be excluded, as butyrate has recently been shown to stimulate epithelial proliferation in short-term organ culture of human colonic mucosa where circulating and neural factors are not operating (Scheppach *et al.*, 1992).

It has been suggested that a deficiency of luminal butyrate leads to an

Table 21.1. *The paradoxical effects of butyrate on cell proliferation and differential of normal and neoplastic colonic epithelial cells*

	Normal cells		Cancer cells	
	In vitro	*In vivo*	*In vitro*	*In vivo*
Cell proliferation	No change[a]/?increased[b]	Increased[c]	Reduced[d]	Probably reduced[e]
Differentiation	Suppressed[f]	No change[g]	Induced[h]	Unknown

[a] Gibson *et al.* (1991*a*); [b] Scheppach *et al.* (1992); [c] Sakata (1984, 1987); [d] Kim *et al.* (1980); Tsao *et al.* (1982); Whitehead *et al.* (1986); Czerniak *et al.* (1987); Colony (1989); Barnard & Warwick (1992); Souleimani & Asselin (1992); [e] De Cosse *et al.* (1989); McIntyre *et al.* (1993); [f] Gibson *et al.* (1991*a*); [g] Young & Gibson (1991); [h] Chung *et al.* (1985); Whitehead *et al.* (1986); Barnard & Warwick (1992).

energy-deficient state, because the cells cannot meet energy demands using alternative sources such as glutamine or glucose (Roediger, 1990). Atrophy would, therefore, ensue and regeneration would be anticipated upon reintroduction of luminal butyrate. *In vitro* studies of isolated, viable colonic epithelial cells, mainly from the macroscopically normal mucosa of cancer-bearing colons, do not, however, support this thesis. These cell populations cultured for 24 h in the absence of butyrate do not exhibit reduction in the rates of energy-consuming processes such as DNA, protein and glycoprotein synthesis and the total DNA content is not altered (Gibson *et al.*, 1991*a*). Furthermore, expression of phenotypic markers of differentiation is significantly decreased following 24-h exposure to butyrate, suggesting that butyrate does not promote but may suppress differentiation of normal colonic epithelial cells (Gibson *et al.*, 1991*a*).

Paradoxical effect of butyrate on normal and neoplastic cells

The effects of butyrate on normal colonic epithelium appear paradoxical when compared with the well-documented effects of butyrate on colon cancer cell lines (for summary, see Table 21.1). These paradoxical observations are unlikely to be artefactual; the *in vitro* effects have been observed at non-toxic concentrations of butyrate, and the enzymatic cell isolation technique used for normal cells does not change responsiveness of cancer cells subsequently exposed to butyrate (Gibson *et al.*, 1991*a*). Yet the paradox is not observed in other tissues. In certain non-colonic epithelia – keratinocytes (Schmidt *et al.*, 1989), hepatocytes (Staecker, Sattler & Pitot, 1988) and rumen epithelial cells (Neogrady, Galfi & Kutas, 1989) – cellular response to butyrate is like that of the corresponding cancer cells. Therefore, it would seem that the paradox is unique to the colon.

The 'normal' human cells used for study of *in vitro* responses to butyrate may not be truly normal, as they have actually been derived from cancer-bearing colons (Gibson *et al.*, 1989; Gibson *et al.*, 1991*a*). Colonic epithelium distant from tumours exhibits abnormal differentiation characteristics in addition to increased proliferative activity (Gibson *et al.*, 1992). We have also observed unusual *in vitro* behaviour of colonic crypt cells from cancer-bearing colons, namely, marked suppression of protein synthesis by serum in a proportion of such populations (Gibson, Rosella & Young, 1994).

The mechanisms underlying the paradox are unclear. The metabolic profile of cancer cells and normal cells might be different. A histochemical study suggested that colon cancer cells *in vivo* switch from principally aerobic to anaerobic metabolism (Jass, Strudley & Faludy, 1984). Failure to oxidize butyrate might lead to higher intracellular butyrate concentrations or greater intracellular acidification in the cancer cells, resulting in exaggerated or different effects on gene expression. Whatever the mechanism, different responses are seen at the two ends of the tumorigenic pathway. At what stage a 'switch' in the pattern of response to butyrate occurs is not known, but such information could be of great relevance to dietary prevention of colorectal neoplasia.

The paradoxical response to butyrate does not, however, apply to all of its effects. For example, butyrate is a potent inhibitor of urokinase secretion by LIM1215 colon cancer cells (G. P. Young & P. R. Gibson, unpublished data) and normal cells. Colon cancer cells both secrete urokinase and express urokinase receptors (Boyd *et al.*, 1988), and cell-surface urokinase activity is greatest at the invading front of the cancer (Kohga *et al.* 1985). The inhibitory effect of butyrate on its secretion may have pathophysiological importance in modulating tissue invasion, especially at an early stage in colorectal tumorigenesis, when the relevant cells are more likely to be exposed to high butyrate concentrations.

Steps in colorectal tumorigenesis

While the multistep process of tumorigenesis has been known for over 20 years, it is only recently that investigators have identified important genetic events and speculated on their significance for each of the phenotypic steps. The progression through hyperproliferative epithelium, formation of aberrant crypts, the various stages of dysplasia seen in adenomas, to preinvasive, invasive and metastatic carcinoma, is now well known and generally accepted (Willson, 1989; Fearon & Vogelstein, 1990; Fig. 21.2). It is generally considered that there is a progressive disorder of growth control in this multistage process. The determinants for each stage are not yet clearly defined and the factors controlling progression from one stage to the next are not yet clear.

Increasing evidence suggests that this multistep process depends upon an accumulation of genetic alterations (Fearon & Vogelstein, 1990). In the development of human colorectal cancer these include the APC (adenomatous polyposis coli) locus on chromosome 5, the p53 gene on chromosome 17, and the DCC (deleted in colorectal cancer) gene on chromosome 18. Another genetic alteration thought to be of importance is mutation of the *ras* proto-oncogene. These genetic events are acquired in random order, although mutations in the APC gene may be inherited. Precisely how these

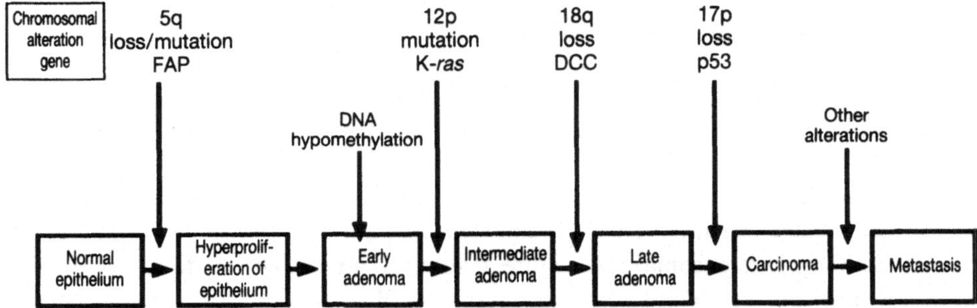

Fig. 21.2. Proposed model for relationship between phenotypic stages and genetic events in colorectal tumorigenesis. Modified from Fearon & Vogelstein (1990) and reproduced from Young (1991) with permission of the publisher.

are acquired and how they relate to the environment is of importance in management and especially prevention of colorectal neoplasia. Genetic disturbances, whether inherited or acquired, become manifest as disorders of synthesis of proteins and both the genetic events and protein synthesis may be subject to environmental control. It is intriguing that butyrate, a colonic factor determined by the dietary and microbial environment, might influence some of these genetic events (see below).

The p53 gene is commonly affected in cancers but not adenomas (Fearon & Vogelstein, 1990) and is thought to function normally as a tumour suppressor gene. Deletion of the allelic pair or mutation to create an oncogenic form might provide a selective growth advantage or ability to invade mucosa (Fearon & Vogelstein, 1990).

Mutation of the *ras* proto-oncogene is relatively common in carcinoma and intermediate to late adenomas (Fig. 21.2). It may be initiating events in a subset of colorectal carcinomas, or else be responsible for increasing dysplasia in adenomas. Both amplification and gene rearrangements have been reported for certain other oncogenes, including c-*myc*, c-*myb* and the *trk* oncogene (see Fearon & Vogelstein, 1990).

Hypomethylation occurs in up to one-third of DNA regions in the epithelium of patients with even small adenomas (Fearon & Vogelstein, 1990). This non-specific change is known to inhibit chromosomal condensation and may lead to mitotic non-disjunction, loss or gain of chromosomes, and allelic losses. As yet, there is no proven link between hypomethylation and the chromosomal changes described above.

Butyrate and its genetic effects

Acetylation and methylation of DNA

Butyrate can have a general influence on cellular DNA in three main ways:

(1) Butyrate induces hyperacetylation of histones by inhibition of histone deacetylase (Kruh, 1982; de Haan, Gevers & Parker, 1986). It is suggested that this alters chromatin structure, leading to a non-specific down-regulation of gene expression and eventual arrest of proliferation (Toscani *et al.*, 1988).
(2) Butyrate prevents phosphorylation of the histones H1 and H2A (see de Haan *et al.*, 1986).
(3) Butyrate hypermethylates pre-existing and newly-synthesized DNA (de Haan *et al.*, 1986). As a generalization, hypermethylation correlates with gene inactivation, again with the possibility of eventual arrest of proliferation. Note that this would tend to correct the hypomethylation observed in colorectal tumorigenesis.

Such effects on DNA would be non-specific and would seem largely to cause down-regulation. Yet, as discussed below, butyrate does induce expression of some genes.

Butyrate, the cell cycle and oncogenes

The effect of butyrate on protein products of some proto-oncogene families has been studied. These products are believed to be important in growth regulation.

Proto-oncogenes in the *ras* family, Ki-*ras*, Ha-*ras* and N-*ras*, have been the most studied. These encode GTP-binding proteins of M_r 21 000, termed p21 (see Czerniak *et al.*, 1987). In some cells (e.g. NIH 3T3), p21 is needed for the cell to move from G_1 into the S-phase of the cell cycle, thus enabling cell division. Mutation of the *ras* proto-oncogene is important in malignant transformation of adult acute non-lymphocytic leukaemias and NIH 3T3 fibroblasts (see Czerniak *et al.*, 1987). Activation of p21 in the murine haematopoietic cell line 32D C13(G) is remarkably reversible by butyrate, which induces a terminal differentiation of these cells into granulocytes. In the HT29 colon cancer cell line (Czerniak *et al.*, 1987), butyrate brings about a dose-dependent reduction in the production of Ha-p21. An inverse relationship between p21 expression and induction of differentiation has been noted in a range of cell types and this genetic effect might be linked to the proliferation-suppressing effect of butyrate.

Foss *et al.* (1989) examined the effect of butyrate on expression of the

Table 21.2. *Summary of effects of butyrate on molecular events relevant to large-bowel neoplasia*

Gene	Chromosome	Effect of butyrate
FAP/MCC	5q	Unknown
p53	17p	Inhibited (NIH 3T3 cells)
DCC	18q	Unknown
c-*ras*	12p	p21 inhibited (HT29 cells)
c-*src*		pp60, p56 inhibited (SW620 cells)
c-*myc*		Inhibited
L/B/K alkaline phosphatase[a]	1p	Activated/induced (many cell lines)

[a] Liver/bone/kidney alkaline phosphatase, the form expressed in the colon.

tyrosine kinases of the *src* family of proto-oncogenes in the SW620 colon cancer cell line. The enzymatic products studied were pp60$^{c\text{-}src}$ (expressed in normal and neoplastic cells) and p56^{lck} (expressed in neoplasms only). They found that butyrate decreased proliferation and contact-independent growth, and increased expression of alkaline phosphatase activity and protein, in parallel with a decrease in protein kinase activity and protein of pp60$^{c\text{-}src}$ and p56^{lck}. The effect of butyrate was specific, as comparable retardation of proliferation induced in deficient media did not decrease pp60$^{c\text{-}src}$ levels, nor increase alkaline phosphatase. They subsequently showed, in a panel of four other lines, that those which were resistant to the differentiating effect of butyrate failed to show a butyrate-mediated decrease in pp60. Foss *et al.* (1989) suggested that down-regulation of the *src* family of oncogenes was important to achieve a differentiated phenotype. Perhaps loss of the ability to develop a differentiated phenotype on exposure to butyrate is an important step on the road to tumorigenesis in the colon.

Butyrate reduces c-*myc* mRNA in CaCo-2 cells by inducing a protein important in its degradation and induces c-*fos* mRNA (Souleimani & Asselin, 1992). In HT-29 cells it induces alkaline phosphatase mRNA and reduces c-*myc* mRNA (Barnard & Warwick, 1992).

From these few studies it is clear that butyrate can modify the expression of certain genes or their products in a relatively specific manner (see Table 21.2). Where oncogenes are affected, there are accompanying effects on markers of cell differentiation. Whether the primary effect of butyrate is on genetic events controlling induction of terminal differentiation of cells already at a late stage in the multistep pathway to carcinoma, or on inhibition of a critical genetic event early in the pathway and linked to loss of growth control, is not yet clear. Nonetheless, butyrate might be one of the keys to understanding the interaction of the environment (dietary) and genetic (often acquired) events in colorectal tumorigenesis.

Acknowledgements

We wish to thank the National Health and Medical Research Council of Australia, the Anti-Cancer Council of Victoria and the Victor Hurley Medical Research Fund for supporting our studies referred to above.

References

Ardawi, M. S. M. & Newsholme, E. A. (1985). Fuel utilization in colonocytes of the rat. *Biochemical Journal*, **231**, 713–19,

Barnard, J. A. & Warwick, G. (1992). Sodium butyrate rapidly induces 'enterocytic-like' differentiation and growth inhibition of HT-29 cells. *Gastroenterology*, **102**, A199.

Bell, L. & Williams, L. (1979). Histochemical demonstration of alkaline phosphatase in human large intestine, normal and diseased. *Histochemistry*, **60**, 84–90.

Bishop, P. R., Warwick, G. J., Gishan, F. K. & Barnard, J. A. (1992). Sodium butyrate upregulates Na^+/H^+ exchanger mRNA and transport activity in CaCo-2 cells. *Gastroenterology*, **102**, A358.

Boyd, D., Florent, G., Kim, P. & Brattain, M. (1988). Determination of the levels of urokinase and its receptor in human colon carcinoma cell lines. *Cancer Research*, **48**, 3112–16.

Butler, R. N., Stafford, I., Triantafillos, E., O'Dee, C. Jarrett, I. G., Fettman, M. J. & Roberts-Thomson, I. R. T. (1990). Pyruvate sparing by butyrate and propionate in proliferating colonic epithelium. *Comparative Biochemistry and Physiology*, **97B**, 333–40.

Chung, Y. S., Song, I. S., Erickson, R. H., Sleisenger, M. H. & Kim, Y. S. (1985). Effect of growth and sodium butyrate on brush border membrane associated hydrolases in human colorectal cancer cell lines. *Cancer Research*, **45**, 2976–82.

Colony, P. C. (1989). The identification of cell types in the normal adult colon. In *Cell and Molecular Biology of Colon Cancer*, ed. L. H. Augenlicht, pp. 2–21. Boca Raton, FL: CRC Press.

Czerniak, B., Herz, F., Wersto, R. P. & Koss, L. G. (1987). Modification of H-*ras* oncogene p21 expression and cell cycle progression in the human colon cancer cell line HT-29. *Cancer Research*, **47**, 2826–30.

De Cosse, J. J., Miller, H. H. & Lesser, M. L. (1989). Effect of wheat fiber and vitamins C and E on rectal polyps in patients with familial adenomatous polyposis. *Journal of the National Cancer Institute*, **81**, 1290–7.

de Haan, J. B., Gevers, W. & Parker, M. I. (1986). Effects of sodium butyrate on the synthesis and methylation of DNA in normal cells and their transformed counterparts. *Cancer Research*, **46**, 713–16.

Fearon, E. R. & Vogelstein, B. (1990). A genetic model for colorectal tumorigenesis. *Cell*, **61**, 759–67.

Foss, F. M., Veillette, A., Sartor, O., Rosen, N. & Bolen, J. B. (1989). Alterations in the expression of pp60$^{c\text{-}src}$ and 056^{lck} associated with butyrate-induced differentiation of human colon carcinoma cells. *Oncogene Research*, **5**, 13–23.

Freeman, H. J. (1986). Effects of differing concentrations of sodium butyrate on 1,2-dimethylhydrazine induced rat intestinal neoplasia. *Gastroenterology*, **91**, 596–602.

Gibson, P. R., Folino, M., Rosella, O., Finch, C. F., Moeller, I., Alexeyeff, M., Lindley, J. & Young, G. P. (1992). Neoplasia and hyperplasia of large bowel – focal lesions in an abnormal epithelium. *Gastroenterology*, **103**, 1452–9.

Gibson, P. R., Folino, M. Rosella, O., McIntyre, A., Finch, C. F. & Young, G. P. (1993*a*). Effects of dietary fibre on colonic mucosal characteristics in rats (abstract). *Gastroenterology*, **104**, A405.

Gibson, P. R., Moeller, I., Kagelari, O., Folino, M. & Young, G. P. (1991*a*). Contrasting effects of butyrate on differentiation of neoplastic and non-neoplastic colonic epithelial cells. *Journal of Gastroenterology and Hepatology*, **7**, 165–72.

Gibson, P. R., Rosella, O., Rosella, G. & Young, G. P. (1993*b*). Butyrate: a potent inhibitor of urokinase secretion by colonic epithelium (abstract). *Gastroenterology*, **104**, A706.

Gibson, P. R., Rosella, O. & Young, G. P. (1994). Serum-free medium increases expression of markers of differentiation in human colonic crypt cells. *Gut*, **35**, 791–7.

Gibson, P. R., van de Pol, E. & Doe, W. F. (1991*b*). Cell associated urokinase activity and colonic epithelial cells in health and disease. *Gut*, **32**, 191–5.

Gibson, P. R., van de Pol, E., Maxwell, L. E., Whitehead, J. S., Arnstein, P., Bennett, J. & Hicks, J. (1989). Isolation of colonic crypts that maintain structural and metabolic viability *in vitro*. *Gastroenterology*, **96**, 283–91.

Goodlad, R. A. & Wright, N. A. (1983). Effects of addition of kaolin or cellulose to an elemental diet on intestinal cell proliferation in the rat. *British Journal of nutrition*, **50**, 91–8.

Higgins, P. J. (1989). Antigenic and cytoarchitectural 'markers' of differentiation pathways in normal and malignant colonic epithelial cells. In *Cell and Molecular Biology of Colon Cancer*, ed. L. H. Augenlicht, pp. 112–32. Boca Raton, FL: CRC Press.

Janne, P., Carpentier, Y. & Willems, G. (1977). Colonic mucosal atrophy induced by a liquid elemental diet in rats. *American Journal of Digestive Diseases*, **22**, 808–12.

Jass, J. R., Strudley, I. & Faludy, J. (1984). Histochemistry of epithelial metaplasia and dysplasia. *Scandinavian Journal of Gastroenterology*, **19** (Suppl. 104), 109–30.

Kashtan, H. Stern, H. S., Jenkins, D. J. A., Jenkins, A. L., Thompson, L. U., Hay, K., Marcon, N., Minkin, S. & Bruce, W. R. (1992). Colonic fermentation and markers of colorectal-cancer risk. *American Journal of Clinical Nutrition*, **55**, 723–8.

Kim, Y. S., Tsao, D., Siddiqui, B., Whitehead, J. S., Arnstein, P., Bennett, J. & Hicks, J. (1980). Effects of sodium butyrate and dimethylsulfoxide on biochemical properties of human colon cancer cells. *Cancer*, **45**, 1185–92.

Kirchheimer, J. C. & Binder, B. R. (1991). Function of receptor-bound urokinase. *Seminars in Thrombosis and Hemostasis*, **17**, 246–50.

Kohga, S., Harvey, S. R., Weaver, R. M. & Markus, G. (1985). Localization of plasminogen activators in human colon cancer by immunoperoxidase staining. *Cancer Research*, **45**, 1787–96.

Kripke, S. A., Fox, A. D., Berman, J. M., Settle, R. G. & Rombeau, J. L. (1989). Stimulation of intestinal mucosal growth with intracolon infusion of short-chain fatty acids. *Journal of Parenteral and Enteral Nutrition*, **13**, 109–19.

Kruh, J. (1982). Effects of sodium butyrate, a new pharmacological agent, on cells in culture. *Molecular and Cellular Biochemistry*, **42**, 65–82.

Lazarus, G. S. & Jensen, P. J. (1991). Plasminogen activators in epithelial biology. *Seminars in Thrombosis and Hemostasis*, **17**, 210–16.

McIntyre, A., Gibson, P. R. & Young, G. P. (1993). Butyrate production from dietary fiber and protection against large bowel cancer in a rat model. *Gut*, **34**, 386–91.

McIntyre, A., Young, G. P., Taranto, T., Gibson, P. R. & Ward, P. (1991). Different fibers have different regional effects on luminal contents of rat colon. *Gastroenterology*, **101**, 1274–81.

Neogrady, S., Galfi, P. & Kutas, F. (1989). Effects of butyrate and insulin and their interaction on the DNA synthesis of rumen epithelial cells in culture. *Experientia*, **45**, 94–6.

Paraskeva, C., Corfield, A. P., Harper, S., Hague, A., Audcent, K. & Williams, A. C. (1990). Colorectal carcinogenesis: sequential steps in the *in vitro* immortalization and transformation of human colonic epithelial cells. *Anticancer Research*, **10**, 1189–200.

Pollanen, J., Saksela, O., Salonen, E. M., Andreasen, P., Nielsen, L., Dano, K. & Vaheri, A. (1987). Distinct localizations of urokinase-type plasminogen activator and its type I inhibitor under cultured human fibroblasts and sarcoma cells. *Journal of Cell Biology*, **104**, 1085–96.

Roediger, W. E. W. (1980). Role of anaerobic bacteria in the metabolic welfare of the colonic mucosa in man. *Gut*, **21**, 793–8.

Roediger, W. E. W. (1982). Utilization of nutrients by isolated epithelial cells of the rat colon. *Gastroenterology*, **83**, 424–9.

Roediger, W. E. W. (1989). Short-chain fatty acids as metabolism regulators of ion absorption in the colon. *Acta Veterinaria Scandinavica*, **S86**, 116–25.

Roediger, W. E. W. (1990). The starved colon: diminished mucosal nutrition, diminished absorption and colitis. *Diseases of the Colon and Rectum*, **33**, 858–62.

Roediger, W. E. W. & Moore, A. (1981). Effect of short-chain fatty acids on sodium absorption in isolated human colon perfused through the vascular bed. *Digestive Disease Science*, **26**, 100–6.

Ruppin, H., Bar-Meir, S. & Soergel, K. H. (1980). Absorption of short-chain fatty acids by the colon. *Gastroenterology*, **78**, 1500–8.

Sakata, T. (1984). Influence of short-chain fatty acids on epithelial cell division of digestive tract. *Journal of Experimental Physiology*, **69**, 639–48.

Sakata, T. (1987). Stimulatory effect of short-chain fatty acids on epithelial cell proliferation in the rat intestine: a possible explanation for trophic effects of fermentable fibre, gut microbes and luminal trophic factors. *British Journal of Nutrition*, **58**, 95–101.

Sakata, T. (1988). Depression of intestinal epithelial cell production rate by hindgut bypass in rats. *Scandinavian Journal of Gastroenterology*, **12**, 1200–2.

Sakata, T. (1989). Stimulatory effect of short-chain fatty acids on epithelial cell proliferation of isolated and denervated jejunal segment of the rat. *Sandinavian Journal of Gastroenterology*, **24**, 886–90.

Sakata, T. & von Engelhardt, W. (1983). Stimulatory effect of short chain fatty acids on the epithelial cell proliferation in rat large intestine. *Comparative Biochemistry and Physiology*, **74A**, 459.

Scheppach, W. Bartram, P. Richter, A., Richter, F., Liepold, H., Dusel, G., Hofstetter, G., Ruthlein, J. & Kasper, H. (1992). Effect of short-chain fatty acids on the human colonic mucosa *in vitro*. *Journal of Parenteral and Enteral Nutrition*, **16**, 43–8.

Schmidt, R., Cathelineau, C. Cavey, M. T., Dionisius, V., Michel, S., Shroot, B. & Riechert, U. (1989). Sodium butyrate selectivity antagonizes the inhibitory effect of retinoids on cornified envelope formation in cultured human keratinocytes. *Journal of Cell Physiology*, **140**, 281–7.

Schmitt, M., Chucholowski, N., Busch, E., Hellmann, D., Wagner, B. Goretzki, L., Janicke, F., Gunzler, W. A. & Graeff, H. (1991). Fluorescent probes as tools to assess the receptor for the urokinase-type plasminogen activator on tumor cells. *Seminars in Thrombosis and Hemostasis*, **17**, 291–302.

Sellin, J. H. & DeSoignie, R. (1992). R. (1991). Short-chain fatty acid regulation of intracellular pH in colonocytes. *Gastroenterology*, **102**, A356.

Souleimani, A. & Asselin, C. (1992). Regulation of proto-oncogene expression by sodium butyrate in the human colon carcinoma cell line CaCo-2. *Gastroenterology*, **102**, A400.

Staecker, J. L., Sattler, C. A. & Pitot, H. C. (1988). Sodium butyrate preserves aspects of the differential phenotype of normal adult rat hepatocytes in culture. *Journal of Cell Physiology*, **135**, 367–76.

Takahashi, K., Ikeo, K., Gojorbori, T. & Tanifuji, M. (1990). Local function of urokinase receptor at the adhesion contact sites of a metastatic tumour cell. *Thrombosis Research*, **10** (Suppl.), 55–61.

Toscani, A., Soprano, D. R. & Soprano, K. J. (1988). Molecular analysis of sodium butyrate-induced growth arrest. *Oncogene Research*, **3**, 223–38.

Tsao, D., Morita, A., Bella, A., Luu, P. & Kim, Y. S. (1982). Differential effects of sodium butyrate, dimethyl sulfoxide, and retinoic acid on membrane-associated antigen, enzymes and glycoproteins of human rectal adenocarcinoma cells. *Cancer Research*, **42**, 1052–8.

Whitehead, R. H., Young, G. P. & Bhathal, P. S. (1986). Effects of short chain fatty acids on a new human colon carcinoma cell line (LIM1215). *Gut*, **27**, 1457–63.

Willson, J. K. V. (1989). Biology of large bowel cancer. *Hematology/Oncology Clinics of North America*, **3**, 19–34.

Young, G. P. (1990). Dietary fibre in the prevention of colorectal cancer: lessons from studies in animal models. *Proceedings of the Nutrition Society of Australia*, **15**, 112–19.

Young, G. P. (1991). Butyrate and the molecular biology of the large bowel. In *Short-chain Fatty Acids: Metabolism and Clinical Importance*, ed. J. L. Rombeau, J. H. Cummings & T. Sakata, pp. 39–44. Columbus, OH: Ross Laboratories.

Young, G. P. & Gibson, P. R. (1991). Contrasting effects of butyrate on proliferation and differentiation of normal and neoplastic cells. In *Short-chain Fatty Acids: Metabolism and Clinical Importance*, ed. J. L. Rombeau, J. H. Cummings & T. Sakata, pp. 50–5. Columbus, OH: Ross Laboratories.

Young, G. P., Macrae, F. A., Gibson, P. R., Alexeyeff, M. & Whitehead, R. (1992). Brush border hydrolases in normal and neoplastic colonic epithelium. *Journal of Gastroenterology and Hepatology*, **7**, 347–54.

22

The place of short-chain fatty acids in colonocyte metabolism in health and ulcerative colitis: the impaired colonocyte barrier

W. E. W. ROEDIGER

Colonic epithelial cells, alternatively termed colonocytes (Roediger & Truelove, 1979), are a functional constituent of the colonic mucosa. In ulcerative and Crohn's colitis, research endeavours have been weighted towards immune studies, with scant regard to colonocytes (Kirsner & Shorter, 1988). This chapter gives an overview of the metabolism and function of colonocytes with reference to short-chain fatty acids (SCFA) both in health and in ulcerative colitis.

Colonic epithelial cell barrier

Colonic epithelial cells form a diaphanous layer between the reductive environment of the lumen and the oxidative environment of the lamina propria. A defensive role has been ascribed to colonocytes based on mucus production and shedding of surface cells, which are replenished by renewal from crypt cells. Former interest in colonocytes was in ion transfer, in which regard analysis of ion pumps and electrophysiological experiments predominated (Powell, 1981).

The barrier function of epithelial cells can, however, be considered in terms of cellular metabolism – substrate breakdown, ability to assemble cell membranes and to detoxify luminal agents. Furthermore, epithelial cells have mechanisms which uphold a redox balance between the adjoining oxidative and reductive environments. In all these functions SCFA play a central metabolic role in upholding a dynamic epithelial-cell barrier in the colon.

SCFA metabolism of colonocytes in health

The first studies with SCFA and the colonic mucosa were carried out in Melbourne, Australia, between 1962 and 1972. Interest originally was in the

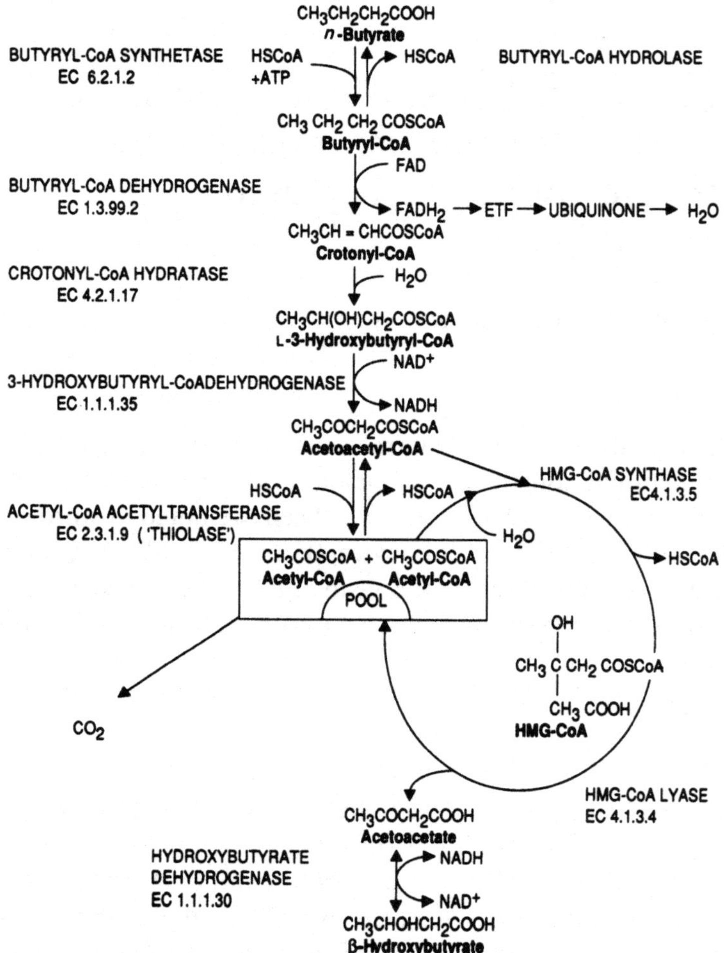

Fig. 22.1. β-Oxidation pathway of *n*-butyrate to acetyl-CoA and ketone bodies. The HMG-CoA pathway is found in colonocytes (Henning & Hird, 1970).

pathway by which ketone bodies were generated in the liver (Hird & Symons, 1962). That led to an analysis of the pathway of ketogenesis from SCFA in fermentative organs of Australian mammals. The first report of ketogenesis from *n*-butyrate in the colon was in 1970 (Henning & Hird, 1970): differential labelling of 1 and 3 carbon atoms of *n*-butyrate showed that ketogenesis in the colonic mucosa occurred via the β-hydroxy-β-methylglutaryl-CoA (HMG-CoA) pathway (Fig. 22.1). Studies of SCFA metabolism along the length of the colon (Henning & Hird, 1972*a*) and transport of SCFA across the caecal mucosa followed (Henning & Hird, 1972*b*).

In 1977 transfer of observations from animals to man with emphasis on mucosal diseases seemed worthwhile, as the role of SCFA in the human colonocyte before 1977 was unknown. The task was tackled by (1) developing an isolated colonic epithelial system for metabolic studies in both animals and man; (2) procuring human colonic tissue for laboratory studies; and (3) evaluating SCFA metabolism in conjunction with that of glucose and glutamine. The procedure was to measure substrate utilization and metabolite appearance rather than to characterize the individual enzymes of metabolic pathways. The historical evaluation of the type of colonic tissue used in the past has been presented elsewhere (Roediger, 1982*b*, 1989) but animal observations now reviewed were almost all derived from isolated colonocytes of the rat.

In rat colonocytes utilization of glucose was at a high rate: 5.57 ± 0.97 to 6.88 ± 0.60 μmol/min per g dry wt (Roediger, 1982*a*; Ardawi & Newsholme, 1985) but some 79–83% of that was converted to lactate. After discounting of lactogenesis and calculation of glucose entry into the Krebs cycle against oygen consumption, only 28–45% of glucose was found to be oxidized to carbon dioxide. Such low oxidative values in the past were attributed to damaged mucosal cells (Krebs, 1972) rather than being accepted as the normal state of metabolic affairs. Glucose oxidation fell to 1–2% in the presence of *n*-butyrate (10 mM) despite an overall increase in total oxygen consumption. These observations led to estimates of substrate contribution to total oxygen consumption by means of substrate labelling of single carbon (not universal carbon) isotopes. Moreover, the effect of one substrate on oxidation of another could be observed and carbon flux into the Krebs cycle measured across pyruvate dehydrogenase ([1-^{14}C]pyruvate), thiolase ([1-^{14}C]butyrate) and glutaminase ([1-^{14}C]glutamine). *n*-Butyrate had a sparing effect on glucose and glutamine oxidation and the labelling of *n*-butyrate revealed that glucose or glutamine did not reduce the entry of fatty-acid carbon into the Krebs cycle. All observations indicated that fatty-acid *n*-butyrate was the premier fuel for colonocytes and that the proportional contribution to total oxygen consumption from *n*-butyrate was over 70% for all oxidation. Colonocytes also oxidize long-chain fatty acids (Roediger & Nance, 1990) but less avidly than water-soluble fatty acids. Similar observations had also been made in the ruminal mucosa (Cook, McGilliard & Richard, 1968).

Observations from animal experiments provided a means to study healthy human colonocytes. To obtain sufficient cells for comparative experiments to be performed simultaneously a large area of mucosa (5×6 cm) was required, though methods using small biopsies have recently been reported (Williams *et*

Table 22.1. *Oxidation of glucose and* n-*butyrate by colonocytes of the proximal and distal human colon. Data collated and recalculated from Roediger (1980*b)

	Observation (μmol/min per g dry wt)	
	Ascending colon ($n = 7$)	Descending colon ($n = 7$)
Glucose alone (10 mM)		
Oxygen consumed	9.29 ± 0.60	7.88 ± 0.83
Glucose removed	5.74 ± 0.97	3.61 ± 0.90
Lactate produced	5.14 ± 0.55	5.36 ± 0.55
Contribution to O_2 consumption	100% (+)	59%
n-*Butyrate alone (10 mM)*		
Oxygen consumed	10.11 ± 0.56	9.30 ± 0.88
CO_2 from butyrate	1.05 ± 0.1	1.09 ± 0.19
Ketogenesis (mean total)	2.31	1.70
Contribution to O_2 consumption	73%	75%
Glucose and n-*butyrate (10 mM)*		
Oxygen consumed	10.97 ± 0.64	9.31 ± 0.58
Glucose removed	[illegible]13 ± 0.51	3.38 ±
Contribution to O_2 consumption	80%	32%
CO_2 from butyrate	1.09 ± 0.19	1.18 ± 0.22
Ketogenesis (mean total)	1.43	1.00
Contribution to O_2 consumption	59%	72%

al., 1992; Chapman *et al.*, 1992). Observations with human colonocytes were regionalized into the proximal and distal colon, because the work of Henning & Hird (1972*a*) showed less potential for ketogenesis and therefore dependence on fatty-acid oxidation in the distal colon. Preference of substrate utilization was similar to that in the rat, but regional variation between the proximal and distal colon was found. Relevant values are given in Table 22.1 with the glucose oxidation recalculated according to Roediger (1982*a*) and not as incorrectly indicated in Roediger (1980*b*). Glucose oxidation in the distal colon was less pronounced than in the proximal colon. No glutamine, measured in its non-radioactive form, was oxidized via ketoglutarate into the Krebs cycle in the distal colon where *n*-butyrate oxidation predominated. Of note in Table 22.1 is that the rates of $^{14}CO_2$ production from *n*-butyrate are equivalent in the proximal and distal human colon, as was subsequently shown by Chapman *et al.* (1992). In determining the main utility of fuels in the proximal and distal colon, consideration should be given not only to the rates of $^{14}CO_2$ production but also to the suppressibility of oxidation of glucose/pyruvate (Roediger, 1979; Butler *et al.*, 1990) and to the comparison of individual substrate oxidation against total oxygen consumption (Roediger, 1980*b*). Another feature of note is that glucose oxidation measured on the basis of glucose removed has great variability (Fleming *et al.*, 1991). Glucose oxidation can be measured more accurately by $^{14}CO_2$ production from [6-^{14}C]glucose rather than [U-^{14}C]glucose, which measures CO_2 production from the number of turns through the Krebs cycle.

Regulation of *β*-oxidation (*n*-butyrate) in colonocytes

Concentration of SCFA does not appear to be a strong regulatory factor in the control of *β*-oxidation, as 1.0–5.0 mmol/l of *n*-butyrate was converted to CO_2 and ketone bodies at equal rates (Roediger & Nance, 1990). Availability of SCFA, on the other hand, very strongly affects *β*-oxidation. Colonocytes, when starved of SCFA, oxidize *n*-butyrate at a drastically reduced rate, with diminished ketogenesis (Roediger *et al.*, 1986; Firmansyah *et al.*, 1989). Glucose oxidation was also reduced, though glucose utilization was not significantly changed (Ardawi & Newsholme, 1985), thereby providing lactate for gluconeogenesis in the liver to maintain the fasting state of metabolism. Ketogenesis in the liver during starvation is markedly increased (Ferre *et al.*, 1983), indicating that regulation of ketogenesis in the liver and colonic mucosa is differently organized. Reduction of *β*-oxidation has marked functional consequences for colonocytes (Fig. 22.2).

Activation of SCFA to their CoA derivatives by short-chain CoA synthetases (Fig. 22.1), each separately for acetate, propionate and butyrate, appears to be the chief means whereby SCFA individually or in combination influence cellular metabolism (Ash & Baird, 1973; Scaife & Tichivangana, 1980). All observations of CoA synthetases have been made in the ruminal mucosa and are assumed to apply to colonocytes. Activation of SCFA occurs in the order of *n*-butyrate > propionate > acetate; acetate is hardly activated and neither acetate nor propionate change the dominance of *n*-butyrate activation, though generation of CO_2 from butyrate diminishes somewhat with addition of acetate and propionate (Roediger, 1982*a*). The prominent activation of *n*-butyrate rather than that of acetate implies that derivation of acetyl-CoA for cellular lipogenesis is mainly from *n*-butyrate (Roediger, Kapaniris & Millard, 1992). The general regulation of lipogenesis in enterocytes and colonocytes is different from hepatocytes, as insulin (Williamson, Ilic & Hughes, 1985) catecholamines, glucagon (Gebhard *et al.*, 1991) and HMG-CoA reductase inhibitors (Shakir, Sundaram & Margolis, 1978) do not affect lipogenesis in epithelial cells as they do in the liver.

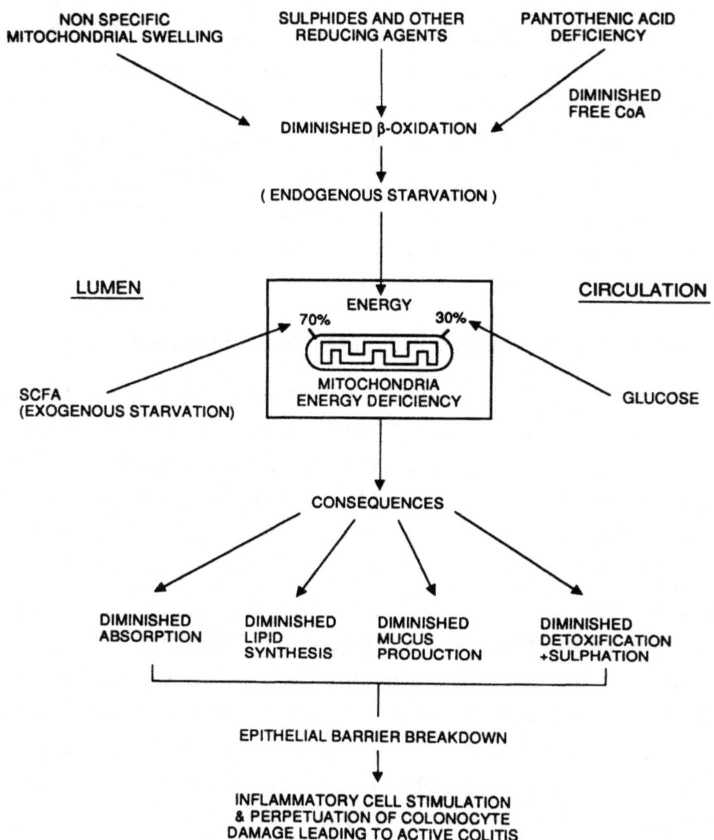

Fig. 22.2. The role of short-chain fatty acids (SCFA) in colonocyte metabolism in health, with hypothetical factors that may impair SCFA metabolism.

The cellular level of free CoA alters the acetyl-CoA/free CoA ratio, which in turn changes thiolase activity (Quandt & Huth, 1985; Randle, 1986), but to date neither free CoA nor acetyl-CoA levels have been measured, in mitochondria or in the cytosol of colonocytes. Glucose and crotonate alter the NAD/NADH ratio, which changes the disposition of ketone bodies (Roediger & Nance, 1990). The presence of exogenous ketone bodies reduces *n*-butyrate oxidation to a small degree (Roediger, 1982*a*).

n-Butyrate added to isolated colonic mitochondria did not alter oxidation ratios measured by an oxygen electrode (Radcliffe, Nance & Roediger, 1986), an observation that was unexpected but may be attributed to swelling or matrix volume changes of mitochondria. Such changes particularly affect *n*-butyrate oxidation (Halestrap & Dunlop, 1986) and swelling of mitochondria *in vivo* may therefore drastically diminish β-oxidation of *n*-butyrate.

Genetic control of the enzymes of butyrate oxidation have been observed in spontaneous mutants of *Escherichia coli.* Enzyme induction of either butyryl CoA-synthetase or thiolase have gene loci (ato A and ato B) that are closely linked to form an operon (Pauli & Overath, 1972; Nunn, 1986). Molecular genetics (Goodridge, 1990) of colonocytes would be a very suitable field in which to study metabolic regulation of β-oxidation, particularly with relevance to mucosal disease.

Colonocytes are continuously exposed to bacteria and bacterial metabolites, some of which have a strong influence on fatty-acid oxidation. Sodium hydrogen sulphide (Roediger *et al.*, 1993*a*), sodium mercaptoacetate (Duncan *et al.*, 1990; Roediger & Nance, 1990) and sodium sulphite (Roediger, 1991) all affect CO_2 generation from *n*-butyrate. Sulphide acts powerfully and selectively on β-oxidation, probably by decreasing butyl-CoA dehydrogenase activity through persulphide formation (Roediger *et al.*, 1993*b*). Persulphides strongly diminish short-chain acyl-CoA dehydrogenase activity (Shaw & Engel, 1987) and the only bodily tissue where short-chain acyl dehydrogenases and sulphides continuously interact are colonocytes. A regulator role involving other bacterial agents is at present unknown.

Fasting, famine, fatty acids and function of colonocytes

Fasting prominently reduced SCFA oxidation in colonocytes without displaying a compensatory increase in metabolism of other substrates (Roediger *et al.*, 1986; Firmansyah *et al.*, 1989). Consequently, colonocyte function was explored under conditions of limited SCFA availability. Fasting greatly limited production of SCFA in the animal colon (Illman, Topping & Trimble, 1986) which would be analogous for humans under fasting and famine conditions. Whenever SCFA have been withheld from the colon, the capacity of the colonic mucosa to absorb sodium and water has been drastically reduced (see Roediger (1990) for review), shown in the dog (Roediger & Rae, 1982), rat (Roediger *et al.*, 1986) and rabbit (Bell *et al.*, 1991), with isolated loops of colon. Starvation of the severest forms may lead to mucosal changes termed 'colitis' (Fig. 22.2), seen particularly in kwashiorkor (Redmond *et al.*, 1971) and famine conditions (Keys *et al.*, 1950; Thaysen & Thaysen, 1952). Some of the effects of fasting on colonocytes can be redressed by the reintroduction of SCFA, as shown in dog colonic loops (Roediger & Rae, 1982) or the human defunctioned colon affected by diversion colitis (Harig *et al.*, 1989).

Table 22.2. *Butyrate metabolism in colonocytes of quiescent and acute ulcerative colitis*

Study	Tissue type and site	Disease category	Cases (*n*)	Healthy controls (*n*)	Disease controls (*n*)	Observations on *n*-butyrate oxidation
Roediger, 1980*a*	Operative; descending colon	Quiescent and acute colitis	10	7	None	Diminished *n*-butyrate oxidation in both quiescent and acute colitis
Ireland & Jewell, 1989	Operative; distal ulcerative colitis	Non-inflamed and inflamed colons	7	13	None	Reduced butyrate oxidation: even in non-inflamed colon
Chapman *et al.*, 1992	Biopsies; non-inflamed areas	Established ulcerative colitis	11	14	None	Diminished *n*-butyrate oxidation
Finnie *et al.*, 1992	Biopsies; ascending and descending colon	Quiescent colitis	7	10	None	No change in *n*-butyrate oxidation
Williams *et al.*, 1992	Biopsies	Established colitis	2	5	3	Diminished *n*-butyrate oxidation

A hypothesis for the disease process of ulcerative colitis

Searches for the cause of ulcerative colitis have converged on cytokines, prostaglandins and other agents considered 'damaging' to the colonic mucosa (Brynskov *et al.*, 1992). The action of these agents on SCFA metabolism and colonocytes has not been investigated in any great detail. A recurrent question in pathogenic studies is what the precise sequence of events is in ulcerative colitis between bacteria, colonocytes and immune cells. The question has been answered theoretically (Roediger, 1988*a*) and the epithelial cell nominated as the key factor in the disease process. The hypothesis is that ulcerative colitis is due either to exogenous or to endogenous starvational factors limiting fatty-acid oxidation in colonocytes (Fig. 22.2). Exogenous starvation can be equated with 'diversion colitis' (Harig *et al.*, 1989) while ulcerative colitis can be equated with endogenous starvation brought about by CoA deficiency (McDowell, 1989) or inhibitors of fatty-acid oxidation (Roediger & Nance, 1986). The following paragraph concerns the effects of altered fatty-acid oxidation in disease and the potential induction of colitis by derangement of SCFA metabolism.

Short-chain fatty acid metabolism in colonocytes of ulcerative colitis

Evaluation of SCFA metabolism in ulcerative colitis seemed a sequitur to the findings in healthy colonocytes; however, studies of the diseased colon were performed concurrently with studies of the healthy colonocytes, so that prior knowledge of the normal/abnormal state of metabolic affairs was not then known (Roediger, 1979). *n*-Butyrate oxidation was very strikingly reduced in colonocytes of acute ulcerative colitis, and as Dr Truelove in 1977 had a number of patients with dysplastic mucosal changes, butyrate oxidation could also be assessed in quiescent colitis. In a comparison between separate groups of acute and quiescent colitis, β-oxidation was found to be significantly reduced in both groups (Roediger, 1980*a*, 1988*b*). Strikingly, glucose and glutamine oxidation was increased. Such a compensation does not occur in starved colonocytes and the observation must either be a chronic regulatory rearrangement of metabolism or be due to therapy, as most patients were on salazopyrin or prednisolone. A disease control group (Crohn's disease) was not included in the study, but β-oxidation in colonocytes of two cases of Crohn's colitis was not reduced. A number of years passed before the above observations were confirmed (Table 22.2). Studies by Ireland & Jewell (1989), with the same colon involved in ulcerative colitis distally and uninvolved proximally, confirmed drastic reduction in β-oxidation in the diseased portion as well as reduction of β-oxidation in the uninvolved segments. These findings suggest that changes in β-oxidation precede the onset of overt colitis. Two further reports (Williams *et al.*, 1992; Chapman *et al.*, 1992) have confirmed diminished β-oxidation in colitis, while another study on quiescent colitis did not confirm altered β-oxidation (Finnie, Taylor & Rhodes, 1992). *In vivo* reduction of CO_2 production from butyrate in colitis was confirmed by noting bicarbonate production generated by β-oxidation in dialysis bags (Roediger *et al.*, 1984). A more detailed study of fatty-acid oxidation in ulcerative colitis should resolve any controversy of fatty-acid oxidation changes in ulcerative colitis.

At a cellular level, fatty-acid oxidation of *n*-butyrate takes place in mitochondria, which histologically do not appear to be impaired in colonocytes of ulcerative colitis (Listrom & Fenoglio-Preiser, 1988). Estimation of cytochrome oxidase and succinate dehydrogenase activity in acute ulcerative colitis did not show impairment and mRNA analysis for NADH dehydrogenases suggested no abnormality in this component of respiratory-chain activity (Mayall *et al.*, 1992), suggesting that the Krebs cycle is not changed in ulcerative colitis. Despite these findings, ATP levels are diminished in quiescent colitis (Kameyama *et al.*, 1984). Most notable is that sulphation of xenobiotics, strongly dependent on ATP levels, and sulphation of mucus is significantly diminished in acute and also quiescent colitis (Ramakrishna *et al.*, 1991; Raouf *et al.*, 1992). Observations of changes of β-oxidation and diminished ATP levels are in line with the proposal that ulcerative colitis is an energy deficiency disease.

Fatty acids and mitochondrial oxidation defects

Observations on inherited defects of mitochondrial fatty acid oxidation (Vianey-Liaud *et al.*, 1987; Scholte, 1988; Turnbull, Shepherd & Aysley-Green, 1988; Rhead, 1991; Hale & Bennett, 1992) would appear to suggest a similarity of metabolic changes in ulcerative colitis. Most inherited conditions of fatty-acid oxidation defects can be related to acyl-CoA dehydrogenase defects of medium- and long-chain acids. Only six cases of short-chain acyl-CoA dehydrogenases have been reported in humans (Hale & Bennett, 1992) and these in very young infants that died soon after birth. Whether short-chain acyl-CoA dehydrogenases are organ-specific (e.g. muscle only) or involve all bodily organs, including the colon has not been evaluated. Nevertheless, the possibility does exist that β-oxidation changes in ulcerative colitis could be due to defects in short-chain acyl-CoA dehydrogenases that are organ-specific. To date no studies have been carried out.

Causes of impaired SCFA oxidation in ulcerative colitis

Either morphological changes such as mitochondrial swelling (Halestrap & Dunlop, 1986) or biochemical inhibitors could bring about impairment of β-oxidation of SCFA. β-Oxidation of SCFA comprises five enzymic steps (Fig. 22.1) and enzyme activity in mitochondria seemed a possible site of action of biochemical inhibitors.

Because mitochondrial NAD/NADH-dependent dehydrogenases were not found deficient in acute colitis (Mayall *et al.*, 1992), this enzyme group was not studied further. Consideration was given to inhibitors of thiolases, such as mercaptoacetate (Sabourault *et al.*, 1979), as this agent was found in the colon (Duncan *et al.*, 1990). Inhibition of CO_2 generation from butyrate by mercaptoacetate led to acetoacetate accumulation (Roediger & Nance, 1990; Roediger *et al.*, 1993*a*), a finding contrary to that observed in active or quiescent ulcerative colitis.

As sulphur is an integral requirement for the production of experimental colitis in animals (Ishioka *et al.*, 1986), the hypothesis was advanced that a sulphur-containing agent was responsible for impaired fatty-acid oxidation (Roediger, 1991). Fermentative products of sulphur-proteins include hydrogen sulphide and methanethiol (Kadota & Ishida, 1972) and these were tested in healthy human and rat colonocytes (Roediger *et al.*, 1993*a*,*b*): sulphides selectively impaired β-oxidation, depending on the concentration of reagents, possibly due to an action on butyryl-CoA dehydrogenase. Action on this enzyme would account for the changes of both CO_2 and ketones observed in active colitis. As free CoA levels appear to be low in colonocytes of active colitis (Ellestad-Sayed *et al.*, 1976) CoA could be bound to other cellular components. The species of sequestered CoA has not yet been identified and further work in this direction is required.

Conclusions

Metabolism of SCFA, mainly *n*-butyrate, is crucial to the metabolic welfare of colonocytes. In colonocytes, fatty-acid oxidation governs processes such as ATP generation, lipogenesis, absorption of sodium, detoxification of xenobiotics and acetylation of histones. An endogenous starvation of colonocytes is postulated to be the cause of ulcerative colitis, possibly related to sulphide inactivation of fatty-acid dehydrogenases or inactivation of butyryl-CoA synthetase. Diminished fatty-acid oxidation would lead to a breached barrier of colonic epithelial cells and subsequent immune changes. The effect of immune cells and therapeutic agents on fatty-acid oxidation and the potential to reverse the inhibition of fatty-acid oxidation need to be investigated by future research.

References

Ardawi, M. S. M. & Newsholme, E. A. (1985). Fuel utilization in colonocytes of the rat. *Biochemical Journal*, **231**, 713–19.

Ash, R. & Baird, G. D. (1973). Activation of volatile fatty acids in bovine liver and rumen epithelium. Evidence for control by autoregulation. *Biochemical Journal*, **136**, 311–19.

Bell, C. J., Hunt, D., Stiel, D. & O'Loughlin, E. V. (1991). Impaired distal colonic electrolyte salvage in chronic malnutrition. *Australian and New Zealand Journal of Medicine*, **21**, 565.

Brynskov, J., Nielsen, O. H., Ahnfelt-Ronne, I. & Bendtzen, K. (1992). Cytokines in inflammatory bowel disease. *Scandinavian Journal of Gastroenterology*, **27**, 897–906.

Butler, R. N., Stafford, I., Triantafillos, E., O'Dee, C. D., Jarrett, I. G., Fettman, N. J. & Roberts-Thomson, I. C. (1990). Pyruvate sparing by butyrate and propionate in proliferating colonic epithelium. *Comparative Biochemistry and Physiology*, **97B**, 333–7.

Chapman, M. A. S., Grahn, M., Rogers, J., Hutton, M., Norton, B. & Williams, N. S. (1992). New technique to measure mucosal metabolism and the characterization of regional metabolism in the large bowel. *British Journal of Surgery*, **79**, 1233–4.

Cook, D. A., McGilliard, D. & Richard, M. (1968). *In vitro* conversion of long-chain fatty acids to ketones by bovine rumen mucosa. *Journal of Dairy Science*, **51**, 715–20.

Duncan, A., Kapaniris, O. & Roediger, W. E. W. (1990). Measurement of mercaptoacetate levels in anaerobic batch culture of colonic bacteria. *FEMS Microbiology and Ecology*, **74**, 303–8.

Ellestad-Sayed, J. J., Nelson, R. A., Adson, M. A., Palmer, W. M. & Soule, E. H. (1976). Pantothenic acid, coenzyme A and human chronic ulcerative and granulomatous colitis. *American Journal of Clinical Nutrition*, **29**, 1333–8.

Ferre, P., Satabin, P., Decaux, J. F., Escriva, F. & Girard, J. (1983). Development and regulation of ketogenesis in hepatocytes isolated from newborn rats. *Biochemical Journal*, **214**, 937–42.

Finnie, I. A., Taylor, B. A. & Rhodes, J. M. (1992). Mucosal metabolism in ulcerative colitis. A reappraisal of the butyrate hypothesis. *Clinical Science*, **83**, 17p–18p.

Firmansyah, A., Penn, D. & Lebenthal, E. (1989). Metabolism of glucose, glutamine, *n*-butyrate, β-hydroxybutyrate in isolated rat colonocyte following acute fasting and chronic malnutrition. *Gastroenterology*, **97**, 622–9.

Fleming, S. E., Fitch, M. D., Devries, S., Liu, M. L. & Kight, C. (1991). Nutrient utilization by cells isolated from rat jejunum, caecum and colon. *Journal of Nutrition*, **121**, 869–78.

Gebhard, R. L., Ewing, S. L., Schlasner, L. A., Hunningmake, D. B. & Prigge, W. F. (1991). Effect of 3-hydroxy-3-methylglutaryl coenzyme A reductase inhibition on human gut mucosa. *Lipids*, **26**, 492–4.

Goodridge, A. G. (1990). The new metabolism: molecular genetics in the analysis of metabolic regulation. *FASEB Journal*, **4**, 3099–110.

Hale, D. E. & Bennett, M. J. (1992). Fatty acid oxidation disorders: a new class of metabolic diseases. *Journal of Paediatrics*, **121**, 1–11.

Halestrap, P. & Dunlop, J. L. (1986). Intramitochondrial regulation of fatty acid β-oxidation occurs between flavoprotein and ubiquinone. *Biochemical Journal*, **239**, 559–65.

Harig, J. M., Soergel, K. H., Komorowski, V. R. A. & Wood, C. M. (1989). Treatment of diversion colitis with short-chain-fatty acid irrigation. *New England Journal of Medicine*, **320**, 23–8.

Henning, S. J. & Hird, F. J. R. (1970). Concentrations and metabolism of volatile fatty acids in the fermentative organs of two species of kangaroo and the guinea pig. *British Journal of Nutrition*, **24**, 145–55.

Henning, S. J. & Hird, F. J. R. (1972*a*). Ketogenesis from butyrate and acetate by the caecum and the colon of rabbits. *Biochemical Journal*, **130**, 785–90.

Henning, S. J. & Hird, F. J. R. (1972*b*). Transport of acetate and butyrate in the hind-gut of rabbits. *Biochemical Journal*, **130**, 791–6.

Hird, F. J. R. & Symons, R. H. (1962). The mechanism of ketone-body formation from butyrate in rat liver. *Biochemical Journal*, **84**, 212–16.

Illman, R. J., Topping, D. L. & Trimble, R. P. (1986). Effects of food restriction and starvation–refeeding on volatile fatty acid concentrations in the rat. *Journal of Nutrition*, **116**, 1694–700.

Ireland, A. & Jewell, D. P. (1989). 5-Aminosalicylic acid (5-ASA) has no effect on butyrate metabolism in human colonic epithelial cells (abstract). *Gastroenterology*, **98**, A176.

Ishioka, T., Kuwabara, N., Oohashi, Y. & Wakabayashi, K. (1986). Induction of colorectal tumours in rats by sulfated polysaccharides. *CRC Critical Review in Toxicology*, **17**, 215–44.

Kadota, H. & Ishida, Y. (1972). Production of volatile sulfur compounds by microorganisms. *Annual Review of Microbiology*, **26**, 127–38.

Kameyama, J., Narui, H., Inui, M. & Sato, T. (1984). Energy level in large intestinal mucosa in patients with ulcerative colitis. *Tohoku Journal of Experimental Medicine*, **143**, 253–4.

Keys, A., Brozek, J., Henschel, A., Mickelsen, O. & Taylor, H. L. (1950). *The Biology of Human Starvation*, vol. 1, pp. 587–601. Minneapolis: The University of Minnesota Press.

Kirsner, J. B. & Shorter, R. G. (eds) (1988). *Inflammatory Bowel Disease*, 3rd edn. Philadelphia: Lea Febiger.

Krebs, H. A. (1972). The Pasteur effect and the relations between respiration and fermentation. *Essays in Biochemistry*, **8**, 1–34.

Listrom, M. B. & Fenoglio-Preiser, C. M. (1988). The colon: normal ultrastructure and pathological patterns. In *Ultrastructure of the Digestive Tract*, ed. P. M. Motta, H. Fujita & S. Correr, pp. 119–44. Boston: Martinus Nijhoff.

Mayall, T., MacPherson, A., Bjarnason, I., Forgacs, I. & Peters, T. (1992). Mitochondrial function of colonic epithelial cells in inflammatory bowel disease (abstract). *Gut*, **33**, S24.

McDowell, L. R. (ed.) (1989). *Vitamins in Animal Nutrition: Comparative Aspects to Human Nutrition*, pp. 256–74. San Diego: Academic Press.

Nunn, W. D. (1986). A molecular view of fatty acid catabolism in *Escherichia coli*. *Microbiological Reviews*, **50**, 179–92.

Pauli, G. & Overath, P. (1972). Ato operon: a highly induceable system for acetoacetate and butyrate degradation in *Escherichia coli. European Journal of Biochemistry*, **29**, 553–62.

Powell, D. W. (1981). Barrier function of epithelia. *American Journal of Physiology*, **241**, G275–G288.

Quandt, L. & Huth, W. (1985). On the mechanism of the chemical modification of the mitochondrial acetyl-CoA acetyltransferase by coenzyme A. *Biochimica et Biophysica Acta*, **829**, 103–8.

Radcliffe, B. C., Nance, S. H. & Roediger, W. E. W. (1986). The isolation of coupled mitochondria from rat colonic mucosa. *Proceedings of the Australian Society of Medical Research*, **19**, 24.

Ramakrishna, B. S., Roberts-Thomson, I. C., Pannall, P. R. & Roediger, W. E. W. (1991). Impaired sulphation of phenol by the colonic mucosa in quiescent and active ulcerative colitis. *Gut*, **32**, 46–9.

Randle, P. J. (1986). Fuel selection in animals. *Biochemical Society Transactions*, **14**, 799–806.

Raouf, A. H., Tsai, H. H., Parker, N., Hoffman, J., Walker, R. J. & Rhodes, J. M. (1992). Sulphation of colonic and rectal mucin in inflammatory bowel disease – reduced sulphation of rectal mucus in ulcerative colitis. *Clinical Science*, **83**, 626–32.

Redmond, A. D. B., Kaschula, R. O. C., Freeseman, C. & Hansen, J. D. L. (1971). The colon in kwashiorkor. *Archives of Disease in Childhood*, **46**, 470–3.

Rhead, W. J. (1991). Inborn errors of fatty acid oxidation in man. *Clincal Biochemistry*, **24**, 319–29.

Roediger, W. E. W. (1979). The functional activity of the colonic mucosa in health and in disease. DPhil thesis, University of Oxford, Oxford.

Roediger, W. E. W. (1980*a*). The colonic epithelium in ulcerative colitis: an energy-deficiency disease? *Lancet*, **2**, 712–15.

Roediger, W. E. W. (1980*b*). Role of anaerobic bacteria in the metabolic welfare of the colonic mucosa. *Gut*, **21**, 793–8.

Roediger, W. E. W. (1982*a*). Utilization of nutrients by isolated epithelial cells of the rat colon. *Gastroenterology*, **83**, 424–9

Roediger, W. E. W. (1982*b*). The effect of bacterial metabolites on nutrition and function of the colonic mucosa. Symbiosis between man and bacteria. In *Colon and Nutrition*, ed. H. Kasper & H. Goebell, pp. 11–25. Lancaster: MTP Press.

Roediger, W. E. W. (1988*a*). What sequence of pathogenetic events leads to acute ulcerative colitis? *Diseases of the Colon and Rectum*, **31**, 482–7.

Roediger, W. E. W. (1988*b*). The role of colonic mucosal metabolism, in the pathogenesis of ulcerative colitis. In *Inflammatory Bowel Diseases – Basic Research and Clinical Implications*, ed. A. Goebell, B. M. Peskar & H. Malchow, pp. 69–78. Lancaster: MTP Press.

Roediger, W. E. W. (1989). Short chain fatty acids as metabolic regulators of ion absorption in the colon. *Acta Veterinaria Scandinavica*, **S86**, 116–25.

Roediger, W. E. W. (1990). The starved colon – diminished mucosal nutrition diminished absorption and colitis. *Diseases of the Colon and Rectum*, **33**, 8558–862.

Roediger, W. E. W. (1991). The role of sulphur metabolism and mercapto fatty acids in the aetiology of ulcerative colitis. In *Inflammatory Bowel Disease. Progress in Basic Research and Clinical Implications*, ed. H. Goebell, K. Ewe, H. Malchow & Ch. Koelbel, pp. 17–27. Dordrecht: Kluwer Academic Press.

Roediger, W. E. W., Deakin, E. J., Radcliffe, B. C. & Nance, S. (1986). Anion control of sodium absorption in the colon. *Quarterly Journal of Experimental Physiology*, **71**, 195–204.

Roediger, W. E. W., Duncan, A., Kapaniris, O. & Millard, S. (1993*a*). Reducing sulfur compounds of the colon impair colonocyte nutrition: implications for ulcerative colitis. *Gastroenterology*, **104**, 802–9.

Roediger, W. E. W., Duncan, A., Kapaniris, O. & Millard, S. (1993*b*). Sulphide impairment of substrate oxidation in rat colonocytes: a biochemical basis for ulcerative colitis? *Clinical Science*, **85**, 623–7.

Roediger, W. E. W., Kapaniris, O. & Millard, S. (1992). Lipogenesis from *n*-butyrate in colonocytes. *Molecular and Cellular Biochemistry*, **118**, 113–18.

Roediger, W. E. W., Lawson, M. J., Kwok, V., Kerr Grant, A. & Pannall, P. R. (1984). Colonic bicarbonate output as a test of disease activity in ulcerative colitis. *Journal of Clinical Pathology*, **37**, 704–7.

Roediger, W. E. W. & Nance, S. (1986). Metabolic induction of experimental colitis by inhibition of fatty acid oxidation. *British Journal of Experimental Pathology*, **67**, 773–82.

Roediger, W. E. W. & Nance, S. (1990). Selective reduction of fatty acid oxidation in colonocytes: correlation with ulcerative colitis. *Lipids*, **25**, 646–52.

Roediger, W. E. W. & Rae, D. A. (1982). Trophic effect of short chain fatty acids on mucosal handling of ions by the defunctioned colon. *British Journal of Surgery*, **69**, 23–5.

Roediger, W. E. W. & Truelove, S. C. (1979). Method of preparing isolated colonic epithelial cells (colonocytes) for metabolic studies. *Gut*, **20**, 484–8.

Sabourault, D., Bauche, F., Giudicelli, Y., Nordmann, J. & Nordmann, R. (1979). Inhibitory effect of 2-mercapto-acetate on fatty acid oxidation in the liver. *FEBS Letters*, **108**, 465–8.

Scaife, J. R. & Tichivangana, J. Z. (1980). Short chain acyl-CoA synthetases in bovine rumen epithelium. *Biochimica et Biophysica Acta*, **619**, 445–50.

Scholte, H. R. (1988). The biochemical basis of mitochondrial diseases. *Journal of Bioenergetics and Biomembranes*, **20**, 161–91.

Shakir, K. M. M., Sundaram, S. G. & Margolis, S. (1978). Lipid synthesis in isolated intestinal cells. *Journal of Lipid Research*, **19**, 433–42.

Shaw, L. & Engel, P. C. (1987). CoA-persulphide: a possible *in vivo* inhibitor of mammalian short-chain acyl-CoA dehydrogenase. *Biochimica et Biophysica Acta*, **919**, 171–4.

Thaysen, E. H. & Thaysen, J. M. (1952). Hunger diarrhoea. *Acta Medica Scandinavica*, **174** (Suppl.), 124–60.

Turnbull, D. M., Shepherd, I. M. & Aynsley-Green, A. (1988). Inherited defects of mitochondrial fatty acid oxidation. *Biochemical Society Transactions*, **16**, 424–7.

Vianey-Liaud, C., Divry, P., Gregersen, N. & Matheu, M. (1987). The inborn errors of mitochondrial fatty acid oxidation. *Journal of Inherited Metabolic Diseases*, **10**, 159–98.

Williams, N. N., Branigan, A., Fitzpatrick, J. M. & O'Connell, P. R. (1992). Glutamine and butyric acid metabolism measurement in biopsy specimens (*in vivo*): a method of assessing treatment on inflammatory bowel conditions (abstract). *Gastroenterology*, **102**, A713.

Williamson, D. H., Ilic, V. & Hughes, J. (1985). Effects of short term insulin deficiency on lipogenesis and cholesterol synthesis in rat small intestine and liver *in vivo*. *Biochemical Journal*, **231**, 221–3.

23

Management of diversion colitis, pouchitis and distal ulcerative colitis

W. SCHEPPACH, P. BARTRAM AND F. RICHTER

There is increasing evidence that short-chain fatty acids (SCFA) are emerging from being a matter of scientific interest to a tool of clinical medicine. Selected inflammatory conditions of the distal alimentary tract seem to respond to SCFA treatment. At present, SCFA have to be administered by rectal irrigation and not by mouth because orally administered SCFA are rapidly and completely absorbed in the jejunum (Schmitt, Soergel & Wood, 1977) and do not reach lower parts of the intestine. A slow-release form of SCFA has not yet been developed. In this chapter clinical trials using SCFA enemas in diversion colitis, pouchitis and distal ulcerative colitis are reviewed.

What is the rationale for using SCFA in inflammatory bowel diseases? It is known from the work of Roediger (1980) that *n*-butyrate is the primary metabolic fuel for colonocytes, predominantly in the distal colon (Fig. 23.1). In ulcerative colitis, a decreased luminal availability (Vernia *et al.*, 1988) and an impaired intracellular oxidation of butyrate (Roediger, 1988) have been described. If this metabolic defect is partial, it could be overcome by 'mass action' (Soergel, 1990), i.e. by raising the luminal butyrate concentration above normal. Thus, the use of SCFA enemas in distal ulcerative colitis and other forms of inflammation is based on the assumption that epithelial energy deficiency may be one factor in the pathogenesis of these diseases and that the supply of the preferred nutrients may ameliorate inflammation (for details see Chapter 22).

Diversion colitis

If colonic epithelial starvation leads, in the short term, to mucosal hypoplasia and, in the long term, to 'nutritional' colitis (Roediger, 1990), this problem should be especially evident in the excluded rectum after complete diversion of the faecal stream. This entity was first described by Glotzer, Glick &

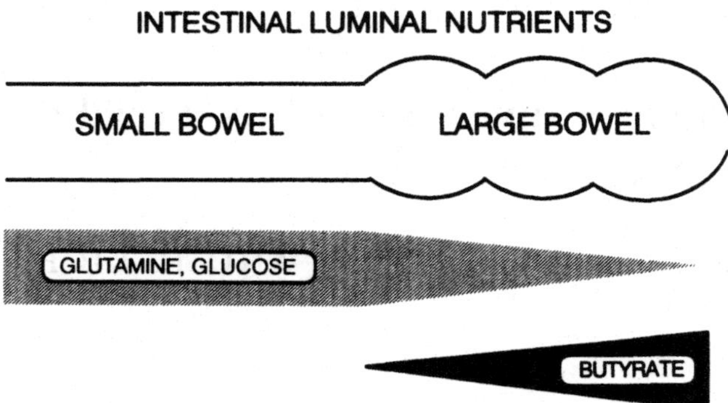

Fig. 23.1. Gut luminal nutrients. Preference of the distal colon for butyrate over the substrates (glutamine, glucose).

Goldman (1981) in the defunctioned distal colon; the colitis subsided after colonic reanastomosis. The endoscopic picture of diversion colitis is characterized by oedema, erythema, granularity, friability and ulcers (Ma, Gottlieb & Haas, 1990). In histology, crypt abscesses, lymphocytic infiltrates, architectural alterations of crypts and regenerative changes simulating mild forms of ulcerative colitis are seen. About one-third of patients complain of mucous discharge, bleeding or anal tenderness (Ma *et al.*, 1990).

Harig *et al.* (1989) were the first to treat diversion colitis with SCFA irrigation. They administered SCFA enemas to five patients twice daily for 2–6 weeks (acetate 60 mmol/l, propionate 30 mmol/l, butyrate 40 mmol/l, sodium salts, pH 7, 280–290 mosm/l, volume 60 ml). For control runs (2–4 weeks) in the same patients, isotonic saline was used. Treatment response was assessed by an endoscopic score ranging from 0 to 10; overall inflammatory change was graded histologically from 0 to 4. As shown in Fig. 23.2(*a*), the endoscopic appearance of the mucosa improved after 2 weeks of SCFA administration and even more after 4–6 weeks. With saline, no consistent change in inflammation was observed (Fig. 23.2(*b*)). Histological findings paralleled endoscopic observations. Two patients, who were placed on maintenance therapy of between one enema per day and two enemas per week, were kept in remission, as judged by endoscopic criteria.

Encouraged by these data, Guillemot *et al.* (1991) performed a double-blind prospective study in 13 patients with diversion colitis for 2 weeks. Seven patients received SCFA enemas (composition as used by Harig *et al.*, 1989) and six received placebo (isotonic saline). No change in the endoscopic and histological scores in the treatment or control group was observed. It has been argued that a positive result may have been missed, due to the short duration of the study (Roediger, 1992). Furthermore, mild forms of colitis

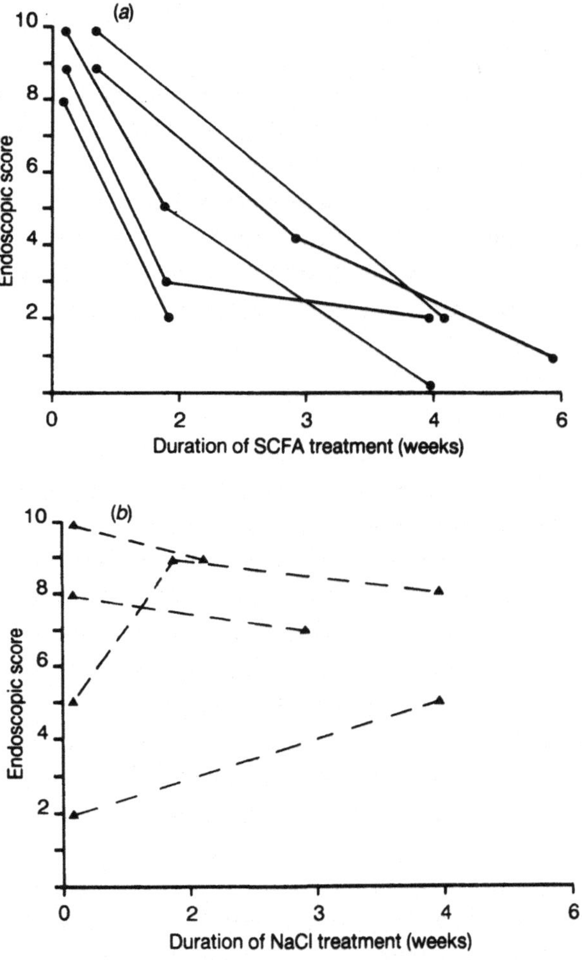

Fig. 23.2. Treatment of diversion colitis with short-chain fatty acid (SCFA) irrigation. Endoscopic score (range 0–10). in patients treated (*a*) for 2–6 weeks with SCFA ($n = 5$) or (*b*) for 2–4 weeks with NaCl ($n = 4$). Data taken from Harig *et al.* (1989).

were included, which may show less marked improvement than severe forms of disease.

In an open-label trial, Körber *et al.* (unpublished data) treated seven patients with diversion colitis and underlying Crohn's disease with SCFA enemas (composition as used by Harig *et al.*, 1989) twice daily for 6 weeks. The endoscopic index (Harig *et al.*, 1989) fell from 7–9 at entry to 4–6 after 2 weeks and further to 1–3 after 6 weeks. This finding emphasizes the need for prolonged (>4–6 weeks) SCFA irrigation to induce remission.

Mortensen *et al.* (1991) showed that SCFA irrigation (acetate 75 mmol/l, propionate 35 mmol/l, butyrate 20 mmol/l) had microcirculatory and trophic effects in the human rectum after Hartmann's procedure: in six patients mucosal blood flow and parameters of cellularity (crypt epithelial and nuclear volumes) increased in the excluded rectosigmoid after 10–14 days of treatment. The question of inflammation was not addressed in this study.

In summary, there is good evidence that diversion colitis is a consequence of luminal nutrient deficiency that is reversed by colonic reanastomosis. SCFA (especially *n*-butyrate) are the preferred mucosal nutrients in the distal colon. It is likely that rectal SCFA irrigation ameliorates inflammation if employed for a sufficient period of time.

Pouchitis

There are preliminary reports on the use of SCFA in pouchitis, another postoperative condition. Pouchitis occurs in about one-third of patients with ileo–anal pouches (IAP) after colectomy for ulcerative colitis (Wischmeyer *et al.*, 1991). Wischmeyer *et al.* (1991) found that SCFA concentrations in the effluent of patients with pouchitis were reduced significantly compared with patients with IAP and without pouchitis. This finding was confirmed by Clausen, Tvede & Mortensen (1992); these authors also described reduced SCFA production by faecal homogenates from patients with pouchitis. However, a reduced SCFA concentration in ileal effluent does not necessarily mean lower production; it could also result from more severe diarrhoea (dilution effect).

De Silva *et al.* (1989) treated two patients with IAP and with pouchitis topically with SCFA enemas (twice daily, composition as used by Harig *et al.*, 1989). After 2 and 4 weeks of treatment, there was no effect on the inflamed ileal mucosa. Wischmeyer *et al.* (1992) used butyrate suppositories (40 mmol twice daily) in pouchitis and found clinical improvement in only three of nine patients after a 3-week period. However, six of ten patients responded to glutamine suppositories (1 g, twice daily); this may indicate a greater importance of glutamine as a nutrient for the ileal mucosa.

On the basis of limited data, there is at present little justification to support a role for SCFA in the treatment of pouchitis.

Distal ulcerative colitis

As there are striking histological similarities between diversion colitis and ulcerative colitis, rectal SCFA irrigation has also been tested in the latter condition. It has been shown by radioactive labelling of mesalamine enemas

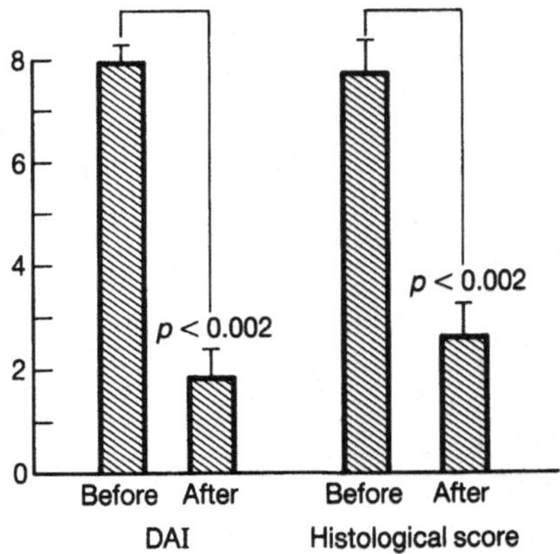

Fig. 23.3. Treatment of distal ulcerative colitis with short-chain fatty acid (SCFA) enemas. Disease activity index (DAI) and histological score before and after 6 weeks of SCFA irrigation. Data taken from Breuer *et al.* (1991).

that the rectum and sigmoid and descending colon can be treated topically by this mode of application (Chapman *et al.*, 1992). Therefore, SCFA trials have been limited to distal ulcerative colitis with a maximum involvement of mucosa from the rectum to the splenic flexure.

Breuer *et al.* (1991) used a combination of SCFA (acetate 80 mmol/l, propionate 30 mmol/l, butyrate 40 mmol/l) in an open-label trial. They treated ten patients with active distal disease for 6 weeks and considered nine patients at least much improved. The mean disease activity index (DAI, covering clinical activity and the endoscopic appearance of the mucosa) and the histological degree of inflammation fell significantly following SCFA irrigation (Fig. 23.3).

Because the evidence from the literature (Roediger, 1988) is strongest for the effect of butyrate on the colonic mucosa, Scheppach *et al.* (1992) have administered butyrate in a higher than physiological concentration (sodium butyrate 100 mmol/l, sodium chloride 40 mmol/l, 280–290 mosm/l, pH 7, volume 100 ml). Ten patients with active distal disease were treated twice daily for 2 weeks. A single-blind crossover design was used and a placebo control (sodium chloride 140 mml/l) included. Clinical symptoms (stool frequency, rectal bleeding) regressed under butyrate but not under placebo. The endoscopic score proposed by Harig *et al.* (1989) and the histological degree of overall inflammation decreased significantly in the butyrate but not the control phase (Fig. 23.4). In three patients with marginal improvement after 2 weeks, the butyrate trial was extended to 4 weeks; at this time a further amelioration of inflammation was noted.

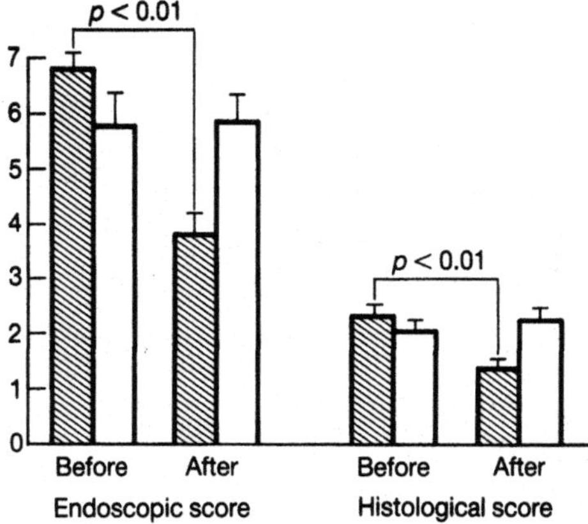

Fig. 23.4. Treatment of distal ulcerative colitis with enemas of butyrate (hatched bars) or NaCl placebo (white bars). Endoscopic score (range 0–10, taken from Harig *et al.*, 1989) and histological score (range 0–3) before and after 2 weeks of treatment. Data taken from Scheppach *et al.* (1992).

Steinhart, Brzezinski & Baker (1992) studied seven patients with distal ulcerative colitis refractory to standard medical therapy (oral and topical 5-aminosalicylic acid, topical corticosteroids) in an open-label trial. Patients were treated with nightly enemas consisting of 60 ml of 80 mmol/l sodium butyrate for a period of at least 6 weeks. Clinical and endoscopic response was seen in three of seven patients after 21–46 days of treatment.

Senagore *et al.* (1992) performed a randomized, prospective comparison of corticosteroid (hydrocortisone, 6 mg), mesalamine (5-aminosalicylic acid, 4 g) and SCFA enemas (composition according to Harig *et al.*, 1989) in patients with proctosigmoiditis. In every group, patients were evaluated (symptoms, endoscopic score, histological score) at entry and after 6 weeks of continuous treatment. Improvement occurred in a similar proportion in the three treatment arms: corticosteroid enemas 10/12 patients, mesalamine 17/19, SCFA 12/14 (no significant difference between the groups). It was emphasized by the authors that SCFA enemas were equally effective as standard drugs at a significant cost saving.

The results obtained with SCFA enemas in distal ulcerative colitis are encouraging and justify the initiation of further controlled trials. First, it will have to be shown in a greater number of patients that SCFA are superior to placebo. It will also be of interest to know if a combination of SCFA (acetate + propionate + butyrate) or a monocomponent enema (butyrate) offers advantages over the other. Furthermore, SCFA will have to show at least equal efficacy as standard drugs used in the topical treatment of ulcerative colitis; the paper by Senagore *et al.* (1992) points in this direction. An advantage of the SCFA approach is the lack of side effects, because SCFA are physiological components of colonic luminal contents.

Conclusion

SCFA are the predominant anions in the colonic lumen and are key regulators of the *milieu interieur*. Their production by bacterial fermentation of carbohydrates, absorption and role as epithelial nutrients are well established. There is information that mucosal energy deficiency may play a role in the pathogenesis of diversion colitis and other inflammatory conditions of the distal alimentary tract. Clinical trials in small numbers of patients are encouraging, but require confirmation by extended studies. In the words of Rabassa & Rogers (1992), 'the welfare of colonic mucosa, as it relates to SCFA metabolism, awaits another exciting decade of investigation'.

References

Breuer, R. I., Buto, S. K., Christ, M. L., Bean, J., Vernia, P., Paoluzi, P., DiPaolo, M. C. & Caprilli, R. (1991). Rectal irrigation with short-chain fatty acids for distal ulcerative colitis. Preliminary report. *Digestive Diseases and Sciences*, **36**, 185–7.

Chapman, N. J., Brown, M. L., Phillips, S. F., Tremaine, W. J., Schroeder, K. W., Dewanjee, M. K. & Zinsmeister, A. R. (1992). Distribution of mesalamine enemas in patients with active distal ulcerative colitis. *Mayo Clinic Proceedings*, **67**, 245–8.

Clausen, M. R., Tvede, M. & Mortensen, P. B. (1992). Short-chain fatty acids in pouch contents from patients with and without pouchitis after ileal pouch–anal anastomosis. *Gastroenterology*, **103**, 1144–53.

De Silva, H. J., Ireland, A., Kettlewell, M., Mortensen, N. & Jewell, D. P. (1989). Short-chain fatty acid irrigation in severe pouchitis (letter). *New England Journal of Medicine*, **321**, 1416–17.

Glotzer, D. J., Glick, M. E. & Goldman, H. (1981). Proctitis and colitis following diversion of the fecal stream. *Gastroenterology*, **80**, 438–41.

Guillemot, F., Colombel, J. F., Neut, C., Verplanck, N., Lecomte, M., Romond, C., Paris, J. C. & Cortot, A. (1991). Treatment of diversion colitis by short-chain fatty acids. *Diseases of the Colon and Rectum*, **34**, 861–4.

Harig, J. M., Soergel, K. H., Komorowski, R. A. & Wood, C. M. (1989). Treatment of diversion colitis with short-chain fatty acid irrigation. *New England Journal of Medicine*, **320**, 23–8.

Ma, C. K., Gottlieb, C. & Haas, P. A. (1990). Diversion colitis: a clinicopathologic study of 21 cases. *Human Pathology*, **21**, 429–36.

Mortensen, F. V., Hessov, I., Birke, H., Korsgaard, N. & Nielsen, H. (1991). Microcirculatory and trophic effects of short chain fatty acids in the human rectum after Hartmann's procedure. *British Journal of Surgery*, **78**, 1208–11.

Rabassa, A. A. & Rogers, A. I. (1992). The role of short-chain fatty acid metabolism in colonic disorders. *American Journal of Gastroenterology*, **87**, 419–23.

Roediger, W. E. W. (1980). Role of anaerobic bacteria in the metabolic welfare of the colonic mucosa in man. *Gut*, **21**, 793–8.

Roediger, W. E. W. (1988). The role of colonic mucosal metabolism in the pathogenesis of ulcerative colitis. In *Inflammatory Bowel Diseases – Basic Research and Clinical Implications*, ed. H. Goebell, B. M. Peskar & H. Malchow, pp. 69–78. Lancaster: MTP Press.

Roediger, W. E. W. (1990). The starved colon – diminished mucosal nutrition, diminished absorption, and colitis. *Diseases of the Colon and Rectum*, **33**, 858–62.

Roediger, W. E. W. (1992). Oxidative and synethetic functions of *n*-butyrate in colonocytes (letter). *Diseases of the Colon and Rectum*, **35**, 511–12.

Scheppach, W., Sommer, H., Kirchner, T., Paganelli, G. M., Bartram, P., Christl, S., Richter, F., Dusel, G. & Kasper, H. (1992). Effect of butyrate enemas on the colonic mucosa in distal ulcerative colitis. *Gastroenterology*, **103**, 51–6.

Schmitt, M. G., Soergel, K. H. & Wood, C. M. (1977). Absorption of short chain fatty acids from the human jejunum. *Gastroenterology*, **70**, 211–15.

Senagore, A. J., MacKeigan, J. M., Schneider, M. & Ebrom, S. (1992). Short-chain fatty acid enemas: a cost-effective alternative in the treatment of nonspecific proctosigmoiditis. *Diseases of the Colon and Rectum*, **35**, 923–7.

Soergel, K. H. (1990). Colitis and short-chain fatty acids. *IBD Forum Symposium, Digestive Disease Week*, San Antonio.

Steinhart, A. H., Brzezinski, A. & Baker, J. P. (1992). Butyrate enemas in the treatment of refractory distal ulcerative colitis: an open label trial. *Gastroenterology*, **102**, A615.

Vernia, P., Gnaedinger, A., Hauk, W. & Breuer, R. I. (1988). Organic anions and the diarrhea of inflammatory bowel disease. *Digestive Diseases and Sciences*, **33**, 1353–8.

Wischmeyer, P., Grotz, R. L., Pemberton, J. H. & Phillips, S. F. (1992). Treatment of pouchitis after ileo–anal anastomosis with glutamine and butyric acid. *Gastroenterology*, **102**, A617.

Wischmeyer, P. E., Tremaine, W. J., Haddad, A. C., Ambroze, W. L., Pemberton, J. H. & Phillips, S. F. (1991). Fecal short chain fatty acids in patients with pouchitis after ileal pouch anal anastomosis. *Gastroenterology*, **100**, A848.

24

The effects of short-chain fatty acids on phagocytic cell function

G. F. BRISSEAU AND O. D. ROTSTEIN

Introduction

The outcome of bacterial infection represents the end result of a complex interaction between invading microbial pathogens and local host defence mechanisms. The recruitment of phagocytic cells to the site of an infecting bacterial inoculum is a crucial component of the early host response to infection. Polymorphonuclear leukocytes (PMNs) arrive within hours and provide an early wave of microbicidal activity (Hau, Hoffman & Simmons, 1978). Reactive oxygen species as well as lysosomal enzymes released by activated PMNs serve to effect bacterial killing. Macrophages are recruited to the inflammatory site somewhat later. In addition to their intrinsic microbicidal activity, macrophages also release a wide array of mediator molecules that heighten the PMNs' bacterial killing capacity, attract more phagocytic cells and initiate local wound repair (Nathan, 1987). Failure of host defence mechanisms to effect complete clearance of bacteria results in the persistence of infection, usually manifested by local abscess formation.

Several local factors may adversely affect the ability of phagocytic cells to ingest and kill bacteria. For example, at sites of surgical trauma, various adjuvant substances such as blood, foreign bodies and necrotic tissue are known to promote infection by impairing local phagocytic cell function (deHoll *et al.*, 1974; Pruett *et al.*, 1984; Zimmererli, Lew & Waldvogel, 1984). Furthermore, most pathogenic bacterial species are armed with virulence factors that are toxic to phagocytic cells or render them ineffective. One area of investigation that has received relatively little attention is the potential influence of the local inflammatory microenvironment on host–pathogen interactions. This milieu is characterized by low pH (Bryant *et al.*, 1980), low oxygen tension (Silver, 1978) and intense fibrin deposition (McRitchie, Cummings & Rotstein, 1989). All three factors are known to impair cell function. The initial report describing very high concentrations of short-chain fatty acids (SCFA) at sites of localized anaerobic infection dates back more than 15 years (Gorbach *et al.*, 1976). Presumably, SCFA accumulate as a result of their production by bacteria engaged in anaerobic metabolism and by phagocytic cells that are metabolically active.

The purpose of this review is to document the effects of SCFA on phagocytic cell function and to describe the presumed mechanisms underlying these effects. The ability of SCFA to impair local host defences represents another means by which the microenvironment of infection may thwart bacterial clearance and lead to persistence of infection.

Effect of SCFA on phagocytic cell function

The concept that SCFA might modulate phagocytic cell function was derived from several areas of investigation. These include periodontal disease (Van Dyke *et al.*, 1982), polymicrobial surgical infections (Rotstein, Pruett & Simmons, 1985*b*) and dermatological studies examining the pathogenesis of comedones (Puhvel & Sakamoto, 1978). The common feature of these processes is the role of anaerobic bacteria in the pathogenesis of the disease. It was postulated that anaerobic bacteria and/or their byproducts might interact with local inflammatory cells, mainly PMNs, and thus contribute to the initiation of the disease. For example, Van Dyke and colleagues showed that culture supernatants and sonic extracts of major bacterial species recovered from the human oral cavity were able to inhibit PMN migration and impaired phagocytosis (Van Dyke *et al.*, 1982). By contrast, comedonal lipids were chemotactic for phagocytic cells, and the fatty-acid extract from this material constituted a significant portion of the chemotactic activity (Puhvel & Sakamoto, 1978). The role of SCFA in polymicrobial surgical infections was examined in part to define the mechanisms underlying the ability of anaerobic bacteria such as *Bacteroides* species to promote the virulence of mixed infections, while themselves lacking significant intrinsic toxicity. Namavar *et al.* demonstrated that a heat-stable factor with molecular weight of <3500 present in the culture supernatant of five *Bacteroides* strains inhibited the bactericidal activity of PMNs (Namavar *et al.*, 1983). These authors suggested a possible role for butyrate but did not directly test this molecule. These studies led to further investigation of the effect of SCFA on phagocytic cell function by our own and other laboratories.

The accumulation of phagocytic cells at the site of inflammation requires diapedesis from the circulation into extravascular sites. Several studies have investigated the ability of SCFA to alter PMN migration. Incubation of PMNs with butyrate, succinate, propionate, isovalerate and isobutyrate has been shown to impair chemotactic migration in response to casein, formyl-methionyl-leucyl-phenylalanine (fMLP) and the complement component C5a (Botta *et al.*, 1985; Rotstein *et al.*, 1985*a*; Eftimiadi *et al.*, 1987). SCFA also reduced random cell migration. In some studies, these effects were augmented by incubation of cells in acid medium, in 5% CO_2 or under anaerobic conditions.

SCFA also alter the phagocytic killing capacity of PMNs (Eftimiadi *et al.*, 1990; Tonetti *et al.*, 1991). Most studies have examined the effect of SCFA with fewer than 5 carbon atoms. These uniformly inhibit phagocytic killing. This effect appears to be mediated by both a reduction in phagocytic uptake of bacteria (Eftimiadi *et al.*, 1990) and a reduction in the microbicidal activity of the phagocytic cell. Studies by Eftimiadi and colleagues (Eftimiadi *et al.*, 1990) demonstrated that butyrate, succinate, and propionate were able to inhibit phagocytic uptake of *Staphylococcus aureus* by human alveolar macrophages, while others have documented the ability of various SCFA, specifically succinate, butyrate, isobutyrate and propionate, to reduce both oxygen-dependent and oxygen-independent killing mechanisms (Rotstein, Nasmith & Grinstein, 1987*a*, 1988; Eftimiadi *et al.*, 1990; Tonetti *et al.* 1991). SCFA induced a significant decrease in superoxide production and chemiluminescence in PMNs in response to the protein kinase C stimulus, phorbol myristate acetate. Some investigators have shown a corresponding reduction in hydrogen peroxide release and in oxygen consumption, while others have not (Rotstein *et al.*, 1988; Tonetti *et al.*, 1991). The precise explanation for this discrepancy is unclear. Release of the granule enzyme, lysozyme, from PMNs following stimulation with fMLP is also impaired, indicating an effect of SCFA on oxygen-independent microbicidal function (Eftimiadi *et al.*, 1987).

Now that it is established that SCFA are able to exert inhibitory effects on phagocytic cell function, it is important to consider whether this observation has any physiological or pathophysiological significance. While SCFA are known to be present at high concentration within abscesses, their ability to alter PMN function *in vivo* is not clear. The addition of SCFA-containing bacterial supernatant to an *Escherichia coli*-infected fibrin clot had no effect on mortality or abscess formation in a rat intra-abdominal infection model (Rotstein & Kao, 1988). However, the likelihood that a sustained elevation of SCFA concentration existed locally within the fibrin mesh is low, due to rapid diffusion out of the clot *in vivo*. The best evidence that SCFA may play a role in modulating PMN activity is derived from *in vitro* studies examining the effect of bacterial supernatants on PMN function. Culture filtrates from various *Bacteroides* species grown *in vitro* were shown to impair a wide range of PMN functions, including migration, phagocytic killing and the respiratory

Table 24.1. *Short-chain fatty acid concentrations (mM) measured in sterile culture medium or the 22-h culture filtrate of* Bacteroides fragilis *9032. The data represent the mean and standard error of three separate samples*

	Culture medium	*Bacteroides* filtrate
Acetic acid	0.7 (0.1)	10.4 (1.0)
Formic acid	0.2 (0.2)	5.8 (0.2)
Lactic acid	0.0	9.2 (1.2)
Succinic acid	5.7 (1.2)	16.0 (1.3)
Fumaric acid	0.0	1.3 (0.1)

From Rotstein *et al.* (1989) with permission.

burst (Rotstein *et al.*, 1987*a*, 1989). Three lines of evidence suggest that this effect was mediated by SCFA released in the filtrate during bacterial growth. First, the SCFA content of *B. fragilis* supernatants derived from stationary phase cultures was measured (Table 24.1). Pure SCFA were then added to sterile medium at the same concentration as that measured and tested for their effect on PMN function. This solution precisely reproduced the ability of the crude filtrate to inhibit phagocytic killing of *E. coli* by PMNs (Rotstein *et al.*, 1987*a*, 1989). Second, the time course of SCFA generation by *B. fragilis* closely mirrored the development of the inhibition of PMN function by the filtrate (Rotstein *et al.*, 1989). Finally, removal of the SCFA-containing fractions of *Bacteroides* filtrates by passage across a Sephadex G-25 column reversed the inhibitory effect of the filtrate. When considered together, these data provide evidence that SCFA produced by bacteria during growth are capable of exhibiting inhibitory effects on PMNs (Rotstein *et al.*, 1987*b*). SCFA may also play a role in promoting the development of peritonitis in patients receiving peritoneal dialysis for end-stage renal failure. Exposure of both PMNs and macrophages to fresh dialysis fluid rendered them unable to undergo a respiratory burst (Topley *et al.*, 1988; Manahan, *et al.*, 1989; Gupta *et al.*, 1990). The inhibitory effect was dependent on both the presence of sodium lactate (35 mM) in the solution and the acidic pH (5.3) of the solution (Topley *et al.*, 1988). Dialysis fluid also has an inhibitory effect on the activation of cells of the monocyte/macrophage lineage (Jorres *et al.*, 1992). Dialysate significantly reduced the release of tumour necrosis factor α and interleukin-6 by lipopolysaccharide-stimulated peripheral blood monocytes. This effect required the simultaneous presence of lactate and low extracellular pH. When considered together, these findings are consistent with the notion that the SCFA composition of dialysate may be responsible for an inhibitory effect on phagocytic cell function.

Cellular effects of SCFA: mechanisms of leukocyte inhibition

Exposure of phagocytic cells, particularly PMNs, to SCFA has been shown to induce several cellular alterations. These include intracellular acidification, a rise in cytoplasmic calcium concentration and the initiation of actin polymerization. This section reviews these alterations and attempts to relate them to SCFA-induced alterations in cell function.

For years, SCFA have been used experimentally to induce cytoplasmic acidification. As they are weak acids (pK_a 4.8–5.2), a significant proportion of these molecules exist in the protonated state at physiological extracellular pH. These hydrophobic molecules traverse the plasma membrane and accumulate intracellularly, thereby equilibrating the SCFA concentration inside and outside the cell. In so doing, these molecules shuttle protons into the cytoplasmic compartment and induce a modest intracellular acidification (Grinstein *et al.*, 1984). The degree of cytoplasmic acid loading can be increased by reducing the extracellular pH. The proposed mechanism is illustrated in Fig. 24.1. Table 24.2 compares cytoplasmic pH levels at various extracellular pH levels in the presence and absence of sodium succinate (30 mM).

Based on the sensitivity of various cellular processes to alterations in pH, we hypothesized that the inhibitory effect of SCFA on PMN function might

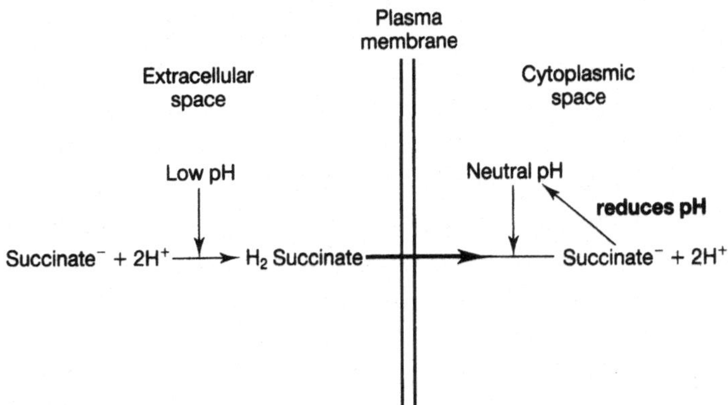

Fig. 24.1. At low extracellular pH, the weak acid succinate is protonated and traverses the plasma membrane. Within the cytoplasmic space, the molecule dissociates and releases H^+ ion, thereby reducing the intracellular pH. Reproduced from Rotstein *et al.* (1988), with permission.

Table 24.2. *Effect of succinate (30 mM) on intracellular pH at various levels of extracellular pH. Polymorphonuclear leukocytes, loaded with 2,7-biscarboxyethyl-5(6)-carboxyfluorescein, were suspended in the indicated medium, and the intracellular pH was determined after a 10-min incubation period*

	Intracellular pH (pH_i)	
Medium pH (pH_o)	Control medium	Succinate medium
7.4	7.16 ± 0.08	7.09 ± 0.08
6.5	6.83 ± 0.05	6.60 ± 0.06
6.0	6.66 ± 0.05	6.11 ± 0.05
5.5	6.32 ± 0.05	5.52 ± 0.02

Adapted from Rotstein *et al.* (1987*a*).

be related to their ability to induce cytoplasmic acidification. By pharmacologically 'clamping' pH_i at levels created by succinate at various pH_o using the K^+/nigericin technique, the effect of altered pH_i on cell function was examined (Rotstein *et al.*, 1987*a*). The respiratory burst of PMNs was evaluated by measuring phorbol ester-induced oxygen consumption and superoxide release. This function was evaluated on the basis of its important contribution to the microbicidal activity of the cell and also because the enzyme responsible for the respiratory burst, NADPH oxidase, is known to be markedly sensitive to pH in cell-free systems (Nasmith & Grinstein, 1986). Incubation of cells in various SCFA at pH_o 7.4 had no effect on superoxide production, while reducing the pH_o to 5.5 resulted in marked inhibition of superoxide release (Fig. 24.2). When the pH_i was clamped at the pH_i levels measured under these conditions (7.10 v. 5.50), the respiratory burst was markedly abrogated at the low, but not the high pH level. Thus, the succinate-mediated reduction in pH_i at low extracellular levels could account entirely for the effect of the SCFA on cell function. Subsequent studies demonstrated that *Bacteroides* culture filtrate effected comparable pH-dependent inhibition of PMN function and that this effect was mediated via the ability of the SCFA in the filtrate to reduce the cytoplasmic pH (Rotstein *et al.*, 1989). In addition to the respiratory burst, SCFA-induced acidification probably contributes to modulation of other cell functions, such as migration. Simchowitz and Cragoe demonstrated a linear correlation between migration and pH_i over an intracellular pH range of 6.8–8.6. Cytoplasmic acidification relative to resting pH_i (7.25) resulted in impaired migration. The authors postulated that this effect was mediated by pH-induced alterations in the

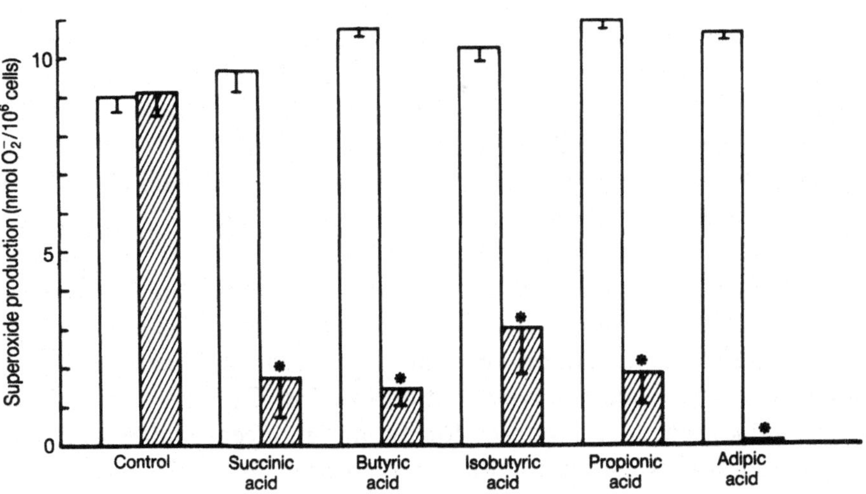

Fig. 24.2. Effect of different short-chain fatty acids (SCFA) on superoxide production by polymorphonuclear leukocytes. Cells were incubated in 30-mM solutions of various SCFA at either pH 5.5 (hatched bars) or pH 7.4 (white bars) for 20 min at 37 °C, washed and resuspended in balanced salt solution at pH 7.4 prior to testing. Results expressed as nanomoles of O_2^- per 10^6 cells per 20 min. Means and standard error of at least two experiments performed in duplicate are shown. * $p < 0.01$ v. control SCFA at pH 7.4. Reproduced with permission from Rotstein *et al.*, 1989.

regulation of actin polymerization (Simchowitz & Cragoe, 1986). Presumably, the effect of dialysis fluid on phagocytic cell function is mediated by a similar mechanism, although this has not been directly tested.

While many of the inhibitory effects of SCFA can be explained by the ability of SCFA to induce a sustained cytoplasmic acidification, other mechanisms are clearly important. For example, Eftimiadi and colleagues demonstrated that butyric, succinic and propionic acids were capable of impairing phagocytic activity by both PMNs and macrophages (Eftimiadi *et al.*, 1987, 1990). At the concentration used (30 mM), there was a modest and transient reduction in pH_i (Rotstein *et al.*, 1987*a*). This degree of acidification per se is unlikely to inhibit cellular function directly. However, as is discussed in the following paragraphs, acidification may influence signal transduction mechanisms in cells and thus cause alterations in their function.

The cytoskeleton plays an important role in normal cell function. For example, activation of the actin-based cytoskeletal network is considered to be responsible for changes in cell shape, membrane ruffling and cell migration following exposure to chemotactic peptides (Fechheimer & Zigmond, 1983;

White, Naccache & Sha'afi, 1983), while movement of lysosomes to the periphery of the cell prior to degranulation is mediated via microtubules (Heuser, 1989). Several lines of evidence suggest that cytoplasmic acidification following exposure of cells to chemoattractants such as fMLP or leukotriene B_4 contributes to cellular activation (Naccache, 1987; Yuli & Oplatka, 1987; Naccache *et al.*, 1989; Tonetti, Budnick & Niederman, 1990). The magnitude of the acidification mimics that induced by various SCFA, such as propionate, and thus suggests that SCFA may modulate cell activation by this mechanism. First, cell acidification initiated by agonists is accompanied by actin polymerization. Second, prevention of agonist-induced acidification with protonophores prevents actin polymerization (Yuli & Oplatka, 1987). Finally, the time course and dose reponses for agonist-induced acidification and actin polymerization are similar (Faucher & Naccache, 1987). Indeed, propionic acid is itself capable of initiating actin polymerization over a range of concentrations from 0.5 to 30 mM (Naccache, 1987).

The mechanism responsible for the ability of chemoattractants and SCFA to induce actin polymerization is not completely defined. Pertussis toxin blocks actin polymerization in response to propionate without inhibiting acidification, indicating a role for G-proteins (Molski & Sha'afi, 1987). Initial studies suggested a role for calcium in the initiation of actin polymerization following cell exposure to both agonists and weak acids, since these treatments were able to induce a rise in cytoplasmic calcium capable of stimulating actin polymerization (Naccache *et al.*, 1988). However, several investigators have subsequently demonstrated that a rise in cytoplasmic calcium is neither necessary nor sufficient for actin polymerization, thus making this mechanism unlikely (Molski & Sha'afi, 1987; Al-Mohanna & Hallett, 1990; Downey *et al.*, 1990). It is noteworthy, however, that even though the SCFA-induced increase in calcium is not vital to actin polymerization, it may act to modulate other cell functions.

The effect of cytoplasmic acidification also does not appear to be mediated through the release of PMN-derived activators, a phenomenon that occurs in response to acid treatment of PMNs (Zigmond & Hargrove, 1981). The propionic acid-induced light-scatter response (a measure of cell shape change) is not affected by treatment of the cells with a leukotriene synthesis inhibitor or an antagonist of platelet activating factor. This suggests that the effect is not mediated by either of these two chemoattractants. In addition, it appears that absolute cytoplasmic acidification is not required for stimulation of the light scatter response by either fMLP or propionic acid. Alkalinization of cells with ammonium chloride prior to their exposure to either of the two stimuli produced a light-scatter response without lowering the cytoplasmic pH below resting levels (Naccache *et al.*, 1989). Thus, a change in pH rather than cytoplasmic acidification per se is the responsible initiating event.

While an association between cytoplasmic acidification and initiation of actin polymerization clearly exists, a causal relationship between the two and their contribution to cell function remains to be defined. The finding that PMNs from patients with chronic granulomatous disease exhibit normal migration in response to chemoattractants, despite their failure to acidify, makes it unlikely that acidification alone is the sole signal for migration (Grinstein, Furuya & Biggar, 1986). Further, the finding that protonophores prevent the light-scatter response to cytoplasmic acidification (Yuli & Oplatka, 1987; Tonetti *et al.*, 1990) has been challenged by a report demonstrating that prevention of agonist-induced acidification with a cytoplasmic calcium buffer did not ablate the cytoskeletal rearrangement in response to cell stimulation (Naccache *et al.*, 1989). When considered together, these data suggest that while acidification per se is not an absolute requirement for actin polymerization, induction of acidification by agents such as SCFA is sufficient to initiate alterations in the cytoskeleton. Recent studies by Brunkhorst and colleagues (Brunkhorst *et al.*, 1992) suggest that this effect may result in an altered response to chemotactic peptides. This may represent one of the mechanisms whereby SCFA may impair phagocytic cell migration at physiological extracellular pH levels (Eftimiadi *et al.*, 1987).

Conclusions

SCFA appear to have a profound influence on phagocytic cell function measured in the *in vitro* setting. Whether this effect occurs *in vivo* remains to be determined. The complexity of the microenvironment at sites of infection and inflammation precludes precise examination of this question. However, the local conditions required for SCFA to exert their effects *in vivo* clearly exist. SCFA have been measured at concentrations greater than 30 mM, while the pH of sites of inflammation has been measured to be as low as 5.7. These data, therefore, provide further evidence for the role of the local milieu in modulating host–pathogen interaction during infection.

References

Al-Mohanna, A. & Hallett, M. B. (1990). Actin polymerization in neutrophils is triggered without a requirement for a rise in cytoplasmic calcium. *Biochemical Journal*, **266**, 669–74.

Botta, G. A., Eftimiadi, C., Costa, A., Tonetti, M., van Steenbergen, T. J. M. & de Graaff, J. (1985). Influence of volatile fatty acids on human granulocyte chemotaxis. *FEMS Microbiology Letters*, **27**, 39–72.

Brunkhorst, B. A., Kraus, E., Coppi, M., Budnick, M. & Niederman, R. (1992). Propionate induces polymorphonuclear leukocyte activation and inhibits formylmethionyl-leucyl-phenylalanine-stimulated activation. *Infection and Immunity*, **60**, 2957–68.

Bryant, R. E., Rashad, A. L., Mazza, J. A. & Hammond, D. (1980). Beta-lactamase activity in human pus. *Journal of Infectious Diseases*, **142**, 594–601.

deHoll, D., Rodeheaver, G. T., Edgerton, M. T. & Edlich, R. F. (1974). Potentiation of infection by suture closure of dead space. *American Journal of Surgery*, **127**, 716.

Downey, G. P., Chan, C. K., Trudel, S. & Grinstein, S. (1990). Actin assembly in electropermeabilized neutrophils: role of intracellular calcium. *Journal of Cell Biology*, **110**, 1975–82.

Eftimiadi, C., Buzzi, E., Tonetti, M., Buffa, P., van Steenbergen, M. T. J., de Graaff, J. & Botta, G. A. (1987). Short-chain fatty acids produced by anaerobic bacteria alter the physiological responses of human neutrophils to chemotactic peptides. *Journal of Infection*, **14**, 43–53.

Eftimiadi, C., Tonetti, M., Cavallero, A., Sacco, O. & Rossi, G. A. (1990). Short-chain fatty acids produced by anaerobic bacteria inhibit phagocytosis by human lung phagocytes. *Journal of Infectious Diseases*, **161**, 138–42.

Faucher, N. & Naccache, P. H. (1987). Relationship between pH, sodium, and shape changes in chemotactic-factor-stimulated human neutrophils. *Journal of Cellular Physiology*, **132**, 483–91.

Fechheimer, H. & Zigmond, S. H. (1983). Changes in cytoskeletal protein of polymorphonuclear leukocytes by chemotactic peptides. *Cell Motility*, **3**, 349–61.

Gorbach, S. L., Mayhew, J. W., Bartlett, J. G., Thadepalli, H. & Onderdonk, A. B. (1976). Rapid diagnosis of anaerobic infections by direct gas–liquid chromatography of clinical specimens. *Journal of Clinical Investigation*, **57**, 478–84.

Grinstein, S., Furuya, W. & Biggar, W. D. (1986). Cytoplasmic pH regulation in normal and abnormal neutrophils. Role of superoxide generation and Na^+/H^+ exchange. *Journal of Biological Chemistry*, **261**, 512–14.

Grinstein, S., Goetz, J. D., Furuya, W., Rothstein, A. & Gelfand, E. W. (1984). Amiloride-sensitive Na^+–H^+ exchange in platelets and leukocytes by electronic sizing. *American Journal of Physiology*, **247**, C293–C298.

Gupta, D. K., Ing, B. L., Manahan, F. J., Zhou, F.-Q., Yu, A. W., Nawab, Z. M. & Rahman, M. A. (1990). Superoxide generation by neutrophils after exposure to conventional peritoneal dialysis solutions for different time periods. *International Journal of Artificial Organs*, **13**, 228–30.

Hau, T., Hoffman, R. & Simmons, R. L. (1978). Mechanisms of the adjuvant effect of hemoglobin in experimental peritonitis. I: *In vivo* inhibition of peritoneal leukocytosis. *Surgery*, **83**, 223–9.

Heuser, J. (1989). Changes in lysosomal shape and distribution correlated with changes in cytoplasmic pH. *Journal of Cell Biology*, **108**, 855–64.

Jorres, A., Topley, N., Steenweg, L., Muller, C., Kottgen, E. & Gahl, G. M. (1992). Inhibition of cytokine synthesis by peritoneal dialysis persists throughout the CAPD cycle. *American Journal of Nephrology*, **12**, 80–5.

Manahan, F. J., Ing, B. L., Chan, J. C., Gupta, D. K., Zhou, F. Q., Pal, I. & Rahman, M. A. (1989). Effects of bicarbonate-containing versus lactate-containing peritoneal dialysis solutions on superoxide production by human neutrophils. *Artificial Organs*, **13**, 495–7.

McRitchie, D. I., Cummings, D. & Rotstein, O. D. (1989). Delayed administration of tissue plasminogen activator reduces intra-abdominal abscess formation. *Archives of Surgery*, **124**, 1406–10.

Molski, T. F. P. & Sha'afi, R. I. (1987). Intracellular acidification, guanine-nucleotide binding proteins, and cytoskeletal actin. *Cell Motility and the Cytoskeleton*, **8**, 1–6.

Naccache, P. H. (1987). Signals for actin polymerization in neutrophils. *Biomedicine and Pharmacotherapy*, **41**, 297–304.

Naccache, P. H., Faucher, N., Caon, A. C. & McColl, S. R. (1988). Propionic acid-induced calcium mobilization in human neutrophils. *Journal of Cellular Physiology*, **136**, 118–24.

Naccache, P. H., Therrien, S., Caon, A. C., Liao, N., Gilbert, C. & McColl, S. (1989). Chemoattractant-induced cytoplasmic pH changes and cytoskeletal reorganization in human neutrophils. Relationship to the stimulated transients and oxidative burst. *Journal of Immunology*, **142**, 2438–44.

Namavar, F., Verweij, A. M. J. J., Bal, M., van Steenbergen, T. J. M., de Graaff, J. & MacLaren, D. M. (1983). Effect of anaerobic bacteria on killing of *Proteus mirabilis* by human polymorphonuclear leukocytes. *Infection and Immunity*, **40**, 930–5.

Nasmith, P. E. & Grinstein, S. (1986). Impairment of Na^+/H^+ exchange underlies inhibitory effects of Na^+-free media on leukocyte function. *FEBS Letters*, **202**, 79–85.

Nathan, C. F. (1987). Secretory products of macrophage. *Journal of Clinical Investigation*, **79**, 319–26.

Pruett, T. L., Rostein, O. D., Fiegel, V. D., Sorenson, J. J., Nelson, R. D. & Simmons, R. L. (1984). Mechanism of the adjuvant effect of hemoglobin in experimental peritonitis: VIII. A leukotoxin is produced by *Escherichia coli* metabolism in hemoglobin. *Surgery*, **96**, 375–83.

Puhvel, S. M. & Sakamoto, M. (1978). The chemoattractant properties of comedonal components. *Journal of Investigative Dermatology*, **71**, 324–9.

Rotstein, O. D. & Kao, J. (1988). The spectrum of *Escherichia coli–Bacteroides fragilis* pathogenic synergy in an intraabdominal infection model. *Canadian Journal of Microbiology*, **34**, 352–7.

Rotstein, O. D., Nasmith, P. E. & Grinstein, S. (1987*a*). The *Bacteroides* by-product succinic acid inhibits neutrophil respiratory burst by reducing intracellular pH. *Infection and Immunity*, **55**, 864–70.

Rotstein, O. D., Nasmith, P. E. & Grinstein, S. (1988). pH-Dependent impairment of the neutrophil respiratory burst by the *Bacteroides* byproduct succinate. *Clinical and Investigative Medicine*, **11**, 259–65.

Rotstein, O. D., Pruett, T. L., Fiegel, V. D., Nelson, R. D. & Simmons, R. L. (1985*a*). Succinic acid, a metabolic by-product of *Bacteroides* species, inhibits polymorphonuclear leukocyte function. *Infection and Immunity*, **48**, 402–8.

Rotstein, O. D. Pruett, T. L. & Simmons, R. L. (1985*b*). Mechanisms of microbial synergy in polymicrobial surgical infections. *Reviews of Infectious Diseases*, **7**, 151–70.

Rotstein, O. D., Vittorini, T., Kao, J., McBurney, M. I., Nasmith, P. E. & Grinstein, S. (1989). A soluble *Bacteroides* by-product impairs phagocytic killing of *Escherichia coli* by neutrophils. *Infection and Immunity*, **57**, 745–53.

Rotstein, O. D., Wells, C. L., Pruett, T. L., Sorenson, J. J. & Simmons, R. L. (1987*b*). Succinic acid production by *Bacteroides fragilis*. A potential bacterial virulence factor. *Archives of Surgery*, **122**, 93–8.

Silver, I. A. (1978). Tissue pO_2 changes in acute inflammation. *Advances in Experimental Medicine and Biology*, **94**, 769–74.

Simchowitz, L. & Cragoe, E. J. Jr (1986). Regulation of human neutrophil chemotaxis by intracellular pH. *Journal of Biological Chemistry*, **261**, 6492–500.

Tonetti, M., Budnick, M. & Niederman, R. (1990). Receptor-stimulated actin polymerization requires cytoplasmic acidification in human PMNs. *Biochimica et Biophysica Acta*, **1054**, 154–8.

Tonetti, M., Cavallero, A., Botta, G. A., Niederman, R. & Eftimiadi, C. (1991). Intracellular pH regulates the production of different oxygen metabolites in neutrophils: effects of organic acids produced by anaerobic bacteria. *Journal of Leukocyte Biology*, **49**, 180–8.

Topley, N., Alobaida, H. M. M., Davies, M., Coles, G. A., Williams, J. D. & Lloyd, D. (1988). The effort of dialysate on peritoneal phagocyte oxidative metabolism. *Kidney International*, **34**, 404–11.

Van Dyke, T. E., Bartholomew, E., Genco, R. J., Slots, J. & Levine, M. J. (1982). Inhibition of neutrophil chemotaxes by soluble bacterial products. *Journal of Periodontology*, **53**, 502–8.

White, J. R., Naccache, P. H. & Sha'afi, R. I. (1983). Stimulation by chemotactic factor of actin association with the cytoskeleton in rabbit neutrophils: effects of calcium and cytochalasin B. *Journal of Biological Chemistry*, **258**, 14041–7.

Yuli, I. & Oplatka, A. (1987). Cytosolic acidification as an early transductory signal of human neutrophil chemotaxis. *Science*, **235**, 340–2.

Zigmond, S. & Hargrove, R. L. (1981). Orientation of PMN in a pH gradient. Acid-induced release of a chemotactic factor. *Journal of Immunology*, **126**, 478–81.

Zimmererli, W., Lew, P. D. & Waldvogel, F. A. (1984). Pathogenesis of foreign body infection. Evidence for a local granulocyte defect. *Journal of Clinical Investigation*, **73**, 1191–200.

25

Short-chain fatty acids, antibiotic-associated diarrhoea, colonic adenomas and cancer

P. B. MORTENSEN AND M. R. CLAUSEN

Diarrhoea associated with the use of antimicrobial agents is a well-recognized problem in clinical medicine. The severity of the diarrhoea ranges from a mild, self-limited process to fulminant necrotizing or pseudomembranous colitis (Viteri, Howard & Dyck, 1974; Neu *et al.*, 1977). *Clostridium difficile* can be detected in the faeces of virtually all patients with pseudomembranous colitis (Bartlett, 1979; Bartlett *et al.*, 1980), and in faeces of some patients with either antimicrobial-associated non-specific colitis or diarrhoea without colitis (Bartlett, 1979; Aronsson, Möllby & Nord, 1981; George, Rolfe & Finegold, 1982). However, *C. difficile* has also frequently been recovered from the faeces of healthy infants (Hall & O'Toole, 1935; Snyder, 1940; Larson *et al.*, 1978; Viscidi, Willey & Bartlett, 1981), occasionally from the faeces of asymptomatic adults (George, Sutter & Finegold, 1978; Larson *et al.*, 1978) and from the faeces of a high percentage of antibiotic-treated patients without diarrhoea (Lishman, Al-Jumaili & Record, 1981; Viscidi *et al.*, 1981; George *et al.*, 1982; Surawicz *et al.*, 1989). Therefore, factors other than an opportunistic colonization of the colon with *C. difficile* must be implicated in many cases of antibiotic-associated diarrhoea (AAD).

Oral administration of certain antibiotics reduces the faecal concentrations of short-chain fatty acids (SCFA) in healthy subjects (Heimdahl & Nord, 1982; Høverstad *et al.*, 1986*a,b*) and clindamycin decreases the bacterial fermentation *in vitro* and increases the residual carbohydrate content of the culture fluid (Edwards, Duerden & Read, 1986). Compared with the ingestion of lactulose alone, the faecal volume, frequency, and carbohydrate excretion increase during the combined administration of lactulose and ampicillin, possibly because of an impaired ability of the colonic flora to ferment carbohydrate, as indicated by a reduction in the breath hydrogen response to lactulose ingestion (Rao *et al.*, 1988). These results, and the increasing awareness of the importance of the bacterial metabolism of carbohydrates

Table 25.1. *Faecal concentrations of short-chain fatty acids (SCFA), L- and D-lactate (L-L and D-L), pH, carbohydrates (CHO),* Clostridium difficile *(CD) and production rates in faecal homogenates of 'endogenous' and 'glucose-stimulated' SCFA ($SCFA_e$ and $SCFA_g$) and L- and D-lactate ($L\text{-}L_g$ and $D\text{-}L_g$) in untreated control subjects, patients with antibiotic-associated diarrhoea (AAD) and patients without diarrhoea treated with the different antibiotics shown*

	n	Total SCFA (mM)	SCFA (% of total) C_2	C_3	C_4	iC_4–C_6	L-L (mM)	D-L (mM)	pH	CHO	Cd	$SCFA_e$ (mmol/h)	$SCFA_g$ (mmol/h)	$L\text{-}L_g$ (mmol/h)	$D\text{-}L_g$ (mmol/h)
Controls	17	60 ± 4	60 ± 6	19 ± 1	11 ± 1	10 ± 1	3 ± 0	4 ± 1	7.1 ± 0.1	3/17	$1^c/17$	12 ± 2	61 ± 7	17 ± 3	15 ± 2
AAD	7	22 ± 4^a	67 ± 5	17 ± 3	11 ± 3	5 ± 1	2 ± 1	2 ± 1	7.1 ± 0.1	0/7	0/7	5 ± 2^b	19 ± 6^a	2 ± 1^a	2 ± 1^a
Penicillin	10	70 ± 4	58 ± 3	21 ± 2	12 ± 1	9 ± 1	2 ± 1	3 ± 1	6.8 ± 0.1^a	1/10	0/10	10 ± 1	87 ± 11^a	21 ± 5	13 ± 3
Pivampicillin	7	67 ± 3	58 ± 2	25 ± 3	10 ± 1	8 ± 1	2 ± 0	3 ± 0	6.9 ± 0.1	2/7	$1^c/7$	15 ± 3	42 ± 5	12 ± 4	8 ± 2^b
Dicloxacillin	10	27 ± 3^a	54 ± 3	34 ± 4^a	5 ± 2^a	7 ± 1	4 ± 1	3 ± 1	7.2 ± 0.1	0/10	1/10	9 ± 1	15 ± 3^a	4 ± 2^a	5 ± 2^a
Erythromycin	8	38 ± 3^a	65 ± 6	16 ± 4	11 ± 2	9 ± 2	2 ± 1	2 ± 1	7.5 ± 0.1^a	0/8	0/8	10 ± 1	34 ± 5^b	3 ± 2^a	4 ± 1^a
IV combination	9	19 ± 2^a	74 ± 7^b	16 ± 4	5 ± 2^a	5 ± 2	4 ± 1	4 ± 1	7.0 ± 0.1	0/9	$1^c/9$	4 ± 1^a	9 ± 5^a	10 ± 4	5 ± 2^a
p (ANOVA)		10^{-4}	0.03	10^{-3}	0.01	ns	ns	ns	10^{-4}			10^{-3}	10^{-5}	10^{-3}	10^{-3}

C_2, acetate; C_3, propionate; C_4, butyrate; iC_4–C_6, isobutyrate, valerate, isovalerate, hexanoate; IV combination, intravenous ampicillin, netilmicin and metronidazole; ANOVA, one-way analysis of variance. Least significant difference compared with untreated controls: $^a p < 0.01$; $^b p < 0.05$; ^{c}cytotoxin-positive.

for colonic function, have lead to the hypothesis that AAD may be caused by a reduced degradation of carbohydrates, leading to an accumulation of osmotically active saccharides in the colon.

Table 25.1 illustrates the faecal concentrations of SCFA and lactate, and the production rates of these organic acids in faecal homogenates from 68 inpatients recruited prospectively (Clausen *et al*., 1991*b*). Seventeen of these patients did not receive any antimicrobial therapy and served as untreated control subjects . Forty-four patients without diarrhoea were treated orally with either penicillin ($n = 10$), pivampicillin ($n = 7$), dicloxacillin ($n = 10$), or erythromycin ($n = 8$), or intravenously with ampicillin, netilmicin and metronidazole in combination ($n = 9$). These patients served as treated control subjects. Seven patients had AAD and were treated orally with pivampicillin ($n = 2$), dicloxacillin ($n = 1$), and erythromycin ($n = 2$), and intravenously with ampicillin and netilmicin in combination ($n = 2$). Freshly passed faeces were collected within half an hour after defecation, homogenized, and either instantly frozen or incubated for *in vitro* determination of organic-acid formation.

Faecal concentrations of SCFA were reduced in all patients with AAD (22 mM) compared with untreated controls (60 mM). However, SCFA were also reduced in patients without diarrhoea treated with dicloxacillin (27 mM) or erythromycin (38 mM), and with ampicillin, netilmicin and metronidazole in combination (19 mM). Neither penicillin nor pivampicillin decreased the faecal concentrations of SCFA. Alterations in the relative distributions of the individual acids (ratios of SCFA) were small and only associated with few of the antimicrobial treatments (Table 25.1), and ratios of acetate, propionate and butyrate remained unchanged during AAD. Concentrations of L- and D-lactate were normal (< 5 mM) in all patients. Faecal pH was, from a clinical point of view, also normal, although statistical analysis showed that the pH was slightly decreased and increased in patients treated with penicillin and erythromycin, respectively.

Saccharides were detected in stools from three of 17 untreated controls, one of ten patients treated with penicillin and two of seven patients treated with pivampicillin, whereas stools from the rest of the investigated subjects, including those with diarrhoea, were devoid of saccharides. None of the patients with AAD were culture-positive for *C. difficile*. One of the untreated controls and three of the patients without diarrhoea had *C. difficile* in their faeces, and three of these four culture-positive subjects were furthermore cytotoxin-positive (Table 25.1).

The colonic capacity of SCFA production was assessed by measuring the 'endogenous' and the 'glucose-stimulated' production of SCFA and L- and

D-lactate in 16.6% faecal homogenates diluted with isotonic NaKCl (150 mM) or glucose (300 mM), respectively, and incubated for 6 h (Table 25.1). The endogenous SCFA formation was reduced in patients with AAD and in patients treated intravenously with ampicillin, netilmicin and metronidazole in combination, but was not influenced by oral treatment with penicillin, pivampicillin, dicloxacillin or erythromycin. Addition of glucose to the homogenates increased the production of organic acids severalfold. However, the glucose-stimulated SCFA production was reduced in patients with AAD (19 mmol/h) and in patients treated with dicloxacillin (15 mmol/h), erythromycin (34 mmol/h) and ampicillin, netilmicin and metronidazole in combination (9 mmol/h), compared with the untreated controls (61 mmol/h), In contrast, oral treatment with pencillin and pivampicillin did not decrease the glucose-stimulated production rates of SCFA. The production of the individual SCFA expressed as percentages of total SCFA production (not shown) did not reveal major differences among the investigated groups, including the production ratio of butyrate. The endogenous productions of L- and D-lactate were negligible in homogenates from all patients. However, the glucose-stimulated lactate production was considerable, but as for SCFA formation, it was clearly reduced in patients with AAD and in some of the patients treated with antibiotics without diarrhoea.

Therefore, AAD was always related to a clear reduction in colonic fermentation measured as faecal concentrations and production rates of SCFA. Conversely, AAD was never observed in antibiotic-treated patients with an unaffected bacterial metabolism, indicating that suppression of the normal colonic fermentation is important in the pathogenesis of AAD. However, the colonic fermentation was severely impaired in several patients during antimicrobial therapy without the development of diarrhoea, and both oral and intravenous administration of antibiotics were able to reduce the colonic degradation of carbohydrates. An association between AAD and the faecal recovery of *C. difficile* was not demonstrated. These results suggest that an impaired colonic fermentation is a precondition for AAD. Other unknown factors must, however, be involved as well, since a reduction in fermentation, as a sole event, did not induce diarrhoea in many patients receiving antibiotics.

Appreciable quantities of carbohydrates reach the colon every day (Cummings, 1984). This has been further emphasized by investigations showing that up to 20% of ingested starch is resistant to absorption in the small bowel (Stephen, Haddad & Phillips, 1983). The degree of carbohydrate malabsorption probably depends on both individual and dietary factors (Anderson, Levine & Levitt, 1981; Levine & Levitt, 1981; Stephen *et al.*, 1983), but in most cases the surplus in the colonic fermentative and absorptive capacity appears to be adequate to avoid diarrhoea. However, impaired fermentation induced by antimicrobial therapy in subjects who depend on a bacterial fermentative capacity near its maximum level may carry an increased risk of AAD, as the ability of the colonic flora to ferment the load of unabsorbed carbohydrate is reduced. The hypothesis that AAD may be a result of impaired fermentation leading to colonic accumulation of unmetabolized carbohydrates, which, by virtue of their osmotic activity, may retain water in the colonic lumen and induce diarrhoea, has also been suggested by other investigators (Caspary, Lembcke & Elsenhans, 1981; Saunders & Wiggins, 1981; Read, 1982; Edwards *et al.*, 1986; Rao *et al.*, 1988), but the antimicrobial therapy did not result in detectable amounts of carbohydrates in faeces, either in patients with AAD or in patients without diarrhoea. However, a reduction in the rate of colonic degradation of incoming carbohydrates may still increase the osmotic load in the more proximal parts of the colon.

A decrease in colonic sodium absorption secondary to reduced SCFA production may also be implicated in the pathogenesis of AAD, as the mucosal absorption of SCFA in the colon provides a stimulus to colonic fluid and electrolyte absorption (Argenzio, Miller & von Engelhardt, 1975; Ruppin *et al.*, 1980; Roediger & Moore, 1981). Butyrate, in particular, increases sodium absorption besides being an important energy source for the colonic mucosa, accounting for the major part of its energy needs (Roediger, 1980). Antibiotics that decrease bacterial SCFA production may consequently compromise the function of the colonic mucosa in its handling of water and electrolytes. The importance of carbohydrate fermentation and production of SCFA in maintaining normal colonic function is supported by studies indicating that a lack of luminal SCFA production may account for the undernourished colonic mucosa and diarrhoea often seen in the terminal stages of malnutrition (Roediger, 1986), starvation (Roediger, 1990) and diversion colitis (Harig *et al.*, 1989). Enteral tube feeding is associated with an increased risk of diarrhoea, and it has been hypothesized that most of the products used for enteral feeding cause 'colonic starvation', due to minimal malabsorption of carbohydrates in the small bowel, resulting in low SCFA production, malnourished colonic mucosa and low sodium and fluid absorption (Silk, 1987; Scheppach *et al.*, 1990). It is interesting that the risk of diarrhoea during tube feeding is further augmented by concomitant therapy with antibiotics (Silk, 1987; Surawicz *et al.*, 1989).

In experimental studies in rats, the association of high intraluminal content of lactate and low pH reduced water and electrolyte absorption and induced colonic mucosal damage (Saunders & Sillery, 1982). Antimicrobial therapy, even in patients with AAD, did not increase faecal lactate or decrease pH.

On the contrary, the production of lactate from glucose was reduced severalfold in patients with AAD, indicating that lactate is not involved in the pathogenesis of AAD.

In conclusion, AAD appears to be associated with a decrease in large bowel fermentation, but additional factors probably have to coexist before a diminished SCFA production leads to AAD. Individuals with either an initial low capacity of colonic carbohydrate degradation or a high pre-existing dependency on SCFA formation may be the only subjects in whom antimicrobial therapy results in AAD.

Short-chain fatty acids and colonic cancer

Epidemiological studies indicate that environmental factors underlie the wide variation in the incidence of colorectal cancer among nations, and nutritional factors seem to be important. Diets high in fat and low in fibre, characteristic of Western countries, are generally associated with a high incidence of colorectal cancer, whereas diets low in fat and high in fibre, which are common in most countries in Africa, Asia and South America, are in most cases associated with a low incidence of large-bowel cancer. Burkitt suggested that dietary fibre may protect against colorectal cancer by decreasing the colonic transit time, thereby reducing the contact between possible carcinogens and colonic epithelium, and by providing bulk to dilute any carcinogens contained within the intestinal lumen. However, the relative importance of dietary fibre in the prevention of colorectal cancer is still not clear, and the way in which fibre may contribute to a lower risk of large-bowel cancer is not known. One of several hypotheses has been that fibre may protect through its fermentation to SCFA.

Several *in vitro* experiments have shown that the rate of fermentation and production of SCFA depends on the polysaccharides fermented. It may, therefore, be possible to select dietary fibre sources and resistant starches in a way that stimulates the production of individual SCFA, e.g. butyrate. A higher colonic level of butyrate may be beneficial, as it provides energy to colonocytes, regulates the differentiation of cultured cells, and has been shown *in vitro* to inhibit tumour growth.

Butyrate and colonic cancer

Butyrate in concentrations of 0.25–5 mM causes reversible growth inhibition in a variety of mammalian tumour cells in culture (Prasad & Hsie, 1971; Macintyre *et al.*, 1972; Sandor, 1973; Helson, Lai & Young, 1974; Leder &

Leder, 1975; Altenburg, Via & Steiner, 1976; Leavitt *et al.*, 1978; Macher *et al.*, 1978; Anderson, Jokinen & Gahmberg, 1979; Chou, 1979; McIntyre & Kim, 1984; Nordenberg *et al.*, 1987; Langdon *et al.*, 1988; Pouillart *et al.*, 1991; Saito *et al.*, 1991). In contrast, the effects of the other SCFA on tissue culture systems have received much less attention. Propionate, valerate and hexanoate may cause morphology changes, induction of alkaline phosphatase activity and growth suppression in certain cell lines (Macher *et al.*, 1978; Reese *et al.*, 1985; Whitehead, Young & Bhathal, 1986; Langdon *et al.*, 1988), although compared with butyrate the effect is modest. During the last decade, studies investigating the effect of sodium butyrate on cultured human colonic adenocarcinoma cells have increased steadily. These *in vitro* studies have demonstrated that exposure to butyrate in concentration of 2–5 mM, well within the range of luminal concentrations found in the human colon, have marked effects on several human colorectal cancer cell lines, all of which are consistent with a more differentiated cell state. The changes include increased doubling times (Kim *et al.*, 1980; Tsao *et al.*, 1982; Dexter *et al.*, 1984; Whitehead *et al.*, 1986; Niles *et al.*, 1988; Foss *et al.*, 1989; Otaka, Singhal & Hakomori, 1989), altered colony-forming abilities in soft agar (Kim *et al.*, 1980; Tsao *et al.*, 1982; Dexter *et al.*, 1984; Whitehead *et al.*, 1986; Niles *et al.*, 1988), changes in morphology (Kim *et al.*, 1980; Tsao *et al.*, 1982; Augeron & Laboisse, 1984; Dexter *et al.*, 1984; Whitehead *et al.*, 1986; Gum *et al.*, 1987; Foss *et al.*, 1989; Otaka *et al.*, 1989), increased activities of certain membrane-associated and cytoplasmic enzymes (Kim *et al.*, 1980; Morita, Tsao & Kim, 1982; Tsao *et al.*, 1982; Chung *et al.*, 1985; Whitehead *et al.*, 1986; Gum *et al.*, 1987; Foss *et al.*, 1989; Otaka *et al.*, 1989; Awad, Horvath & Andersen, 1991), increased expression of carcinoembryonic antigen (Tsao *et al.*, 1982, 1983; Whitehead *et al.*, 1986; Niles *et al.*, 1988; Toribara *et al.*, 1989) and modification of other oncogene markers (Czerniak *et al.*, 1987; Foss *et al.*, 1989), and potentiation of X-ray cell killing (Arundel, Glicksman & Leith, 1985; Arundel *et al.*, 1986; Leith, 1988; Leith *et al.*, 1988). The mode of action of butyrate is still unclear. One suggested mechanism is inhibition of histone deacetylase (Boffa *et al.*, 1978; Candido, Reeves & Davie, 1978; Sealey & Chalkley, 1978; Vidali *et al.*, 1978; Cousens, Gallwitz & Alberts, 1979; Kruh, 1982), which contributes to the regulation of acetylation of histones, a post-translational modification considered to be important in gene regulation.

Knowledge of the effects of butyrate on colonic carcinogenesis *in vivo* is limited. In a study on dimethylhydrazine-treated rats, Freeman (1986) found no reduction in colonic tumour frequency by oral intake of butyrate, which is absorbed in the proximal parts of the intestine, probably not reaching the large bowel. Otaka *et al.* (1989) found that sodium butyrate encapsulated in

Table 25.2. *Concentrations (mM) and ratios (%) of short-chain fatty acids (SCFA) in gut contents from healthy individuals, and adenoma and carcinoma patients*

	Sample	n	Total SCFA (mM)	SCFA (% of total)			Reference
				C_2	C_3	C_4	
Faecal concentration							
Healthy	Faeces	32	142	54	19	11	Vernia *et al.* (1989)
Colonic adenoma[a]	Faeces	8	147	54	24	14	
Colonic cancer[a]	Faeces	20	110	63	14	14	
Healthy	Enema	35		61	16	17	Weaver *et al.* (1988)
Colonic adenoma and/or cancer[b]	Enema	18		69[f]	15	12[f]	
Healthy	**Faeces**	**16**	**91**	**65**	**16**	**12**	**Clausen** *et al.* (1991*b*)
Colonic adenoma[c]	Faeces	17	86	68	15	9	
Colonic cancer[c]	Faeces	17	115	64	16	12	
Healthy	Faeces	33	73			22	Kashtan *et al.* (1992)
Colonic adenoma[c]	Faeces	20	71			8[f]	
24-h faecal production							
Healthy	Homogenate[d]	16	120	45	25	20	Clausen *et al.* (1991*b*)
Colonic adenoma[c]	Homogenate[d]	17	118	47	26	15[f]	
Colonic cancer[c]	Homogenate[d]	17	139	49	26	15[f]	
Healthy	Homogenate[e]	16	242	53	27	15	Clausen *et al.* (1991*b*)
Colonic adenoma[c]	Homogenate[e]	17	252	53	32	10[f]	
Colonic cancer[c]	Homogenate[e]	17	302	56	31	9[f]	

C_2, acetate; C_3, propionate; C_4, butyrate. [a] Before; [b] before and after; and [c] after polypectomy or colonic resection. [d] Faecal homogenates without substrate addition; and [e] with added ispaghula husk. [f] $p < 0.05–0.01$ compared with healthy individuals.

liposomes injected intravenously to athymic mice inhibited the growth of tumours from inoculated human colonic adenocarcinoma HRT-18 or HT-29 cells. Boffa *et al.* (1992) concluded that colonic butyrate levels can be modulated by addition of wheat bran to the diet of rats and that the butyrate produced *in vivo* was linearly correlated with DNA synthesis modulated by colonocyte histone acetylation.

Based on the above-mentioned studies, it might be suggested that a role of dietary fibre is to raise the colonic levels of butyrate, thus increasing the differentiation pressure in colonic enterocytes. This theory would provide a link between dietary fibre and prevention of colonic cancer. Therefore, a diminished supply of carbohydrates for colonic fermentation, either due to the ingestion of a low-fibre diet or due to a more efficient small-intestine absorption of carbohydrates, may increase the risk of colonic neoplasia. Starch absorption has indeed been claimed to be more efficient in patients with colonic adenomas compared with controls (Thornton *et al.*, 1987), but the intestinal malabsorption of starch (evaluated by breath hydrogen excretion) was later reported to be identical in patients with colonic cancer compared with healthy controls (Nordgaard *et al.*, 1992).

Four studies have investigated faecal levels of butyrate in patients with colonic neoplasia (Table 25.2). Vernia *et al.* (1989) compared 20 patients with colorectal cancer, eight patients with colonic polyps and 32 healthy controls. No significant differences were found, although patients with rectal cancers showed slightly lower levels of propionate and butyrate than did those with more proximal cancers. Weaver *et al.* (1988) investigated SCFA distributions in enema samples from a sigmoidoscopy population and found a significantly lower ratio of butyrate to total SCFA and a higher ratio of acetate in colonic polyp/cancer patients (evaluated as one group) compared with normal subjects. Faecal concentrations of butyrate were also significantly lower in patients with previous colonic adenomas compared with controls in a study by Kashtan *et al.* (1992). The difference disappeared when the subjects were placed on a balanced diet, suggesting that the initial low values in the patients with polyps were a consequence of their dietary habits. No differences in faecal concentrations or molar ratios of SCFA were found by Clausen *et al.* (1991*a*) between healthy subjects and patients with former colonic adenomas or former colonic cancer.

An increased production of SCFA in the colonic lumen results in an almost equivalent increased absorption, and the production and absorption of SCFA are presumably more important to mucosal metabolism than the luminal concentrations, which often respond with small changes when fermentation is increased. Since production rates are difficult to measure in humans *in vivo*, an alternative approach is to use a faecal incubation system. Clausen *et al.* (1991*a*) found that the production ratio of butyrate was decreased in faecal homogenates from patients with colonic cancer and adenomas in contrast to the production ratios of other SCFA. Furthermore, the relative production of butyrate remained reduced in faeces from cancer and adenoma patients after the overall SCFA formation was increased by addition of the fibre, ispaghula husk, to homogenates. Therefore, subjects harbouring a colonic flora producing relatively small quantities of butyrate may be at greater risk of developing colonic neoplasia, and may benefit from a diet high in unabsorbable carbohydrates fermented preferably to butyrate.

pH and colonic cancer

Fermentation and production of SCFA also affects intestinal pH, especially in the caecum. Colonic secretion of bicarbonate and other buffers increases the pH in colonic contents along the large bowel, and faecal pH is usually higher and changes less than pH in the proximal parts of the colon (Bown *et al.*, 1974; Cummings *et al.*, 1987; Patil *et al.*, 1987). Epidemiological studies have shown an association between high faecal pH and cancer risk in both population and case–control studies (Macdonald, Webb & Mahony, 1978; Malhotra, 1982; Pietroiusti *et al.*, 1985; Walker, Walker & Walker, 1986). In 1981 Thornton proposed that a high colonic pH promoted, or at least facilitated, colonic bacterial degradation of primary bile acids and cholesterol to carcinogens and that intraluminal pH was influenced by the acidifying effect of dietary fibre fermentation. The hypothesis was supported by Pietroiusti *et al.* (1985), who found a significantly higher faecal pH in patients with colorectal cancer compared with healthy subjects and patients with irritable bowel syndrone (Table 25.2). Further support was drawn from a study performed by Macdonald *et al.* (1978), in which faecal pH was higher in patients with colorectal cancer than in Seventh-Day Adventists, a population at low risk for the development of large bowel cancer (Phillips, 1975). However, in a comparison of cancer patients and healthy controls, no differences in faecal pH were found (Macdonald *et al.*, 1978), and general acceptance of an association between faecal pH and risk of colonic cancer must be tempered by recently reported data. Although Vernia *et al.* (1989) and Bech *et al.* (1990) did find a higher faecal pH in patients with colorectal cancer, the faecal pH in patients with colonic polyps did not differ from that of controls. A normal faecal pH in patients with previous colonic adenomas was also found by Clausen *et al.* (1991*a*) and Kashtan *et al.* (1992). If colonic pH plays a role in the initiation or promotion of neoplastic changes in the mucosa, differences might have been expected between normal subjects and subjects with adenomas, as the adenoma–carcinoma sequence is accepted as the natural developmental pathway for most cases of colorectal cancer.

Clausen *et al.* (1991*a*) found no differences between faecal pH in normal subjects and patients with previous colonic cancer and no signs of recurrence. This was further confirmed by Hove, Clausen & Mortensen (1993) as the study was extended to preoperative patients, who were selected as patients without complaints of appetite reduction or weight loss, and in whom metastasis were absent and surgery feasible and later elective. Charalambides & Segal (1992) reported that patients with colostomies due to either trauma or colorectal cancer had similar mucosal and luminal values of pH. By use of pH-sensitive radiotelemetry capsules, Pye *et al.* (1990) measured the intestinal intraluminal pH in healthy subjects, patients with colorectal adenomas and unresected colorectal cancer and found no differences in luminal pH among these groups. Therefore, the alkaline faecal pH found in the earlier studies in patients with colorectal cancer may be secondary to the inclusion of severely ill patients with anorexia, colonic obstruction, bleeding, secretion, etc., with subsequent diminished or altered colonic fermentation. In this light, an increased faecal pH per se may not be related to an increased risk of colorectal cancer.

References

Altenburg, B. C., Via, D. P. & Steiner, S. H. (1976). Modification of the phenotype of murine sarcoma virus-transformed cells by sodium butyrate. Effects of morphology and cytoskeletal elements. *Experimental Cell Research*, **102**, 223–31.

Anderson, I. H., Levine, A. S. & Levitt, M. D. (1981). Incomplete absorption of the carbohydrate in all-purpose wheat flour. *New England Journal of Medicine*, **304**, 891–2.

Anderson, L. C., Jokinen, M. & Gahmberg, C. G. (1979). Induction of erythroid differentiation in the human leukaemia cell line K562. *Nature*, **278**, 364–5.

Argenzio, R. A., Miller, N. & von Engelhardt, W. (1975). Effect of volatile fatty acids on water and ion absorption from the goat colon. *American Journal of Physiology*, **229**, 997–1002.

Aronsson, B., Möllby, R. & Nord, C. E. (1981). Occurrence of toxin-producing *Clostridium difficile* in antibiotic-associated diarrhoea in Sweden. *Medical Microbiology and Immunology*, **170**, 27–35.

Arundel, C. M., Glicksman, A. S. & Leith, J. T. (1985). Enhancement of radiation injury in human colon tumor cells by the maturational agent sodium butyrate (NaB). *Radiation Research*, **104**, 443–8.

Arundel, C. M., Kennedy, S. M., Leith, J. T. & Glicksman, A. S. (1986). Contrasting effects of the differentiating agent sodium butyrate on recovery processes after X-irradiation in heterogeneous human colon tumor cells. *International Journal of Radiation Onocology, Biology, Physics*, **12**, 959–68.

Augeron, C. & Laboisse, C. L. (1984). Emergence of permanently differentiated cell clones in a human colonic cancer cell line in culture after treatment with sodium butyrate. *Cancer Research*, **44**, 3961–9.

Awad, A. B., Horvath, P. J. & Andersen, M. S. (1991). Influence of butyrate on lipid metabolism, survival, and differentiation of colon cancer cells. *Nutrition and Cancer*, **16**, 125–33.

Bartlett, J. G. (1979). Antibiotic-associated pseudomembranous colitis. *Reviews of Infectious Diseases*, **1**, 530–9.

Bartlett, J. G., Taylor, N. S., Chang, T. & Dzink, J. (1980). Clinical and laboratory observations in *Clostridium difficile* colitis. *American Journal of Clinical Nutrition*, **33**, 2521–6.

Bech, K., Kronborg, O., Engel, K. & Kildleberg, P. (1990). pH og aciditet i faeces ved kolorektal neoplasi. *Ugeskrift for Laeger*, **152**, 161–2.

Boffa, L. C., Lupton, J. R., Mariani, M. R., Ceppi, M., Newmark, H. L., Scalmati, A. & Lipkin, M. (1992). Modulation of colonic epithelial cell proliferation, histone acetylation, and luminal short chain fatty acids by variation of dietary fiber (wheat bran) in rats. *Cancer Research*, **52**, 5906–12.

Boffa, L. C., Vidali, G., Mann, R. S. & Allfrey, V. G. (1978). Suppression of histone deacetylation *in vivo* and *in vitro* by sodium butyrate. *Journal of Biological Chemistry*, **253**, 3364–6.

Bown, R. L., Gibson, J. A., Sladen, G. E., Hicks, B. & Dawson, A. M. (1974). Effects of lactulose and other laxatives on ileal and colonic pH as measured by a radiotelemetry device. *Gut*, **15**, 999–1004.

Candido, E. P. M., Reeves, R. & Davie, J. R. (1978). Sodium butyrate inhibits histone deacetylation in cultured cells. *Cell*, **14**, 105–13.

Caspary, W. F., Lembcke, B. & Elsenhans, B. (1981). Bacterial fermentation of carbohydrates within the gastrointestinal tract. *Clinical Research Reviews*, **1** (Suppl. 1), 107–17.

Charalambides, D. & Segal, I. (1992). Colonic pH: a comparison between patients with colostomies due to trauma and colorectal cancer. *American Journal of Gastroenterology*, **87**, 74–8.

Chou, J. Y. (1979). Regulation of the induction of alkaline phosphatase in choriocarcinoma cells by sodium butyrate. *In Vitro*, **15**, 789–95.

Chung, Y. S., Song, I. S., Erickson, R. H., Sleisinger, M. H. & Kim, Y. S. (1985). Effect of growth and sodium butyrate on brush border membrane-associated hydrolases in human colorectal cancer cell lines. *Cancer Research*, **45**, 2976–82.

Clausen, M. R., Bonnen, H. & Mortensen, P. B. (1991*a*). Colonic fermentation of dietary fibre to short chain fatty acids in patients with adenomatous polyps and colonic cancer. *Gut*, **32**, 923–8.

Clausen, M. R., Bonnen, H., Tvede, M. & Mortensen, P. B. (1991*b*). Colonic fermentation to short-chain fatty acids is decreased in antibiotic-associated diarrhoea. *Gastroenterology*, **101**, 1497–504.

Cousens, L. S., Gallwitz, D. & Alberts, B. M. (1979). Different accessibilities in chromatin to histone acetylase. *Journal of Biological Chemistry*, **254**, 1716–23.

Cummings, J. H. (1984). Colonic absorption: the importance of short chain fatty acids in man, *Scandinavian Journal of Gastroenterology*, **93**, (Suppl.), 89–99.

Cummings, J. H., Pomare, E. W., Branch, W. J., Naylor, C. P. E. & Macfarlane, G. T. (1987). Short chain fatty acids in the human large intestine, portal, hepatic and venous blood. *Gut*, **28**, 1221–7.

Czerniak, B., Herz, F., Wersto, R. P. & Koss, L. G. (1987). Modification of Ha-*ras* oncogene p21 expression and cell cycle progression in the human colonic cancer cell line HT-29. *Cancer Research*, **47**, 2826–30.

Dexter, D. L., Lev, R., McKendall, G. R., Mitchell, P. & Calabres, P. (1984). Sodium butyrate-induced alteration of growth properties and glycogen levels in cultured human colon carcinoma cells. *Histochemical Journal*, **16**, 137–49.

Edwards, C. A., Duerden, B. I. & Read, N. W. (1986). The effect of clindamycin on the ability of a continuous culture of colonic bacteria to ferment carbohydrate. *Gut*, **27**, 411–17.

Foss, F. M., Veilette, A., Sartor, O., Rosen, N. & Bolen, J. B. (1989). Alterations in the expression of $pp60^{c\text{-}src}$ and $p56^{lck}$ associated with butyrate-induced differentiation of human colon carcinoma cells. *Oncogene Research*, **5**, 13–23.

Freeman, H. J. (1986). Effects of differing concentrations of sodium butyrate on 1,2-dimethylhydrazine-induced rat intestinal neoplasia. *Gastroenterology*, **91**, 596–602.

George, W. L., Rolfe, R. D. & Finegold, S. M. (1982). *Clostridium difficile* and its cytotoxin in feces of patients with antimicrobial agent-associated diarrhea and miscellaneous conditions. *Journal of Clinical Microbiology*, **15**, 1049–53.

George, W. L., Sutter, V. L. & Finegold, S. M. (1978). Toxigenicity and antimicrobial susceptibility of *Clostridium difficile*, a cause of antimicrobial agent-associated colitis. *Current Microbiology*, **1**, 55–8.

Gum, J. R., Kam, W. K., Byrd, J. C., Hicks, J. W., Sleisinger, M. H. & Kim, Y. S. (1987). Effects of sodium butyrate on human colonic adenocarcinoma cells. Induction of placental-like alkaline phosphatase. *Journal of Biological Chemistry*, **262**, 1092–7.

Hall, I. C. & O'Toole, E. (1935). Intestinal flora in new-born infants with a description of a new pathogenic anaerobe, *Bacillus difficilis*. *American Journal of Diseases of Children*, **49**, 390–402.

Harig, J. M., Soergel, K. H., Komorowski, R. A. & Wood, C. M. (1989). Treatment of diversion colitis with short-chain fatty acid irrigation. *New England Journal of Medicine*, **320**, 23–8.

Heimdahl, A. & Nord, C. E. (1982). Effect of erythromycin and clindamycin on the indigenous human anaerobic flora and new colonization of the gastrointestinal tract. *European Journal of Clinical Microbiology*, **1**, 38–48.

Helson, L., Lai, K. & Young, C. W. (1974). Papaverine-induced changes in cultured human melanoma cells. *Biochemical Pharmacology*, **23**, 2917–20.

Hove, H., Clausen, M. R. & Mortensen, P. B. (1993). Lactate and pH in faeces from patients with colonic adenomas or cancer. *Gut*, **34**, 625–9.

Hoverstad, T., Carlstedt-Duke, B., Lingaas, E., Midtvedt, T., Norin, K. E., Saxerholt, H. & Steinbakk, M. (1986*a*). Influence of ampicillin, clindamycin, and metronidazole on faecal excretion of short-chain fatty acids in healthy subjects. *Scandinavian Journal of Gastroenterology*, **21**, 621–6.

Hoverstad, T., Carlstedt-Duke, B., Lingaas, E., Norin, E., Saxerholt, H., Steinbakk, M. & Midtvedt, T. (1986*b*). Influence of oral intake of seven different antibiotics on faecal short-chain fatty acid excretion in healthy subjects. *Scandinavian Journal of Gastroenterology*, **21**, 997–1003.

Kashtan, H., Stern, H. S., Jenkins, D. J. A., Jenkins, A. L., Thompson, L. U., Kay, K., Marcon, N., Minkin, S. & Bruce, W. R. (1992). Colonic fermentation and markers of colorectal-cancer risk. *American Journal of Clinical Nutrition*, **55**, 723–8.

Kim, Y. S., Tsao, D., Siddiqui, B., Whitehead, J. S., Arnstein, P., Bennett, J. & Hicks, J. (1980). Effects of sodium butyrate and dimethylsulfoxide on biochemical properties of human colon cancer cells. *Cancer*, **45**, 1185–92.

Kruh, J. (1982). Effects of sodium butyrate, a new pharmacological agent, on cells in culture. *Molecular and Cellular Biochemistry*, **42**, 65–82.

Langdon, S. P., Hawkes, M. M., Hay, F. G., Lawrie, S. S., Schol, D. J., Hilgers, J., Leonard, R. C. F. & Smyth, J. F. (1988). Effect of sodium butyrate and other differentiation inducers on poorly differentiated human ovarian adenocarcinoma cell lines. *Cancer Research*, **48**, 6161–5.

Larson, H. E., Price, A. B., Honour, P. & Borriello, S. P. (1978). *Clostridium difficile* and the aetiology of pseudomembranous colitis. *Lancet*, **1**, 1063–6.

Leavitt, J., Barrett, J. C., Crawford, B. D. & Ts'o, P. O. P. (1978). Butyric acid suppression of the *in vitro* neoplastic state of Syrian hamster cells. *Nature*, **271**, 262–5.

Leder, A. & Leder, P. (1975). Butyric acid, a potent inducer of erythroid differentiation in cultural erythroleukemic cells. *Cell*, **5**, 319–22.

Leith, J. T. (1988). Potentiation of X-ray sensitivity by combinations of sodium butyrate and buthionine sulfoximine. *International Journal of Radiation Oncology, Biology, Physics*, **15**, 949–51.

Leith, J. T., Hallows, K. T., Arundel, C. M. & Bliven, S. F. (1988). Changes in X-ray sensitivity and glutathione content of human colon tumor cells after exposure to the differentiation-induced agent sodium butyrate. *Radiation Research*, **114**, 579–88.

Levine, A. S. & Levitt, M. D. (1981). Malabsorption of starch moiety of oats, corn and potatoes (abstract). *Gastroenterology*, **80**, 1209.

Lishman, A. H., Al-Jumaili, I. J. & Record, C. O. (1981). Spectrum of antibiotic-associated diarrhoea. *Gut*, **22**, 34–7.

Macdonald, I. A., Webb, G. R. & Mahony, D. E. (1978). Fecal hydroxysteroid dehydrogenase activities in vegetarian Seventh Day Adventists, control subjects, and bowel cancer patients. *American Journal of Clinical Nutrition*, **31**, S233–S238.

Macher, B. A., Lockney, M., Moskai, J. R., Fung, Y. K. & Sweeley, C. C. (1978). Studies on the mechanism of butyrate-induced morphological changes in KB cells. *Experimental Cell Research*, **117**, 95–102.

Macintyre, E. H., Wintersgill, C. J., Perkins, J. P. & Vatter, A. E. (1972). The responses in culture of human tumour astrocytes and neuroblasts to N^6, $O^{2'}$- dibutyryl adenosine 3',5'-monophosphoric acid. *Journal of Cell Science*, **11**, 639–67.

Malhotra, S. L. (1982). Faecal urobilinogen levels and pH of stools in population groups with different incidence of cancer of the colon, and their possible role in its aetiology. *Journal of the Royal Society of Medicine*, **75**, 709–14.

McIntyre, L. J. & Kim, Y. S. (1984). Effect of sodium butyrate and dimethyl sulfoxide on human pancreatic tumor cell lines. *European Journal of Cancer and Clinical Oncology*, **20**, 265–71.

Morita, A., Tsao, D. & Kim, Y. S. (1982). Effect of sodium butyrate on alkaline phosphatase in HRT-18, a human rectal cancer cell line. *Cancer Research*, **42**, 4540–5.

Neu, H. C., Prince, A., Neu, C. O. & Garvey, G. J. (1977). Incidence of diarrhea associated with clindamycin therapy. *Journal of Infectious Diseases*, **135** (Suppl.), S120–S125.

Niles, R. M., Wilhelm, S. A., Thomas, P. & Zamcheck, N. (1988). The effect of sodium butyrate and retinoic acid on growth and CEA production in a series of human colorectal tumor cell lines representing different states of differentiation. *Cancer Investigation*, **6**, 39–45.

Nordenberg, J., Wasserman, L., Peled, A., Malik, Z., Stenzel, K. H. & Novogrodsky, A. (1987). Biochemical and ultrastructural alterations accompany the anti-proliferative effect of butyrate on melanoma cells. *British Journal of Cancer*, **55**, 493–7.

Nordgaard, I., Rumessen, J. J., Damgaard Nielsen, Aa. & Gudmand-Hoyer, E. (1992). Absorption of wheat starch in patients resected for left-sided colonic cancer. *Scandinavian Journal of Gastroenterology*, **27**, 632–4.

Otaka, M., Singhal, A. & Hakomori, S. (1989). Antibody-mediated targeting of differentiation inducers to tumor cells: inhibition of colonic cancer cell growth *in vitro* and *in vivo*. A preliminary note. *Biochemical and Biophysical Research Communications*, **158**, 202–8.

Patil, D. H., Westaby, D., Mahida, Y. R., Palmer, K. R., Rees, R., Clark, M. L., Dawson, A. M. & Silk, D. B. A. (1987). Comparative modes of action of lactitol and lactulose in the treatment of hepatic encephalopathy. *Gut*, **28**, 255–9.

Phillips, R. L. (1975). Role of life-style and dietary habits in risk of cancer among Seventh-Day Adventists. *Cancer Research*, **35**, 3513–22.

Pietroiusti, A., Caprilli, R., Giuliano, M., Serrano, S. & Vita, S. (1985). Faecal pH in colorectal cancer. *Italian Journal of Gastroenterology*, **17**, 88–91.

Pouillart, P., Cerutti, I., Ronco, G., Villa, P. & Chany, C. (1991). Butyric monosaccharide ester-induced cell differentiation and anti-tumor activity in mice. Importance of their prolonged biological effect for clinical applications in cancer therapy. *International Journal of Cancer*, **49**, 89–95.

Prasad, K. N. & Hsie, A. W. (1971). Morphologic differentiation of mouse neuroblastoma cells induced *in vitro* by dibutyryl adenosine 3′,5′-cyclic monophosphate. *Nature New Biology*, **233**, 141–2.

Pye, G., Evans, D. F., Ledingham, S. & Hardcastle, J. D. (1990). Gastrointestinal intraluminal pH in normal subjects and those with colorectal adenoma or carcinoma, *Gut*, **31**, 1355–7.

Rao, S. S. C., Edwards, C. A., Austen, C. J., Bruce, C. & Read, N. W. (1988). Impaired colonic fermentation of carbohydrate after ampicillin. *Gastroenterology*, **94**, 928–32.

Read, N. W. (1982). Diarrhoea: the failure of colonic salvage. *Lancet*, **2**, 481–3.

Reese, D. H., Gratzner, H. G., Block, N. L. & Politano, V. A. (1985). Control of growth, morphology, and alkaline phosphatase activity by butyrate and related short-chain fatty acids in the retinoid-responsive 9-1C rat prostatic adenocarcinoma cell. *Cancer Research*, **45**, 2308–13.

Roediger, W. E. W. (1980). Role of anaerobic bacteria in the metabolic welfare of the colonic mucosa in man. *Gut*, **21**, 793–8.

Roediger, W. E. W. (1986). Metabolic basis of starvation diarrhoea: implications for treatment. *Lancet*, **1**, 1082–4.

Roediger, W. E. W. (1990). The starved colon – diminished mucosal nutrition, diminished absorption, and colitis. *Diseases of the Colon and Rectum*, **33**, 858–62.

Roediger, W. E. W. & Moore, A. (1981). The effect of short-chain fatty acids on sodium absorption in the isolated human colon perfused through the vascular bed. *Digestive Diseases and Sciences*, **26**, 100–6.

Ruppin, H., Bar-Meir, S., Soergel, K. H., Wood, C. M. & Schmitt, M. G. (1980). Absorption of short-chain fatty acids by the colon. *Gastroenterology*, **78**, 1500–7.

Saito, H., Morizane, T., Watanabe, T., Kagawa, T., Miyaguchi, S., Kumagai, N. & Tsuchiya, M. (1991). Differentiating effect of sodium butyrate on human hepatoma cell lines PLC/PRF/5, HCC-M and HCC-T. *International Journal of Cancer*, **48**, 291–6.

Sandor, R. (1973). Inhibition of human rhabdomyosarcoma-cell growth in agar by dibutyryl cyclic AMP. *Journal of the National Cancer Institute*, **51**, 257–60.

Saunders, D. R. & Sillery, J. (1982). Effect of lactate and H^+ on structure and function of rat intestine. Implications for the pathogenesis of fermentative diarrhea. *Digestive Diseases and Sciences*, **27**, 33–41.

Saunders, D. R. & Wiggins, H. S. (1981). Conservation of mannitol, lactulose, and raffinose by the human colon. *American Journal of Physiology*, **241**, G397–G402.

Scheppach, W., Burghardt, W., Bartram, P. & Kasper, H. (1990). Addition of dietary fiber to liquid formula diets: the pros and cons. *Journal of Parenteral and Enteral Nutrition*, **14**, 204–9.

Sealy, L. & Chalkley, R. (1978). The effect of sodium butyrate on histone modification. *Cell*, **14**, 115–21.

Silk, D. B. A. (1987). Towards the optimization of enteral nutrition. *Clinical Nutrition*, **6**, 61–74.

Snyder, M. L. (1940). The normal fecal flora of infants between two weeks and one year of age. *Journal of Infectious Diseases*, **66**, 1–16.

Stephen, A. M., Haddad, A. C. & Phillips, S. F. (1983). Passage of carbohydrate into the colon. Direct measurements in humans. *Gastroenterology*, **85**, 589–95.

Surawicz, C. M., Elmer, G. W., Speelman, P., McFarland, L. V., Chinn, J. & van Belle, G. (1989). Prevention of antibiotic-associated diarrhea by *Saccharomyces boulardii*: a prospective study. *Gastroenterology*, **96**, 981–8.

Thornton, J. R. (1981). High colonic pH promotes colorectal cancer. *Lancet*, **1**, 1081–2.

Thornton, J. R., Dryden, A., Kelleher, J. & Losowsky, M. S. (1987). Super-efficient starch absorption – a risk factor for colonic neoplasia? *Digestive Diseases and Sciences*, **32**, 1088–91.

Toribara, N. W., Sack, T. L., Gum. J. R., Ho, S. B., Shively, J. E., Willson, J. K. V. & Kim, Y. S. (1989). Heterogeneity in the induction and expression of carcinoembryogenic antigen-related antigens in human colon cancer cell lines. *Cancer Research*, **49**, 3321–7.

Tsao, D., Morita, A., Bella, A., Luu, P. & Kim, Y. S. (1982). Differential effects of sodium butyrate, dimethyl sulfoxide, and retinoic acid on membrane-associated antigen, enzymes, and glycoproteins of human rectal adenocarcinoma cells. *Cancer Research*, **42**, 1052–8.

Tsao, D., Shi, Z. R., Wong, A. & Kim, Y. S. (1983). Effect of sodium butyrate on carcinoembryonic antigen production by human colonic adenocarcinoma cells in culture. *Cancer Research*, **43**, 1217–22.

Vernia, P., Ciarniello, P., Cittadini, M., Lorenzotti, A., Alessandrini, A. & Caprilli, R. (1989). Stool pH and SCFA in colorectal cancer and polyps. *Gastroenterology*, **96**, A528.

Vidali, G., Boffa, L. C., Bradbury, E. M. & Allfrey, V. G. (1978). Butyrate suppression of histone deacetylation leads to accumulation of multiacetylated forms of histones H3 and H4 and increased DNase I sensitivity of the associated DNA sequences. *Proceedings of the National Academy of Sciences of the USA*, **75**, 2239–43.

Viscidi, R., Willey, S. & Bartlett, J. G. (1981). Isolation rates and toxigenic potential of *Clostridium difficile* isolates from various patient populations. *Gastoenterology*, **81**, 5–9.

Viteri, A. L., Howard, P. H. & Dyck, W. P. (1974). The spectrum of lincomycin-clindamycin colitis. *Gastroenterology*, **66**, 1137–44.

Walker, A. R. P., Walker, B. F. & Walker, A. J. (1986). Fecal pH, dietary fibre intake, and proneness to colon in four South African populations. *British Journal of Cancer*, **53**, 489–95.

Weaver, G. A., Krause, J. A., Miller, T. L. & Wolin, M. J. (1988). Short chain fatty acid, distributions of enema samples from a sigmoidoscopy population: an association of high acetate and low butyrate ratios with adenomatous polyps and colon cancer. *Gut*, **29**, 1539–43.

Whitehead, R. H., Young, G. P. & Bhathal, P. S. (1986). Effects of short chain fatty acids on a new human colon carcinoma cell line (LIM1215). *Gut*, **27**, 1457–63.

26

In vivo and *in vitro* effects of short-chain fatty acids on intestinal blood circulation

F. V. MORTENSEN AND H. NIELSEN

General concepts

Intestinal blood flow is under both extrinsic and intrinsic regulation. Extrinsic regulation is mostly maintained by parasympathetic and sympathetic nerves. Parasympathetic nerve stimulation produces vasodilatation and sympathetic nerve stimulation produces vasoconstriction. Intrinsic vascular control is mainly exerted by metabolic and myogenic mechanisms. Metabolic vascular control is exerted by the vasodilator action of tissue metabolites, whereas myogenic control is triggered by transmural pressure stimuli on the smooth muscle. Instillation of nutrients, including short-chain fatty acids (SCFA), in the intestinal lumen has been reported to improve the blood flow autoregulatory capacity (Kvietys & Granger, 1981). SCFA, acetic, propionic and butyric acid have been shown to be trophic to the mucosa of the small and large intestine (Koruda *et al.*, 1988, 1990; Kripke *et al.*, 1989). This effect can be demonstrated even after intravenous administration in totally parenterally fed rats and in amounts that make it impossible to explain their action as due to caloric supplementation. The mechanism by which SCFA are trophic to the intestinal mucosa remains unclear. One possibility concerns the stimulatory effects of these compounds on the microcirculation in the small and large intestine. These considerations prompted us to examine whether SCFA have relaxant effects on isolated resistance arteries from the human small and large intestines. The reason that we chose to examine resistance arteries is related to the fact that these vessels are the main regulators of blood flow to an organ. We also examined the *in vivo* effects of SCFA on the microcirculation in the human rectum after Hartmann's procedure.

Methods

Patients undergoing surgery for carcinoma of the rectum and patients who had undergone a restorative proctocolectomy with ileal reservoir because of ulcerative colitis served as artery donors. Small pieces of large- or small-intestinal bowel wall (2 × 3 cm) were isolated immediately after resection of the affected segment and placed in cold physiological salt solution. Within 1 h, small arteries (normalized internal diameters approximately 200 μm) were dissected out from each biopsy under the microscope and mounted as ring segments (approximately 2 mm long) in a microvascular myograph capable of measuring isometric tension development (Mulvany & Halpern, 1976). After equilibration for approximately 1 h at 37 °C, the arteries were set to a normalized internal circumference L_1, estimated to be 0.9 times the circumference they would maintain if relaxed and exposed to a transmural pressure of 13.3 kPa (100 mmHg). At L_1, the contraction produced was close to maximal. The effective active pressure (P) was calculated using the law of Laplace (Mulvany & Halpern, 1977):

$$P = (\pi \times F)/(a \times L)$$

where F is the force produced, a is the segment length, and L is the internal circumference.

The arteries were precontracted with K50 (physiological salt solution with 50 mM KCl substituted for NaCl on an equimolar basis), and tested for possible relaxant effects of acetate, propionate, butyrate and the three compounds in mixture according to the proportions of Sakata and Engelhardt (1983).

Six patients who had undergone Hartmann's procedure for perforated diverticulitus were included in a study where we examined *in vivo* micro-circulatory effects of SCFA. Colon continuity was restored after a priod of 4–11 months. For a period of 10–14 days before restoration of bowel continuity, 100 ml SCFA (150 mM) in the proportions described by Sakata and Engelhardt (1983), were installed into the rectum twice daily. Rectal mucosal blood flow was measured by a laser Doppler flow technique with a differential detector system (Periflux, Perimed, Stockholm, Sweden) (Ahn, Lindhagen & Lundgren, 1986). A probe was placed on the rectal mucosa through a proctoscope. Measurements were made on the anterior and posterior wall approximately 10 cm from the linea dentata. A minimum of 4 h had elapsed between the last instillation of SCFA and the taking of the measurements.

Results

The sodium salts of the SCFA dilated the colonic resistance arteries in a concentration-dependent manner after precontraction with K50, as did a

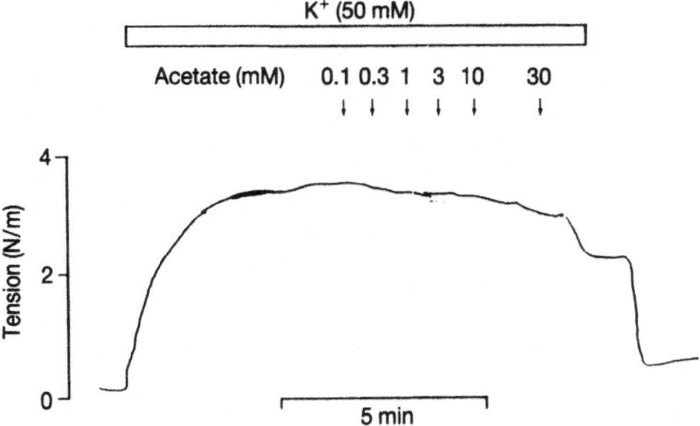

Fig. 26.1. Vasodilatation produced by acetate in a human colonic resistance artery (internal diameter 218 μm) precontracted with 50 mM KCl. Acetate was added cumulatively as indicated.

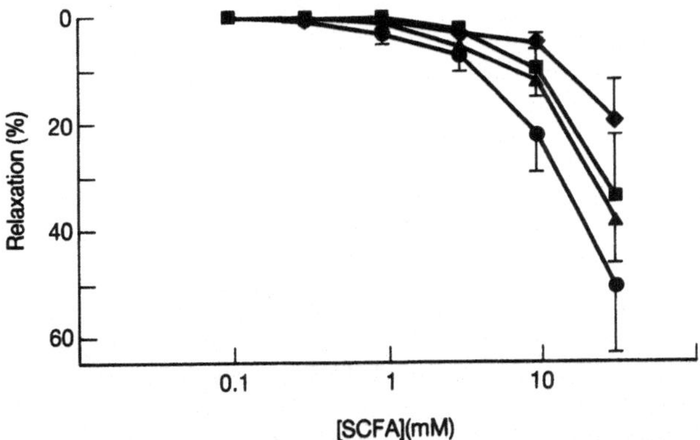

Fig. 26.2. Effects of SCFA on human colonic resistance already contracted with 50 mM KCl: triangles, acetate; squares, propionate; diamonds, butyrate; circles, mixtures ([acetate]:[propionate]:[butyrate] = 60:35:25) (eight arteries). Note the logarithmic division of the abscissa. Values are mean ± SEM.

mixture of acetate, propionate and butyrate in the proportions of Sakata and Engelhardt (Mortensen *et al.*, 1990; Figs. 26.1 and 26.2). The relaxation produced by acetate, propionate and butyrate was for all compounds significant at 3 mM; in mixture the relaxation was significant at 1 mM ($p < 0.05$). Mechanical removal of the endothelium or the addition of indomethacin, propranolol or phentolamine did not affect the relaxant effects of SCFA. Precontraction with vasopressin instead of K50 was also without effect on the relaxing properties of SCFA. SCFA relaxed isolated resistance

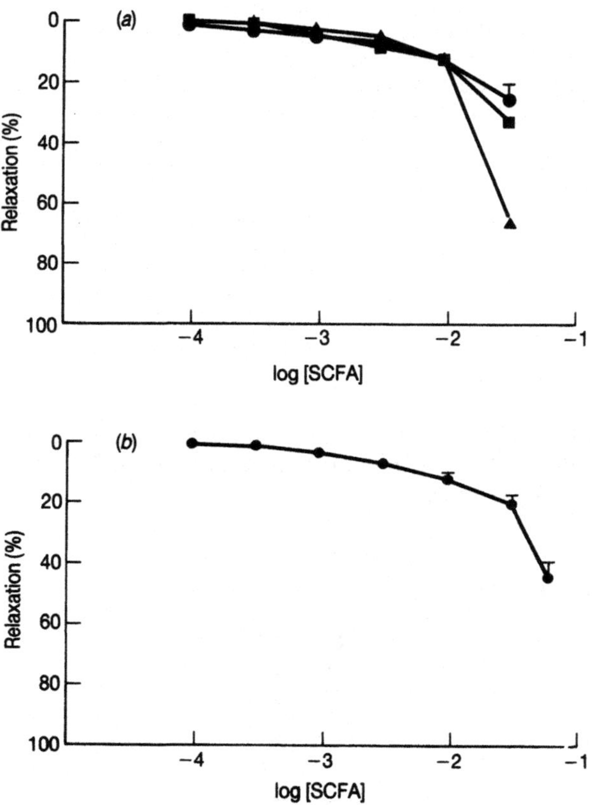

Fig. 26.3. (*a*) Effects of acetate (circles; 10 vessels), propionate (triangles; 8 vessels) or butyrate (squares; 6 vessels) alone on human resistance arteries isolated from the small intestine. (*b*) Effects of acetate, propionate and butyrate in the proportions 60:35:25 on isolated resistance arteries from the human small intestine (10 vessels). Vessels in (*a*) and (*b*) were precontracted with 50 mM KCl. Values are mean ± SEM.

arteries from the human ileum in a qualitatively and quantitatively similar way to isolated resistance arteries from the human colon (Mortensen *et al.*, 1994; Fig. 26.3). Addition of the anion transport inhibitor DIDS (200 μM) to resistance arteries from the human ileum caused a significant reduction in the relaxant properties of SCFA, both alone and in combination (Mortensen *et al.*, 1994; Fig. 26.4). Addition of 60 mM of the sodium salts of the three SCFA in the proportions noted above caused an increase in pH in the physiological salt solution of 0.08 ± 0.03. Addition of 10 mM acetate only caused minor changes in intracellular pH, indicating that this is not the mechanism by which relaxation is produced. In the same study we showed that simultaneously with acetate-induced relaxation (at 10 mM), there was a

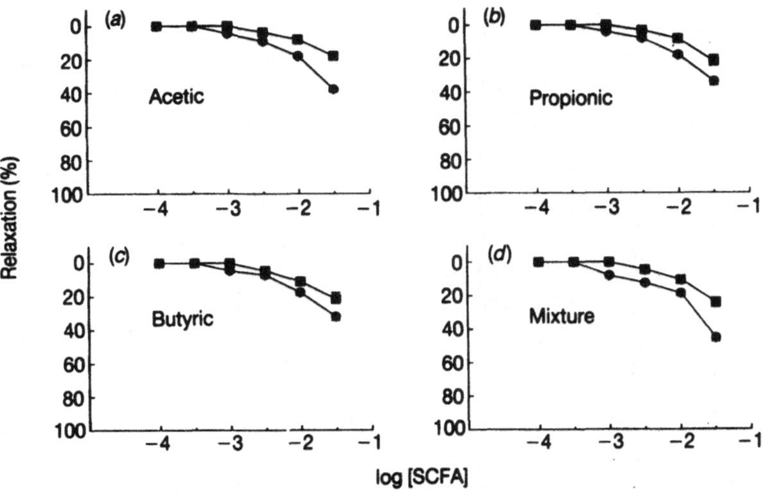

Fig. 26.4. Effects of acetate (*a*), propionate (*b*), and butyrate (*c*), both alone and in combination (*d*), on isolated resistance arteries from the human small intestine before (circles, 4 vessels) and after (squares, 4 vessels) addition of 200 μM DIDS. The vessels were precontracted with 50 mM KCl. Values are mean ± SEM.

significant fall in intracellular calcium level (C. Aalkjaer & F. V. Mortensen, unpublished data).

Instillation of SCFA into the rectum of patients who had undergone Hartmann's procedure caused a significant increase in blood flow, ranging from a 1.5-fold increase to a 5-fold increase, highest for the patients with the lowest starting values (Mortensen *et al.*, 1991; Fig. 26.5).

Discussion

The sodium salts of SCFA, both separately and in mixture, had relaxant effects on colonic resistance arteries *in vitro*. The relaxation was concentration-dependent. In mixture, the relaxation produced by SCFA was significant from 1 mM and above; separately, acetate, propionate and butyrate all produced significant relaxation from 3 mM and above (Mortensen *et al.*, 1990). There are several reasons for believing that the concentrations necessary to produce significant relaxation are reached under physiological circumstances in the environment of colonic resistance arteries. Firstly, the total concentration of SCFA in the healthy human colon ranges from 131 mmol/kg in the caecum to 80 mmol/kg in the descending colon (Cummings *et al.*, 1987), and they are readily transported across the intestinal epithelium in the colon in both ionic

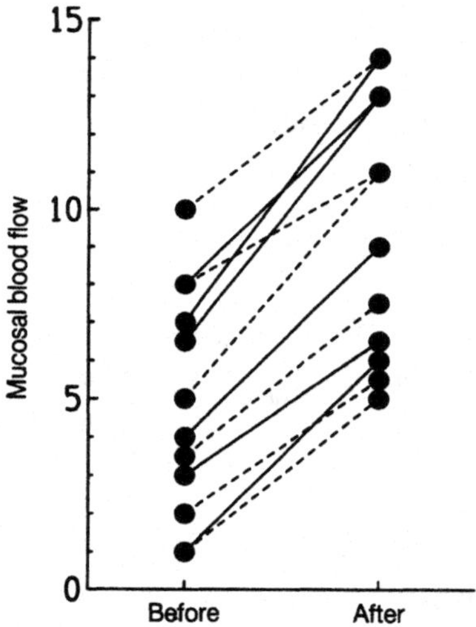

Fig. 26.5. Relative mucosal blood flow (arbitrary units) before and after a 10–14-day period with SCFA instillation into the human rectum. Dashed lines show measurements from the anterior wall, unbroken lines from the posterior wall. All patients showed an increase in mucosal blood flow, both on the anterior and posterior wall.

and non-ionic forms (Ruppin *et al.*, 1980). Concentrations in the millimolar range are therefore likely in the interstitial phase of the colonic wall. Secondly, SCFA are mainly produced in the colon (Cummings, 1981), but only a minor fraction of the portal vein emanates from this organ. Nevertheless, concentrations of SCFA of 0.4 mmol/l have been reported in the human portal vein (Cummings *et al.*, 1987), and the concentration must therefore be well above this level in the capillaries of the colonic wall and, if anything, higher in the interstitial tissue surrounding the arteries. Thus the concentrations needed to produce relaxation (Figs. 26.1, 26.2) are probably reached in the environment of the colonic resistance arteries *in vivo*.

SCFA relaxes isolated resistance arteries from the human ileum in a qualitatively and quantitatively similar way to isolated resistance arteries from the human colon (F. V. Mortensen *et al.*, unpublished data; Fig. 26.3). Under physiological conditions, SCFA could have an important effect on the microcirculation in the terminal ileum, where the number of bacteria is as high as 10^8/ml, most of these being anaerobic (Draser & Hill, 1974). These bacteria provide a solid basis for the production of SCFA by anaerobic fermentation. Autopsy of sudden-death victims has shown SCFA concentrations of 13 ± 6 mmol/kg in the terminal ileum (Cummings *et al.*, 1987). As in the colon, absorption of SCFA in the ileum is concentration-dependent in both ionic and non-ionic forms (Buguat, 1987). Concentrations of SCFA in the millimolar range in the interstitial tissue surrounding the resistance arteries in the ileal wall are possible. SCFA could be of even greater importance for the microcirculation in patients with an ileal pouch, where it is known that the bacterial flora and characteristics are more similar to those in the colon (Nasmuth *et al.*, 1989).

SCFA *in vivo* stimulated the mucosal blood flow in the rectum of patients who had undergone Hartmann's procedure (Mortensen *et al.*, 1990; Fig. 26.5). These findings are in agreement with a study on autoperfused denervated dog colon showing that SCFA after instillation in the lumen increased colonic blood flow (Kviety's & Granger, 1981). A likely explanation for this increase in mucosal blood flow after instillation of SCFA could be by a direct action on the resistance arteries, i.e. relaxation. Another explanation could be an increased blood flow secondary to increased metabolism, in that SCFA are the preferred oxidative fuel for the colonic mucosa. A third and less likely explanation is that SCFA stimulate angiogenesis in the atrophic rectum to increase the total number of capillaries. Bearing in mind that SCFA stimulated the blood flow in the denervated dog colon preparations, neural reflexes do not seem to be involved in their mechanism of action.

The relaxation produced by SCFA in the above mentioned *in vitro* studies was not due to a time-dependent loss of contractility, because compounds such as glutamine were without effect on vessel tone, both in relaxed and precontracted resistance arteries. Mechanical removal of the endothelium, the inhibition of prostaglandin production (indomethacin), propranolol (β-adrenoceptor antagonist) or phentolamine (α-adrenoceptor antagonist) did not affect the relaxing properties of the SCFA. These observations indicate that the relaxant effects of SCFA are not mediated by endothelium-derived relaxing factors, prostaglandins, α- or β-adrenoceptors. Addition of 60 mmol/l of the sodium salts of the three SCFA in the proportions of Sakata and Engelhardt only caused an increase of the pH in the physiological salt solution of 0.08 ± 0.03, making it unlikely that the vasorelaxant effects were mediated through this increase. DIDS, an anion exchange inhibitor known to inhibit the transport of HCO_3^- and Cl^- in small arteries significantly inhibited the relaxant effects of SCFA (Aalkjaer & Hughes, 1991). These results lead to the following possibilities with respect to the site of action of SCFA. One possibility is that SCFA mediate their action via a receptor on the cell surface and the binding site is DIDS-sensitive. Another possibility is that SCFA traverse the cell membrane by an anion-transport-protein system and bring about relaxation by an intracellular mechanism. The latter possibility is in agreement with a study showing that propionate transport by human ileal brush-border membrane vesicles takes place via a specific anion-exchange mechanism that also transports HCO_3^- and which is attenuated by DIDS. Addition of 10 mM acetate to the physiological salt solution only causes minor changes in intracellular pH in the resistance vessels, indicating that this is not the mechanism by which SCFA produce relaxation. In the same study we showed that simultaneously with acetate-induced relaxation (10 mM acetate) there was a major fall in free intracellular calcium (C. Aalkjaer & F. V. Mortensen, unpublished data). A decreased availability of intracellular Ca^{2+} is known to be associated with relaxation in resistance arteries (Rasmussen & Barrett, 1984).

A stimulation of the microcirculation in the intestinal wall could, at least in part, explain the trophic effect of SCFA in the small and large intestine. Such an action might also explain how SCFA, after intravenous administration in small doses, can be trophic to the intestine in rats (Koruda *et al.*, 1988, 1990).

Three processes are necessary to transfer a solute from the gastrointestinal lumen to the blood. Intestinal motility stirs the contents, allowing the solute to approach the absorptive epithelium. Diffusion and active transport conduct it through the epithelium, and capillary blood flow removes it from the site of absorption. The blood flow results in the solutes being transported to the target organs and a concentration gradient over the epithelium being maintained. SCFA stimulate gastrointestinal motility (Kamath, Philips & Zinsmeister, 1988) and they are readily transported across the intestinal epithelium throughout the gastrointestinal tract (Ruppin *et al.*, 1980; Buguat, 1987). They also relax isolated resistance arteries from the ileum and colon (Mortensen *et al.*, 1990) as they stimulate the microcirculation in the human rectum after Hartmann's procedure (Mortensen *et al.*, 1991). By these means, SCFA control their own absorption, i.e. if the concentration of SCFA increases in the gastrointestinal tract they stimulate both the motility and the circulation, thereby facilitating their own absorption. This is in agreement with a study showing that colonic capacity for SCFA absorption can increase considerably if the production increases (Rasmussen *et al.*, 1987).

In many critical clinical conditions, the welfare of the gastrointestinal tract, especially that of the mucosa is of great importance. Unfortunately, many patients suffering from one of these conditions are unable to take sufficient food orally, which in many studies has been shown to cause atrophy throughout the gastrointestinal tract. In the future, a way to maintain the intestinal mucosa in such patients could be by enteral administration of SCFA by tube or even by parenteral administration. Another future indication for therapy with SCFA could be ischaemic disorders in the gastrointestinal tract, to improve the circulation in the intestinal wall. Instillation of SCFA after colorectal anastomoses could also be of benefit in an attempt to reduce the high incidence of leakage, bearing in mind that microcirculatory failure seems to be the main determining factor in this (Taggart, 1981).

References

Aalkjaer, C. & Hughes, A. (1991). Chloride and bicarbonate transport in rat resistance arteries. *Journal of Physiology*, **436**, 57–73.

Ahn, H., Lindhagen, J. & Lundgren, O. (1986). Measurements of colonic blood flow with laser doppler flowmetry. *Scandinavian Journal of Gastroenterology*, **21**, 861–80.

Buguat, M. (1987). Occurrence, absorption and metabolism of short chain fatty acids in the digestive tract of mammals. *Comparative Biochemistry and Physiology*, **86B**, 439–72.

Cummings, J. H. (1981). Dietary fibre. *British Medical Bulletin*, **37**, 65–70.

Cummings, J. H., Pomare, E. W., Branch, W. J., Nagler, C. P. E. & Macfarlane, G. T. (1987). Short chain fatty acids in human large intestinal, portal, hepatic and venous blood. *Gut*, **28**, 1221–7.

Draser, B. S. & Hill, M. J. (1974). *Human Intestinal Flora.* London: Academic Press.

Kamath, P. S., Philips, S. F. & Zinsmeister, A. R. (1988). Short chain fatty acids stimulate ileal motility in humans. *Gastroenterology*, **95**, 1496–502.

Koruda, M. J., Rolando, H. R., Bliss, D. Z., Hastings, J. & Rombeau, J. L. (1990). Parenteral nutrition supplemented with short chain fatty acids: effects on the small-bowel mucosa in rats. *American Journal of Clinical Nutrition*, **51**, 685–9.

Koruda, M. J., Rolando, R. H., Settle, R. G., Zimmaro, D. M. & Rombeau, J. L. (1988). Effect of parenteral nutrition supplemented with short chain fatty acids on adaptation to small bowel resection. *Gastroenterology*, **95**, 715–20.

Kripke, S. A., Fox, A. D., Berman, J. M., Settle, G. R. & Rombeau, J. L. (1989). Stimulation of intestinal mucosal growth with intracolonic infusion of short chain fatty acids. *Journal of Parenteral and Enteral Nutrition*, **95**, 109–16.

Kvietys, P. R. & Granger, D. N. (1981). Effect of volatile fatty acids on blood flow and oxygen uptake by the dog colon. *Gastroenterology*, **80**, 962–9.

Mortensen, F. V., Hessov, I., Birke, H., Korsgaard, N. & Nielsen, H. (1991). Microcirculatory and trophic effects of short chain fatty acids in the human rectum after Hartmann's procedure. *British Journal of Surgery*, **78**, 1208–11.

Mortensen, F. V., Nielsen, H., Aalkjaer, C., Mulvany, M. J. & Hessov, I. (1994). Short chain fatty acids relax isolated resistance arteries from the human ileum by a mechanism dependent on anion exchange. *Pharmacology and Toxicology*, **75**, 181–5.

Mortensen, F. V., Nielsen, H., Mulvany, M. J. & Hessov, I. (1990). Short chain fatty acids dilate isolated human colonic resistance arteries. *Gut*, **31**, 1391–4.

Mulvany, M. J. & Halpern, W. (1976). Mechanical properties of vascular smooth muscle cells *in situ*. *Nature*, **260**, 617–19.

Mulvany, M. J. & Halpern, W. (1977). Contractile properties of small resistance vessels in spontaneously hypertensive and normotensive rats. *Circulation Research*, **41**, 19–26.

Nasmuth, D. G., Godwin, P. G. R., Dixon, M. F., Williams, N. S. & Johnston, D.

(1989). Ileal ecology after pouch–anal anastomosis or ileostomi. *Gastoenterology*, **96**, 817–24.

Rasmussen, H. & Barrett, R. Q. (1984). Calcium messenger system: an integrated review. *Physiological Reviews*, **64**, 938–84.

Rasmussen, H. S., Holtug, K., Andersen, J. R., Krag, E. & Mortensen, P. B. (1987). The influence of isapaghula husk and lactulose on the *in vivo* and the *in vitro* production capacity of short chain fatty acids. *Scandinavian Journal of Gastroenterology*, **22**, 406–10.

Ruppin, H., Bar-Meir, S., Soergel, K. H., Wood, G. M. & Schmitt, M. G. (1980). Absorption of short chain fatty acids by the colon. *Gastroenterology*, **78**, 1500–7.

Sakata, T. & Engelhardt, W v. (1983). Stimulatory effect of short chain fatty acids on epithelial cell proliferation in rat large intestine. *Comparative Biochemistry and Physiology*, **74A**, 459–62.

Taggart, R. E. B. (1981). Colorectal anastomosis: factors reflecting success. *Journal of the Royal Society of Medicine*, **74**, 111–18.

27

Short-chain fatty acids and intestinal surgery: rationale and clinical implications

J. L. ROMBEAU, K. J. REILLY
AND R. H. ROLANDELLI

Introduction

Colonic surgery is associated with a higher morbidity and mortality than are other gastrointestinal operations, because of infectious complications resulting, in part, from impaired anastomotic healing. The incidence and severity of infectious complications is significantly reduced by preoperative cleaning of the colon and administration of perioperative antibiotics; however, reducing the faecal mass and bacterial content of the colon has not reduced the incidence of anastomotic leakage. Short-chain fatty acids (SCFA) are normally produced by colonic bacteria and are important stimulators of colonocyte growth and absorptive function. The lack of SCFA can lead to colonic inflammation, such as diversion colitis and pseudomembranous colitis. Moreover, other types of colonic inflammation, such as ulcerative colitis, may be associated with a mucosal defect in the metabolism of SCFA (Roediger, 1990). Therefore, investigations of SCFA, as an adjuvant therapy with surgery, appear warranted in treating certain colonic diseases.

The provision of appropriate cellular nutrients is particularly important to improve wound healing in intestinal surgery, support collagen synthesis, enhance epithelial proliferation and differentiation, and improve absorptive function. Examples of nutrients that improve intestinal structure and function include glutamine for the small bowel (Souba, Smith & Wilmore, 1985) and SCFA, especially butyrate, for the colon (Roediger, 1982). Moreover, it has been hypothesized that under selected surgical conditions of intestinal dysfunction, it might be preferable to feed into the intestine those fuels, such as SCFA, that are preferentially utilized by its epithelial cells rather than provide bowel rest, which produces intestinal atrophy and hypofunction (Rolandelli *et al.*, 1986*a*). This chapter reviews the rationale and potential clinical implications for the use of SCFA in intestinal surgery.

Rationale for the provision of SCFA in intestinal surgery

The rationale for providing SCFA in intestinal (small intestine and colon) surgery is based upon their confirmed enhancement of intestinal growth and function in animal models of resection (Kripke, Fox & Berman, 1987) and in human conditions of intestinal inflammation (Scheppach *et al.*, 1992). To fully appreciate the effects of SCFA on the postoperative intestine, it is important to review the processes of growth and regeneration of the gut epithelium. The mucosa of the small intestine and colon have rapid epithelial cell turnover rates, which are dependent in part upon the incessant division of proliferating cells located deep within mucosal crypts. Rapid growth of mucosa is especially important to the intestinal anastomosis, because its strength is determined in part by the comparative rates of proliferation and exfoliation of epithelial cells. When proliferation is balanced by exfoliation of mature or senescent epithelial cells from the villous tip in the small intestine, mucosal structure is maintained at a steady state. In order for mucosal growth to occur, the rate of cell proliferation must exceed the rate of cell loss. This growth may occur when the rate of proliferation increases but the rate of loss remains constant, or when proliferation remains constant but exfoliation decreases. When cell proliferation is insufficient or cell loss increases, mucosal atrophy or hypoplasia results. In contrast, when cell production increases or cell life is prolonged, mucosal hyperplasia occurs. Thus, the rate of intestinal cell turnover determines mucosal growth, and significant alterations in these processes will result in physiological changes (Johnson, 1987). These concepts are particularly relevant to the postoperative effects of SCFA, because of their marked enhancement of postresectional epithelial proliferation in both the small bowel and colon (Kripke *et al.*, 1989).

To measure intestinal epithelial growth, an increased number of cells in the mucosa must be determined. Increased DNA synthesis, determined by measurements of tritiated thymidine or bromodeoxyuridine and DNA tissue content are used in mucosal growth analysis and are indicators of epithelial cellularity (Johnson, 1987). Other measures of proliferation include the rate of crypt cell production and the content of stem proliferative enzymes, such as ornithine decarboxylase. Postoperative infusions of SCFA enhance DNA content in the intestinal epithelium in animal models (Sakata, 1987; Kripke *et al.*, 1989), although the extent of these proliferative effects in postoperative patients is unknown.

Mechanisms by which SCFA may mediate postoperative intestinal proliferation and function are shown in Fig. 27.1. These include the following: (1) provision of energy; (2) stimulation of blood flow; (3) production of

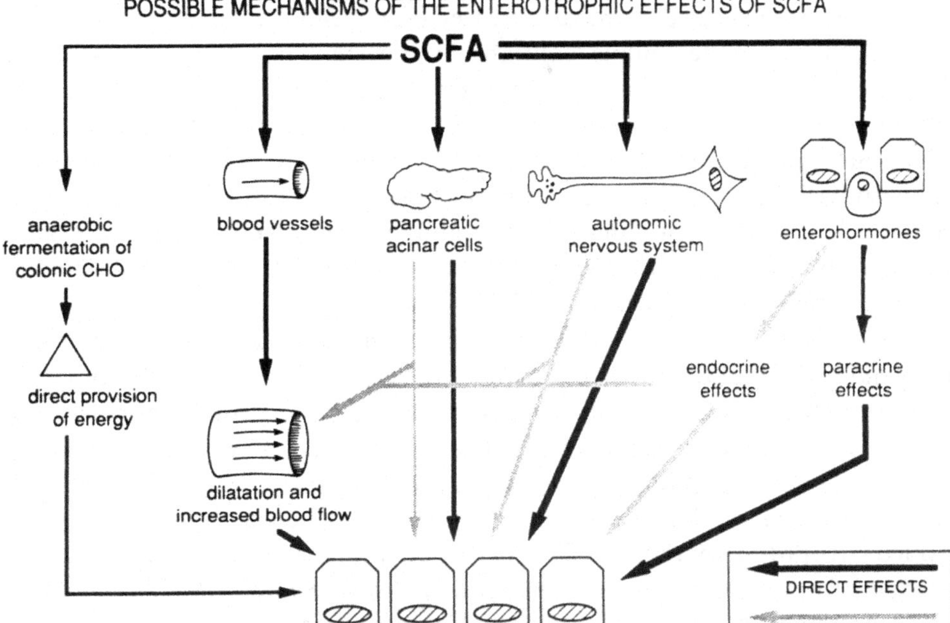

Fig. 27.1. Possible mechanisms by which short-chain fatty acids (SCFA) may mediate postoperative intestinal proliferation and function.

exocrine pancreatic secretions; (4) stimulation of the autonomic nervous system; and (5) production of enterotrophic gastrointestinal hormones.

Direct luminal contact of SCFA and local provision of energy

SCFA are produced in humans by bacterial fermentation, in the lumen of the colon, of polysaccharides such as soluble fibre and undigested starch. Luminal nutrition is defined as the presence of digestible or indigestible nutrients within the intestine. Several studies have demonstrated the importance of luminal nutrition in the maintenance of intestinal mucosal growth, especially after surgical resection (Feldman *et al.*, 1976; Ryan *et al.*, 1979; Ecknauer, Sircar & Johnson, 1981). Luminal nutrition primarily affects mucosal growth by direct physical contact rather than by indirect systematic factors. The addition of luminal nutrients, such as soluble dietary fibre, to liquid diets has been proposed as a means to increase the production of SCFA and improve postoperative proliferation of the colonic epithelium (Rolandelli *et al.*, 1986*b*). Proliferation studies with [^{3}H] thymidine show that animals on fibre-supplemented diets have increased crypt cell turnover and accelerated cell migration to the villous columns in the small intestine (Vahouny & Cassidy, 1986). Examples of soluble fibres that alter the rate of cell turnover in the small intestine and colon are pectin and guar gum. Rats fed pectin- or guar gum-supplemented diets demonstrated faster rates of intestinal epithelial cell turnover than did those fed with oat bran and fiber-free diets (Jacobs & White, 1983). In the jejunum, pectin stimulated cell proliferation more than did guar gum. Similar effects were noted in the ileum but not in the duodenum (Jacobs & White, 1983; Jacobs, 1989).

Other studies have shown that fibre ingestion is important in the maintenance and growth of the epithelial mass in the colon (Jacobs & Lupton, 1984). Low-fibre diets produce colonic atrophy as noted by mucosal hypoplasia and a decreased rate of epithelial cell renewal (Bristol & Williamson, 1988). Although other dietary components are important in sustaining colonic mucosal integrity (Cameron *et al.*, 1990), it is believed that the nutrient-induced trophism in the colon is mediated primarily by the fermentation products from dietary fibre and undigested starch (Sakata, 1987; Cummings, 1991). Whether the effects of undigested polysaccharide on colonic epithelial proliferation are primarily due to the direct provision of SCFA or are the result of indirect, systematic factors is currently being investigated.

SCFA may directly stimulate intestinal cell growth by providing energy from the anaerobic fermentation of colonic carbohydrates. The exact amount of energy produced from colonic fermentation in humans is unknown; however, it is largely dependent upon the quality and quantity of dietary carbohydrate. If undigested dietary carbohydrate is the primary substrate for colonic fermentation and 70% of the potential energy is available for absorption as SCFA, the theoretical yield in a patient ingesting a balanced diet is equivalent to about 5% of total energy requirements with a possible range (based on 20–60 g substrate fermented) of 3–9% in people consuming Western diets. A considerably higher percentage is likely in populations existing primarily on starch-based staples. This energy is targeted to the colonic epithelium, which comprises a very small percentage of the total body weight. Theoretically, SCFA could therefore provide a substantial amount of energy for the colon (Cummings, Gibson & Macfarlane, 1989).

Stimulation of intestinal blood flow

The trophic effects of SCFA on the intestinal mucosa are probably mediated in part by increased mesenteric blood flow. Infused physiological concentrations of SCFA into dog colons produced a 24% increase in mesenteric blood flow, suggesting that these substances directly dilate the colonic vasculature (Kvietys & Granger, 1981). Of the three most abundant SCFA, acetate produced a greater increase of blood flow than did either propionate or *n*-butyrate. More recently, it was demonstrated that SCFA individually and in combination produced a significant and concentration-dependent dilatation of resistant arteries in isolated human colons (Mortensen *et al.*, 1990). This vasodilatory effect suggests that SCFA may improve the colonic microcirculation *in vivo*, thus providing an explanation for their trophic effect on colonic mucosa. Such results might explain how modest doses of SCFA have trophic effects on intestinal mucosa even after parenteral administration (Koruda *et al.*, 1991).

The aforementioned studies suggest that the enterotrophic effects of SCFA may be due in part to increased blood flow to the intestinal mucosa; however, the magnitude of these effects in either the normal or the stressed state remain to be investigated. Studies are needed to determine if the vascular dilatation is caused directly by SCFA or indirectly by either production of gastrointestinal hormones or stimulation of the autonomic nervous system.

Increased production of pancreatobiliary secretions

Another possible explanation for the enterotrophic effects of SCFA is the enhanced stimulation of pancreatic exocrine secretions and bile acids. Intravenous infusion of SCFA directly stimulate pancreatic acinar secretions and enhance glucagon and insulin secretion in a dose-dependent manner in sheep (Harada & Kato, 1983; Katoh, 1991). Both pancreatic and biliary secretions stimulate intestinal growth in animal models (Altman, 1971). Moreover, pancreatic exocrine secretions stimulate mucosal proliferation in rats after bowel resections (Weser, Heller & Tawil, 1977; Al-Mukhter, Sago & Ghatei, 1983). Further studies are needed to define the association between SCFA-induced pancreatic exocrine secretions and intestinal trophism.

Stimulation of the autonomic nervous system

There is evidence for a role of the autonomic nervous system in the mediation of the enterotrophic effects of SCFA. When SCFA were perfused at a rapid rate into the colon of fasted anaesthetized rats, increases in the mitotic index and the labelling index of the large intestinal epithelial cells were noted (Sakata & Engelhardt, 1983). The acute trophic stimulation was abolished by preceding surgical vagotomy or chemical sympathectomy with guanethidine sulfate (Sakata & Engelhardt, 1983; Sakata & Yajima, 1984).

Table 27.1. *Effects of short-chain fatty acids (SCFA) and the autonomic nervous system on jejunal morphometrics. Values expressed as mean ± SEM*

	Villous height (μm)	Crypt depth (μm)	Surface area (mm^2)
Innervated			
Saline	465 ± 8	117 ± 1	0.155 ± 0.004
SCFA	564[a] ± 29	127[a] ± 4	0.204[a] ± 0.017
Denervated			
Saline	481 ± 8	117 ± 3	0.152 ± 0.008
SCFA	447 ± 18	113 ± 2	0.146 ± 0.010

[a] Innervated SCFA v. all groups, $p < 0.05$ by ANOVA and protected least significant difference. From Frankel *et al.* (1992).

The role of efferent autonomic innervation in mediation of the acute effects of SCFA was also evaluated in a subsequent study (Sakata, 1989). A segment of jejunum was transplanted under the skin with or without its mesenteric connection and the acute trophic effects of caecally infused SCFA were evaluated. SCFA infusion significantly increased the crypt cell production rate in both normally innervated and extrinsically denervated jejunal segments. These results indicate that SCFA can systemically stimulate jejunal epithelial cell proliferation in the acute setting, and this effect does not require efferent autonomic nervous connections (Sakata, 1989).

The results of the previous acute study differ from studies of chronic infusions (Frankel *et al.*, 1992), where SCFA administration for 10 days into a normally innervated caecum out of intestinal continuity produced trophic changes in the jejunum. When extrinsic denervation of the caecum was performed, the jejunotrophic effects of caecally infused SCFA were abolished (Table 27.1). Moreover, rats with denervated caeca had significantly less SCFA-mediated jejunotrophism when compared to animals with normal caecal innervation. However, in this experiment, the *afferent* innervation (i.e. from the caecum to the central nervous system) was essential for the jejunotrophic effects of caecal SCFA, while in the previous study, transection of the *efferent* pathway did not alter the trophic effects.

Another chronic infusion experiment was recently performed to determine which branch of the autonomic nervous system (i.e. the parasympathetic or the sympathetic) was important in the signalling mechanism of caecal SCFA to the jejunum (Reilly *et al.*, 1993). After surgical vagotomy, chemical sympathectomy with guanethidine, or sham operation, rats were given a caecal infusion of either SCFA or saline for 10 days. The effects of SCFA on

Table 27.2. *Effects of short-chain fatty acids (SCFA) on jejunal morphometrics in normally innervated, vagotomized and sympathectomized rats. Values expressed as mean ± SEM*

	[^{14}C]Glucose absorption (μmol/cm^2 per h)	Surface area (mm^2)	Villous height (μm)	Crypt depth (μm)	Protein (mg/cm)
Control					
Saline	1.59 ± 0.55	0.20 ± 0.01	523 ± 21	143 ± 8	2.68 ± 0.42
SCFA	4.46 ± 0.52[a]	0.25 ± 0.01[a]	589 ± 18[a]	166 ± 7	3.20 ± 0.38
Vagotomy					
Saline	2.85 ± 0.50	0.18 ± 0.01	501 ± 17	142 ± 7	2.42 ± 0.37
SCFA	2.34 ± 0.56	0.18 ± 0.01	519 ± 17	140 ± 7	2.40 ± 0.39
Sympathectomy					
Saline	2.45 ± 0.72	0.19 ± 0.01	512 ± 21	144 ± 8	1.52 ± 0.53
SCFA	3.09 ± 0.69	0.16 ± 0.01	510 ± 21	145 ± 8	1.41 ± 0.48

[a] SCFA v. saline, $p < 0.03$ by ANOVA and least significant difference.
From Reilly *et al.* (1993).

jejunal structure and function were measured at sacrifice. While both the parasympathetic and sympathetic nervous systems were important in mediating trophic effects of caecal SCFA on jejunal structure (morphometrics, protein), only disruption of the parasympathetic connections fully abolished the effects on jejunal function (glucose absorption, disaccharidase activity), as shown in Table 27.2 (Reilly *et al.*, 1993). When considered together, these findings strongly suggest that autonomic receptors play an important role in SCFA-induced regulation and proliferation of epithelial cells in the small-intestinal mucosa.

Increased production of enterotrophic gastrointestinal hormones

Stimulation of gastrointestinal hormones may be an important mechanism by which SCFA produce their enterotrophic effects. Gastrin, enteroglucagon and peptide YY (PYY) are the three hormones most often implicated in mediation of intestinal epithelial cell proliferation and growth (Goodlad *et al.*, 1983).

Gastrin is trophic to several segments of the intestinal tract. For example, gastrin stimulates epithelial cell proliferation and increases levels of DNA, RNA and protein content of duodenal, ileal and proximal colonic mucosa (Johnson, Aures & Yuen, 1969; Johnson, 1977). Removal of the antrum and its gastrin-producing G cells in animal models resulted in decreased DNA content in the colon (Dembinski & Johnson, 1979). Exogenous administration of pentagastrin caused a fivefold increase in cell number in *in vitro* studies with normal human colonic epithelial cells (Sirinek, Levin & Moyer, 1985). In further studies of cultured enterocytes, administration of gastrin increased ^{3}H-thymidine incorporation into DNA (Conteas & Majumdar, 1987).

The compensatory responses in rat gastrointestinal epithelium to starvation and their association with plasma levels of gastrin and enteroglucagon have been investigated (Goodlad *et al.*, 1983). Plasma gastrin levels increased slowly after refeeding and only correlated with crypt cell production rate in the duodenum. Plasma levels of enteroglucagon, however, rapidly returned to above control levels, and correlated positively with crypt cell production rate in several intestinal sites. These findings indicate that enteroglucagon may be important in generalized control of epithelial cell renewal (Goodlad *et al.*, 1983).

Fermentable fibre may serve as a substrate precursor for SCFA production in the postabsorptive intestine. The effects on plasma hormone levels of an elemental diet, supplemented with various types of fibre, were examined in the same starvation model (Goodlad *et al.*, 1987). Fermentable fibre stimulated colonic epithelial cell proliferation, especially in the distal colon, but mechanical bulk alone (kaolin) did not. This increased cell turnover with fermentable fibre was closely associated with increased plasma levels of enteroglucagon throughout the gastrointestinal tract, with PYY only in the colon, and there was no significant correlation with levels of plasma gastrin.

Most enteroglucagon-producing cells are present in the terminal ileum and proximal colon, although they are found throughout the gastrointestinal tract (Bloom, 1980). These cells are therefore in a good position to 'monitor' the digesta for the presence of SCFA or unabsorbed nutrients. This milieu provides a potential feedback mechanism to regulate SCFA production. Studies have shown a positive correlation between intestinal cell proliferation and plasma levels of enteroglucagon in a variety of experimental models (Sagor *et al.*, 1981).

PYY is produced mainly in the small bowel and colon in rats and humans and its receptors are localized primarily in the small bowel (Goodlad *et al.*, 1987; Calam *et al.*, 1989; Hill *et al.*, 1991). Luminal SCFA increase PYY release in an isolated perfused rabbit colon model (Longo *et al.*, 1990). The interaction of the autonomic nervous system and PYY and gastrin or jejunal trophism was recently investigated in rats receiving caecally infused SCFA (Frankel *et al.*, 1992). In rats with a normally innervated caecum, SCFA had a systemic jejunotrophic effect, which was associated with significantly

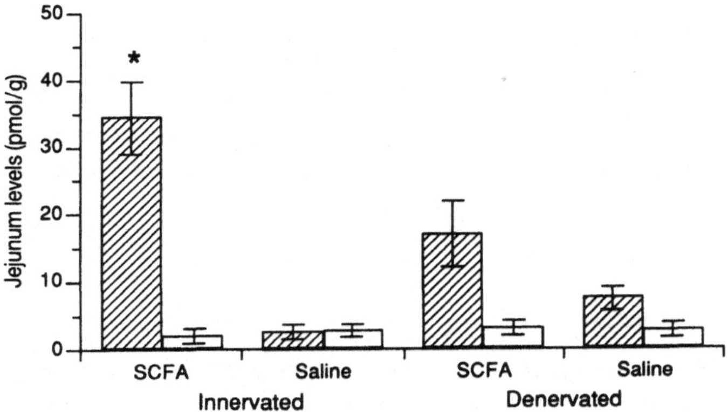

Fig. 27.2. Effects of ten days of infusion of short-chain fatty acids (SCFA) into normally innervated or surgically denervated caeca on jejunal concentrations of gastrin (hatched bars) and peptide YY (white bars). Asterisk, $p < 0.05$ between innervated and denervated caeca. From Frankel *et al.* (1992), with permission.

elevated levels of jejunal tissue gastrin (Fig. 27.2). When the caecum was denervated by transection of the nerves accompanying the mesenteric vessels, both the jejunal trophic effects and the elevated tissue gastrin levels were abolished. Jejunal PYY levels did not increase significantly with caecal SCFA infusions in either innervated or denervated rats. Studies utilizing gastrin antagonists are ongoing to clarify the relationship between SCFA-induced jejunotrophism and jejunal gastrin levels.

Summary

The mechanism(s) of action for the enterotrophic effects of SCFA are complex and probably multifactorial. The direct addition of energy to the intestinal mucosa is a moderate contributor, while the increase in blood flow may provide a slightly larger contribution to enterotrophism. Locally mediated mechanisms alone, as described previously, cannot account for the trophic effects of SCFA, because intestinal trophism occurs both locally and distantly from the site of infusion of SCFA. As noted, SCFA stimulate growth in the small intestine as well as the large bowel when infused into the colons of rats. Increased pancreatic exocrine secretions, stimulation of enterotrophic gastro-intestinal hormones and incitement of the autonomic nervous system may be additional mediators of both the local and systemic enterotrophic effects of SCFA. Defining the specific hormonal messengers and the cellular processes by which they are released are active areas of ongoing research.

Potential clinical indications – intestinal surgery

Potential indications for the use of SCFA in intestinal surgery include the following: colonic anastomosis, postcolostomy colonic diversion, caecectomy, ileal pouch–post total protocolectomy, short-bowel syndrome and total parenteral nutrition (TPN)-induced bowel rest.

Colonic anastomosis

The leakage of colonic anastomosis is associated with a twofold increase in hospital stay and a threefold increase in mortality (Koruda & Rolandelli, 1990). To reduce postoperative infectious complications, the colon is prepared with laxatives, enemas and intestinal antibiotics. These again effectively reduce the number of bacteria as well as faecal mass in the colonic lumen while depriving the colonic mucosa of SCFA.

Intraluminal SCFA increase epithelial proliferation and may facilitate anastomotic healing in patients after colonic surgery. These findings have important implications for the postoperative management of patients with colonic resections who generally are not given solid oral nutrition for several days. The effect of adding a highly fermentable fibre, such as citrus pectin, to an elemental diet as a precursor for SCFA production was investigated, to determine if the integrity and strength of the colonic anastomosis in the rat might be enhanced (Rolandelli *et al.*, 1986*b*). Transection and anastomosis in the rat was selected as a paradigm of colonic injury because of extensive validation of this model and the proximity of the anastomosis to fibre fermentation and caecal production of SCFA (Jiborn, Ahonen & Zedesfeldt, 1978; Hesp *et al.*, 1984). A feeding gastrostomy was inserted concurrently, and rats were fed continuously with either an elemental diet alone or the same elemental diet supplemented with 1% citrus pectin. Continuous feeding was used to ensure a uniform supply of substrate for bacterial fermentation in the colon. Study variables included the measurements of bursting pressure, bowel wall tension and hydroxyproline content at the anastomotic site, as well as mucosal pH. Bursting pressure was measured by infusing saline continuously into the excised anastomotic segment until leakage occurred. Bowel wall tension was determined by Laplace's equation using bursting pressure and bowel radius (Jiborn *et al.*, 1978):

$$\text{Bowel wall tension (dyne/cm)} = \text{pressure (dyne/cm}^2) \times \text{radius (cm)}$$

Hydroxyproline, an amino acid present almost exclusively in collagen, was

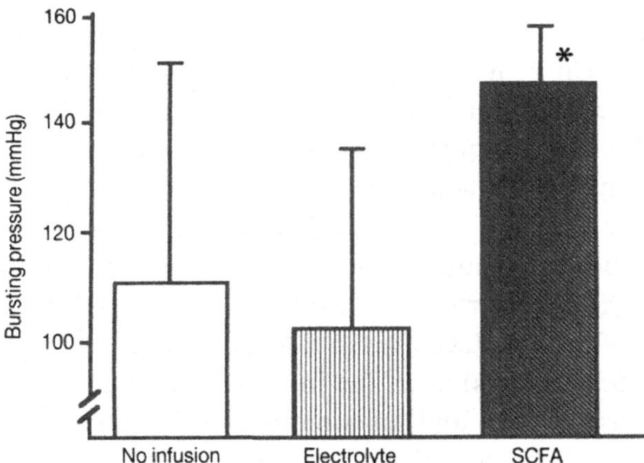

Fig. 27.3. Bursting pressures of colonic anastomoses in the rat following infusion with electrolyte vehicle or combined short-chain fatty acids (SCFA: sodium acetate 75 mM, sodium propionate 35 mM, *n*-butyric acid 20 mM). Adapted from Rolandelli *et al.* (1986*b*).

measured to provide an indirect index of collagen content. Significantly greater bursting pressure, bowel-wall tension, and hydroxyproline content were found in the pectin-fed rats when compared to rats fed solely an elemental diet. Inasmuch as pectin is largely fermented to SCFA, it was hypothesized that SCFA might be responsible for the healing effects on the colonic anastomosis.

To isolate the effects of SCFA on colonic anastomotic healing, a subsequent study investigated the direct intracolonic infusion of SCFA (Rolandelli *et al.*, 1986*b*). Rats were fed a fibre-free diet for 4 days and underwent transection and anastomosis of the descending colon. An infusion catheter was placed into the colon proximal to the anastomosis and tunnelled out of the dorsum of the animal in a swivel apparatus for continuous infusion of SCFA. An end colostomy was performed proximal to the anastomosis and infusion catheter to totally divert the proximal enteric contents and eliminate the local effects of endogenously produced SCFA. Rats received no infusion, infusion with a balanced salt solution, or infusion of combined SCFA (sodium acetate 75 mM, sodium propionate 35 mM, *n*-butyric acid 20 mM). The bursting pressure (Fig. 27.3) and bowel wall tension were significantly greater in the SCFA group than in the two groups. Spontaneous anastomotic dehiscence occurred only in the non-infusion group, demonstrating that complete colonic division had an adverse effect on anastomotic healing (data not shown).

Although these are useful models to describe the effects of pectin and SCFA on anastomotic healing, they are not particularly relevant to the postoperative clinical setting. For example, patients frequently receive antibiotics in the postoperative period which reduces fermentation in the colon. Thus, if a soluble fibre such as pectin is not fermented, it may function as a bulking agent and increase intraluminal pressure before the anastomosis can resist such pressure. Additionally, intracolonic infusions of SCFA require the placement of a catheter into the colon which adds a potential source for postoperative complications. Because of these concerns, the parenteral route as an alternative for SCFA delivery to the colon was investigated.

The same mixture of SCFA (acetate 75 mM, propionate 35 mM, and *n*-butyrate 20 mM as sodium salts) as in the intracolonic infusion study was used. Rats underwent transection and anastomosis of the descending colon and placement of a silastic catheter in the superior vena cava. Postoperatively, rats were randomly assigned to receive TPN (1.4 g of nitrogen and 230 non-protein kilocalories per kilogram body weight per day, respectively) or the same TPN with SCFA. The control TPN group received 130 mM sodium chloride to control for the sodium load delivered with the SCFA salts. Neither the mechanical strength (bursting pressure and bowel wall tension) nor the hydroxyproline content were enhanced by the addition of SCFA (J. L. Rombeau *et al.*, unpublished data). In an attempt to explain these negative results, it was postulated that the amount of SCFA reaching the colon was insufficient to enhance healing.

The colon receives only 8–9% of the cardiac output; therefore, any of the other tissues receiving the remaining 91–92% of the cardiac output can theoretically extract and metabolize SCFA. Therefore, if the same formula used for intracolonic infusion of SCFA is infused intravenously, the amount received by the colon is less than one-tenth of the quantity infused into the lumen. Since the sodium content of the formula limits the amount of SCFA to be infused, it was decided to use all 130 mM sodium as a vehicle to infuse *n*-butyrate. Using the methodology as described previously, a significantly higher bursting pressure (107 ± 30.3 v. 83 ± 41.0) and bowel wall tension (20.7 ± 7.6 v. 14.1 ± 9.9) was demonstrated in the animals receiving 130 mM sodium *n*-butyrate added to the TPN solution (Rolandelli *et al.*, 1994).

Postcolostomy colonic diversion

Emergency surgery is often performed on patients with acute colonic diseases without preoperative bowel preparation. This type of surgery may occur in patients with obstructing carcinomas, massive bleeding from angiodysplasia or diverticular disease, acute diverticulitis, severe colitis with systemic toxicity (e.g. ulcerative, granulomatous, pseudomembranous) and traumatic injuries.

In these circumstances, leakage from suture lines and ensuing morbidity are more frequent when compared to elective colon surgery with preoperative bowel preparation. To potentially reduce the possibility of leakage from the colon, a colostomy can be constructed proximal to the surgical site (repair or anastomosis). Another option is to remove or exteriorize the diseased segment of colon without anastomosing the bowel. In this setting, the proximal end of transected colon is exteriorized as a colostomy, while the distal end is either exteriorized as a mucous fistula, or closed as a Hartmann's procedure. The patient is allowed to recover from the initial surgery before operative re-establishment of colonic continuity in approximately 3 months. Before this second operation, some patients will develop an acute inflammation of the diverted colon, which is termed 'diversion colitis'. The clinical manifestations vary from mild bloody diarrhoea to a febrile syndrome with malaise and abdominal pain. Histologically, diversion colitis is almost indistinguishable from acute ulcerative colitis with crypt microabscesses. The clinical manifestations and histological features often resolve with the administration of SCFA enemas (see Chapter 23). Although this type of colitis is usually a minor side effect of a proximal colostomy, the structural and functional changes occurring in the colonic wall during diversion seem to retard the healing of a colonic anastomosis. A multicentre controlled study is currently under way to further investigate the effects of SCFA in this condition. If the results confirm that the deprivation of SCFA is directly related to diversion colitis, it may be efficacious to add SCFA to the preoperative bowel preparation of patients undergoing a colostomy takedown.

One of us (R.H.R.) treated an unusual form of diversion colitis in a patient with bloody vaginal discharge. The patient had undergone a transsexual operation in which part of the sigmoid colon was used to construct a neovagina. At physical examination the mucosa of the neovaginal transposed colon had the typical appearance of diversion colitis. The patient was treated with douches of SCFA, and the inflammation subsided in 72 h.

As the result of the frequent use of perioperative broad-spectrum antibiotics, surgeons are very familiar with antibiotic-induced colitis (Morris, Zollinger & Stellato, 1990). Most patients with this condition have mild diarrhoea that responds to discontinuation of antibiotics and dietary adjustments. In the most severe form of pseudomembranous colitis, which is often caused by *Clostridium difficile*, the disease may progress to toxic megacolon and colonic perforation. Even if the diagnosis of pseudomembranous colitis is well established, surgery is indicated for refractoriness to medical treatment with progressive sepsis. When the colon is congested and oedematous, but without dilatation or perforation, the surgeon must decide whether or not to proceed

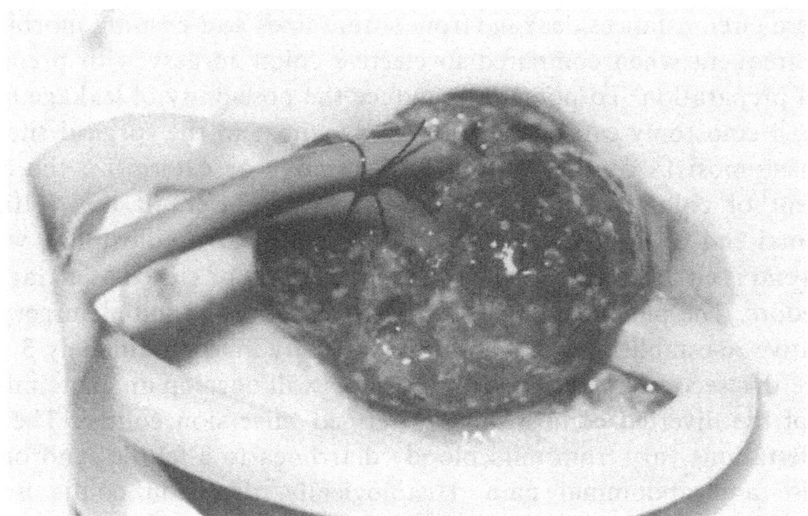

Fig. 27.4. Colostomy with irrigation catheter. Note plaques on colonic mucosa.

with a colectomy. A recent review reported a mortality of 38% in patients who underwent colectomies for pseudomembranous colitis (Morris *et al.*, 1990). If no perforation is found and the bowel is viable, some surgeons advocate a conservative non-operative approach; however, this conservative approach can lead to a fulminant course. Recently, a patient with this condition underwent a loop colostomy for colonic decompression and to provide access for intraluminal infusions of SCFA. Although the diagnosis of pseudomembranous colitis was established, and appropriate treatment was promptly instituted preoperatively, the patient developed septic shock and an acute abdomen. After fluid resuscitation, a laparotomy was performed and findings included ascites, mild dilatation of the small bowel, and congestion of the colon without perforation or dilatation. A loop of transverse colon was exteriorized and the abdomen was closed. The colostomy was matured, an ellipse of colonic wall was excised, and rubber catheters were passed into the ascending and transverse colon (see Fig. 27.4). Beginning on the first postoperative day, the colonic lumen was irrigated with a solution of SCFA including acetate, propionate and butyrate. During the first four post-operative days, there was liquid bloody stool through the stoma and per rectum. The diarrhoea then subsided and tube feedings were initiated. The colostomy was subsequently closed without complications.

The rationale for this therapy is based upon several findings. Colostomy irrigations restore antegrade flow with cleansing of the colonic lumen and eliminate bacteria and enterotoxins. The addition of SCFA to the irrigant solution lowers the luminal pH, inhibiting the growth of *Clostridium difficile* and its production of enterotoxins (Gurian, Ward & Katon, 1982; Ramakrishna *et al.*, 1990). Finally, SCFA provides a fuel for the colonocytes, reduces inflammation and promotes healing of the injured mucosa.

Caecectomy

Caecectomy is commonly performed for patients with villous tumours or inflammatory masses. Postoperatively, these patients frequently have diarrhoea, which may be due to removal of caecal fermentation. The potential trophic effects of intracolonic infusions of SCFA on the colonic mucosa were investigated in the rat following caecectomy (Kripke *et al.*, 1989). Rats were deprived of their usual exogenous SCFA source (fibre) and endogenous site of SCFA production (caecum). Caecectomy, ileocolonic anastomosis and placement of an infusion catheter into the proximal colon were performed. Postoperatively rats were assigned to receive a continuous infusion of one of these butyrate concentrations (20 mM, 40 mM, 150 mM SCFA, 7 mM acetate plus 35 mM propionate plus 20 mM butyrate), saline or no infusion. The SCFA infusion approximated the intracaecal concentration of SCFA in a rat consuming a regular chow diet (Remesy & Demigné, 1976; Demigné & Remesy, 1985). Butyrate concentrations were chosen to be equal to (20 mM) or greater than (40 mM then 50 mM) the butyrate concentration in the normal rat caecum. Mucosal weights, protein, DNA and RNA contents were measured in the small intestine and colon. In the colon, the 40-mM butyrate infusion resulted in significant increases in all mucosal parameters (DNA, RMA, mucosal mass and protein) when compared to the control groups. Butyrate (20 mM) and SCFA infusions significantly increased colonic mucosal DNA when compared to the control goups (Fig. 27.5). Increasing the butyrate concentration to above-normal physiological levels did not significantly increase the mucosal indices. Jejunal (Fig. 27.6) and ileal mucosal DNA contents were also significantly increased in the SCFA group when compared with the control groups. It was concluded that colonic infusions of SCFA produce trophism throughout the intestine while the trophic effect of butyrate was most pronounced in the colon.

Ileal pouch–post total proctocolectomy

Patients with chronic ulcerative colitis and familial polyposis are at risk of developing colon carcinoma. A total proctocolectomy is the best prevention

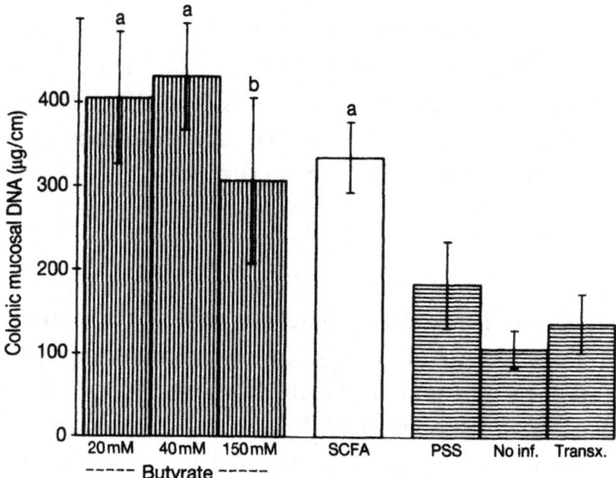

Fig. 27.5. Effects of seven days of intracolonic infusion of butyrate or short-chain fatty acids (SCFA) on colonic mucosal DNA (μg/cm). Butyrate infusions, 20 mM, 40 mM or 150 mM; SCFA, infusion of 70 mM acetate + 35 mM propionate + 20 mM butyrate; PSS, saline infusion; No inf, no infusion; Transx, transection and reanastomosis of proximal colon with caecectomy or infusion. a, p < 0.05 v. PSS, No inf, Transx; b, $p < 0.05$ v. No inf, Transx. From Kripke, *et al.* (1989), with permission.

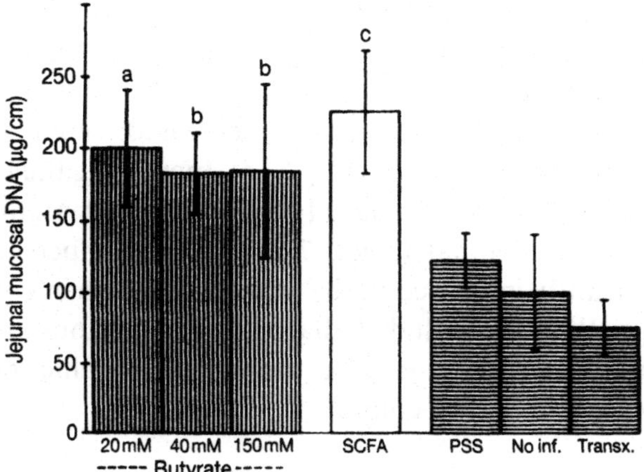

Fig. 27.6. Effects of seven days of intracolonic infusion of butyrate or short-chain fatty acids (SCFA) on jejunal mucosal DNA (μg/cm). a, $p < 0.05$ v. PSS, No inf, Transx; b, $p < 0.05$ v. Transx; c, $p < 0.05$ v. PSS, No inf, Transx (see Fig. 27.3 for group definition).

of cancer in these patients. The traditional permanent ileostomy following total proctocolectomy has now been replaced by the creation of a pelvic ileal reservoir connected to the anus: ileal-pouch–anal anastomosis (IPAA). The terminal ileum is folded over and connected to itself in two limbs ('J' pouch), three limbs ('S' pouch), or four limbs ('W' pouch). This creates a reservoir which, over time, adapts to compensate for the lack of a rectum. The IPAA operation involves multiple suture and staple lines in patients who may have impaired healing from malnutrition and chronic corticosteroid therapy. Therefore, this surgery is usually performed in separate operative stages, with a diverting ileostomy constructed until healing of the IPAA is complete. Similar to diverting colostomies, diverting ileostomies result in atrophy and decreased reservoir capacity. In addition, anal strictures are common with both diverting colostomies and diverting ileostomies after IPAA. During the phase of diversion, the ileal reservoir becomes colonized with aerobic bacteria, particularly *Pseudomonas aeruginosa.* Once the ileostomy is closed, the ileal reservoir develops a flora similar to the normal colon, which allows for fermentation of dietary fibre and undigested starch and provides consistency to the stool. Patients with well-functioning ileal reservoirs have a pattern of SCFA in the stool similar to that of normal stool. A prospective randomized study is at present being conducted at the University of California at Los Angeles to investigate the effect of SCFA infusion into the pouch during the phase of diversion. The hypothesis is that SCFA infusions will prevent atrophy of the pouch and IPAA strictures, and will promote faster adaptation of the ileal reservoir to function as a neorectum.

Pouchitis is an acute inflammation of the mucosa of the ileal reservoir following total proctocolectomy, and symptoms include diarrhoea, bloody rectal discharge and fever. The incidence of pouchitis varies between 6 and 50% (Madden, Farthing & Nicholls, 1990; Rabassa & Rogers, 1992). Pouchitis usually occurs in patients with ulcerative colitis and is infrequently seen in patients following IPAA for familial polyposis (Gustavsson, Weiland & Kelly, 1987; Dozois *et al.*, 1989). Bacterial overgrowth has been postulated to be a contributory factor; however, no clear correlation has been established. More recently, SCFA levels have been found to be significantly reduced in patients with pouchitis when compared to patients with normal pouches (Wischmeyer *et al.*, 1991). Further investigations have shown that both concentration and production of SCFA are decreased in faecal homogenates from patients with pouchitis. Administration of fermentable saccharides to patients with pouchtis improves SCFA concentrations indicating, perhaps, a lack of fermentable substrates in diseased ileal pouches. Interestingly, the faecal microflora and pH are not significantly altered (Clausen, Tvede & Mortensen, 1982). In a brief report of two patients with pouchitis, pouch irrigation with SCFA appeared to potentiate the disease during treatment (DeSilva *et al.*, 1989). The role of SCFA in ileal pouchitis needs further investigation, and perhaps glutamine should be added to the infusate (Rabassa & Rogers, 1992). While butyrate is the most important oxidative fuel for the colonocyte, glutamine is preferred by the small-bowel mucosa and may be more appropriate for the ileal–anal pouch.

Short-bowel syndrome

The short-bowel syndrome is characterized by decreased mucosal surface area causing malabsorption, diarrhoea and body-weight loss. Following massive small-bowel resection, the remaining intestine dilates and lengthens in an adaptive response, to increase its absorptive capacity (Wilmore *et al.*, 1971). Nutritional treatment for patients with short-bowel syndrome is usually provided by TPN, despite its atrophic effects on the bowel. The administration of TPN and the lack of oral intake inhibit intestinal adaptation in rats and this inhibition is largely reversed by enteral feeding (Ford *et al.*, 1984). Inasmuch as fibre is trophic to the colonic mucosa, it was hypothesized that providing soluble fibre, such as citrus pectin, might enhance intestinal adaptation to massive small-bowel resection.

The effect of a pectin-supplemented elemental diet on intestinal adaptation following massive small-bowel resection was investigated (Koruda *et al.*, 1986). Rats underwent an 80% small-bowel resection and were fed either an elemental diet alone or the same elemental diet supplemented with 2% pectin. The pectin-supplemented group had significantly greater intestinal adaptation and maintenance of body weight than did the non-supplemented group. Postresectional colonic mucosal DNA was significantly increased in the pectin-supplemented group when compared to the control animals. Inasmuch as pectin is completely fermented to SCFA, it was hypothesized that the pectin-induced trophism might be mediated by SCFA.

Most patients with massive small-bowel resection required TPN; therefore, an ensuing study was undertaken to determine whether TPN supplemented with SCFA might enhance intestinal adaptation after massive small-bowel resection (Koruda *et al.*, 1988). Rats underwent 80% small-bowel resection and received TPN either with or without SCFA for 7 days. The SCFA-supplemented rats had significantly less postresection jejunal mucosal atrophy than did rats receiving TPN without SCFA (Fig. 27.7). It was concluded that the mucosal atrophy in the small intestine induced by TPN was partially reduced by the addition of intravenous SCFA.

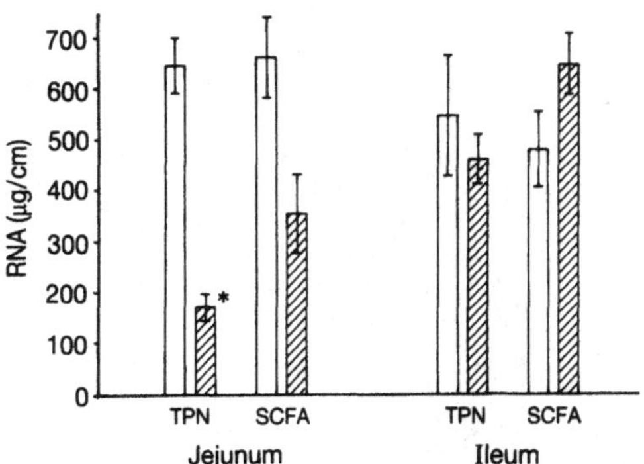

Fig. 27.7. Effect of seven days of short-chain fatty acids (SCFA: sodium acetate 36 mequiv/l, sodium propionate 15 mequiv/l, sodium butyrate 9 mequiv/l) added to total parenteral nutrition (TPN) on mucosal RNA concentration in rats before (white bars) and after (hatched bars) 80% small-bowel resection. Asterisk, $p < 0.001$, pre- v. postresection; values are means ± SEM. Adapted from Koruda *et al.*, (1988).

TPN-induced bowel rest

As part of the therapy plan for patients with gastrointestinal dysfunction, many hospitalized patients are given TPN. As mentioned previously, TPN and bowel rest deprive the intestinal mucosa of its preferred fuels and produce atrophy and hypofunction. This atrophy can be both prevented and reversed by enteral alimentation (Levine *et al.*, 1974). Fibre-free diets produce distal small-bowel and colonic atrophy that can be prevented by adding fibre to the diets (Ryan *et al.*, 1979). All of the above would indicate that bowel rest deprives the intestinal mucosa of its essential fuels, producing hypofunctions, atrophy and diarrhoea. Rapid refeeding clearly worsens the diarrhoea, as the absorptive capacity of the mucosal cells is insufficient to adapt to acutely increased nutrient demands. Prevention and treatment of 'nutritional colitis' and diarrhoea is possible by provision of SCFA or fibre as a substrate for bacterial production of SCFA (Roediger, 1990).

Since the provision of enteral nutrients is not always possible for post-operative patients, it was hypothesized that intravenous supplementation with intestinal fuels such as SCFA might reduce the mucosal atrophy induced by TPN and bowel rest. The effect of TPN supplementation with SCFA was investigated to determine if mucosal atrophy could be prevented or reduced in the normal rat (Koruda *et al.*, 1990). Rats were assigned randomly and equally to one of four dietary groups for seven days: (1) intravenous saline and rat chow; (2) TPN alone; (3) TPN with intravenous SCFA; and (4) TPN

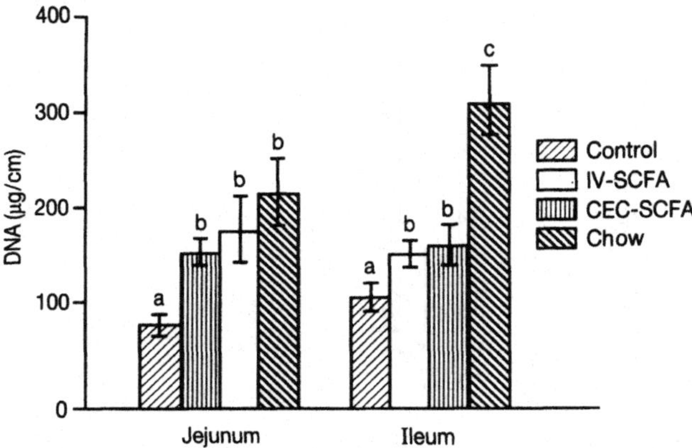

Fig. 27.8. Effects of seven days of dietary infusion on jejunal and ileal mucosal DNA. Control, standard total parenteral nutrition (TPN); IV SCFA, standard TPN + intravenous short-chain fatty acids (SCFA: sodium acetate 36 mM, sodium propionate 15 mM, sodium butyrate 9 mM); CEC-SCFA, standard TPN + intracaecally infused SCFA. For each segment, a v. b, $p < 0.05$; a v. c, $p < 0.005$; b v. c, $p < 0.001$. From Koruda *et al.* (1990), with permission.

supplemented with intracaecal infusion of SCFA. All animals underwent superior vena cava cannulation with swivel placement. Sham laparotomy and caecal catheter insertion were performed concurrently. The intestines of those rats given TPN demonstrated significant atrophy of the ileal and jejunal mucosa when compared to controls. This atrophy was significantly decreased by both the intracaecal and intravenous infusion of SCFA when compared to control groups, as demonstrated in Fig. 27.8. Interestingly, there was no significant difference in small bowel mucosal DNA when the SCFA were delivered either into the caecum or intravenously.

Practical aspects of administering SCFA

The first problem the surgeon encounters when considering the administration of SCFA is the route of delivery to the colon. Short-chain fatty acids are effectively absorbed by the gastric and small-bowel mucosa by passive diffusion; therefore, they will not reach the human colon when infused into the stomach or small bowel. This leaves very few options for delivery. One of the methods of delivery is the retrograde perfusion by enemas. Enemas have been successfully used in patients with diversion colitis, non-specific procto-sigmoiditis, ulcerative proctocolitis, and ileal pouchitis (see Chapter 23). However, substances administered by enemas only reach the descending colon, and the exposure of the total colonic mucosa to such substances is not uniform. Antegrade perfusion offers more uniform exposure and a constant rate; however, it requires the placement of a catheter into the distal ileum or proximal colon. Long nasoenteric tubes are difficult to position in the terminal ileum, particularly in patients affected by diseases requiring surgical intervention. Additionally, direct placement of a tube across the bowel wall during laparotomy creates a potential source for complications. Another possible solution is the administration of a fermentable, non-absorbable carbohydrate source for bacterial fermentation, such as lactulose or pectin. The problems with this approach are that it relies upon bacterial metabolism, which is significantly reduced by preoperative colonic cleansing and antibiotic therapy, and the production of gas, which increases intraluminal pressure in the colon.

Parenteral infusion is an alternative route to intraluminal infusion (see Chapter 33). As discussed previously, significant enterotrophic affects of SCFA have been obtained by parenteral infusions in animals. Unfortunately, the parenteral route of delivery is associated with some problems. If SCFA are infused as salts, the quantity to be infused is limited by the cation, e.g. sodium. As mentioned previously, the extraction of parenteral SCFA by the colon is proportional to the inflow of blood, which is poor in the colon, consisting of only 8–9% of the cardiac output. The development of structured lipids with triglycerides containing SCFA would theoretically allow the infusion of larger quantities (see Chapter 33).

Conclusion

Studies in postoperative animals and humans have confirmed the enterotrophic effects of SCFA. These effects are presumably mediated in many ways, such as providing local energy, increasing the production of pancreatic and biliary secretions, stimulating intestinal blood flow, inciting the automatic nervous system, and increasing the production of enterotrophic gastrointestinal hormones. Current nutritional prescriptions for patients undergoing intestinal surgery deprive the small bowel and colon of SCFA. The intestine is therefore iatrogenically depleted of potentially important fuels at a time of increased nutrient demands. Potential indications for the use of SCFA in intestinal surgery include colonic anastomosis, postcolostomy diversion colitis, caecectomy, pouchitis following total proctocolectomy, short-bowel syndrome and TPN-induced bowel rest. Controlled clinical studies are needed to investigate the therapeutic effects of the SCFA in patients with these conditions.

References

Al-Mukhter, M. Y., Sago, G. R. & Ghatei, M. A. (1983). The role of pancreaticobiliary secretions in intestinal adaptation after resection and its relationship to plasma enteroglucagon. *British Journal of Surgery*, **70**, 398–400.

Altman, G. C. (1971). Influence of bile and pancreatic secretions on the size of the intestinal villi in the rat. *American Journal of Anatomy*, **132**, 167–78.

Bloom, S. R. (1980). Gut and brain-endocrine connections. The Gaulstonian Lecture, 1979. *Journal of the Royal College of Physicians London*, **14**, 51–7.

Bristol, J. B. & Williamson, R. C. N. (1988). Nutrition, operations, and intestinal adaptation. *Journal of Parenteral and Enteral Nutrition*, **12**, 299–309.

Calam, J., Ghatei, M. A., Domin, J. *et al.* (1989). Regional differences in concentrations of regulatory peptides in human colon mucosal biopsy. *Digestive Diseases and Sciences*, **34**, 1193–8.

Cameron, I. L., Ord, V. A., Hunter, K. E., Van Nguyen, M., Padilla, G. M. & Heitman, D. W. (1990). Quantitative contribution of factors regulating rat colonic crypt epithelium: role of parenteral and enteral feeding, caloric intake, dietary cellulose level, and the carcinogen DMH. *Cell Tissue Kinetics*, **23**, 227–35.

Clausen, M. R., Tvede, M. & Mortensen, P. B. (1992). Short-chain fatty acids in pouch contents from patients with and without pouchitis after ileal pouch–anal anastomosis. *Gastroenterology*, **103**, 1144–53.

Conteas, C. N. & Majumdar, A. P. (1987). The effects of gastrin, epidermal growth factor, and somatostatin on DNA synthesis in a small intestinal crypt cell line (IEC-6). *Proceedings of the Society of Experimental Biological Medicine*, **184**, 307–11.

Cummings, J. H. (1991). Production and metabolism of short-chain fatty acids in humans. *Short-chain Fatty Acids: Metabolism and Clinical Importance. Report of Tenth Ross Conference on Medical Research*, pp. 11–17.

Cummings, J. H., Gibson, G. R. & Macfarlane, G. T. (1989). Quantitative estimates of fermentation in the hindgut of man. *Acta Veterinaria Scandinavica*, **86**, 76–82.

Dembinski, A. B. & Johnston, L. R. (1979). Stimulation of pancreas and gastrointestinal mucosa in antrectomized and gastrin-treated rats. *Endocrinology*, **105**, 769–73.

Demigné, C. & Remesy, C. (1985). Stimulation of absorption of volatile fatty acids and minerals in the cecum of rats adapted to a very high fiber diet. *Journal of Nutrition*, **115**, 53–60.

DeSilva, H. J., Ireland, A., Kettlewell, M. *et al.* (1989). Short-chain fatty acid irrigation in severe pouchitis, letter to editor, *New England Journal of Medicine*, **321**, 1416–17.

Dozois, R. R., Kelly, K. A., Welling, D. R. *et al.* (1989). Ileal pouch–anal anastomosis: comparison of results in familial adenomatous polyposis and chronic ulcerative colitis. *Annals of Surgery*, **210**, 268–73.

Ecknauer, R., Sircar, B. & Johnson, L. R. (1981). Effect of dietary bulk on small intestinal morphology and cell renewal in the rat. *Gastroenterology*, **81**, 781–6.

Feldman, E. J., Dowling, R. H. *et al.* (1976). Effects of oral versus intravenous nutrition on intestinal adaptation after small bowel resection in the dog. *Gastroenterology*, **70**, 712–19.

Ford, W. D. A., Boelhaower, R. U., King, W. W. K. *et al.* (1984). Total parenteral nutrition inhibits intestinal adaptive hyperplasia in young rats: reversal by feeding. *Surgery*, **96**, 527–34.

Frankel, W., Zhang, W., Singh, A. *et al.* (1992). Stimulation of the autonomic nervous system mediates short-chain fatty acid induced jejunotrophism. *Surgical Forum*, **43**, 24–6.

Goodlad, R. A., Al-Mukhtar, M. Y., Ghatei, M. A., Bloom, S. R. & Wright, N. A. (1983). Cell proliferation, plasma enteroglucagon and plasma gastrin levels in starved and refed rats. *Vichows Archives* (*Cell Pathology*) **43**, 55–62.

Goodlad, R. A., Lerton, W., Ghatei, M. A., Adrian, T. E., Bloom, S. R. & Wright, N. A. (1987). Effects of an elemental diet, inert bulk, and different types of dietary fibre on the response of the intestinal epithelium to refeeding in the rat and relationship to plasma gastrin, enteroglucagon, and PYY concentrations, *Gut*, **28**, 171–80.

Gurian, L., Ward, T. T. & Katon, R. M. (1982). Possible food-borne transmission in a case of pseudomembranous colitis due to *Clostridium difficile*. *Gastroenterology*, **83**, 465–9.

Gustavsson, S., Weiland, L. H. & Kelly, K. A. (1987). Relationship of backwash ileal pouchitis after ileal pouch–anal anastomosis. *Diseases of the Colon and Rectum*, **30**, 25–8.

Harada, E. & Kato, S. (1983). Effect of short-chain acids on the secretory response of the ovine exocrine pancreas. *American Journal of Physiology*, **244**, G284–G290.

Hesp, F. L., Hendriks, T., Libbers, E.-J. C. & Deboes, H. (1984). Wound healing in the intestinal wall: a comparison between experimental ileal and colonic anastomoses. *Diseases of the Colon and Rectum*, **27**, 99–104.

Hill, F. L. C., Zhang, T., Gomez, G. *et al.* (1991). Peptide YY, a new gut hormone (a mini-review). *Steroids*, **56**, 77–82.

Jacobs, L. R. (1989). Dietary fiber and the intestinal mucosa. In *The Role of Dietary Fiber in Enteral Nutrition*, ed. J. H. Cummings, pp. 14–35. Chicago: Abbott International.

Jacobs, L. R. & Lupton, J. R. (1984). Effect of dietary fibers on rat large bowel mucosal growth and cell proliferation. *American Journal of Physiology*, **246**, G378–G385.

Jacobs, L. R. & White, F. A. (1983). Modulation of mucosal cell proliferation in the intestine of rats fed a wheat bran diet. *American Journal of Clinical Nutrition*, **37**, 945–53.

Jiborn, H. Ahonen, J. & Zedesfeldt, B. (1978). Healing of experimental colonic anastomoses. 1. Bursting strength of the colon after left colon resection and anastomosis. *American Journal of Surgery*, **136**, 587–94.

Johnson, L. R. (1977). New aspects of the trophic action of gastrointestinal hormones. *Gastroenterology*, **72**, 788–92.

Johnson, L. R., (1987). Regulation of gastrointestinal growth. In *Physiology of the Gastrointestinal Tract*, 2nd edn, vol. 1, ed. L. R. Johnson, pp. 301–33. New York: Raven Press.

Johnson, L. R. Aures, D. & Yuen, L. (1969). Pentagastrin-induced stimulation of protein synthesis in the gastrointestinal tract. *American Journal of Physiology*, **217**, 251–4.

Katoh, K. (1991). The effect of short-chain fatty acids on the pancreas: endocrine and exocrine. *Short-chain Fatty Acids: Metabolism and Clinical Importance. Report of the Tenth Ross Conference on Medical Research*, pp. 74–7.

Koruda, M. J. & Rolandelli, R. H. (1990). Experimental studies on the healing of colonic anastomosis. *Journal of Surgical Research*, **48**, 504–16.

Koruda, M. J., Rolandelli, R. H., Settle, R. G. *et al.* (1986). The effect of pectin-supplemented elemental diet on intestinal adaptation to massive small bowel resection in the rat. *Journal of Parenteral and Enteral Nutrition*, **10**, 343–50.

Koruda, M. J., Rolandelli, R. H. Settle, R. G. *et al.* (1988). The effect of parenteral nutrition supplemented with short-chain fatty acids on adaptation to massive small bowel resection. *Gastroenterology*, **95**, 710–20.

Koruda, M. J., Rolandelli, R. H., Zimmaro-Bliss., D. *et al.* (1990). Parenteral nutrition supplemented with short-chain fatty acids: effect on the small bowel mucosa in normal rats. *American Journal of Clinical Nutrition*, **51**, 685–9.

Kripke, S. A., Fox, A. D. & Berman, J. M. (1987). Stimulation of mucosal growth with intracolonic butyrate infusion. *Surgical Forum*, **38**, 47–9.

Kripke, S. A., Fox, A. D., Berman, J. M. *et al.* (1989). Stimulation of intestinal mucosal growth with intracolonic infusion of short-chain fatty acids. *Journal of Parenteral and Enteral Nutrition*, **13**, 109–16.

Kvietys, P. R. & Granger, N. D. (1981). Effect of volatile fatty acids on blood flow and oxygen uptake by the dog colon. *Gastroenterology*, **80**, 962–9.

Levine, G. M., Deren, J. J., Steiger, E. *et al.* (1974). Role of oral intake in maintenance of gut mass and disaccharidase activity. *Gastroenterology*, **67**, 975–82.

Longo, W. E., Ballantyne, G. H., Savoca, P. E. *et al.* (1990). Short-chain fatty acids release of peptide YY in the isolated rabbit distal colon. *Scandinavian Journal of Gastroenterology*, **26**, 442–8.

Madden, M. V., Farthing, M. J. G. & Nicholls, R. D. (1990). Inflammation in ileal reservoirs: 'pouchitis'. *Gut*, **31**, 247–9.

Morris, J. B., Zollinger, R. M. & Stellato, T. A. (1990). Role of surgery in antibiotic-induced pseudomembranous enterocolitis. *American Journal of Surgery*, **160**, 553–9.

Mortensen, F. V., Nielsen, H., Mulvany, M. J. & Hessov, I. (1990). Short-chain fatty acids dilate isolated human colonic resistance arteries. *Gut*, **31**, 1391–4.

Rabassa, A. O. & Rogers, A. I. (1991). The role of short-chain fatty acid metabolism in colonic disorders. *American Journal of Gastroenterology*, **87**, 419–23.

Ramakrishma, B. S., Nance, S. H., Roberts-Thomson, I. C. & Roediger, W. E. W. (1990). The effects of enterotoxins and short-chain fatty acids on water and electrolyte fluxes in ileal and colonic loops *in vivo* in the rat. *Digestion*, **45**, 93–101.

Reilly, K., Frankel, W., Klurfeld, D., Choi, D. & Rombeau, J. L. (1993). The parasympathetic (PSNS) and sympathetic (SNS) nervous systems mediate the systemic effects of short-chain fatty acid (SCFA) on jejunal structure and function. *Surgical Forum*, **44**, 20–2.

Remesy, C. & Demigné, C. (1976). Partition and absorption of volatile fatty acid in the alimentary canal of the rat. *Annales Recherche Vétérinaire*, **7**, 39–55.

Roediger, W. E. W. (1982). Utilization of nutrients by isolated epithelial cells of the rat colon. *Gastroenterology*, **83**, 424–9.

Roediger, W. E. W. (1990). The starved colon – diminished mucosal nutrition, diminished absorption and colitis. *Diseases of the Colon and Rectum*, **33**, 858–62.

Rolandelli, R. H., Berstein, K. A., Hiyama, P. *et al.* (1994). Intravenous butyrate and the healing of colonic anastomosis in the rat. *American Journal of Surgery*, in press.

Rolandelli, R. H., Koruda, M. J., Settle, R. G. *et al.* (1986*a*). Effects of intraluminal infusion of short-chain fatty acids on the healing of colonic anastomosis in the rat. *Surgery*, **100**, 198–203.

Rolandelli, R. H., Koruda, M. J., Settle, R. G. *et al.* (1986*b*). The effect of enteral feedings supplemented with pectin on the healing of colonic anastomoses in the rat. *Surgery*, **99**, 703–7.

Ryan, G. P., Dudrick, S. J., Copeland, E. M. *et al.* (1979). Effects of various diets on colonic growth in rats. *Gastroenterology*, **77**, 658–63.

Sagor, G. R., Al-Mukhtar, M. Y., Ghatei, M. A. *et al.* (1981). Enteroglucagon and intestinal adaptation. *Gut*, **22**, 439–45.

Sakata, T. (1987). Stimulatory effect of short-chain fatty acids on epithelial cell proliferation in the rat intestine: a possible explanation for trophic effects of fermentable fibre, gut microbes, and luminal trophic factors. *British Journal of Nutrition*, **58**, 95–103.

Sakata, T. (1989). Stimulatory effect of short-chain fatty acids on epithelial cell proliferation of isolated and denervated jejunal segment of the rat. *Scandinavian Journal of Gastroenterology*, **24**, 886–90.

Sakata, T. & Engelhardt, W. v. (1983). Stimulatory effect of short-chain fatty acids on the epithelial cell proliferation in the rat large intestine. *Comparative Biochemistry and Physiology*, **74A**, 459–62.

Sakata, T. & Yajima, T. (1984). Influence of short-chain fatty acids on the epithelial cell division of the digestive tract. *Quarterly Journal of Experimental Physiology*, **69**, 639–48.

Scheppach, W. M., Sommer, H., Kirchner, T. *et al.* (1992). Effect of butyrate enemas on the colonic mucosa in distal ulcerative colitis. *Gastroenterology*, **193**, 51–6.

Sirinek, K. R., Levin, B. A. & Moyer, M. P. (1985). Pentagastrin stimulates *in vitro* growth of normal and malignant human colon epithelial cells. *American Journal of Surgery*, **147**, 35–9.

Souba, W. W., Smith, R. J. & Wilmore, D. W. (1985). Glutamine metabolism by the intestinal tract. *Journal of Parenteral and Enteral Nutrition*, **9**, 608–16.

Vahouny, G. V. & Cassidy, M. M. (1986). Dietary fiber and intestinal adaptation. In *Dietary Fiber: Basic and Clinical Aspects*, ed. G. B. Vahouny and D. Kritchevsky, pp. 181–209. New York: Plenum Press.

Weser, E., Heller, R. & Tawil, T. (1977). Stimulation of mucosal growth in the rat ileum by bile and pancreatic secretions after jejunal resection. *Gastroenterology*, **73**, S24–S29.

Wilmore, D. W., Dudrick, S. J., Daly, J. M. *et al.* (1971). The role of nutrition in the adaptation of the small intestine after massive resection. *Surgery, Gynecology and Obstetrics*, **132**, 673–80.

Wischmeyer, P. E., Tremaine, W. J., Haddad, A. C. *et al.* (1991). Fecal short-chain fatty acids after ileal pouch anal anastomosis. *Gastroenterology*, **100**, 2.

28

Short-chain fatty acids as an energy source in the colon: metabolism and clinical implications

G. LIVESEY AND M. ELIA

Introduction

Short-chain fatty acids (SCFA) are saturated aliphatic monocarboxylic acids and include acetic, propionic and butyric acids. Some 60% of a ruminant's energy requirement can be met by SCFA, which are produced by anaerobic fermentation of carbohydrate and protein (Armstrong & Blaxter, 1961). Although it was known that anaerobic fermentation occurred in the hindgut of humans (and of non-ruminant herbivores) the absorption of SCFA by the human colon was initially doubted (McCance & Lawrence, 1929; McCance & Widdowson, 1940). However, the studies of McNeil, Cummings & James (1978) and Ruppin *et al.* (1980) showed conclusively that the human large intestine absorbs these acids. Their quantitative contribution to energy metabolism in humans has since been in debate. In the field of artificial nutritional support, there has been a growing interest in the use of SCFA as an alternative or additional energy source to the long- and medium-chain lipids (Campos & Meguid, 1988). In a variety of clinical conditions, at least butyric acid may be a conditionally essential nutrient for the colon, just as glutamine may be conditionally essential for the small intestine (Evans & Shronts, 1992; Elia, 1992*a*); and absence of butyrate may lead to suboptimal colonic function (Roediger, 1980).

The aims of this chapter are threefold. The first aim is to assess the extent of SCFA production in the human colon, the contribution the gut makes to total SCFA production (endogenous and exogenous), and the contribution that SCFA make to energy expenditure by the whole body and by individual tissues. Such an evaluation involves consideration of the supply of fermentable substrate to the colon, the stoichiometry of anaerobic fermentation in colonic micro-organisms, and the stoichiometry of oxidative catabolism in mammalian tissues. Secondly, the chapter aims to assess the physiological implications of the fermentation process with respect to the possible energy cost of absorption of SCFA, acid–base balance and the calculation of fuel utilization by indirect calorimetry. Thirdly, the chapter aims to access the possible benefits to patients with gastrointestinal disease that might arise when SCFA are used to meet some of the patients' energy requirements.

Sources of short-chain fatty acids

SCFA are present in the diet in small amounts, for example acetic acid in vinegar and butyric acid in milk and butter (Paul & Southgate, 1978). They may also be present in fermented foods, and propionic acid may be added to foods in small amounts as an antimicrobial food additive (Elund, 1987). Acetic, propionic and butyric acids are produced by fermentation of dietary carbohydrates in the human hindgut, where they are the predominant intraluminal organic anions (Cummings *et al.*, 1987). The metabolism of ethanol in the liver gives rise to much circulating acetate (Lundquist *et al.*, 1962, 1973), and substantial amounts of circulating acetate arise both during ketogenesis associated with starvation (Scheppach *et al.*, 1991) and in diabetes mellitus (Smith, Humphreys & Hockaday, 1986). Acetate is the major anion buffer in many total parenteral nutrition regimens (Lazarus & Stein, 1988), and kidney-dialysis patients metabolize very large quantities of the acetate used to buffer dialysis solutions (Weiner, 1982; Skutches *et al.*, 1983). Acetate may also be used pharmocologically for the correction of acidosis due to diarrhoeal disorders (Cash *et al.*, 1969; Ekblad, Kero & Takala, 1985), to balance the acidity of cysteine-HCl when this is added to parenteral nutrition regimens (Laine *et al.*, 1991), and to prevent the urinary loss of calcium (Berkelhammer, Wood & Sitrin, 1988). With the rise in interest in the possible clinical applications of SCFA as modifiers of gut function, they are likely to become used more frequently in metabolic studies, and perhaps become developed commercially as components of enteral and parenteral feeds; for example as monoacyl glycerol (e.g. monobutyryl glycerol; Birkhahn, McMenamy & Border, 1977), as triacyl glycerols (e.g. triacetin; Bailey, Haymon & Miles, 1991) and as sodium or calcium salts.

Unavailable carbohydrates in mixed diets as a source of SCFA and energy

There is now an overwhelming body of evidence showing that carbohydrates undigested by enzymes of the human small intestine become extensively fermented in the large intestine, and supply systemic metabolism with energy as SCFA. For the purpose of this chapter, such carbohydrates are termed 'unavailable carbohydrates'. This evidence conflicts with present food-labelling regulations in Europe, the USA (now under review) and elsewhere, which assume that humans obtain no energy from such carbohydrates, an assumption that is partly based on the early doubts about SCFA absorption and partly based on the studies of metabolizable energy balance in men and women performed by Southgate & Durnin (1970). These studies were consistent with a lack of energy being obtained from these carbohydrates. However, more evidence from this type of study has been obtained, and shows (Livesey, 1990*a*, 1991) the unavailable carbohydrates of mixed diets to contribute an average of about 8.4 kJ (2 kcal)/g at all levels of intake. A similar amount of energy is calculated to be made available on the basis of the extent to which the unavailable carbohydrate is fermented.

The disposition of energy from the unavailable carbohydrates in mixed diets is known only approximately. In these diets the fraction of unavailable carbohydrate that is fermented in humans is about 0.7, irrespective of whether intake is low (9 g daily), medium (25 g daily) or very high (77 g daily) (Livesey, 1990*a*). Of the carbohydrate energy that is fermented, a fraction, about 0.3, is lost to faeces, mainly as bacterial matter (Livesey, 1990*a*, 1991). Since the heat of combustion of unavailable carbohydrate is about 17.2 kJ/g, the amount of energy made available can be calculated (Livesey, 1993) to be 8.4 kJ/g [i.e. $17.2 \times 0.7 \times (1 - 0.3)$]. This amount of energy is essentially identical to that determined in the energy balance studies mentioned above, and is released mainly in the form of SCFA ($\approx$7.2 kJ/g), and partly as heat fermentation ($\approx$0.6 kJ/g) and as the combustible gases, hydrogen and methane ($\approx$0.6 kJ/g), which are lost in breath and flatus. This distribution of energy from unavailable carbohydrate in mixed diets eaten by humans is summarized in Fig. 28.1. The figure also indicates that SCFA are less efficient systematic fuels than is glucose in generating ATP (see both the legend to Fig. 28.1 and the stoichiometry of ATP production from SCFA, p. 454). Once this inefficiency is accounted for, the net energy available for metabolism is about 6.2 kJ/g (1.5 kcal/g) of unavailable carbohydrate. It should be remembered that this value applies to the unavailable carbohydrates in mixed diets, and so a different disposition might occur when plant cell-wall polysaccharides are included in polysaccharide-free enteral feeds.

The amounts of energy made available as SCFA from carbohydrates undergoing colonic fermentation in normal humans eating conventional diets or diets enriched with cell-wall polysaccharides, oligosaccharides and sugar alcohols have now been evaluated elsewhere in detail (Livesey, 1993).

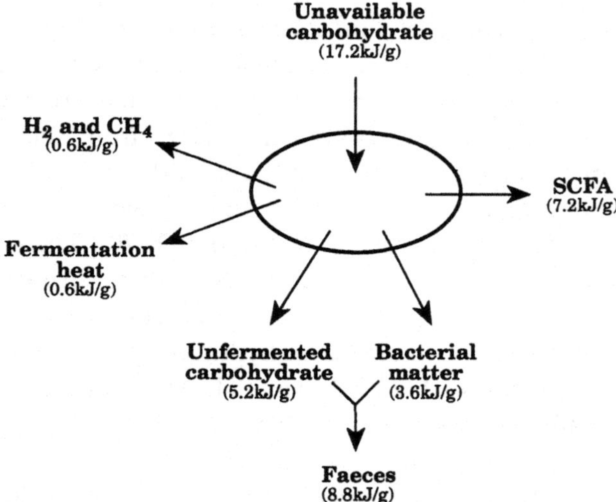

Fig. 28.1. Carbohydrate fermentation in the human colon: distribution of energy between end products and the supply of energy to human tissues from the unavailable carbohydrates of mixed Western-style diets, where about 70% is fermented (Livesey, 1993), with heat of combustion 17.2 kJ/g. Of the unavailable carbohydrate, 30% (5.2 kJ/g) is unfermented and so becomes a component of faeces. Of the 70% that is fermented, 30% is recovered as bacterial matter in faeces (3.6 kJ/g), about 5% as combustible gases (0.6 kJ/g) and about 5% as heat of fermentation. Absorbed energy is in the form of short-chain fatty acids (SCFA; 7.2 kJ/g). For substrates with a different extent of fermentation from 70%, the disposition of energy would differ. As SCFA are not metabolized for maintenance with the same efficiency as glucose, about 15% (i.e. 1 kJ/g out of the 7.2 kJ/g) more energy is released as heat than if glucose were the substrate, so leaving 6.2 kJ/g as the net energy available from the carbohydrates of mixed diets.

Other unavailable carbohydrates as a source of SCFA

In addition to the unavailable carbohydrates, in the form of plant cell walls, and some starch that resists digestion in the small intestine, a variety of other carbohydrates enter the colon (Table 28.1). The exact quantities of each varies with the diet. Moreover, the methods used to quantify the escape of substrates from the small to the large intestine are far from precise (EURESTA, 1991; Livesey, 1992).

A recent survey showed that intake of dietary fibre in several European countries was about 20 g daily per head, the amount being remarkably similar in each country (European Commission contract, COST 92). Individual intakes are likely to vary at least twofold. Some starch may escape to the large intestine and is termed resistant starch. The origins, nature and

Table 28.1. *Substrates fermented in the large intestine*

Substrate	Amount (g) Approximate mean[a]	Possible range[b]
Dietary fibre	20	8–30
Resistant starch	3	1–40
Oligosaccharides	•	2–5
Inulin and natural fructo-oligosaccharides	3	2–8
Artificial polysaccharides	•	Unknown
Commercial oligosaccharides	•	Unknown
Sugar alcohols[c]	2	0–20[c]
Dietary protein	•	3–9
Pancreatic and small-intestinal secretions	•	4–6
Desquamated cells	•	Unknown
Bacterial population turnover	•	Unknown
Mucus	•	2–3
Organic acids	•	Unknown
Therapeutics, e.g. ispaghula, lactulose	•	Unknown

[a] Based on information from surveys in European countries during the years approaching 1991 (see text).
[b] Based on information from Cummings (1991).
[c] Data for diabetic subjects in the UK (MAFF, 1990).
• Values are not known precisely (see text).

physiological effects of resistant starch have been discussed in the proceedings of a recent meeting (EURESTA, 1992). Estimates of the intake of resistant starch in several European countries (European Commission contract, COST 911) suggest a remarkably small but similar value of about 3 g daily per head in each country. The validity of this estimate is uncertain, since Cummings *et al.* (1990) reported that more starch than plant-wall polysaccharide exists in the colon of sudden-death victims. It is an intriguing possibility that such starch may accumulate in the large intestine because of an inhibition of amylolysis by propionate produced there. Oral propionate inhibits starch digestion and very markedly lowers the postprandial blood glucose response to starch (Todesco *et al.*, 1991).

Other carbohydrates escape the small intestine (and sometimes the food analyst). Inulin and oligofructose, which are energy stores in onions, Jerusalem and globe artichokes, leeks, asparagus and garlic, and which are present in small amounts in cereals, may contribute 2–8 g of additional unavailable carbohydrate daily (Egan & Petersen, 1992). Milk contains appreciable amounts of oligogalactose, beans contain oligosaccharides of the raffinose family and sugar beet contains ethanol-soluble arabinogalactans, etc. The quantities of oligosaccharides ingested is unknown and probably variable. Some oligosaccharides are developed commercially as alternative bulk sweeteners, e.g. the fructo-oligosaccharide called neosugar (Hidaka *et al.*, 1982), and several sugar alcohols are consumed, usually by diabetic populations in which the average intake is small, but widely variable between individuals (MAAF, 1990). Polydextrose® was one of the first artificial polysaccharides used in human nutrition and is a randomly linked polymer of glucose and sorbitol (10:1). Cell-wall polysaccharides, e.g. ispaghula, sterculia, wheat bran and psyllium, may be used therapeutically for constipation. The synthetic disaccharide lactulose, which is used as a laxative, escapes digestion in the small intestine but is completely fermented in the large intestine.

Dietary carbohydrates are not the only source of substrates for fermentation; others are remnants of dietary protein, pancreatic and small-intestinal secretions and sloughed mucosal cells. Mucus secreted by the alimentary tract and mucopolysaccharides produced by bacteria will also make a contribution, as will bacterial cell autolysis. Dietary organic acids, e.g. oxalate, also contribute substrate to the fermentation process (Florin, Neale & Cummings, 1990).

The efficiency with which carbohydrates are converted to SCFA in humans varies, as is shown in Table 28.2. Carbohydrates, such as guar gum, which are completely fermented, contribute about 60% of their gross energy as SCFA. Pectin is about 95% fermented and so about 57% is converted to SCFA. Some unavailable carbohydrates are poorly fermented, for example Solka-floc® cellulose, and so contributes little to SCFA production.

Other unavailable carbohydrates such as Polydextrose manufactured by industry, as distinct from those prepared in the laboratory (Figdor & Bianchine, 1983), are fermented to an uncertain extent. In the rat about 75% of this carbohydrate is fermented when it is included in a fibre-free diet, and about the same amount is fermented *in vitro* by human faecal microorganisms (Livesey *et al.*, 1993). Furthermore, about 5% of Polydextrose is free glucose, which will be absorbed in the small intestine. Therefore, a likely high estimate of the percentage conversion of Polydextrose to SCFA is $\approx 42\%$ $[(0.75 - 0.05) \times 0.6]$.

It has not been possible to give any precise values for SCFA availability from the sugar alcohols in Table 28.2. This is partly because the amount reaching the large intestine may depend on whether intake is with food or with drink alone (Beaugerie *et al.*, 1990; Livesey, 1990*b*) and partly because of the scant information available on their utilization from solid foods. With

Table 28.2. *Heats of combustion of carbohydrates and percentage of energy available as carbohydrate and short-chain fatty acids (SCFA). Based on data from Livesey (1993)*

Substrate	Heat of combustion (ΔH) (kJ/g)	Available as carbohydrate (%)	Available as SCFA (%)[a]
Polysaccharides			
Average for the unavailable carbohydrates of mixed diets	17.2	0	40
Sokla-floc cellulose	17.5	0	6
Psyllium gum	15.5	0	20
Guar gum	17.5	0	60
Gum arabic	17.2	0	60
Pectin	16.5	0	57
Sugar-beet fibre	17.6	0	44
Oligosaccharides			
Polydextrose®	17.0	≈ 5	≤ 45
Polyfructose	16.9	0	60
Soya bean OS	16.8	0–0.2	≤ 65
Sugar alcohols			
Xylitol	17.0	>50	≤ 29
Mannitol	16.7	0	≤ 48
Sorbitol	16.7	≤ 80	≥ 12
Lactitol	17.0	0	58
Maltitol	17.0	≤ 80	≥ 12

[a] Calculated as 0.60 times the proportion of the dose fermented in the large intestine (Livesey, 1993), the remainder being the heat of fermentation (0.05), hydrogen and methane production (0.05) and bacteria production (0.30).
Based on data from Livesey (1993).

drinks, intestinal hurry may increase the proportion of the ingested dose that escapes small-intestinal digestion. All the values in Table 28.2 are for consumption with solid foods. It is likely that different values would be obtained for some sugar alcohols, particularly sorbitol, maltitol and isomalt, should they be included in liquid enteral feeds. All sugar alcohols in current use are easily fermented anaerobically, but not all the ingested dose reaches the colon. Some is absorbed in the small intestine and excreted in the urine (e.g. mannitol) or metabolized in the tissues (e.g. sorbitol and maltitol). Some sugar alcohols, such as lactitol, almost completely escape digestion and absorption in the small intestine (>98%), and so are efficiently converted to SCFA in the colon. The disposition of sugar alcohols has recently been reviewed (Livesey, 1993).

The contribution of SCFA to energy requirements

Since SCFA are almost completely absorbed in the human large intestine (McNeil *et al.*, 1978; Ruppin *et al.*, 1980), a question arises as to how much of the human energy requirement is made available from these acids. There is little quantiative information in the literature that answers this question, so we have made calculations based on the intakes and faecal losses of energy, carbohydrates and nitrogen and other calculations based on differences of arterial and portal venous concentrations.

SCFA production based on the intake and fermentability of unavailable carbohydrates

For mixed Western-style diets the ratio of SCFA (kJ) production from unavailable carbohydrates to total metabolizable energy (ME) intake is shown in Fig. 28.2. Data in this figure are based on information collected (Livesey, 1990*a*) from the literature on 17 diets, and the following formulae:

$$SCFA\ (\text{kJ}) = \Delta H \times UC \times D_{UC} \times 0.6 \tag{28.1}$$

$$ME\ (\text{kJ}) = 0.96 \times E - 9UC - 30N_{\text{d}} \tag{28.2}$$

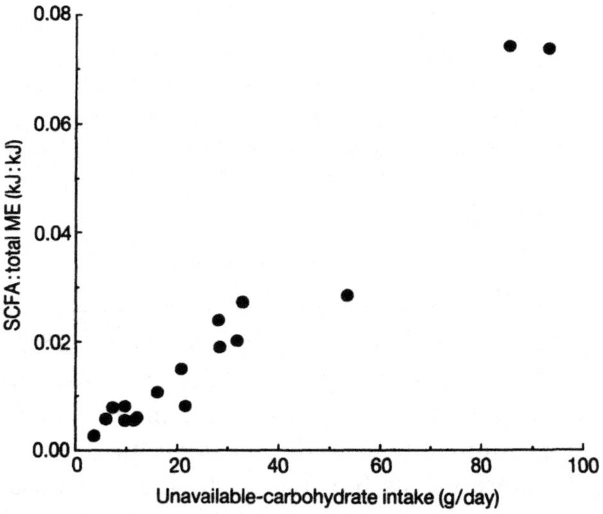

Fig. 28.2. Production of short-chain fatty acids (SCFA) with increasing daily intake of unavailable carbohydrate: data based on the intake and apparent digestibility of unavailable carbohydrate (ME, metabolizable energy), estimated using eqs. 28.1 and 28.2 (see text) with inputs for mixed diets from Livesey (1990*a*). Linear regression indicated $SCFA{:}ME = -0.002$ (SD 0.002, NS) + 0.00081 (SD 0.00004, $p < 0{\cdot}001$) UC; residual SD = 0.047; $r^2 = 0.957$.

SCFA in eq. 28.1 is the energy made available daily as SCFA, ΔH is the heat of combustion of unavailable carbohydrate (on average 17.2 kJ/g), *UC* is the unavailable carbohydrate intake from mixed diets (g daily), D_{UC} is the apparent digestibility [(intake – faecal loss)/intake] of the unavailable carbohydrate, 0.6 is the fraction of energy in a carbohydrate that is fermented to SCFA (Livesey, 1993), *ME* is the metabolizable energy intake from the whole diet, *E* is the corresponding daily gross energy from the whole diet (kJ), and N_d is the daily dietary nitrogen (protein) intake (g). The equation for calculating *ME* was derived from a detailed analysis of results involving the use of over 30 diets with varying unavailable carbohydrate content (Livesey, 1991).

At a daily intake of 20 g unavailable carbohydrate (as measured in various energy-balance studies; Livesey, 1990*a*), which is typical of intake in Western society, the contribution of SCFA to energy requirements on the basis of eqs. 28.1 and 28.2 is about 1.5% of *ME* (Fig. 28.2). This amount corresponds to about 150 kJ on a 10-MJ diet. Assuming molar proportions of SCFA of 0.60 : 0.24 : 0.14 for acetic, propionic and butyric acids, respectively (Cummings, 1981), which corresponds to energy proportions of 0.43 : 0.30 : 0.27 (Livesey, 1993), there are daily productions of 65 kJ or 74 mmol acetic acid, 46 kJ or 30 mmol propionic acid, and 38 kJ or 18 mmol butyric acid. The total SCFA production from the daily intake of 20 g unavailable carbohydrate is, therefore, about 122 mmol. It is possible that more carbohydrate is fermented than is indicated for the various assays of unavailable carbohydrate that have been applied to mixed diets. Thus according to Table 28.1 it may be as high as 28 g. The additional 8 g is of material that is easily fermented and would supply an additional 70 kJ of SCFA energy, making a total SCFA production of about 180 mmol/day. Therefore, in normal Western individuals, SCFA uptake would correspond to about 2.5% of energy requirement. As described below, other estimates are possible too. Also, the intake of unavailable carbohydrates might be 2–4 times greater for some traditional Asian and African diets.

SCFA production based on faecal protein excretion

A different approach to calculating the amount of SCFA produced in the colon considers the expected production of one fermentation product relative to another. For example, bacterial mass excreted in faeces can be used to estimate the extent of fermentation. In humans the faecal loss of bacteria (Stephen & Cummings, 1980) and non-carbohydrate (Livesey, 1990*a*; Wisker & Feldheim, 1992) is greater than expected from the amounts of unavailable carbohydrate apparently fermented. To account for this discrepancy, it has been postulated that more starch reaches the large intestine than is evident from the various assays for unavailable carbohydrate (see Livesey, 1990*a*). Additionally, other carbohydrates enter the colon and are not usually measured, for example polyfructose (inulin), oligofructose, the raffinose family of saccharides from beans, oligogalactose in milk, etc. (Tables 28.1 and 28.2).

Since the efficiency of conversion of carbohydrate to bacterial energy is about 30 kJ/100 kJ of carbohydrate fermented (Livesey, 1993), and since bacteria consist largely of protein, so accounting for most of the nitrogen present in faeces (highly indigestible protein sources are atypical for subjects in Western societies), an upper estimate to total SCFA production can be made from the following equation:

$$SCFA\ (\mathrm{kJ}) = 6.25 \times N_{\mathrm{f}} \times 23.6 \times 1.85 \tag{28.3}$$

In this equation, $6.25 \times N_{\mathrm{f}}$ is faecal protein, measured as nitrogen N_{f} (g) and is approximate, since some faecal nitrogen will be in the form of ammonia; 23.6 is the heat of combustion of protein (kJ/g) and 1.85 is the ratio of SCFA production to bacterial protein production expected during fermentation (Livesey, 1993). As shown in Fig. 28.3 the estimate of total SCFA production, expressed as a proportion of total *ME* intake, increases with increasing intake of unavailable carbohydrate. Unlike in Fig. 28.2, where the intercept is near zero, a positive intercept is found in Fig. 28.3. As intake of unavailable carbohydrate approaches zero, the data tend to fall towards zero SCFA production, i.e. fall from the intercept towards the origin. What happens to total SCFA production in this region of the curve is uncertain, as the approach to the origin may result not from a change in total SCFA production, but from a resorption of bacterial protein due to long transit times through the colon on low-residue diets. Such resorption would lead to an underestimation of SCFA production.

Fig. 28.3 indicates that at a daily intake of 20 g unavailable carbohydrate and 10 MJ metabolizable energy, typical of that eaten in Western societies, 4% of the energy requirement is met by SCFA. On a 10-MJ diet this corresponds to about 400 kJ of SCFA daily. Again assuming an energy ratio of 0.43 : 0.30 : 0.27 for the acetic : propionic : butyric acids (Livesey, 1993), this quantity of energy amounts to 172 kJ or 196 mmol acetic, 120 kJ or 78 mmol propionic and 108 kJ or 49 mmol butyric acids, totalling 323 mmol SCFA daily. The amount of SCFA produced (323 mmol/day) would require the fermentation of 54 g of carbohydrate, assuming this as the only substrate.

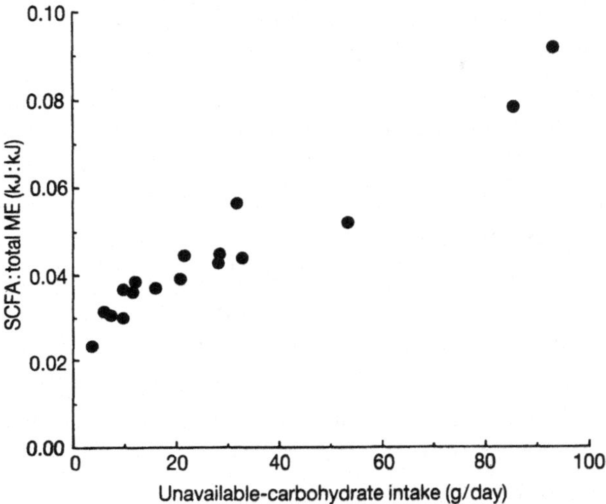

Fig. 28.3. Production of short-chain fatty acids (SCFA) with increasing daily intake of unavailable carbohydrate: data based on the faecal loss of nitrogen. Data are estimated using eqs. 28.2 and 28.3 (see text) with inputs for mixed diets from Livesey (1990*a*). Linear regression indicated $SCFA{:}ME = 0.027$ (SD 0.002, $p < 0.001$) + 0.00063 (SD 0.00004, $p < 0.001$) UC; residual SD = 0.046; $r^2 = 0.933$.

SCFA production based on arterio-venous exchanges

Another way of estimating the extent of SCFA absorption is from measurements of differences in arterio-portal venous (A-PV) concentration. In one study carried out in Philadelphia, USA (Skutches *et al.*, 1979) the plasma A-PV concentration difference of acetate was measured in patients undergoing elective surgery, and found to be 73 μmol/l. This corresponds to an uptake of 105 mmol/day, if it is assumed that the blood-flow rate is 1 l/min. Unfortunately, no details were given of the period that had elapsed since the last meal, or possible bowel preparation prior to surgery. Nevertheless, the value is very similar to that calculated from A-PV plasma measurements made on a group of patients undergoing cholecystectomy (Dankert, Zijlstra & Wolthers, 1981) and virtually identical to the calculated value in Fig. 28.2. In another study (Peters, Pomare & Fisher, 1992) of A-PV plasma measurements in patients undergoing cholecystectomy, lower results were obtained (A-PV, 51 μmol/l), which can be explained by the ingestion of a polysaccharide-free diet for 24 h prior to surgery. In yet another study carried out in Soweto, South Africa, the plasma A-PV concentration difference in subjects undergoing surgery following trauma or accidental injury was 137 μmol/l for acetate, and

262 μmol/l for total SCFA (acetate, propionate and butyrate). This has been calculated to correspond to 337 mmol/day, assuming blood flow was 1 l/min (Cummings, Gibson & Macfarlane, 1989). The value, which is twofold higher than obtained in the Philadelphia subjects, may overestimate SCFA uptake in subjects eating a Western-style diet, partly because the estimated exchange has been based on measurements made on plasma and not whole blood, and partly because the study was in black Africans. The concentration of acetate in red cells is only 40–80% of that in plasma (Neilsen, Owen-Ash & Thor, 1978; Akanji, 1987) and that in whole blood about 80–85% of that in plasma, and the intake of unavailable carbohydrate in black Africans is usually greater than for subjects eating a Western-style diet. Furthermore, the estimates for SCFA uptake from A-PV measurements alone are only approximate, partly because blood flow rate is needed to convert A-PV measurements into the rates of flux (blood flow was not measured in any of the above studies and its prediction must depend on haemodynamic stability of the patient which is affected by injury, blood loss and drug administration) and partly because of the obvious difficulty in extrapolating from a single A-PV difference to 24-h values (especially in patients whose recent dietary intake was not controlled or assessed). The effects of surgical or accidental injury on the exchange of various metabolites, including the SCFA across the gut and portal-drained viscera (A-PV exchange) and their effects on blood flow remain uncertain.

SCFA supply limits their metabolism

Both Figs. 28.2 and 28.3 suggest that up to 8% of the energy requirements of humans can be met by SCFA derived from fermentation in the gut, but normally it is 2–4%. These rates are small by comparison with the possible rates at which SCFA can be used when they are administered directly. In both normal and type II diabetic subjects studied by Akanji, Bruce & Frayn (1989), infusions of intravenous sodium acetate were used at a rate equal to 40% of the non-protein energy expenditure, and in uraemic subjects undergoing renal dialysis, the utilization of acetate reached 40% of energy expenditure (Skutches *et al.*, 1983). In the last study there was no indication that the limit of acetate utilization had been reached, although the rate of acetate utilization from the circulation may be limited by simultaneous provision of glucose (Akanji & Hockaday, 1990). Up to 60% of total energy requirement of the rat can be supplied by SCFA substrates (Birkhahn *et al.*, 1977; Birkhahn & Border, 1978; Kirvela & Takala, 1986; Kripke *et al.*, 1988). In sheep adapted to high rates of SCFA utilization, butyric and propionic acids were each capable of meeting the maintenance energy requirements, at least in the short term (see Blaxter, 1989). It seems that it is the production and not the utilization of SCFA that limits their contribution to energy metabolism.

Stoichiometry of fermentation

The stoichiometry of anaerobic fermentation in humans is uncertain and probably varies in different situations with time. It is affected by the subtrate fermented, the microbial population present in the colon, the rate of fermentation, transit time through the colon, accumulation of end products, and the presence of other dietary constituents, for example sulphate (Macfarlane, 1991). Nevertheless, an attempt is made below to obtain an insight into the stoichiometry of fermentation from the point of view of energy. There is particular concern over the disposal of the hydrogen donated from carbohydrates during the fermentation. It must be remembered that about half of the energy in carbohydrate is associated with its hydrogen content, and, therefore, knowledge of the disposition of hydrogen is crucial to a precise understanding of the consequences of fermentation, including the provision of energy to humans.

Hydrogen sinks during anaerobic fermentation

Fermentation in the large intestine is exclusively anaerobic. In order to obtain energy in an environment without oxygen, electrons from oxidizable substrates must be transferred to electron acceptors other than oxygen. Consequently, the fermentation products are highly reduced. When carbohydrate is fermented anaerobically, acetic acid is usually the major SCFA end product, though this acid has an oxidation state similar to that of carbohydrate. Not surprisingly, therefore, other end products are more reduced than is carbohydrate, as is shown in Table 28.3. In this table the relative oxidation states are expressed as the ratio of oxidizable to oxidized electrons in the substrate and products. Bacterial cells (consisting mainly of protein) and butyric acid are more reduced than carbohydrate and constitute important hydrogen sinks, as is made evident further below. Other hydrogen sinks are hydrogen gas, methane and hydrogen sulphide (and water where the oxygen is donated from sulphate). These sinks are considered in detail in other chapters, and, therefore, here we are only concerned with the stoichiometric implications.

If it is assumed that each day about 35 g carbohydrate is fermented in humans (Cummings, Allison & Macfarlane, 1986; Table 28.1) and 150 ml of methane and 600 ml hydrogen gas are produced (Marthinsen & Flemming,

Table 28.3. *The ratio of oxidizable to oxidized electrons in carbohydrate and the products of anaerobic fermentation*

Substrate	Formula	Oxidizable electrons	Oxidized electrons	Oxidizable/ oxidized
Glucose	$C_6H_{12}O_6$	36	12	3
Acetic acid	$C_2H_4O_2$	12	4	3
Propionic acid	$C_3H_6O_2$	18	4	4.5
Butyric acid	$C_4H_8O_2$	24	4	6
Bacterial cells	$C_6H_{12}O_3$	36	6	6
Methane	CH_4	8	0	∞
Hydrogen gas	H_2	2	0	∞
Hydrogen sulphide	H_2S	2[a]	0	∞

[a] Sulphur not included, otherwise 8.

1982; Flemming & Calloway, 1983), then 1 mol of methane and 4 mol of hydrogen gas are produced for each 29 mol of carbohydrate fermented (see Livesey & Elia, 1988). The proportion of carbohydrate energy converted to combustible gases is possibly an overestimate if more carbohydrate enters the colon, a possibility argued in the foregoing. Together the gaseous products use up only a small number of hydrogen atoms [H], at most 16 g-atoms per 29 mol monosaccharide (or 0.55 g-atom/mol), about equally divided between the two gases:

$$H_2CO_3 + 8[H] \rightarrow CH_4 + 3H_2O \quad (28.4)$$

$$8[H] \rightarrow 4H_2 \quad (28.5)$$

Thirty-hour studies in an enclosed respiratory chamber (indirect calorimetry) have shown that within those subjects who excrete methane, the hydrogen and methane production may be inversely related across time (S. Poppitt, M. Elia and G. Livesey, unpublished data). Between subjects, hydrogen sulphide production tends to be inversely related to methane production (Gibson, Cummings & Macfarlane, 1988; Christl, Gibson & Cummings, 1992). Dietary sulphate is a significant oxidant for sulphate-reducing bacteria that produce hydrogen sulphide (Florin *et al.*, 1991), but has been reported not to affect breath hydrogen concentrations (Christl *et al.*, 1992). Mucin, a source of sulphate, depressed methanogenesis *in vitro* (Demeyer *et al.*, 1989) and dietary sulphate depressed methane production in volunteers (Christl *et al.*, 1992). The physiology and ecology of sulphate reducing bacteria have recently been reviewed (Gibson, 1990). The presence of sulphate in the colon, and in faecal incubations *in vitro*, decreased methane production and appears, therefore, to be an alternative rather than an additional hydrogen sink:

$$H_2SO_4 + 8[H] \rightarrow H_2S + 4H_2O \qquad (28.6)$$

Possible stoichiometry of fermentation

Based on the usual ratios of SCFA produced, anaerobic fermentation appeared to progress with the production of a large excess of [H]; it was 256 g-atoms per 58 mol monosaccharide fermented and was much in excess of the hydrogen used for combustible gas production (approximately 32[H], i.e. 58 × 0.55) in this instance (Livesey & Elia, 1988):

$$58C_6H_{12}O_6 + 36H_2O \rightarrow 60CH_3\text{—}CO_2H + 24C_2H_5\text{—}CO_2H + 16C_3H_7\text{—}CO_2H + 92CO_2 + 256[H] \qquad (28.7)$$

When bacterial cells ($C_6H_{12}O_3$) are produced in amounts equivalent to 30% of the energy in the carbohydrate fermented, which is consistent with observations in humans (Livesey, 1990*a*, 1991), the production of excess hydrogen atoms is less (172 g-atom per 72 mol glucose fermented), but still in excess of that expected to be used for gas production (approximately 40[H], i.e. 72 × 0.55):

$$72C_6H_{12}O_6 \rightarrow 60CH_3\text{—}CO_2H + 24C_2H_5\text{—}CO_2H + 16C_3H_7\text{—}CO_2H + 92CO_2 + 6H_2O + 14C_6H_{12}O_3 + 172[H] \qquad (28.8)$$

Stoichiometry with butyrate as a major hydrogen sink

The proportions of SCFA produced during fermentation are dependent on the nature of the substrate being fermented. These ratios are commonly expressed on a molar basis, but in Table 28.4 values are given on an energy (kJ) basis. Acetate, propionate and butyrate contribute ≈90% of total SCFA in the colon (Cummings, 1981) and faecal incubation systems (Mortensen, Holtung & Rasmussen, 1988*a*). It seems that butyrate may contribute from below 10 to about 50% of the energy made available from these acids (Table 28.4). Large amounts of butyrate are produced when starch is fermented, when it accounts for almost 50% of the SCFA production (Table 28.4). Comparisons between substrates in Table 28.4 are based on studies with human faecal incubations carried out in several laboratories. The extent of interlaboratory variation is not yet known and could be high.

Table 28.4. *Proportion of SCFA energy (kJ) made available as butyrate, propionate and acetate, based on studies* in vitro. *Sum of proportions approximates unity*

Substrate	Butyric acid	Propionic acid	Acetic acid	Reference
Pectin	0.04	0.21	0.74	Englyst *et al.* (1987)
Xylan	0.06	0.23	0.71	Englyst *et al.* (1987)
Arabinogalactan	0.14	0.51	0.35	Englyst *et al.* (1987)
Gum arabic	0.17	0.28	0.56	Adiotomre *et al.* (1990)
Arabinogalactan	0.30	0.27	0.42	Vince *et al.* (1990)
Pectin	0.32	0.17	0.51	Vince *et al.* (1990)
Cellulose	0.33	0.24	0.43	Vince *et al.* (1990)
Wheat bran	0.34	0.23	0.42	McBurney & Thompson (1987)
Lactulose	0.36	0.16	0.48	Vince *et al.* (1990)
Oat bran	0.38	0.24	0.38	McBurney & Thompson (1987)
Starch	0.45	0.24	0.31	Englyst *et al.* (1987)
Resistant starch	0.55	0.21	0.24	Englyst & Macfarlane (1986)

Since butyrate is more reduced than is carbohydrate, it may be regarded as an important hydrogen sink. The molar ratio of acetate : propionate : butyrate with resistant starch as the fermentation substrate was 41:21:38 (Englyst & Macfarlane, 1986). With this ratio the following stoichiometry applies, which is again associated with [H] production in excess of expectations (36[H], i.e. 66 × 0.55):

$$66C_6H_{12}O_6 + 2H_2O \rightarrow 41CH_3\text{—}CO_2H + 21C_2H_5\text{—}CO_2H + 38C_3H_7\text{—}CO_2H + 99CO_2 + 202[H] \quad (28.9)$$

Once more considering bacterial cell ($C_6H_{12}O_3$) production as a hydrogen sink, with cell production equalling 30% of the carbohydrate fermented, the following stoichiometry is derived when butyrate production is high, as with resistant starch (Table 28.4):

$$82C_6H_{12}O_6 \rightarrow 41CH_3\text{—}CO_2H + 21C_2H_5\text{—}CO_2H + 38C_3H_7\text{—}CO_2H + 99CO_2 + 16C_6H_{12}O_3 + 46H_2O + 106[H] \quad (28.10)$$

In eq. 28.10, virtually all the hydrogen in the carbohydrate would be accounted for by the end products of fermentation. Acetogenesis provides a further hydrogen sink (Demeyer *et al.*, 1989), but its activity in humans is uncertain. In any event, acetogenic activity is accounted for in the above stoichiometries as one of the processes that contributes to acetic acid production:

$$2CO_2 + 4H_2 \rightarrow CH_3—CO_2H + 2H_2O \qquad (28.11)$$

Inferences from the stoichiometric considerations

Five inferences can be drawn from eqs. 28.4–28.11. First: unlike sulphate reduction and methane production which deacidify the colon (cf. eqs. 28.5 and 28.6), acetogenesis (eq. 28.11) should lead to acidification. Lactulose, 20 g twice weekly for 1 week, leads to acidification of the stool in non-methane excreters more than in methane excreters (Flick & Perman, 1989). Acidification may be protective against colorectal cancer (Kritchevsky, 1986), a disorder more prevalent in methane-producers than in non-methane-producers (Hains *et al.*, 1977; Piqué *et al.*, 1984). In this context, the occurrence of acetogenesis in the colon might not be beneficial as a hydrogen sink, although it does salvage energy that would otherwise be wasted.

Second: a consequence of the production of butyric acid and bacterial cell mass is that less hydrogen is available for the production of hydrogen gas, methane and hydrogen sulphide. The last may be toxic to the colonocyte (Aslam *et al.*, 1992). Additionally, butyric acid is an important substrate in colonocyte respiration (Roediger, 1980) and is likely to enhance the repair of any chemically induced damage (as discussed in subsequent sections). A higher bacterial cell production would also suggest that nitrogen is incorporated into bacterial protein rather than released as ammonia, which is toxic at high concentrations, and an inhibitor of mitochondrial respiration and cellular function, e.g. pinocytic and lysosomal activity (Livesey *et al.*, 1980).

Third: the conversion ratio of carbohydrate utilized to CO_2 produced during fermentation varies in eqs. 28.7–28.10, being 1.59, 1.27, 1.51 and 1.21 mol CO_2/mol monosaccharide, respectively. Preferential production of bacterial mass during fermentation decreases the gas production, both in terms of [H] excess (hence potential for H_2 and methane production) and in terms of CO_2. It might be predicted that bloating, due to fermentation of carbohydrates, may depend not only on the amount of substrate undergoing fermentation but also on the stoichiometry of the fermentation process.

Fourth: a consequence of bacterial cell production is the recovery of less carbohydrate energy as SCFA, 61% v. 76% for the usual ratio of SCFA produced (eqs. 28.8 and 28.7) and 65% and 81% when butyric acid is produced in high proportion relative to other SCFA (eqs. 28.10 and 28.9). For the purpose of calculating the energy values of fermentable carbohydrates in humans, it is the 61% value that best fits the experimental data for mixed diets (Livesey, 1990*a*, 1991) and appears to be applicable to most fermentable carbohydrates (Livesey, 1993).

Fifth: in eq. 28.10, which shows the fermentation of starch, only 6[H] are produced, so there is no excess hydrogen, and the hydrogen sinks appear to be fully accounted for. However, for production of the usual amounts of hydrogen gas, methane and bacterial matter and ratios of SCFA produced in humans, eq. 28.8 is more likely to apply. In this equation (eq. 28.8) no more than 80% of the hydrogen entering the fermentation process is accounted for. It is possible that the ratios of SCFA produced are different from what is currently believed. A higher proportion of acetate and butyrate relative to propionate implies a greater disposal of [H]. Finally, the complex fermentation process may involve other substrates (e.g. protein) and end products (other hydrogen sinks, e.g. conversion of unsaturated to saturated fatty acids), and there may be some absorption of intermediates, such as lactic acid. The contribution of luminally derived lactic acid to human metabolism is unknown, and may be significant, especially during gastrointestinal disease. The absorption of lactic acid would imply an increased efficiency with which energy is salvaged from the carbohydrate that is fermented, but it is possible that less carbohydrate is fermented when lactic acid becomes a major end product.

SCFA uptake from the colon

SCFA may enter colonocytes by at least two mechanisms. Their relative importance seems to depend on animal species, site of large-intestinal absorption and concentration of SCFA (Engelhardt & Rechkemmer, 1982; Holtug, 1989; Engelhardt *et al.*, 1991). At the pH in the intestinal lumen, mucosal tissue and plasma, >97% of SCFA is unprotonated and so is hydrophilic and unable to pass through cell membranes. Equilibrium with the protonated form allows SCFA movement from the lumen to the circulation via cellular and paracellular routes (Rechkemmer & Engelhardt, 1982; Holtug, 1989).

$$R{-}CO_2^- + H^+ \Leftrightarrow RCO_2H \xleftarrow[\text{Lumen}]{} \| \xrightarrow[\text{Cytoplasm}]{} \| \xrightarrow[\text{Circulation}]{} R{-}CO_2H$$

$$\Leftrightarrow R{-}CO_2^- + H^+$$

The higher concentration of SCFA in the lumen than in the circulation creates a concentration gradient along which SCFA flow. The higher concentration of protons (lower pH) in the lumen compared with the cytosol and plasma must also drive the absorption of organic anions. A linear dependence of SCFA absorption is expected under this circumstance and is observed for acetic, propionic and butyric acids in the range 0–90 mmol/l in the human colon (Ruppin *et al.*, 1980). The whole process, being a displaced equilibrium, requires no energy expenditure to move the SCFA from the lumen to the circulation.

SCFA uptake is thought to be made more rapid by a luminal cell membrane Na^+/H^+ antiport (Binder & Rawlins, 1973). Entry of a proton into the lumen in exchange for a sodium ion also contributes to sodium absorption. The increase in proton concentration at the luminal surface increases further the concentration of the protonated SCFA at the luminal surface and so increases its rate of uptake. However, a lower concentration in the cytoplasm causes the SCFA to dissociate there, replacing the proton ejected at the Na^+/H^+ antiport. When in operation, this mechanism must result in the net absorption of the solution salt of the SCFA, acidification of the colon and alkalinization of mucosal cells and the circulation.

Potentially the colon could make a contribution to the regulation of acid–base balance if it could switch between uptake of the salts of SCFA. This is analogous to the pharmacological use of acetate salt for the treatment of acidosis (Cash *et al.*, 1969; Ekblad *et al.*, 1985).

It is possible that the major function of the Na^+/H^+ antiport is to protect the colonocyte from becoming as acidic as the colonic lumen. There is also discussion of a K^+/H^+ antiport that may operate in the same way as the Na^+/H^+ antiport. Absorption of the sodium salt of the SCFA would influence systemic acid–base balance, respiratory compensation and the interpretation of the respiratory exchange ratio (discussed further below). Acidification of the cell cytoplasm by SCFA might also drive sodium absorption. When sodium transport is abolished, SCFA anion and proton uptake are the same (Engelhardt & Rechkemmer, 1982), which might suggest that the protonated SCFA freely pass through the cell membrane. However, an alternative mechanism exists.

The luminal cell surface also appears to carry a SCFA anion/HCO_3^- antiport. HCO_3^- and H^+ are produced in the cytoplasm from CO_2 and water, and catalysed by carbonic anhydrase, to be exchanged through the antiport with the negatively charged SCFA anion. The net result is that the absorption of SCFA as the anion may accompany the H^+ generated by the carbonic anhydrase, so that SCFA appear to be absorbed in the protonated form. By this mechanism an elevated concentration of CO_2 in the cytoplasm could drive absorption of the SCFA. Carbon dioxide could be derived from fermentation in the colonic lumen. Moreover, the mechanism of SCFA uptake may operate secondarily to the facilitation of CO_2 absorption from the colon by carbonic anhydrase, the latter process perhaps being the principal function of this enzyme. It is notable that HCO_3^- accumulation in the lumen is not stoichiometric with SCFA absorption (Umesaki *et al.*, 1979), suggesting that the bicarbonate exchange mechanism is not the only mechanism of SCFA uptake.

The involvement of the above antiports, or transporters, could explain the observation of saturation kinetics in SCFA uptake in certain tissue preparations and cells (Holtug, 1989). It should be noted that acidification of the colon, due principally to the Na^+/H^+ antiport, is contrary to the general view that the SCFA anion/HCO_3^- exchange results in deacidification of the colon by HCO_3^- released into the lumen. This stresses the poor state of knowledge about the precise mechanism of uptake of SCFA in the colon.

Sodium entering the colonocyte in association with SCFA anions may enter the circulation via the basement membrane driven by the Na^+/K^+ ATPase, thus short chain fatty anion absorption might stimulate sodium absorption with an associated energy cost. However, this cost is associated with sodium uptake, not SCFA uptake. Through this mechanism it may appear that SCFA absorption is actively supported. Such has been observed in the rat distal colon at low butyrate concentrations, but diffusion appears to be most important at concentrations near those found *in vivo* (Rabbani & Binder, 1989). The principal conclusion to be drawn here is that there is no evidence of energy expenditure being obligatory for the absorption of SCFA.

Interorgan transport and systemic metabolism of SCFA

Not all the energy in butyric acid entering the colonocyte is transferred to the circulation. This is because this SCFA is the preferred fuel of the colonic mucosal tissue (Roediger, 1980, 1982). For their metabolism, SCFA (like the long-chain fatty acids) require activation with coenzyme-A (CoA). This is energetically expensive, requiring the equivalent of two molecules of ATP (1 ATP to 1 AMP + PP_i). Butyryl-CoA may be partially oxidized to acetyl-

CoA via β-oxidation. Some acetic acid produced in the gut lumen by fermentation might also be used to form acetyl-CoA in human colonocytes. Mitochondrial acetyl-CoA is used in the citric acid cycle for ATP production, for the synthesis of ketone bodies (Henning & Hird, 1972) and, after transfer to the cytosol, for the synthesis of lipid (Strange & Dietschy, 1983). The ketones enter the circulation principally as β-hydroxybutyric acid, but the lipids may become incorporated into the colonocytes (e.g. membranes), some of which are lost into the colon during exfoliation.

Circulating butyric acid is partly bound to albumin (Rémésy & Demigné, 1974). Propionic acid may also be slightly bound, as it displaces from this protein the branched-chain oxo-acids, the transamination products of the amino acids leucine, valine and isoleucine, though less powerfully than butyric acid (Livesey & Lund, 1982). The interaction of acetic and β-hydroxybutyric acids with albumin is almost negligible. In addition, peripheral human blood has low concentrations of butyrate and propionate. All the SCFA (acetate, propionate and butyrate) are more abundant in portal blood.

Based on the concentrations in peripheral and portal blood, about 75% of acetate, 90% of propionate and 95% of butyrate are extracted during a single pass of blood through the human liver (Dankert *et al.*, 1981; Peters *et al.*, 1992). If such fractional extractions apply to the quantities of SCFA that are considered to be produced in normal humans (see Figs. 28.2 and 28.3 for their energy content), it can be calculated that their complete oxidation in the liver could account for more than a third of the energy expenditure there (Elia, 1992*b*). However, not all the SCFA taken up by the liver are oxidized there (see below). Furthermore, after ethanol administration, studies in arteriovenous difference show the liver to be a net producer of acetic acid (Lundquist *et al.*, 1962). Under these conditions a variety of human tissues, including skeletal muscle (Lindeneg *et al.*, 1964; Jorfeldt & Juhlin-Dannfelt, 1978) and brain (Juhlin-Dannfelt, 1977) utilize considerable quantities of acetate (see below).

In humans, the only SCFA to reach the circulation beyond the liver in appreciable quantity is acetate. The peripheral venous plasma concentration of acetate in normal humans, as measured by gas–liquid chromatography, is about 50 μmol/l in the 12-h fasting state, rising to 114 μmol/l after 108 h of fasting (Scheppach *et al.*, 1991). Propionate and butyrate, in contrast, were found to be below the detection limit (2 μmol/l) in forearm arterial and venous blood in the studies of Pomare, Branch & Cummings (1985), and 4 μmol/l for propionate and only trace quantities for butyrate were found in peripheral venous blood in the studies of Peters *et al.* (1992). The low concentrations of propionate and butyrate in peripheral venous blood serve to demonstrate the efficiency of the liver in extracting these substrates. Indeed, 10 mmol propionate and 10 mmol butyrate administered by mouth with 30 mmol acetate in water failed to render peripheral propionate and butyrate concentrations detectable, whereas the acetate concentration increased by about 150 μmol/l (Pomare *et al.*, 1985). In this instance the SCFA were considered to be absorbed from the stomach largely in the protonated form, due to the low pH there.

Acetate in peripheral blood is not entirely derived from the colon, since several tissues both produce and consume acetate simultaneously, as demonstrated in the dog (Bleiberg *et al.*, 1992). Butyrate may reach the peripheral circulation in patients with liver disease (Muto & Takahasi, 1964; Muto, 1966) and in hepatectomized dogs (Zieve & Nicoloff, 1976). Elevated plasma concentrations of butyrate and propionate have been suggested to be partly responsible, along with ammonia, for the development of hepatic coma (Zieve *et al.*, 1974), which is due to toxicity to the central nervous system (Samson, Dahl & Dahl, 1956). It is interesting that a change from butyrate fermentation to acetate fermentation using lactulose (Mortensen *et al.*, 1988*a*,*b*, 1990*a*) may be one mechanism by which this disaccharide acts to rouse patients from hepatic coma. Starch in the colon (Cummings *et al.*, 1990), as a producer of butyrate (Table 28.4), might, therefore, be damaging in this condition.

Because a large variety of methods have been used to assay acetate, it is not possible to state precisely how the circulating concentration of acetate differs in the variety of circumstances examined (see Chapter 3). Therefore, incremental values or multiples of basal values for healthy people may be more reliable than absolute values, especially at low concentrations. After 20 g of pectin was fed to normal volunteers, the peripheral venous concentration of acetate increased twofold, and after 20 g lactulose, it increased fourfold, each due to large intestinal fermentation (Pomare *et al.*, 1985). The plasma concentration of acetate is reported to increase about 1.3 times normal in severely ill patients and to increase further to twice normal in severely ill patients receiving total parenteral nutritional solutions buffered with acetate (Lazarus & Stein, 1988). In kidney dialysis patients, and in normal subjects ingesting ethanol, acetate concentrations may rise to more than 1 mmol/l (Lundquist *et al.*, 1962, 1973; Juhlin-Dannfelt, 1977; Tollinger, Vreman & Weiner, 1979; Weiner, 1982; Skutches *et al.*, 1983). In experimental studies in humans, a plasma concentration of 0.5–1 mmol/l may be reached by intravenous acetate feeding (Akanji *et al.*, 1989; Akanji & Hockaday, 1990) and a value as high as 2.0–2.5 mmol/l has been obtained for a period of about 1 h (Weiner, 1982).

Arteriovenous difference studies show that beyond the liver, acetic acid is used by the human forearm, where it may contribute about 1–5% of energy expenditure of resting muscle (Coppack *et al.*, 1990; M. Elia, unpublished data), and about 3% of the energy expenditure of the human heart (Lindeneg *et al.*, 1964). When the circulating acetate concentration is increased to 0.8–1.1 mmol/l by the consumption of alcohol (typically about 25 g), acetate taken up by the tissues contributes 12–22% of energy expenditure of muscle both at rest and during exercise (Lundquist *et al.* 1973; Jorfeldt & Juhlin-Dannfelt, 1978), 15–20% of energy expenditure of the heart (Lindeneg *et al.*, 1964), and about 6% of energy expenditure of the brain (Juhlin-Dannfelt, 1977). In these calculations, we have assumed that the acetate taken up by the tissues is completely oxidized, that the whole-blood concentration of acetate is 85% of the plasma concentration, and that the fractional extraction of acetate from whole blood is similar to that in plasma. The above results are not too surpising since 60–100% of the ethanol metabolized in human liver is released as acetate (Lundquist *et al.*, 1962). Acetate uptake by human adipose tissue accessed by arteriovenous differences is small after an overnight fast, and surprisingly shows no increase after ethanol ingestion (Frayn *et al.*, 1990).

The utilization of acetate by a variety of tissues such as in the heart, brain, forearm and leg is dependent on the circulating concentration of acetate, both before and after ethanol ingestion (e.g. see Lindeneg *et al.*, 1964; Lundquist *et al.*, 1973; Juhlin-Dannfelt, 1977). Furthermore, under normal circumstances, the uptake of acetate by the liver is dependent on the portal blood concentration. Therefore, the tissues or sites that produce acetate (e.g. bacteria in the gut or liver after ethanol ingestion), can be regarded as providing the flux-generating step for the uptake and metabolism of acetate in other tissues, just as the small intestine is flux-generating for glucose metabolism after ingestion of sucrose, glucose or starch.

When the arterial concentration of acetate falls below approximately 80 μmol/l (as assayed by a type 3 enzymatic method; see Chapter 3) human liver and skeletal muscle may release acetate into the circulation (Skutches *et al.*, 1979); other tissues must then dominate acetate utilization. Potentially this circumstance operates at all times in ileostomies in which the peripheral venous concentration is very low, at about 20 μmol/l (Scheppach *et al.*, 1991). Animal studies also show that in addition to the small intestine and brain, acetate is also a fuel of both cardiac and smooth muscle and to a small extent the kidneys (Bleiberg *et al.*, 1992). As in humans, acetate is released by the rat liver, provided portal blood concentrations are low and β-oxidation is active (Buckley & Williamson, 1977). It is possible that efflux of acetate is normally related to ketogenic activity in the liver, whereas simultaneous uptake into the liver is dependent on plasma concentrations. Thus, acetate uptake by the liver is expected to be concentration-dependent, since the liver contains a high K_m ($\approx$10 mM) mitochrondrial acetyl-CoA synthetase. In animals the liver also contains a low K_m ($\approx$0.1 mM) cytosolic acetyl-CoA synthetase, which is said to be inducible by insulin (Rémésy, Demigné & Morand, 1991).

Acetate utilization by the liver contributes to ketogenesis. Administration of labelled acetate can result in the release of labelled glutamine by the liver (Desmoulin, Canioni & Cozzone, 1985). Both the ketone bodies and glutamine are preferred respiratory fuels of the small intestine (Windmueller & Spaeth, 1978; Souba, Scott & Wilmore, 1985). However, the major sources of these fuels are glutamine release by skeletal muscle and ketogenesis from non-esterified fatty acids in the liver. At least some muscle glutamine may be produced from circulating glutamate (Elia & Livesey, 1983; Elia, 1992*c*) and labelled acetate increases labelled glutamate release from the liver, at least in rats (Desmoulin *et al.*, 1985). In these animals, acetic acid, ketone bodies and glutamine are fuels for the small intestine, where they have trophic effects (Sakata, 1987; Grant & Snyder, 1988; Klimberg *et al.*, 1990). Diabetic rats, which have high concentrations of circulating ketone bodies and acetate, also show hypertrophy of the small bowel mucosa (Schedl & Wilson, 1971; Miller *et al.*, 1977; Schedl *et al.*, 1982). Furthermore, monoacetoacetin inhibits the mucosal atrophy associated with total parenteral nutrition in the rat (Kripke *et al.*, 1988), and triacetin reduces small- and large-bowel mucosal atrophy seen in burned rats (Karlstrad *et al.*, 1992).

The utilization and metabolic effects of SCFA may depend on the rate and route of administration. Under normal circumstances the peripheral tissues use virtually no propionic or butyric acids, because they are removed from the circulation during their first pass through the liver. However, these substrates may be used differently or may have different metabolic effects depending on whether they are given orally, intravenously or rectally. For example, a greater proportion of acetate is expected to be used by peripheral tissues when given parenterally than when given enterally. Furthermore, acetate given orally appears to have no effect on the plasma concentration of pancreatic glucagon (Scheppach *et al.*, 1988*a*), but given rectally it has repeatedly been shown to increase the concentration of this peptide hormone in the circulation (Stephen *et al.*, 1989; Wolever, Spadafora & Eshuis, 1991). In contrast, rectal, oral and intravenous acetate each lower the concentration of plasma non-esterified fatty acids in humans (Crouse *et al.*, 1968; Scheppach *et al.*, 1988*b*; Akanji *et al.*, 1989; Akanji & Hockaday, 1990). The observation is consistent with the effect of SCFA in sparing long-chain fatty acids from oxidation in humans (Lundquist *et al.*, 1962; Crouse *et al.*, 1968; Skutches *et al.*, 1983; Akanji *et al.*, 1989; Akanji & Hockaday, 1990) and in reducing lipolysis in rat adipocytes *in vitro* (Nilsson & Belfrage, 1978). The antilypolytic effect involved may be mediated by the same mechanism that occurs when ketone bodies reduce lipolysis in adipose tissue (Robinson & Williamson, 1980; Balasse, 1986).

Insulin resistance, glucose intolerance and coronary heart disease arise in part from raised plasma non-esterified fatty acids (Kaplan, 1989; Vague, 1990). Although acetate might contribute to a reversal of this trend, it is also a substrate for cholesterol synthesis, and may elevate circulating total and low-density lipoprotein cholesterol concentrations, as observed when acetate is infused rectally (Wolever *et al.*, 1991). Lactulose fermentation, which produces a large proportion of SCFA as acetate (Mortensen *et al.*, 1988*b*), has also been found to elevate plasma total and low-density lipoprotein cholesterol concentrations, and to elevate plasma apolipoprotein B and serum triglycerides in healthy subjects (Brighenti & Jenkins, 1990; Jenkins *et al.*, 1991). Acetate might, therefore, have some implications for risk of cardiovascular disease, but the position is unclear, and the effect may not be substantial. The effects of dietary and colonically derived propionate on lipid metabolism may counter this possible effect of acetate, but again the position is unclear (Venter, Vorster & Cummings, 1990; Wolever, 1991). The possibility that acetate metabolism during haemodialysis further increases an already high risk of atherosclerosis in uraemic subjects has been considered, and the problem is thought not to be exacerbated (Weiner, 1982). However, whether rectal or even caecal acetate absorption at lower rates under more physiological conditions would be without effect is unclear.

Lipogenesis in humans is considered to be predominantly a hepatic activity and proceeded at a negligible rate from glucose in fasted and fed (not overfed) volunteers (Hellerstein *et al.*, 1991). In contrast up to 10% of lipid in very-low-density lipoproteins secreted by the liver is reported to be derived from ethanol metabolism (Koziet *et al.*, 1991). The reason for low rates of hepatic lipogenesis from glucose in humans is not known, although two possibilities are a limitation of flux through hepatic pyruvate dehydrogenase (perhaps by inhibition due to acetyl-CoA generated from acetate and fatty-acid oxidation) and inhibition of glycolysis (e.g. citrate accumulation inhibits phosphofructokinase activity). If these were the explanations then circulating acetate may be lipogenic in the human liver and may contribute to raised levels of plasma triglycerides (and possibly cholesterol). The influence of acetate on thermogenesis in normal and diabetic subjects when fed at near maintenance-energy intakes is not consistent with high rates of lipogenesis from high (1–1.5 mmol/l) plasma acetate concentrations (Akanji *et al.*, 1989). Nevertheless, more definitive studies are required and it is possible that acetate could have a role in nutritional repletion by total parenteral nutrition when acetate production from the gut is likely to be small, and when lipogenesis from glucose is evident in humans (Pullicino & Elia, 1991).

The antilipolytic effect of acetate complements the observed (Del Boca & Flatt, 1969) enhancement of lipogenesis from glucose in adipocytes in the presence of acetate. The latter arises because lipogenesis from glucose produces ATP (Elia & Livesey, 1988) and when the amount of ATP produced is more than adipocytes can use, lipogenesis is limited. In contrast, lipogenesis from acetate is a process that consumes ATP, and, therefore, it allows lipogenesis to operate at higher rates. The synergism between acetate and glucose might be expected to be of significance only when carbohydrate intake is high and the non-protein respiratory exchange ratio (CO_2/O_2) is greater than unity. It is notable that on conventional foods a high intake of complex carbohydrate foods is accompanied by a high intake of starch and fermentable plant cell-wall carbohydrates. This synergism may once have had survival value (and may still do so in some species), but Western humans ingest a high-fat diet, and so rarely achieve a non-protein respiratory quotient above unity.

It may be that the potential advantages of acetate suggested for insulin sensitivity and coronary heart disease risk are countered at high food intake by acetate, favouring fat storage due to antilipolytic and lipogenic effects. The suggested benefits of high fibre in a diet might then be realized only when food intake is limited.

It is possible that acetate with other SCFA act as a feedback signal influencing digestion and metabolism over the longer term, but are without effect in the short term. In ruminant animals the SCFA are acute stimulants of insulin release, but this does not seem to occur in non-ruminant animals (Manns & Bode, 1967; Horino *et al.*, 1968; Katoh, 1991), although acetate has been reported to potentiate glucose-stimulated insulin release from the rat islet cell *in vitro* and to improve glucose tolerance in the rat (Patel & Singh, 1979). Acute studies in humans in which oral acetate has been administered to achieve high physiological concentrations of acetate in peripheral blood, affect neither glucose tolerance nor glucose turnover (Scheppach *et al.*, 1988*a,b*). However, these findings do not exclude the possibility that increased availability of acetate and other SCFA may in the long term increase the absorptive capacity of the small intestine through their trophic effects there, either directly (Schedl & Wilson, 1971; Miller *et al.*, 1977; Kripke *et al.*, 1988) or indirectly mediated via secondary signals from the large intestine (Sakata, 1991). It has even been suggested that SCFA may stimulate pancreatic exocrine secretions, which also have trophic effects (Weser, Heller & Tawil, 1977). A very high dose of a triacetin and tributyrin mixture has also been shown to increase the weight of pancreatic tissue in the rat (Al-Mukhtar *et al.*, 1983).

Endogenous versus exogenous (colonic) production of acetate and energy expenditure on acetyl-CoA–acetate recycling

With knowledge of the turnover of acetate in the human body and the rate at which acetate is produced from the gut, the rate of endogenous acetate production can be calculated. The turnover of endogenously derived acetate results from the simultaneous production and utilization of acetate by several tissues, as demonstrated in animal studies (Bleiberg *et al.*, 1992). Acetate production from non-colonic tissues is made possible by the occurrence of acetyl-CoA hydrolase and utilization by acetyl-CoA synthetase. The synthesis is fuelled by the hydrolysis of ATP to PP_i and AMP, the equivalent of 2 ATP to 2 ADP. Together these reactions constitute an energy-dissipating substrate cycle. If under normal circumstances gut-derived acetate production is about 196 mmol/day, then for a subject with a body weight of 70 kg the rate is equivalent to about 2 μmol/kg body weight per min. This contribution to the acetate pool by the colon is much less than the turnover of acetate in the total body pool, for which remarkably similar values are reported from three different laboratories. A value of 8.2 μmol/kg per min was obtained in normal young adult humans infused with [1-^{14}C]acetate (Skutches *et al.*, 1979). The turnover of acetate in the basal state in normal subjects in the study of Akanji & Hockaday (1990) was 8.6 μmol/kg per min and a value of 9.4 μmol/kg per min for normal humans using [1-^{13}C]acetate infusions was reported verbally (see discussion by Kein, after the paper of Wolever *et al.*, 1991). The implication is that colonically derived acetate contributes to only about 25% of acetate turnover in normal circumstances. This figure should be regarded as tentative, since estimates of acetate turnover are dependent on the method for the determination of circulating acetate concentration (see Chapter 3). When using labelled acetate, the specific activity or enrichment may decrease as blood perfuses the peripheral tissues, since acetate can be produced and used simultaneously. Therefore, derived values for acetate turnover are expected to be dependent on whether arterial or venous blood is used to calculate turnover. In a steady-state isotope-dilution study with [2-^{13}C]acetic acid in a single 50-kg young adult after a 12-h fast, an acetate turnover rate of 54.3 μmol/kg per min was reported (Rocchiccioli, Lepetit & Bougnéres,

1989). This value is extremely high compared with previously reported values, and would imply acetyl-CoA–acetate recycling at a rate of about 5% of total energy expenditure. With acetate turnover studies it is clearly important to validate the methodology.

Nevertheless, based on the turnover of acetate of 8 μmol/kg per min and a colonic production of 2 μmol/kg per min, the cycle must involve 6 μmol/kg per min, with the equivalent expenditure of 12 μmol ATP/kg per min. As the energy equivalent of ATP is approximately 80 kJ/mol (Livesey, 1984, 1987), the cost of this cycle is 96 kJ per 70-kg subject per day. This is about 1% of daily energy expenditure. The value compares with 0.5% of energy expenditure in the overnight fasted state for another substrate cycle, in which long-chain fatty acids are continually produced by triglyceride hydrolysis and reactivated by long-chain acyl-CoA synthetase, i.e. the triglyceride–fatty acid cycle (Elia *et al.*, 1987; Livesey, 1987). The same authors showed that energy expenditure on the triglyceride–fatty-acid cycle during starvation for four days increased to 3% of energy expenditure. Although there is little understanding of the regulation of acetate turnover, it is possible that energy expenditure on the acetyl-CoA–acetate cycle also increases in starvation as circulating concentrations of acetate rise, possibly in association with ketogenesis. Acetate turnover is positively correlated with acetate concentrations in humans (Skutches *et al.*, 1979), and raised acetate concentrations and turnover may also occur in obese subjects due to raised conversion of non-esterified fatty acids to acetate (Skutches *et al.*, 1979; Seufert, Mewes & Soeling, 1984). On the other hand, circulating concentrations may arise because utilization and turnover of acetate are decreased, as in type II diabetic subjects (Akanji & Hockaday, 1990). In the last circumstance, gut-derived acetate probably explains about half of the acetate turnover, which is about 4 μmol/kg per min, and the cost of acetate recycling then falls to about 0.25% of energy expenditure in diabetes mellitus. Interestingly, acetate turnover decreases with age, falling to 4 μmol/kg per min by about the age of 50 years (Skutches *et al.*, 1979).

Stoichiometry of ATP production from SCFA

The efficiency with which SCFA are used as fuels in systemic metabolism can be determined in two ways. The first is to determine experimentally the amount of substrate that needs to be administered to an organism to spare endogenous fuels and maintain energy balance. Here, efficiency can be defined as the amount of energy needed relative to the amount of glucose needed to achieve the same effect. There are few experimental studies that address this issue, though one or two are of note. Mixtures of acetic, propionic and butyric acids, infused into the spare body fat of sheep, gave an efficiency close to 0.85 times the energy supplied from glucose (Blaxter, 1989); similar results were obtained for propionic and butyric acids supplied alone. In a different type of study in the growing pig (Roth, Kirchgessner & Müller, 1988) the change in deposition of lean tissue and fat due to administration of acetic and propionic acids gave results consistent with the findings in sheep, discussed by Blaxter (1989).

The second method is to calculate the net amount of ATP gained from the standard oxidative metabolic pathways. Since ATP is both produced and used in many metabolic pathways (e.g. ATP is used in the activation of SCFA), ATP gain is defined as the net ATP made available during complete oxidation of the fuels (Livesey & Elia, 1988). With this method, efficiency can be defined as the amount of a substrate needed to give the same ATP yield as glucose (ATP/kJ substrate per ATP/kJ glucose). Computations of the yield of ATP from the SCFA vary to some degree. Bär (1990) indicated an ATP gain of 10, 17 and 27 mol/mol acetic, propionic and butyric acids, respectively; whereas Blaxter (1967) gave values of 10, 18 and 27, respectively. These values differ for propionic acid, and examination of several biochemical texts suggests that 18 ATP/mol is correct. Neither Bär nor Blaxter take account of the current view that mitochondrial stoichiometries are fractional (Livesey, 1984); i.e. ATP generated at the substrate level intramitochondrially (ATP_{mit}) is worth only 0.67 times the value of cytosolic ATP (ATP_{cyt}), since there is a cost of moving ATP from the mitochondrial matrix to the cytosol where it is used. Similarly, there is a cost of $\frac{1}{3}$ ATP (i.e. one proton) associated with moving NADH from the cytosol to the mitochondrial matrix for ATP generation. Table 28.5 shows the calculation of cytosolic ATP gain from the SCFA and glucose. In this table, information is provided for when activation of SCFA to its CoA derivative is cytosolic and when it is mitochondrial. In the latter case there is one ATP produced at the substrate level in mitochondria, and activation takes the equivalent of two ATP (ATP to AMP + PP_i); therefore, the net ATP_{mit} is -1.00. Previously it had been thought that activation of SCFA, including acetic acid, may be cytosolic, though recent evidence suggests that it may be mitochondrial (Crabtree, Gordon & Christie, 1990). The relative importance of the two *in vivo* is not known. The calculations show ATP_{cyt} gains of 10.3, 18 and 27 for acetic, propionic and butyric acids, respectively, when activation is mitochondrial, but smaller values of 9.7, 17.3 and 26.3, respectively, when activation is cytosolic (Table 28.5). When compared with glucose, the SCFA are oxidized with efficiencies of 0.91, 0.91 and 0.97 for acetic, propionic and butyric acids, respectively when

Table 28.5. *Calculation of ATP gain from the direct oxidation of short-chain fatty acids (SCFA) and glucose, with the assumption of no cost for absorption of either glucose or SCFA*

Substrate	New cofactor production and its cytoplasmic ATP equivalent					ATP gain	ΔH (kJ)	ATP/J	Efficiency relative to glucose
	ATP_{cyt} 1.00	ATP_{mit} 0.67	$NADH_{cyt}$ 2.67	$NADH_{mit}$ 3.00	$FADH_2$ 2.00				
Glucose	2.00	2.00	2.00	8.00	2.00	36.7	2803	13.0	1.00
Glycerol	1.00	1.00	2.00	4.00	1.00	21.0	1655	12.7	0.98
Cytosolic activation									
Acetic acid	−2.00	1.00	0.00	3.00	1.00	9.7	875	11.1	0.85
Propionic acid	−2.00	1.00	1.00	4.00	2.00	17.3	1527	11.3	0.87
Butyric acid	−2.00	2.00	0.00	7.00	3.00	26.3	2184	12.0	0.92
Mitochondrial activation									
Acetic acid	0.00	−1.00	0.00	3.00	1.00	10.3	875	11.8	0.91
Propionic acid	0.00	−1.00	1.00	4.00	2.00	18.0	1527	11.8	0.91
Butyric acid	0.00	0.00	0.00	7.00	3.00	27.0	2184	12.6	0.97

cyt, cytosolic; mit, mitochondrial.

activation is mitochondrial, but 0.85, 0.87 and 0.93, respectively, when it is cytosolic (Table 28.5). If it is assumed that the SCFA are activated in the cytosol rather than in mitochondria, then these coefficients are more in keeping with the results of both the animal studies mentioned and a human study discussed below. For comparison, long-chain triglycerides are oxidized with an efficiency of about 0.97 relative to glucose (Livesey, 1984).

It is perhaps worth noting that some authors assume all SCFA to produce ATP with an efficiency of 0.69 compared with glucose (see e.g. Iwakawa, 1989). The basis for this low conversion efficiency is obscure, but appears to rely on poorly documented studies on the metabolism of acetic acid in animals. Values as low as 0.60 have been found for acetic acid administered to sheep under non-physiological conditions, in which a supplementary thermogenesis was induced, a process which is poorly understood (Blaxter, 1967). Studies on the metabolism of acetate in the rat heart (Randle, England & Denton, 1970) and in the rat hind quarter (Karlsson, Fellenius & Keissling, 1977) showed that acetate did not significantly affect tissue oxygen consumption when it replaced other substrates as fuels, findings that would not be expected if acetate was usually oxidized with efficiencies as low as 0.6 or 0.69.

A study in humans where sodium acetate was infused at about 40% of the non-protein energy expenditure reports no significant effects of acetate on energy expenditure (Akanji *et al.*, 1989). However, close inspection shows that after data were combined from normal and diabetic subjects, there was a small increase in energy expenditure, from 4.700 to 5.005 kJ/min, due to a constant infusion of 2.186 kJ/min of acetate. The increase in expenditure, 0.305 kJ/min, was 0.14 times the rate of acetate infusion (0.305/2.186). If all the acetate was oxidized, which seems likely, the efficiency of oxidation would have been 0.86. This value is essentially identical to the findings with sheep mentioned above (Blaxter, 1989), though it is not definitive, since the exact rate of acetate oxidation was assumed and the variation in energy expenditure was rather high, corresponding to a mean standard error of 0.20 times the rate of acetate infusion. Furthermore, some acetate may have been used for lipogenesis (Skutches *et al.*, 1983).

Acid–base regulation, ammoniagenesis, ureagenesis, heat production and interpretation of respiratory gas measurements

The choice of SCFA substrate for metabolic studies and for enteral and parenteral feeds has implications for acid–base balance, heat production and assessment of substrate utilization by indirect calorimetry (Elia & Livesey, 1988, 1992; Livesey & Elia, 1988).

The calculation by classic indirect calorimetry for fuel selection in humans usually assumes that only three substrates are oxidized (fat, carbohydrate and protein) and that the end products are carbon dioxide, water and the nitrogenous products in urine. Fermentation can invalidate these calculations to some extent, since the end products include methane and hydrogen gas, which in human studies are not normally taken into consideration. However, the effect of these on the calculated energy expenditure in humans is often negligible, and by ignoring these gases the error in the calculated contribution of carbohydrate and fat to energy expenditure is only about 3% (Livesey & Elia, 1988). Larger errors can occur when fermentation is more active, as in ruminants. Procedures for making corrections to the indirect calorimetry calculations when fermentation uses a significant amount of the respiratory fuels are described elsewhere (Elia & Livesey, 1992). A different problem arises when SCFA are administered, because specific amounts of heat and carbon dioxide are released during their oxidation, i.e. their specific respiratory quotients (CO_2/O_2) and energy equivalents of oxygen (kJ/l O_2) need to be taken into account.

The heat released during the metabolism of the various forms of SCFA may be calculated using information on heats of combustion (Dolmalski, 1972) and formation (Wilhout, 1969) of the reactants and products of oxidation. In the case of the salts of SCFA, bicarbonate is a product that may either temporarily accumulate in plasma and perturb acid–base balance or be lost to urine. For example, with salts of acetate and without consideration of any perturbation of acid–base balance:

Conversion of the anionic to the acidic form:

$$CH_3—CO_2^- + H_2O + CO_2 \rightarrow CH_3—CO_2H + HCO_3^-$$

$$\Delta H = +3.0\ \text{kJ} \quad (28.12)$$

Oxidation of the acidic form:

$$CH_3—CO_2H + 2O_2 \rightarrow 2CO_2 + 2H_2O$$

$$\Delta H = -874.5\ \text{kJ}; \quad RQ = 1 \quad (28.13)$$

Overall oxidation of the anionic form:

$$CH_3—CO_2^- + 2O_2 \rightarrow CO_2 + H_2O + HCO_3^-$$

$$\Delta H = -871.5\ \text{kJ}; \quad RQ = 0.5 \quad (28.14)$$

Infusion studies in humans show a 1:1 production ratio of bicarbonate from acetate (Weiner, 1982). Three kilojoules of heat are absorbed when one mole each of the aqueous anion (e.g. acetate), carbon dioxide and water are converted to the aqueous acid (e.g. acetic) and bicarbonate. The trapping of CO_2 as bicarbonate affects the interpretation of respiratory gas exchange during indirect calorimetry; thus with acetic acid the respiratory quotient (RQ) is 1.0 and with acetate the RQ is 0.5. These values compare with the range of RQ in humans of ≈ 0.71 when oxidizing fats, to 1.3 when oxidizing carbohydrate and at the same time maximally converting carbohydrate to fat. Computed values of the heat, oxygen and carbon dioxide exchanges are given in Table 28.6 for the major short-chain fatty substrates.

Bicarbonate production may induce alkalosis, which may be regulated by diversion of nitrogen excretion further towards urea excretion and less towards ammonia excretion (Atkinson & Bourke, 1982).

Bicarbonate-induced shift from ammoniagenesis to ureagenesis:

$$2HCO_3^- + 2NH_4^+ \rightarrow NH_2CONH_2 + CO_2 + 3H_2O \qquad \Delta H = -19\ \text{kJ} \quad (28.15)$$

New overall oxidation of the anionic form:

$$2CH_3\text{—}CO_2^- + 4O_2 + 2NH_4^+ \rightarrow 3CO_2 + 5H_2O + NH_2CONH_2 \qquad \Delta H = 1762\ \text{kJ}; \quad RQ = 0.75 \quad (28.16)$$

The overall RQ is now 0.75, compared with the previous 1.0 (eq. 28.14) and 0.5 (eq. 28.15). There is no obvious information on how salts of SCFA affect the pattern of nitrogen excretion.

Use of SCFA as the acid rather than as the salt may, in contrast, induce a temporary acidosis. Respiratory compensation for the acidosis may increase both ventilation and CO_2 loss, but as the SCFA are removed by oxidation, the acidosis and hyperventilation disappear. These temporary ventilatory effects change the respiratory exchange ratio (CO_2 excretion to O_2 consumption) which then provides misleading information about the fuels oxidized, as assessed by classical indirect calorimetry (Livesey & Elia, 1988). Large doses of SCFA in the acid form can be tolerated in ruminants, provided there is a supply of glucose. However, attempts to meet energy expenditure with acetic acid alone induces a severe acidosis, hypoglycaemia and increased gluconeogenesis, and elevates both nitrogen excretion and energy expenditure (Blaxter, 1967). Interestingly, ethanol administration, which inhibits gluconeogenesis, also produces hypoglycaemia, elevates the plasma acetate concentration, and increases energy expenditure (Akanji *et al.*, 1989).

Table 28.6. *Short-chain fatty acid substrates used or potentially useful in metabolic studies*

Substrate	Formula	Heat released in metabolism					
		kJ/mol	kJ/g	kJ/l O_2	O_2/mol	CO_2/mol[a]	RQ[a]
Acetic acid[b]	CH_3—CO_2H	874.5	14.56	19.51	2	2	1.0
Sodium acetate[b]	CH_3—$CO_2^-Na^+$	871.5	10.62	19.44	2	1	0.5
Calcium acetate[b]	$(CH_3$—$CO_2^-)_2Ca^{2+}$	1743	11.02	19.44	4	2	0.5
Triacetin[b]	$(CH_3$—$CO)_3C_3H_5O_3$	4281.5	19.62	20.01	9.5	9	0.947
Propionic acid[b]	C_2H_5—CO_2H	1527	20.61	19.47	3.5	3	0.857
Sodium propionate[b]	C_2H_5—$CO_2^-Na^+$	1524	15.86	19.43	3.5	2	0.571
Calcium propionate[b]	$(C_2H_5$—$CO_2^-)_2Ca^{2+}$	3048	16.36	19.43	7	4	0.571
Tripropionin	$(C_2H_5$—$CO)_3C_3H_5O_3$	6239	23.97	19.88	14	12	0.818
Butyric acid[b]	C_3H_7—CO_2H	2183.5	24.78	19.48	5	4	0.80
Sodium butyrate[b]	C_3H_7—$CO_2^-Na^+$	2180.5	19.80	19.45	5	3	0.60
Calcium butyrate[b]	$(C_3H_7$—$CO_2^-)_2Ca^{2+}$	4361	20.35	19.45	10	6	0.60
Tributyrin	$(C_3H_7$—$CO)_3C_3H_5O_3$	8208.5	27.15	19.79	18.5	15	0.81
Monoacetoacetin	C_3H_5O—CO—$C_3H_7O_3$	3047	17.32	18.10	7.5	7	0.933
Monobutyrin	C_3H_7—CO—$C_3H_7O_3$	3836	23.68	20.13	8.5	7	0.824

[a] Assumes no perturbation of the acid–base status.
[b] Water soluble.
RQ, respiratory quotient.

Perturbation of acid–base regulation and problems of interpretation of measurements of respiratory gas exchange are largely reduced when the mono- or triglycerides, or possibly other esters, of the SCFA are used.

When the salts are used as fuels, the rate of SCFA utilization and oxidation must be measured or assumptions must be made about these rates if indirect calorimetry is to be used to estimate the proportions of long-chain triglyceride and carbohydrate to substrate utilization. Without these corrections, errors will occur to an extent that can be calculated according to procedures outlined elsewhere (Elia & Livesey, 1992). In their studies of acetate metabolism in humans assessed by indirect calorimetry, Akanji *et al.* (1989) made the assumption that 90% of the infused acetate was used. The infusion rate was high, at 40% of the non-protein energy expenditure. Acetate utilization and infusion rates were the same as judged from the steady-state plasma acetate levels, so a 100% utilization rate is justified, though slightly less may be oxidized, since some lipogenesis from acetate may occur simultaneously (Weiner, 1982).

The anaerobic fermentation of carbohydrates may also give rise to lactic and succinic acids, and the anaerobic fermentation of protein may give rise to the branched-chain fatty acids, isobutyric (C4), isovaleric (C5) and isocaproic (C6) (Mortensen *et al.*, 1990*b*). These acids are present in small amounts in the human large intestine by comparison with acetic, propionic and butyric acids ($\approx$10% of total SCFA; Cummings *et al.*, 1987), and since they are unlikely substrates for enteral and parenteral feeds, they have not been included in Table 28.6. Moreover, there is concern about the possible toxicity of some triglycerides, mostly with C4, C5 and C6 fatty acids, which may penetrate the blood–brain barrier (Campos & Meguid, 1988). In the free-acid form, these acids are implicated in the induction of hepatic coma (Zieve *et al.*, 1974). These low-molecular-weight hydrophobic triglycerides potentially may enter the circulation in the unesterified form. The risk of possible toxicity is less with oral administration of the SCFA-triglycerides. Thus although these triglycerides are readily digested by salivary lipase of the stomach (Hamosh & Burns, 1977; Tiruppathi & Balasubramanian, 1982), pancreatic lipase (Erlanson & Bergstrom, 1970; Lairon *et al.*, 1980), intracellular mucosal lipases (Barry, Jackson & Smith, 1966) and serum lipase (Nath & Debnath, 1968), the hydrolytic products are removed by the intestinal tissues and liver. Therefore, although tributyrin (Table 28.6) has a potential for safe administration via the enteral route, the administration of butyrate esters by the parenteral route, which bypasses the splanchnic tissues, is more likely to be associated with potential hazards.

SCFA in colonic disease

There is scanty information about clinical effects and possible benefits of SCFA administration, but a number of conditions are considered below in relation to the absorption, energy supply and metabolic effects of SCFA in patients with colonic disease.

Diarrhoea

A major function of the large intestine is the absorption of sodium ions. Sodium absorption is stimulated by luminal SCFA in humans and several animal species (Engelhardt & Rechkemmer, 1982). Butyric acid provides the colonocyte with three factors to support Na^+ absorption (Roediger, 1986, 1989): a preferred fuel for the generation of ATP used for the transport and absorption of sodium; increased intracellular CO_2 for carbonic acid production catalysed by carbonic anhydrase, and so the supply of protons for sodium absorption at the Na^+/H^+ antiport at the luminal surface of the epithelium; and protons for this antiport generated by diffusion of the SCFA into the colonocyte cytosol on its dissociation into the anionic form. Additionally, SCFA have been reported to dilate human colonic resistance arteries *in vitro* (Mortensen *et al.* 1990*b*). A mixture of SCFA stimulates blood flow and oxygen consumption in the mucosa of dogs; however, only acetic acid is effective when given alone (Kvietys & Granger, 1981). An elevated blood-flow rate might also increase the availability of other nutrients to the mucosa from the circulation, and thus contribute to normalization of colonic function.

Impaired fermentation and butyric acid production leading to reduced sodium absorption have been implicated in the cause of diarrhoea due to refeeding after chronic starvation, and to feeding of germ-free animals (Thaysen & Thaysen, 1952; Loeschke & Gordon, 1969). Furthermore, diarrhoea is an important adverse effect of the administration of broad-spectrum antibiotics. The mechanism is not fully understood, although it has been suggested that inhibition of fermentation by antibiotics is an important contributory factor. Interestingly, the risk may be higher in subjects on diets high in unavailable carbohydrates (Rao *et al.*, 1988). An overly active colonic fermentation has been suggested to be a cause of functional constipation (Bond *et al.*, 1980); but it may be associated with diarrhoea in malabsorption syndromes, e.g. short-bowel syndrome (see below).

The incidence of diarrhoea in patients receiving enteral nutrition in hospital practice is as high as 30% (Wilcock *et al.*, 1991). The mechanism is poorly understood, and, therefore, several factors have been implicated, including osmotic load of the feed, lactose intolerance, lack of dietary fibre, gastrointestinal disease, bacterial overgrowth, and neuroendocrine changes. Recent studies have suggested that fibre-free intragastric enteral feeding produces fluid secretion in the ascending colon (Silk, 1993). It is possible that a greater production of SCFA in the colon may reduce diarrhoea in some patients. However, clinical trials on the effects of dietary fibre have not provided consistent results, because the multiple clinical variables that affect colonic function have not always been adequately controlled, and because studies have usually been carried out with a single source of dietary fibre. However, in some studies diarrhoea was present in about 60% of critically ill patients (Kelly & Hillman, 1983; Flynn, Norton & Fisher, 1987) and the incidence was reported to be reduced by incorporation of pectin, which is rapidly fermented to SCFA (Zimmaro *et al*., 1989). Assuming the importance of butyric acid in the prevention of diarrhoea, pectin may be a poor choice of non-starch polysaccharide, as other substrates may yield more butyrate (Table 28.4).

Bowel rest

Total parenteral nutrition during bowel rest for gastrointestinal dysfunction produces intestinal atrophy and hypofunction. Rapid enteral feeding after bowel rest may induce or aggravate the diarrhoea in this condition. In animal studies both enteral and parenteral SCFA prevented colonic atrophy (Sakata & Yajima, 1984; Koruda *et al*., 1988, 1990; Kripke, Fox & Berman, 1989; Sakata, 1991). The extent to which this is due to absence of fuels such as butyric acid remains to be established. Clinical studies in this area are notably lacking.

Ulcerative colitis

The cause of ulcerative colitis remains unknown, although Roediger (1980) has described the condition as an energy-deficiency disease. This is based on the finding of an impaired ability of the affected mucosa to utilize and oxidize butyric acid. This finding by itself does not necessarily indicate that an energy deficiency is causative; however, a mucosal lesion in rats similar to ulcerative colitis is produced on inhibition of β-oxidation of fatty acids, including butyric, with 2-bromooctanoate (Roediger & Nance, 1986). Further, activation of butyric acid with coenzyme A is needed for its metabolism, and coenzyme -A depletion also produces lesions similar to those seen in ulcerative colitis (Rabassa & Rogers, 1992). In addition, a low coenzyme-A level has been reported in the mucosa in this condition (Ellestad-Sayed *et al*., 1976). Finally, in a chemical model of colitis, the risk of developing colitis was found to be reduced by addition of pectin to an enteral feed – i.e. by addition of a substrate that can be fermented to SCFA (Rolandelli *et al*., 1988).

Butyric acid concentrations in the stools of patients with ulcerative colitis are decreased compared with concentrations in healthy subjects (Vernia *et al.*, 1988*a*). Interestingly, enemas of sodium butyrate in patients unresponsive to standard therapy have been reported to decrease both stool frequency and blood loss, and to increase both endoscopic and histological grading of inflammation compared to a control group (Scheppach *et al.*, 1992). This successful treatment was achieved with a total dose of 20 mmol sodium butyrate daily, which is 2–3-fold less than the estimated total production in normal subjects. The administered dose perhaps restored a deficiency in this condition. However, peak concentration of butyrate may have been 'pharmacological', particularly since the administration was directly onto the distal colonic mucosa, a site usually affected by the colitic process. Under normal circumstances only a fraction of a the butyrate produced by anaerobic fermentation would reach the dixtal colon.

It there was a failure of butyrate absorption in active ulcerative colitis, this would decrease HCO_3^- excretion, acidify the colon, reduce faecal HCO_3^- and acidify stools in this condition (Roediger *et al.*, 1984; Caprilli *et al.*, 1986). Lactic acid is a normal intermediate in anaerobic fermentation, its production is favoured over the SCFA at low pH, and it is found in considerable amounts in the stool of patients with severe ulcerative colitis (Vernia *et al.*, 1988*a*).

Diversion colitis

Diversion colitis results when the proximal bowel is separated from the colon so that luminal nutrients do not reach the distal colonic segment. When colorectal continuity is restored, the inflammatory condition is improved (Glotzer, Glick & Goldman, 1981; Korelitz *et al.*, 1985; Roediger, 1988). SCFA enemas in the excluded colonic segment improve both endoscopic and histological grading of the inflammation, as judged from preliminary studies on four people (Harig *et al.*, 1989).

Crohn's colitis

Faecal SCFA appear normal in this condition and lactate concentrations are high. Abnormalities of SCFA production and utilization are not as yet evident. It has been suggested that diarrhoea in this condition may be osmotic in origin, due to the poor absorption of carbohydrates (Vernia *et al.*, 1988*b*). It is unclear whether high faecal lactate concentrations are due to increased production or decreased removal due to impaired conversion to SCFA.

Ileal pouchitis

An unnatural metabolic juxtaposition arises when an ileal pouch is constructed after colectomy to act as an artificial colon. The principal fuels made available in the lumen of the pouch are the SCFA; however, glutamine is the preferred fuel of the ileal tissue from which the pouch is constructed. Potentially, glutamine may reduce inflammation in this condition (Rabassa & Rogers, 1992). Glutamine has also been reported to reduce or prevent the development of inflammatory conditions of the gut in animals (Rombeau, 1990), where instillation of SCFA has not been reported to produce improvements and in one study SCFA appeared to enhance the development of ulceration (De Silva *et al.*, 1989).

Short-bowel syndrome

Massive small-bowel removal and resection results in malabsorption, diarrhoea and weight loss, due to the extreme decrease in digestive and absorptive capacity. The remaining intestine adapts by increasing its absorptive capacity (Wilmore *et al.*, 1971; Weser, 1983). Small-animal studies suggest nutrition with SCFA should have a beneficial outcome. Postsurgical total parenteral nutrition is associated with pancreatic atrophy (Kripke *et al.*, 1991) and SCFA are reported to stimulate pancreatobiliary secretions that facilitate the adaptive changes (Weser *et al.*, 1977; Hughes, Price & Dowling, 1980; Al-Mukhtar *et al.*, 1983). Mucosal adaptation is impaired by total parenteral nutrition without SCFA (Ford *et al.*, 1984) and stimulated by parenteral feeding with SCFA (Koruda *et al.*, 1988), and by oral feeding (Levine, Deren & Yezdimir, 1976). An equal mixture of triacetin and tributyrin, fed to rats intragastrically at 40% of non-protein calories, resulted in significantly enhanced jejunal and mucosal adaptation towards increased absorptive capacity, when compared with a control without lipids, and with a control with 40% non-protein calories as medium-chain triglycerides (Kripke *et al.*, 1991). It has not been resolved whether the changes produced by SCFA and their triglycerides are due to the supply of a preferred fuel or whether these substrates act principally as signals to regulate the functional capacity of the intestine.

Colonic anastomosis

Rolandelli *et al.* (1986) have demonstrated improved bursting strengths of colonic anastomoses in rats given intraluminal SCFA. This beneficial outcome presumably results from enhanced collagen formation. Influences of SCFA on fibroblasts or on fibroblast–enterocyte interaction may be implicated. Stimulation of blood flow by SCFA (Kvietys & Granger, 1981; Mortensen *et al.*, 1990*b*) may be important.

Bacterial translocation and sepsis

By preventing mucosal atrophy, parenteral SCFA (Levine, Deren & Steiger, 1974; Johnson, Copeland & Castro, 1975; Koruda *et al.*, 1988) might help to maintain the gut barrier, which is important in the prevention of sepsis and endotoxaemia in critically ill patients (Alexander, 1990; Evans & Shronts, 1992). Bacterial translocation occurs in animals on enteral feeds less commonly than in those on parenteral feeds (Alverdy, Aoys & Moss, 1988). After abdominal surgery or trauma, the early use of enteral feeding is reported to decrease the incidence of major infections significantly (Moore *et al.*, 1989). However, variable results have been obtained in animal studies in which a variety of dietary fibre source were used in the feeds. The addition of cellulose to an orally administered solution reduced the incidence of bacterial translocation (Sherman, Soni & Karmali, 1988), but in similar studies, in which citrus pectin was used, no beneficial effects were reported (Spaeth *et al.*, 1990). Again, protection against bacterial translocation has been reported for corn cobs added to a fibre-free diet in animal studies (Alverdy, Aoys & Moss, 1990), but no protection was offered with soy fibre (Alverdy *et al.* 1990) or psyllium fibre (Barber *et al.*, 1990). To what extent the variable results were due to different degrees and patterns of fermentation is unclear. Bulk in the intestinal lumen may be important in preventing bacterial translocation, since indigestible kaolin and poorly fermented cellulose are reported to reduce bacterial translocation in animals (Spaeth *et al.*, 1990). Moreover, the influence of SCFA on immune cells of the gut barrier is unknown, and SCFA in the colon potentially might spare glutamine utilization by the colonocytes in favour of immune cells.

Colorectal polyps and cancer

Colon cancer incidence decreases with increasing stool bulk (Cummings & Bingham, 1992) and epidemilogical evidence suggests an inverse association with increasing intake of dietary fibre (Trock, Lanza & Greenwood, 1990). A relationship between SCFA supply and colon cancer incidence would therefore seem possible. A low faecal butyrate: total SCFA ratio has been found in patients with adenomas and cancers when compared with healthy controls (Clausen, Bonnen & Mortensen, 1991). Butyrate has a differentiating effect on human cancer cells grown *in vitro* and increases the doubling time in induced colonic tumours (Augeron & Laboisse, 1984; Whithead, Young & Bhathal, 1986; Jacobs, 1986; Niles *et al.*, 1988). Expansion of the proliferative zone to the crypt surface is suggested as a biomarker for susceptibility to cancer formation (Lipkin, 1988) and is observed (Biasco *et al.*, 1984) independently of inflammation in patients with ulcerative colitis, a condition with an increased risk of colon cancer (Langholz *et al.*, 1992). Butyrate enemas in distal ulcerative colitis slow the proliferation in this marker zone by 60% (Scheppach *et al.*, 1992). These observations go some way towards refuting the hypothesis that butyrate acts as a tumour promoter on epithelial cells that have a reduced response to terminal differentiation signals (Berry & Paraskeva, 1988). While cell proliferation is dependent on an adequate energy supply, the stimulus to differentiation may depend more on the effects of butyrate on gene expression (Kruh, Defer & Tichonicky, 1991; Young, 1991). It remains to be discovered whether increasing the supply of butyrate will reduce the incidence of any colon cancer.

Summary

Short-chain fatty acids (SCFA) are produced by bacteria within the lumen of the caecum and colon, as well as endogenously by human tissues. The quantities of SCFA produced and absorbed depends on the amount and type of substrates reaching the colon, their extent of fermentation and the stoichiometry of the fermentation process, the details of which remain uncertain and are probably variable. It is estimated that only about 60% of the energy of a carbohydrate that is fermented in the large intestine is absorbed as SCFA, and that the absorption and subsequent oxidation of SCFA from the colon may contribute up to 8% of total energy expenditure or 12% of basal metabolic rate. However, in normal humans eating a Western-style diet, it is estimated that SCFA contribute 2–4% of total energy expenditure. The absorption of SCFA from the large intestine appears not to be an energy-dependent process.

SCFA derived from the colon are largely taken up by the liver during their first pass through this organ, although some acetate ($\approx$25%) escapes into the systemic circulation for metabolism by a variety of peripheral tissues. SCFA are metabolized less efficiently than glucose or long-chain triglycerides, since more energy (kilojoules) is expended ($\approx$15%) per mole of ATP gained. There is no established upper limit to the capacity of the human body to metabolize SCFA, but for acetate alone it is at least 40% of resting energy expenditure. The endogenous production and simultaneous use of acetate by the human body in an energy-requiring substrate cycle may explain about 1% of total energy expenditure in normal humans, but this value probably varies with age and clinical condition and with the method used to assay acetate turnover. Interest in the use of SCFA as energy substrates and as possible metabolic signals has led to a review of their potential benefits in a variety of clinical situations, especially in gastrointestinal diseases. Animal studies support the view that SCFA might be used beneficially in a variety of circumstances, while clinical studies remain small in number and principally involved with colitic diseases where benefit may be gained from the mucosal application of butyrate. It is not established whether the possible clinical benefits of SCFA are achieved at pharmacological or physiological concentrations at the tissue level, nor whether SCFA act as metabolic signals in addition to increasing the supply of preferred fuels for both the small and large intestine.

References

Adiotomre, J., Eastwood, M. A., Edwards, C. A. & Brydon, W. G. (1990). Dietary fibre: *in vitro* methods that anticipate nutrition and metabolic activities in humans. *American Journal of Clinical Nutrition*, **52**, 128–34.

Akanji, O. A. (1987). Measurement of plasma acetate concentrations in humans with reference to diabetes, dietary composition and bowel function. DPhil thesis, University of Oxford, Oxford.

Akanji, O. A., Bruce, M. A. & Frayn, J. N. (1989). Effect of acetate infusion on energy expenditure and substrate oxidation rates in non-diabetic and diabetic subjects. *European Journal of Clinical Nutrition*, **43**, 107–15.

Akanji, O. A. & Hockaday, T. D. R. (1990). Acetate tolerance and the kinetics of acetate utilisation in diabetic and non-diabetic subjects. *American Journal of Clinical Nutrition*, **51**, 112–18.

Alexander, J. W. (1990). Nutrition and translocation. *Journal of Enteral and Parenteral Nutrition*, **14**, 237–43S.

Al-Mukhtar, M. Y. T., Sagor. G. R., Ghatei, M. A., Bloom, S. R. & Wright, N. A. (1983). The role of pancreatobiliary secretions in intestinal adaptation after resection and its relationship to plasma enteroglucagon. *British Journal of Surgery*, **70**, 398–400.

Alverdy, J. C., Aoys, E. & Moss, G. S. (1988). Total parenteral nutrition promotes bacterial translocation from the gut. *Surgery*, **104**, 185–90.

Alverdy, J. C., Aoys, E. & Moss, G. S. (1990). Effects of commercially available chemically defined liquid diets on the intestinal microflora and bacterial translocation from the gut. *Journal of Enteral and Parenteral Nutrition*, **14**, 442–7.

Armstrong, D. G. & Blaxter, K. L. (1961). The utilisation of energy of carbohydrates by ruminants. In *2nd Symposium on Energy Metabolism*, ed. E. Brouwer & A. J. van Es, pp. 187–97. Wageningen: European Association for Animal Production.

Aslam, M., Batten, J. J., Florin, T. H. J., Sidebotham, R. L. & Baron, J. H. (1992). Hydrogen sulphide induced damage to the colonic mucosal barrier in the rat. *Gut*, **33** (Suppl. 2), F274.

Atkinson, D. E. & Bourke, E. (1982). The role of ureagenesis in pH homeostasis. *Current Topics in Cell Regulation*, **21**, 261–302.

Augeron, C. & Laboisse, C. L. (1984). Emergence of permanently differentiated cell clones in a human colonic cancer cell line in culture after treatment with sodium butyrate. *Cancer Research*, **44**, 3961–9.

Bailey, J. W., Haymon, W. & Miles, J. M. (1991). Triacetin: a potential parenteral nutrient. *Journal of Parenteral and Enteral Nutrition*, **15**, 32–6.

Balasse, E. O. (1986). Importance of ketone bodies in endogenous fat transport. *Clinical Nutrition*, **5**, 73–80.

Bär, A. (1990). Factorial calculation model for the estimation of the physiological caloric values of polyols. In *Caloric Evaluation of Carbohydrates*, ed. N. Hosoya, pp. 209–57. Tokyo: Research Foundation for Sugar Metabolism.

Barber, A. E., Jones, W. G., Minei, J. P., Fahey, T. J., Moldawer, L. L., Rayburn, J. L., Fisher, E., Keogh, C. V., Shires, G. T. & Lowrey, S. F. (1990). Glutamine or fibre supplementation of a defined formula diet: impact on bacterial translocation, tissue composition and response to endotoxin. *Journal of Parenteral and Enteral Nutrition*, **14**, 335–43.

Barry, R. J. C., Jackson, M. J. & Smith, D. H. (1966). Handling of glycerides of acetic acid by rat small intestine *in vitro*. *Journal of Physiology (London)*, **152**, 48–66.

Beaugerie, L., Flourié, B., Marteau, P., Pellier, P., Franchisseur, C. & Rambaud, J.-C. (1990). Digestion and absorption in the human intestine of three sugar alcohols. *Gastroenterology*, **99**, 717–23.

Berkelhammer, C. H., Wood, R. J. & Sitrin, M. D. (1988). Acetate and hypercalciuria during total parenteral nutrition. *American Journal of Clinical Nutrition*, **48**, 1482–9.

Berry, R. D. & Paraskeva, C. (1988). Expression of carcinoembryonic antigens by adenoma and carcinoma derived epithelial cell lines, possible marker of tumour progression and modulation of expression by sodium butyrate. *Carcinogenesis*, **9**, 447–50.

Biasco, G., Lipkin, M., Minarini, A., Higgins, P., Miglioli, M. & Barabara, L. (1984). Proliferative and antigenic properties of rectal cells in patients with chronic ulcerative colitis. *Cancer Research*, **44**, 5450–4.

Binder, H. J. & Rawlins, C. L. (1973). Electrolyte transport across isolated large intestinal mucosa. *American Journal of Physiology*, **225**, 1232–9.

Birkhahn, R. H. & Border, J. R. (1978). Intravenous feeding of the rat with short chain fatty acid esters. II. Monoacetoacetin. *American Journal of Clinical Nutrition*, **31**, 436–44.

Birkhahn, R. H., McMenamy, R. H. & Border, J. R. (1977). Intravenous feeding of rats with short chain fatty acid esters I: Glycerol monobutyrate. *American Journal of Clinical Nutrition*, **30**, 2078–82.

Blaxter, K. L. (1967). *The Energy Metabolism of Ruminants*. London: Hutchinson Scientific Press.

Blaxter, K. L. (1989). *Energy Metabolism in Animals and Man*. Cambridge: Cambridge University Press.

Bleiberg, B., Beers, B. Persson, M. & Miles, J. M. (1992). Systemic and regional acetate kinetics in dogs. *American Journal of Physiology*, **262**, E197–E202.

Bond, J. H., Currier, B. E., Buchwald, H. & Levitt, M. D. (1980). Colonic conservation of malabsorbed carbohydrate. *Gastroenterology*, **78**, 444–7.

Brighenti, F. & Jenkins, D. J. A. (1990). Lactulose: understanding the bacterially-mediated health effects of unavailable carbohydrates. *Annals of Microbiology*, **40**, 261–70.

Buckley, B. M. & Williamson, D. H. (1977). Origin of blood acetate in the rat. *Biochemical Journal*, **166**, 539–45.

Campos, A. C. L. & Meguid, M. M. (1988). Short chain fatty acids: present prospects – future alternative. *Journal of Enteral and Parenteral Nutrition*, **12**, 985–1015.

Caprilli, R., Frieri, G., Latella, G., Santoro, M. L. & Vernia, P. (1986). Faecal excretion of bicarbonate in ulcerative colitis. *Digestion*, **35**, 136–42.

Cash, R. A., Toha, K. M., Nalin, D. R., Huq, Z. & Phillips, R. A. (1969). Acetate in the correction of acidosis secondary to cholera. *Lancet*, **2**, 302–3.

Christl, S. U., Gibson, G. R. & Cummings, J. H. (1992). Role of dietary sulphate in the regulation of methanogenesis in the human large intestine. *Gut*, **33**, 1234–8.

Clausen, M. R. Bonnen, H. & Mortensen, P. B. (1991). Colonic fermentation of dietary fibre to short-chain fatty acids in patients with adenomatous polyps and colon cancer. *Gut*, **32**, 923–8.

Coppack, S. W., Frayn, K. N., Humphreys, S. N., Whyte, P. L. & Hockaday, T. D. R. (1990). Arteriovenous differences across human adipose and forearm tissues after an overnight fast. *Metabolism, Clinical and Experimental*, **39**, 384–90.

Crabtree, B., Gordon, M.-J. & Christie, M. L. (1990). Measurement of the rate of acetyl-CoA hydrolysis and synthesis from acetate in rat hepatocytes and the role of these fluxes in substrate cycling, *Biochemical Journal*, **270**, 219–25.

Crouse, J. R., Gerson, C. D., Descari, L. M. & Leiber, C. S. (1968). Role of acetate in the reduction of plasma free fatty acids produced by ethanol in man. *Journal of Lipid Research*, **9**, 509–12.

Cummings, J. H. (1981). Short chain fatty acids in the human colon. *Gut*, **22**, 762–79.

Cummings, J. H. (1991). Production and metabolism of short-chain fatty acids in humans. In *Short-chain Fatty Acids: Metabolism and Clinical Importance*, pp. 11–16. Columbus, OH: Ross Laboratories.

Cummings, J. H., Allison, C. & Macfarlane, G. T. (1986). Significance of fermentation in the large intestine of man. *Journal of Applied Bacteriology*, **61**, 17.

Cummings, J. H., Banwell, J. G., Segal, I., Colman, H., Englyst, H. N. & Macfarlane, G. T. (1990). The amount and composition of large bowel contents in man. *Gastroenterology*, **98**, A408.

Cummings, J. H. & Bingham, S. A. (1992). Towards a recommended intake of dietary fibre. In *Human Nutrition: a Continuing Debate*, ed. M. Eastwood, C. Edwards & D. Parry, pp. 107–20. London: Chapman & Hall.

Cummings, J. H., Gibson, G. R. & Macfarlane, G. T. (1989). Quantitative estimates of fermentation in the hindgut of man. In *Comparative Aspects of Physiology of Digestion in Ruminants and Hindgut Fermenters*, Suppl. 86, pp. 76–81. Copenhagen: Acta Veterinaria Scandinavica.

Cummings, J. H., Pomare, E. W., Branch, W. J. & Naylor, C. P. E. (1987). Short chain fatty acids in the human large intestine, portal hepatic and venous blood. *Gut*, **28**, 1221–7.

Dankert, J., Zijlstra, J. B. & Wolthers, B. G. (1981). Volatile fatty acids in human peripheral and portal blood: quantitative determination by vacuum distillation. *Clinica Chimica Acta*, **110**, 301–7.

Del Boca, J. & Flatt, J. P. (1969). Fatty acid synthesis from glucose and acetate and the control of lipogenesis in adipose tissue. *European Journal of Biochemistry*, **11**, 127–34.

Demeyer, D., De Grave, K., Durand, M. & Sevani, J. (1989). Acetate, hydrogen sink in hindgut fermentation as opposed to rumen fermentation. In *Comparative Aspects of the Physiology of Digestion in Ruminants and Hindgut Fermenters*, Suppl. 86, pp. 68–75. Copenhagen: Acta Veterinaria Scandinavica.

De Silva, H. J., Ireland, A., Kettlewell, M., Mortensen, N. & Jewel, D. P. (1989). Short chain fatty acid irrigation in severe pouchitis. *New England Journal of Medicine*, **321**, 1416–17.

Desmoulin, F., Canioni, P. & Cozzone, P. J. (1985). Glutamate–glutamine metabolism in the perfused rat liver: ^{13}C-NMR study using (2-^{13}C)-enriched acetate. *FEBS Letters*, **185**, 29–32.

Dolmalski, E. S. (1972). Selected values of heats of combustion and heats of formation of organic compounds containing the elements C, H, N, O, P, and S. *Journal of Physical Chemistry Reference Data*, **1**, 221–77.

Egan, S. K. & Petersen, B. J. (1992). *Estimated Consumption of Inulin and Oligofructose by the US Population.* Washington, DC: Technical Assessment Systems.

Ekblad, H., Kero, P. & Takala, J. (1985). Slow sodium acetate infusion in the correction of metabolic acidosis in premature infants. *American Journal of Disease of Childhood*, **139**, 708–10.

Elia, M. (1992*a*). Glutamine in parenteral nutrition. *International Journal of Food Science and Nutrition*, **43**, 47–59.

Elia, M. (1992*b*). Organ and tissue contribution to metabolic rate. In *Energy Metabolism: Tissue Determinants and Cellular Corollaries*, ed. J. M. Kinney, pp. 61–79, New York: Raven Press.

Elia, M. (1992*c*). The interorgan flux of substrates in fed and fasted man as measured by arteriovenous balance studies. *Nutrition Research Reviews*, **4**, 3–31.

Elia, M. & Livesey, G. (1983). Effects of ingested steak and infused leucine on forelimb metabolism in man and the fate of the carbon skeletons and amino groups of branched chain amino acids. *Clinical Science*, **64**, 517–26.

Elia, M. & Livesey, G. (1988). The theory and validity of indirect calorimetry during net lipogenesis. *American Journal of Clinical Nutrition*, **47**, 591–607.

Elia, M. & Livesey, G. (1992). Energy expenditure and fuel selection in biological systems: the theory and practice of calculations based on indirect calorimetry and tracer methods. *World Review of Nutrition and Dietetics*, **70**, 68–131.

Elia, M., Zed, C., Neal, G. & Livesey, G. (1987). The energy cost of triglyceride–fatty acid recycling in non-obese subjects after an overnight fast and four days of starvation. *Metabolism*, **3**, 251–5.

Ellestad-Sayed, J. J., Nelson, R. A., Addison, M. A., Palmer, M. & Soule, E. (1976). Pantothenic acid, coenzyme A, and human chronic ulcerative and granulomatous colitis. *American Journal of Clinical Nutrition*, **29**, 1333–8.

Elund, T. (1987). Organic acid and ester. In *Mechanisms of Food Preservation Procedures*, pp. 170–99. London: Elsevier Applied Sciences.

Engelhardt, W. v., Busche, R., Gros, G. & Rechkemmer, G. (1991). Absorption of short-chain fatty acids: mechanism and regional differences in the large intestine. In *Short-chain Fatty Acids: Metabolism and Clinical Importance*, pp. 60–2. Columbus, OH: Ross Laboratories.

Engelhardt, W. v. & Rechkemmer, G. (1982). The physiological effects of short chain fatty acids in the hind gut. In *Fibre in Human and Animal Nutrition*, ed. G. Wallace & L. Bell, pp. 149–55. Auckland: The Royal Society of New Zealand.

Englyst, H. N., Hay, S. & Macfarlane, G. T. (1987). Polysaccharide breakdown by mixed populations of human faecal bacteria. *Microbial Ecology*, **95**, 161–71.

Englyst, H. N. & Macfarlane, G. T. (1986). Breakdown of resistant and readily digestible starch by human gut bacteria. *Journal of the Science of Food and Agriculture*, **37**, 699–706.

Erlanson, C. & Bergstrom, B. (1970). Tributyrin as a substrate for the determination of lipase activity of pancreatic juice and small intestinal contents. *Scandinavian Journal of Gastroenterology*, **5**, 293–5.
EURESTA (1991). *Methodological Aspects of* in vivo *Methods for Measurement of Starch Digestibility*, AGRF/0027, ed. E. Gudmand-Høyer. Copenhagen: European Flair – Concerted Action on Resistant Starch.
EURESTA (1992). Resistant starch. *European Journal of Nutrition*, **46** (Suppl. 2).
Evans, M. A. & Shronts, E. P. (1992). Intestinal fuels: glutamine, short-chain fatty acids and dietary fibre. *Journal of the American Dietetic Association*, **92**, 1239–49.
Figdor, S. K. & Bianchine, J. R. (1983). Caloric utilisation and disposition of Polydextrose in man. *Journal of Agricultural and Food Chemistry*, **31**, 389–93.
Flemming, S. E. & Calloway, D. H. (1983). Determination of intestinal gas excretion. In *Dietary Fibre*, ed. G. G. Birch & K. J. Parker, pp. 221–54. London: Applied Science Publishers.
Flick, J. A. & Perman, J. A. (1989). Non-absorbed carbohydrate: effect on fecal pH in methane excreting and nonmethane excreting individuals. *American Journal of Clinical Nutrition*, **49**, 1252–7.
Florin, T. H. J., Neale, G. & Cummings, J. H. (1990). Dietary organic anions can make a significant contribution to the total fermentable material in the human large intestine. *Proceedings of the Nutrition Society*, **49**, 226A.
Florin, T. H. J., Neal, G., Gibson , G. R., Christl, S. U. & Cummings, J. H. (1991). The metabolism of dietary sulphate: absorption and excretion in man. *Gut*, **32**, 766–73.
Flynn, K. T., Norton, C. C. & Fisher, R. L. (1987). Enteral tube feeding: indications, practices and outcomes. *Image: Journal of Nursing Scholarship*, **19**, 16–19.
Ford, W. D. A., Boelhaower, R. U., King, W. W. K., de Veris, J. E., Ross, J. S. & Malt, R. A. (1984). Total parenteral nutrition inhibits intestinal adaptive hyperplasia in young rats: reversal by feeding. *Surgery*, **96**, 527–34.
Frayn, K. N., Coppack, S. W., Walsh, P. E., Butterworth, H. C., Humphreys, S. M. & Pedrosa, H. C. (1990). Metabolic response of forearm and adipose tissue to acute ethanol ingestion. *Metabolism*, **39**, 958–66.
Gibson, G. R. (1990). Physiology and ecology of sulphate reducing bacteria. *Journal of Applied Bacteriology*, **69**, 769–97.
Gibson, G. R., Cummings, J. H. & Macfarlane, G. T. (1988). Competition for hydrogen between sulphate-reducing bacteria and methanogenic bacteria from the human large intestine. *Journal of Applied Bacteriology*, **65**, 241–7.
Glotzer, D. J., Glick, M. E. & Goldman, H. (1981). Proctitis and colitis following diversion of the faecal stream. *Gastroenterology*, **80**, 438–41.
Grant, J. & Snyder, P. J. (1988). Use of L-glutamine in total parenteral nutrition. *Journal of Surgical Research*, **44**, 506–13.
Hains, A., Metz, G., Dilawari, J. Blendis, L. & Wiggins, H. (1977). Breath methane in patients with cancer of the large bowel. *Lancet*, **2**, 481–3.
Hamosh, M. & Burns, W. A. (1977). Lipolytic activity of human linguinal glands (Ebner). *Laboratory Investigations*, **37**, 603–8.
Harig, J. M., Soergel, K. H., Komorowski, R. A. & Wood, C. M. (1989). Treatment of diversion colitis with short-chain-fatty acid irrigation. *New England Journal of Medicine*, **320**, 23–8.
Hellerstein, M. K., Christiansen, M., Kaempfer, S., Kletke, C., Wu, K., Reid, S., Mulligan, K., Hellerstein, N. S. & Shackleton, C. H. L. (1991). Measurement

of *de novo* hepatic lipogenesis in humans using stable isotopes. *Journal of Clinical Investigation*, **87**, 1841–52.

Henning, S. J. & Hird, F. J. R. (1972). Ketogenesis from butyrate and acetate by the caecum and colon of rabbits. *Biochemical Journal*, **130**, 785–90.

Hidaka, H., Adachi, T., Tokunaga, T., Niimoto, H. & Nakajima, Y. (1982). Production and characterisation of a new sweetener synthesised from sucrose by the action of fructosyltransferase, abstract 42, *Annual Food Technologists Meeting*, p. 195. Chicago, IL: Institute of Farm Technology.

Holtug, K. (1989). Mechanisms of absorption of short chain fatty acids – coupling to intracellular pH regulation. In *Comparative aspects of the Physiology of Digestion in Ruminants and Hindgut Fermenters*, Suppl. 86, pp. 126–33. Copenhagen: Acta Veterinaria Scandinavica.

Horino, M., Macklin, L. J., Hertelendy, F. & Kipnis, D. M. (1968). Effect of short-chain fatty acids on plasma insulin in ruminant and non-ruminant species. *Endocrinology*, **83**, 118–28.

Hughes, C. A., Price, A. & Dowling, R. H. (1980). Speed of change in pancreatic cell mass and in intestinal bacteriology of parenterally fed rats. *Clinical Science*, **59**, 329–6.

Iwakawa, T. (1989). On the energy value of saccharides that are hard to digest. *New Food Industry*, **31**, 42–7.

Jacobs, L. R. (1986). Relationship between dietary fibre and cancer: metabolic, physiologic and cellular mechanisms. *Proceedings of the Society for Experimental Biology and Medicine*, **183**, 299–310.

Jenkins, D. J. A., Wolever, T. M. S., Jenkins, A., Brighenti, F., Vulcsan, U., Rao, A. V., Cunnane, S. C., Olava, A., Corev, P., Vezina, C., Conelly, P., Buckley, G. & Patten, R. (1991). Specific types of colonic fermentation may raise low-density lipoprotein cholesterol concentratrations. *American Journal of Clinical Nutrition*, **54**, 141–7.

Johnson, L. R., Copeland, E. M. & Castro, G. A. (1975). Structural and hormonal alterations in the gastrointestinal tract of parenterally fed rats. *Gastroenterology*, **168**, 1177–83.

Jorfeldt, L. & Juhlin-Dannfelt, A. (1978). The influence of ethanol on splanchnic and skeletal muscle metabolism in man. *Metabolism: Clinical and Experimental*, **27**, 97–106.

Juhlin-Dannfelt, A. (1977). Ethanol effects on substrate utilization by the human brain. *Scandinavian Journal of Clinical Laboratory Investigations*, **37**, 443–9.

Kaplan, N. M. (1989). The deadly quartet: upper body obesity, glucose intolerance, hypertriglyceridaemia and hypertention. *Archives of Internal Medicine*, **149**, 1514–20.

Karlsson, N., Fellenius, E. & Keissling, K. H. (1977). Influence of acetate on the metabolism of β-hydroxybutyric acid in the perfused hind-quarter of the rat. *Acta Physiologica Scandinavica*, **99**, 113–22.

Karlstrad, M. D., Killeffer, J. A., Bailey, J. W. & Demichele, S. J. (1992). Parenteral nutrition with short and long chain triglycerides – triacetin reduces atrophy of small and large bowel mucosa and improves protein metabolism in burned rats. *American Journal of Clinical Nutrition*, **55**, 1005–11.

Katoh, K. (1991). The effect of short-chain fatty acids on the pancrease: endocrine and exocrine. In *Short-chain Fatty Acids: Metabolism and Clinical Importance*, pp. 74–7. Columbus, OH: Ross Laboratories.

Kelly, T. W. & Hillman, K. M. (1983). Study of diarrhea in critically ill patients. *Critical Care Medicine*, **11**, 7–9.

Kirvela, O. K. & Takala, J. A. (1986). Comparison of monoglyceryl acetoacetate and glucose as parenteral energy substrates after experimental trauma. *European Surgical Journal*, **18**, 80–5.

Klimberg, V. S., Souba, W. W., Dolson, D. J., Salloum, R. M., Hautamaki, R. D., Plumley, D. A., Mendenhall, W. M., Bova, F. J., Khan, S. R., Hackett, R. L., Bland, K. I. & Copeland, E. M. (1990). Prophylactic glutamine protects the mucosa from radiation injury. *Cancer Research*, **66**, 62–8.

Korelitz, B. I., Cheskin, L. J., Sohn, N. & Sommers, S. C. (1985). The fate of the rectal segment after diversion of the faecal stream in Crohn's disease: its implications for surgical management. *Journal of Clinical Gastroenterology*, **7**, 37–43.

Koruda, M. J., Rolandelli, R. H. & Settle, R. G. (1988). Effect of parenteral nutrition supplemented with short-chain fatty acids on adaptation to massive small bowel resection. *Gastroenterology*, **95**, 715–20.

Koruda, M. J., Rolandelli, R. H. & Settle, R. G. (1990). Parenteral nutrition supplemented with short chain fatty acids: effect on the small bowel mucosa in normal rats. *American Journal of Clinical Nutrition*, **51**, 685–9.

Koziet, J., Gross, P., Debry, G. & Royer, M. J. (1991). Evaluation of (^{13}C)ethanol incorporation into very-low density lipoprotein triglycerides using gas chromatography/isotope ratio mass spectrometry coupling. *Biological Mass Spectrometry*, **20**, 777–82.

Kripke, S. A., De Paula, J. A., Berman, J. M., Fox, A. D., Rombeau, J. L. & Settle, R. G. (1991). Experimental short-bowel syndrome: effect of an elemental diet supplemented with short-chain triglycerides. *American Journal of Clinical Nutrition*, **53**, 954–62.

Kripke, S. A., Fox, A. D. & Berman, J. M. (1989). Stimulation of intestinal mucosal growth with intracolonic infusion of short chain fatty acids. *Journal of Parenteral and Enteral Nutrition*, **13**, 109–16.

Kripke, S. A., Fox, A. D., Berman, J. M., De Paula, J., Birkhahn, R. H., Rombeau, J. L. & Settle, R. G. (1988). Inhibition of TPN-associated intestinal mucosal atrophy with monoacetoacetin. *Journal of Surgical Research*, **44**, 436–44.

Kritchevsky, D. (1986). Diet, nutrition and cancer. The role of fibre. *Cancer*, **58**, 1830–6.

Kruh, J., Defer, N. & Tichonicky, L. (1991). Molecular and cellular effects of sodium butyrate. In *Short-chain Fatty Acids: Metabolism and Clinical Importance*, pp. 45–50. Columbus, OH: Ross Laboratories.

Kvietys, P. R. & Granger, D. N. (1981). Effects of volatile fatty acids on blood flow and oxygen uptake by the dog colon. *Gastroenterology*, **80**, 962–9.

Laine, L., Shulman, R. J., Pitre, D., Lifschitz, C. H. & Adams, J. (1991). Cysteine usage increases the need for acetate in neonates who receive total parenteral nutrition. *American Journal of Clinical Nutrition*, **54**, 565–7.

Lairon, D., Nalbone, D., Lafont, H., Leonardi, J., Vigne, J.-L. Chabert, C., Hauton, J. C. & Verger, R. (1980). Effects of bile lipids on the absorption and activity of pancreatic lipase on triacylglycerol emulsion. *Biochimica et Biophysica Acta*, **618**, 119–28.

Langholz, E., Mumkholm, P., Davidsen, M. & Binder, V. (1992). Colorectal cancer risk and mortality in patients with ulcerative colitis. *Gastroenterology*, **103**, 1444–51.

Lazarus, D. D. & Stein, T. P. (1988). Use of acetate in total parenteral nutrition solutions. *Journal of Parenteral and Enteral Nutrition*, **12**, 108S–110S.

Levine, G. M., Deren, J. J. & Steiger, E. (1974). Role of oral intake in the maintenance of gut mass and disaccharidase activity. *Gastroenterology*, **67**, 975–82.

Levine, G. M., Deren, J. J., Yezdimir, E. (1976). Small bowel resection: oral intake is the stimulus for hyperplasia. *Digestive Disease Science*, **21**, 542–6.

Lindeneg, O., Mellemgaard, K., Fabricius, J. & Lundquist, F. (1964). Myocardial utilization of acetate, lactate and free fatty acid after ingestion of ethanol. *Clinical Science*, **27**, 427–35.

Lipkin, M. (1988). Biomarkers of increased susceptibility to gastrointestinal cancer: new application to studies of cancer prevention in human subjects. *Cancer Research*, **48**, 235–45.

Livesey, G. (1984). The energy equivalents of ATP and the energy values of food proteins and fats. *British Journal of Nutrition*, **51**, 15–28.

Livesey, G. (1987). ATP yields from proteins, fats and carbohydrates and mitochondrial efficiency *in vivo*. *Recent Advances in Obesity Research*, **5**, 131–43.

Livesey, G. (1990*a*). Energy values of unavailable carbohydrates and diets: an inquiry and analysis. *American Journal of Clinical Nutrition*, **51**, 617–37.

Livesey, G. (1990*b*). The impact of the concentration and dose of Palatinit® in foods and diets on energy value. *Food Science and Nutrition*, **42F**, 223–43.

Livesey, G. (1991). Calculating the energy values of foods: towards new empirical formulae based on diets with varied intakes of unavailable complex carbohydrates. *European Journal of Clinical Nutrition*, **45**, 1–12.

Livesey, G. (1992). Methodology for the caloric evaluation of fibre and bulking agents. In *Chemistry and Nutritional Effects of Dietary Fibre*, ed. S. Samman & G. Annison, pp. 57–9, Sydney: University of Sydney.

Livesey, G. (1993). The energy values of dietary fibre and sugar alcohols for man. *Nutrition Research Reviews*, **5**, 61–84.

Livesey, G. & Elia, M. (1988). Estimation of energy expenditure, net carbohydrate utilisation, and net fat oxidation and synthesis by indirect calorimetry: evaluation of errors with special reference to the composition of fuels. *American Journal of Clinical Nutrition*, **47**, 608–28.

Livesey, G., Johnson, I. T., Gee, J., Smith, T., Hillan, K. A., Meyer, J. & Turner, S. C. (1993). 'Determination' of sugar alcohol and polydextrose absorption in humans by the breath hydrogen (H_2) technique: the stoichiometry of hydrogen production and the interaction between carbohydrates assessed *in vivo* and *in vitro*. *European Journal of Clinical Nutrition*, **47**, 419–30.

Livesey, G. & Lund, P. (1982). Binding of branched-chain 2-oxo acids to bovine serum albumin. *Biochemical Journal*, **204**, 265–72.

Livesey, G., Williams, K. E., Knowles, S. E. & Ballard, F. J. (1980). Effect of weak bases on the degradation of endogenous and exogenous proteins by rat yolk sacs. *Biochemical Journal*, **188**, 895–903.

Loeschke, K. & Gordon, H. A. (1969). Water movement across the cecal wall of the germfree rat. *Proceedings of the Society for Experimental Biology and Medicine*, **133**, 1217–22.

Lundquist, F., Sestoft, L., Damgaard, S. E., Clausen, J. P. & Trap-Jensen, J. (1973). Utilisation of acetate in the human forearm during exercise after ethanol ingestion. *Journal of Clinical Investigation*, **52**, 3231–5.

Lundquist, F., Tygstrup, N., Winkler, K., Mellemgaard, K. & Munck-Petersen, S. (1962). Ethanol metabolism and production of free acetate in the human liver. *Journal of Clinical Investigation*, **41**, 955–61.

Macfarlane, G. T. (1991). Fermentation reactions in the large intestine. In *Short-chain Fatty Acids: Metabolism and Clinical Importance*, pp. 5–10. Columbus, OH: Ross Laboratories.

MAFF (1990). Intakes of intense and bulk sweeteners in the UK 1987–1988. *Food Surveillance*, paper no. 29. Norwich: Her Majesty's Stationery Office.

Manns, J. G. & Bode, J. M. (1967). Insulin, release by acetate, propionate, butyrate and glucose in lambs and adult sheep. *American Journal of Physiology*, **212**, 747–55.

Marthinsen, D. & Flemming, S. E. (1982). Excretion of breath and flatus gasses by humans. *Journal of Human Nutrition*, **112**, 1133–43.

McBurney, M. I. & Thompson, L. U. (1987). Effect of human faecal inoculum on *in vitro* fermentation variables. *British Journal of Nutrition*, **58**, 233–43.

McCance, R. A. & Lawrence, R. D. (1929). *The Carbohydrate Content of Foods.* Special Report Series of the Medical Research Council, no. 135. London: Her Majesty's Stationery Office.

McCance, R. A. & Widdowson, E. M. (1940). *The Chemical Composition of Foods.* Special Report Series of the Medical Research Council, no. 235. London: Her Majesty's Stationery Office.

McNeil, N. I., Cummings, J. H. & James, W. P. T. (1978). Short chain fatty acid absorption by the human large intestine. *Gut*, **19**, 819–22.

Miller, D. L., Hanson, W., Schedl, H. P. & Osborne, S. W. (1977). Proliferation rate and transit time of mucosal cells in small intestine of diabetic rat. *Gastroenterology*, **73**, 1326–32.

Moore, F. A., Moore, E. E., Jones, T. N. & McKroskey, B. L. (1989). TEN versus TPN following major abdominal trauma – reduced septic morbidity. *Journal of Trauma*, **28**, 916–23.

Mortensen, P. B., Holtung, K., Bonnen, H. & Clausen, M. R. (1990*a*). The degradation of amino acids, protein and blood to short-chain fatty acids in the colon is prevented by lactulose. *Gastroenterology*, **98**, 353–60.

Mortensen, P. B., Holtung, K. & Rasmussen, H. S. (1988*a*). Short chain fatty acid production from mono and dissacharides in faecal incubation systems: implications for colonic fermentation of dietary fibre in humans. *Journal of Nutrition*, **118**, 321–5.

Mortensen, P. B., Nielsen, H., Mulvany, M. J. & Hessov, I. (1990*b*). Short-chain fatty acids dilate isolated human colonic arteries. *Gut*, **31**, 1391–4.

Mortensen, P. B., Rasmussen, H. S. & Holtug, K. (1988*b*). Lactulose detoxifies *in vitro* short-chain fatty acid production in colonic contents induced by blood: implications for hepatic coma. *Gastroenterology*, **94**, 750–4.

Muto, Y. (1966). Clinical study on the relationship of short-chain fatty acids and hepatic encephalopathy. *Japanese Journal of Gastroenterology*, **63**, 19–31.

Muto, Y. & Takahasi, Y. (1964). Gas chromatographic short-chain fatty acids in disease of the liver. *Journal of the Japanese Society of Internal Medicine*, **53**, 828–40.

Nath, R. L. & Debnath, H. (1968). Studies on serum lipase against different triglycerides in some clinical conditions: study on triacetinase and tributyrinase. *Bulletin of the Calcutta School of Tropical Medicine*, **16**, 45–6.

Neilsen, L. G., Owen-Ash, K. & Thor, E. (1978). Gas chromatographic method for plasma acetate analysis in acetate intolerance studies. *Clinical Chemistry*, **24**, 348–50.

Niles, R. M., Willhelm, S. A., Thomas, P. & Zamcheck, N. (1988). The effect of sodium butyrate and retinoic acid on growth and CEA production on a series of human colorectal tumour cell lines representing different states of differentiation. *Cancer Investigation*, **6**, 39–45.

Nilsson, N. O. & Belfrage, P. (1978). Effect of acetate, acetaldehyde and ethanol on lipolysis in isolated rat adipocytes. *Journal of Lipid Research*, **19**, 737–41.

Patel, D. G. & Singh, S. P. (1979). Effect of ethanol and its metabolites on glucose mediated insulin release from isolated islets of rats. *Metabolism*, **28**, 85–8.

Paul, A. A. & Southgate, D. A. T. (1978). *McCance and Widdowson's Composition of Foods*. London: Her Majesty's Stationery Office.

Peters, S. G., Pomare, E. W. & Fisher, C. A. (1992). Portal and peripheral blood short-chain fatty acid concentrations after caecal lactulose instillation at surgery. *Gut*, **33**, 1249–52.

Piqué, K. M., Pallarés, M., Cusó, E., Vilar-Bonet, J. & Gassull, M. A. (1984). Methane production and colon cancer. *Gastroenterology*, **87**, 601–5.

Pomare, E. W., Branch, W. J. & Cummings, J. H. (1985). Carbohydrate fermentation in the human colon and its relation to acetate concentration in venous blood. *Journal of Clinical Investigations*, **75**, 1448–54.

Pullicino, E. & Elia, M. (1991). Intravenous carbohydrate overfeeding: method for rapid nutritional repletion.*Clinical Nutrition*, **10**, 1146–54.

Rabassa, A. O. & Rogers, A. I. (1992). The role of short chain fatty acid metabolism in colonic disorders. *American Journal Gastroenterology*, **87**, 419–23.

Rabbani, G. H. & Binder, H. J. (1989). Evidence for active butyrate absorption by rat distal colon. In *Comparative Aspects of the Physiology of Digestion in Ruminants and Hindgut Fermenters*, Suppl. 86, p. 195. Copenhagen: Acta Veterinaria Scandinavica.

Randle, P. J., England, P. J. & Denton, R. M. (1970). Control of the carboxylate cycle and its interactions with glycolysis during acetate utilisation in rat heart. *Biochemical Journal*, **117**, 677–95.

Rao, S. S. C., Edwards, C. J., Bruce, C. & Read, N. W. (1988). Impaired colonic fermentation of carbohydrate after ampicillin. *Gastroenterlogy*, **94**, 928–32.

Rechkemmer, G. & Engelhardt, W. v. (1982). Absorptive processes in different colonic segments of the guinea pig and the effect of short chain fatty acids. In *Colon and Nutrition*, ed. H. Kasper & H. Goebell, pp. 61–7. Lancaster: MTP Press.

Rémésy, C. & Demigné, C. (1974). Determination of volatile fatty acids in plasma after ethanol extraction. *Biochemical Journal*, **141**, 86–91.

Rémésy, C., Demigné & Morand, C. (1991). Metabolism and utilisation of short-chain fatty acids produced by colonic fermentation. In *Dietry Fibre: A Component of Food*, ed. T. F. Schweizer & C. A. Edwards, pp. 137–50. London: Springer-Verlag.

Robinson, A. M. & Williamson, D. H. (1980). Physiological roles of ketone bodies as substrates and signals in mammalian tissues. *Physiological Reviews*, **60**, 143–87.

Rocchiccioli, F., Lepetit, N. & Bougnéres, P. F. (1989). Capillary gas–liquid chromatography/mass spectrometric measurement of plasma acetate content and (2-^{13}C)acetate enrichment. *Biomedical and Environmental Mass Spectrometry*, **18**, 816–19.

Roediger, W. E. W. (1980). Role of anaerobic bacteria in the metabolic welfare of the colonic mucosa in man. *Gut*, **21**, 793–8.

Roediger, W. E. W. (1982). Utilisation of nutrients by isolated epithelial cells of the rat colon. *Gastroenterology*, **83**, 424–9.

Roediger, W. E. W. (1986). Metabolic basis of starvation diarrhoea: implications for treatment. *Lancet*, **1**, 1088–4.

Roediger, W. E. W. (1988). Short chain fatty acids and mucosal disease. *British Journal of Surgery*, **75**, 346–8.

Roediger, W. E. W. (1989). Short chain fatty acids as metabolic regulators of ion absorption in the colon. In *Comparative Aspects of the Physiology of Digestion in Ruminants and Hindgut Fermenters*, Suppl. 86, pp. 116–25. Copenhagen: Acta Vetrinaria Scandinavica.

Roediger, W. E. W., Lawsong, M. J., Kwok, V., Kerr Grant, A. & Pannall, P. R. (1984). Colonic bicarbonate output as a test of disease activity in ulcerative colitis. *Journal of Clinical Pathology*, **37**, 704–7.

Roediger, W. E. W. & Nance, S. (1986). Metabolic induction of experimental ulcerative colitis by inhibition of fatty acid oxidation. *British Journal of Experimental Pathology*, **67**, 773–82.

Rolandelli, R. H., Koruda, M. J., Settle, R. G. & Rombeau, J. L. (1986). Effects of intraluminal infusion of short chain fatty acids on the healing of colonic anastomosis in the rat. *Surgery*, **100**, 198–203.

Rolandelli, R. H., Saul, S. H., Settle, R. G., Jacobs, D. O., Trevotola, S. O. & Rombeau, J. L. (1988). Comparison of parenteral nutrition and enteral feeding with pectin in experimental colitis in the rat. *American Journal of Clinical Nutrition*, **47**, 715–21.

Rombeau, J. L. (1990). A review of the effects of glutamine-enriched diets on experimentally induced enterocolitis. *Journal of Parenteral and Enteral Nutrition*, **14**, 100S–105S.

Roth, F. X., Kirchgessner, M. & Müller, H. L. (1988). Energetic utilisation of intraceacally infused acetic and propionic acids in sows. *Journal of Animal Physiology and Animal Nutrition*, **59**, 211–17.

Ruppin, H., Bar-Meir, S., Soergel, K. H., Wood, C. M. & Schmitt, M. G. (1980). Absorption of short chain fatty acids by the colon. *Gastroenterology*, **78**, 1500–7.

Sakata, T. (1987). Stimulatory effects of short-chain fatty acids on epithelial cell proliferation in the rat intestine. A possible explanation of the trophic effects of fermentable fibre, gut microbes and trophic factors. *British Journal of Nutrition*, **58**, 95–103.

Sakata, T. (1991). Effects of short chain fatty acids on epithelial cell proliferation and mucus release in the intestine. In *Short-chain Fatty Acids: Metabolism and Clinical Importance*, Report of the Tenth Ross Conference on Medical Research, ed. A. F. Roche, pp. 63–7. Columbus, OH: Ross Laboratories.

Sakata, T. & Yajima, T. (1984). Influence of short chain fatty acids on the epithelial cell division of the digestive tract. *Quarterly Journal of Experimental Physiology*, **69**, 639–48.

Samson, F. E., Dahl, N. & Dahl, D. R. (1956). A study of the narcotic action of the short chain fatty acids. *Journal of Clinical Investigation*, **35**, 1291–8.

Schedl, H. P. & Wilson, H. D. (1971). Effect of diabetes on intestinal growth in the rat. *Journal of Experimental Zoology*, **176**, 487–96.

Schedl, H. P., Wilson, H. D., Ramaswamy, K. & Lichenberger, L. (1982). Gastrin and growth of the alimentary tract in the streptozotocin-diabetic rat. *American Journal of Physiology*, **242**, G460–G463.

Scheppach, W., Cummings, J. H., Branch, W. J. & Schrezenmeir, J. (1988*a*). Effect of gut-derived acetate on oral tolerance in man. *Clinical Science*, **75**, 355–61.

Scheppach, W., Pomare, E. W., Elia, M. & Cummings, J. H. (1991). The contribution of the large intestine to blood acetate in man. *Clinical Science*, **80**, 177–82.

Scheppach, W., Sommer, H., Kirchner, T., Paganelli, G. M., Bartram, P., Christl, S., Richter, F., Dusel, G. & Kasper, H. (1992). Effect of butyrate enemas on colonic mucosa in distal ulcerative colitis. *Gastroenterology*, **103**, 51–6.

Scheppach, W., Wiggins, S., Halliday, D., Self, R., Howard, J., Branch, W. Y., Schrezenmeir, J. & Cummings, J. H. (1988*b*). Effect of gut-derived acetate on glucose turnover in man. *Clinical Science*, **75**, 363–70.

Seufert, C. D., Mewes, W. & Soeling, H. D. (1984). Effect of long-term starvation on acetate and ketone body metabolism in obese patients. *European Journal of Clinical Investigation*, **14**, 163–70.

Sherman, P., Soni, R. & Karmali, M. (1988). Attaching and effacing adherence of vero cytotoxin-producing *Escherichia coli* to rabbit intestinal epithelium *in vivo*. *Infection and Immunity*, **56**, 756–61.

Silk, D. B. E. (1993). Fibre and enteral nutrition. *Clinical Nutrition*, 12 (Suppl. 1), S106–S113.

Skutches, C. L., Holroyde, C. P., Myers, R. W., Paul, P. & Reichard, G. A. (1979). Plasma acetate turnover and oxidation. *Journal of Clinical Investigation*, **64**, 708–13.

Skutches, C. L., Sigler, M. H., Teehan, B. P., Cooper, J. H. & Reichard, G. A. (1983). Contribution of dialysate acetate to energy metabolism: metabolic implications. *Kidney International*, **23**, 57–63.

Smith, R. F., Humphreys, S. & Hockaday, T. D. R. (1986). The measurement of plasma acetate by a manual and automated technique in diabetic and non-diabetic subjects. *Annals of Clinical Biochemistry*, **23**, 285–91.

Souba, W. W., Scott, T. E. & Wilmore, D. W. (1985). Intestinal consumption of intravenously administered fuels. *Journal of Parenteral and Enteral Nutrition*, **9**, 18–22.

Southgate, D. A. T. & Durnin, J. V. G. A. (1970). Calorie conversion factors. An experimental reassessment of the factors used in the calculation of the energy value of human diets. *British Journal of Nutrition*, **24**, 517–35.

Spaeth, G. Specian, R. D., Berg, R. D. & Deitch, E. A. (1990). Bulk prevents bacterial translocation induced by the oral administration of total parenteral nutrition solution. *Journal of Enteral and Parenteral Nutrition*, **44**, 442–7.

Strange, E. F. & Dietschy, J. (1983). Absolute rates of cholesterol synthesis in rat intestine *in vitro* and *in vivo*: a comparison of different substrates in sliced and isolated cells. *Journal of Lipid Research*, **24**, 72–82.

Stephen, A. M., Bagby, B., Hoppel, C. & Banwell, J. (1989). Effect of colonic infusion of short-chain fatty acids on human glucose and fatty acid metabolism. *Federation of American Societies for Experimental Biology*, **3**, A942.

Stephen, A. M. & Cummings, J. H. (1980). The microbial contribution to human faecal mass. *Journal of Medical Microbiology*, **13**, 45–56.

Thaysen, E. H. & Thaysen, J. H. (1952). Hunger diarrhoea. In *Famine Disease*, ed. P. Helweg-Larsen, H. Hoffmeyer, J. Keiler, E. H. Thaysen, J. H. Thaysen, P. Thygesen & M. H. Wulff, Suppl. 274, pp. 124–60. Copenhagen: Acta Medica Scandinavica.

Tiruppathi, C. & Balasubramanian, K. A. (1982). Purification and properties of pancreatic lipase from human gastric juice. *Biochimica et Biophysica Acta*, **712**, 692–7.

Todesco, T., Rao, A. V., Bosello, O. & Jenkins, D. J. A. (1991). Propionate lowers blood glucose and alters lipid metabolism in healthy subjects. *American Journal of Clinical Nutrition*, **54**, 860–5.

Tollinger, C. D., Vreman, J. & Weiner, M. W. (1979). Measurement of acetate in human blood by gas chromatography: effect of sample preparation and various diseases. *Clinical Chemistry*, **25**, 1787–90.

Trock, B., Lanza, E. & Greenwood, P. (1990) Dietary fibre, vegetables and colon cancer: critical review and meta-analysis of the epidemiological evidence. *Journal of the National Cancer Institute*, **82**, 650–61.

Umesaki, Y., Yajima, T., Yokokura, T. & Mutai, M. (1979). Effects of organic acid absorption on bicarbonate transport in the colon. *Pflügers Archiv*, **379**, 43–7.

Vague, J. (1990). Willendorf lecture: diabetogenic and atherogenic fat. In *Progress in Obesity Research*, ed. Y. Oomura, S. Tarui, S. Inoue & T. Shimazu, pp. 343–58. London: John Libbey.

Venter, C. S., Vorster, H. H. & Cummings, J. H. (1990). Effects of dietary propionate on carbohydrate and lipid metabolism in healthy volunteers. *American Journal of Gastroenterology*, **85**, 549–52.

Vernia, P., Caprilli, R., Latella, G., Berbetti, F., Magliocca, F. M. & Cittadini, M. (1988*a*). Faecal lactate and ulcerative colitis. *Gastroenterology*, **95**, 1564–8.

Vernia, P., Gnaedinger, A., Hauck, W. & Breuer, R. I. (1988*b*). Organic anions and the diarrhea of inflammatory bowel disease. *Digestive Diseases Science*, **33**, 1353–8.

Vince, A. J., McNeil, N. I., Wager, J. & Wrong, D. M. (1990). The effect of lactulose, pectin, arabinogalactan and cellulose on the production of organic acids and metabolism of ammonia by intestinal bacteria in a faecal incubation system. *British Journal of Nutrition*, **63**, 17–26.

Weiner, M. W. (1982). Acetate metabolism during hemodialysis. *Artificial Organs*, **6**, 370–7.

Weser, E. (1983). Nutritional aspects of malabsorption: short-gut adaptation. *Clinical Gastroenterology*, **12**, 443–61.

Weser, E., Heller, R. & Tawil, T. (1977). Stimulation of mucosal growth in the rat ileum by bile and pancreatic secretions after jejunal resection. *Gastroenterology*, **73**, 524–9.

Whithead, R. H., Young, G. B. & Bhathal, B. S. (1986). Effects of short chain fatty acids on a new human colon carcinoma cell line (LIM 1215). *Gut*, **27**, 1457–63.

Wilcock, H., Armstrong, J., Cottee, J., Neale, G. & Elia, M. (1991). Artificial nutritional support for patients in the Cambridge Health District. *Health Trends*, **23**, 93–100.

Wilhout, R. C. (1969). Selected values of thermodynamic properties. In *Biochemical Microcalorimetry*, ed. D. H. Brown, pp. 305–17. London: Academic Press.

Wilmore, D. W., Dudrick, S. J., Daly, J. M. & Vors, H. M. (1971). The role of nutrition in the adaptation of the small intestine after massive resection. *Surgery, Gynaecology and Obstetrics*, **132**, 673–80.

Windmueller, H. G. & Spaeth, A. E. (1978). Identification of ketone bodies and glutamine as the major respiratory fuels *in vivo* for postabsorptive rat small intestine. *Journal of Biological Chemistry*, **253**, 69–76.

Wisker, E. & Feldheim, W. (1992). Faecal bulking and energy value of dietary fibre. In *Dietary Fibre – a Component of Food*, ed. T. F. Schweizer & C A. Edwards, pp. 233–46. New York: Springer-Verlag.

Wolever, T. M. S. (1991). Effects of short-chain fatty acids on carbohydrate and lipid metabolism. In *Short-chain Fatty Acids: Metabolism and Clinical Importance*, pp. 24–8. Columbus, OH: Ross Laboratories.

Wolever, T. M. S., Spadafora, P. & Eshuis, H. (1991). Interaction between colonic acetate and propionate in man. *American Journal of Clinical Nutrition*, **53**, 681–7.

Young, G. P. (1991). Butyrate and the molecular biology of the large bowel. In *Short-chain Fatty Acids: Metabolism and Clinical Importance*, pp. 39–44. Columbus, OH: Ross Laboratories.

Zieve, F. J., Zieve, L., Doizaki, W. M. & Gilsdorf, R. B. (1974). Synergism between ammonia and fatty acids in the production of coma: implications for hepatic coma. *Journal of Pharmacology and Experimental Therapeutics*, **191**, 10–16.

Zieve, L. & Nicoloff, D. (1976). Alterations in volatile fatty acids of blood after hepatectomy. *Surgery*, **80**, 554–7.

Zimmaro, D. M., Rolandelli, R. H., Koruda, M. J., Settle, R. G., Stein, P. & Rombeau, J. L. (1989). Isotonic tube feeding formula induces liquid stool in normal subjects: reversal by pectin. *Journal of Enteral and Parenteral Nutrition*, **13**, 117–23.

29

Short-chain fatty acids and carbohydrate metabolism

T. M. S. WOLEVER

Introduction

Interest in the effects of short-chain fatty acids (SCFA) on carbohydrate metabolism in humans was prompted by the suggestion that they may play a role in mediating the effects of dietary fibres that improve blood glucose control in patients with diabetes (Anderson & Bridges, 1984). Acetate, propionate and butyrate are the major SCFA produced during colonic fermentation, and all three have been shown to influence carbohydrate metabolism in cells and organs *in vitro* (Anderson & Bridges, 1984). However, there is evidence that butyrate is virtually completely extracted by the colon, with very little appearing in portal blood for delivery to the liver (Cummings *et al.*, 1987). In addition, acetate is the only SCFA that appears in peripheral blood to any significant extent (Cummings *et al.*, 1987). This chapter will therefore focus on the effects of acetate and propionate on carbohydrate metabolism in humans and non-ruminant animal models.

Carbohydrate metabolism in the liver

The liver has a central role in carbohydrate metabolism, having the unique ability both to take up and store glucose from the bloodstream, and to release glucose into the circulation. In the fed state, the liver takes up glucose from the portal blood and either stores it as glycogen, or converts it to fatty acids, which are incorporated into very-low-density lipoprotein (VLDL), secreted into the blood and ultimately stored in adipose tissue. Under conditions in which the body's demand for glucose exceeds the rate of absorption from the gut (e.g. starvation, low-carbohydrate diet, prolonged exercise) the liver produces glucose from lactate, glycerol or amino acids.

Effects of acetate

It has been appreciated for many years that the oxidation of fatty acids, including acetate, inhibits glycolysis and stimulates gluconeogenesis in muscle (Williamson, 1964; Newsholme & Start, 1973), kidney cortex (Underwood & Newsholme, 1967) and colonic mucosa (Roediger, 1980), as well as the liver (Anderson & Bridges, 1984). Acetate is rapidly activated to acetyl-CoA by acetate thiokinase, which is present in most mammalian tissues in both the cell mitochondria and the cytoplasm (Ballard, 1972). The intracellular concentration of citrate is increased by acetate (Garland & Randle, 1964). Fatty-acid oxidation also increases levels of intracellular acetyl-CoA and citrate (Garland & Randle, 1964). An increased citrate concentration inhibits glycolytic flux by inhibiting phosphofructokinase (PFK) activity (Newsholme & Start, 1973; Anderson & Bridges, 1984; Fig. 29.1). Gluconeogenesis may be stimulated by the high concentration of acetyl-CoA, which inhibits pyruvate oxidation to acetyl-CoA and stimulates pyruvate carboxylation to oxaloacetate (Fig. 29.1).

It is worth noting here that carbon atoms from acetate may appear in glucose (Consoli *et al.*, 1987) but that no *net* glucose production can be obtained from acetate. This is because two carbon atoms from acetyl-CoA enter the tricarboxylic acid (TCA) cycle by condensing with oxaloacetate to form citrate, and two carbon atoms are lost as two molecules of carbon dioxide during each turn of the TCA cycle. However, the carbon atoms lost as carbon dioxide are not the same carbon atoms that were obtained from acetate (Wolfe & Jahoor, 1990). Thus, carbon atoms from acetate are recycled to oxaloacetate, which can be transported across the mitochondrial membrane via the malate shuttle and become a glucose precursor (Fig. 29.1).

Glucose taken up by the liver can be disposed of by three routes: conversion to glycogen, the glycolytic pathway, or the pentose phosphate pathway (Fig. 29.2). There is evidence that acetate, in the presence of insulin, enhances the activity of the pentose phosphate pathway (Flatt & Ball, 1966). This has the effect of providing the reducing equivalents necessary to synthesize fatty acids from acetate. This is consistent with the results of a recent study which showed that the addition of 25 g/day of lactulose, a non-absorbed sugar that is fermented to yield a high proportion of acetate (Mortensen, Holtug & Rasmussen, 1988), to the metabolically controlled diets of healthy subjects for 2 weeks resulted in a significant increase in serum triglyceride levels (Jenkins *et al.*, 1990). Thus, acetate, despite reducing glucose flux through the glycolytic pathway, may increase net glucose utilization by the liver (Flatt

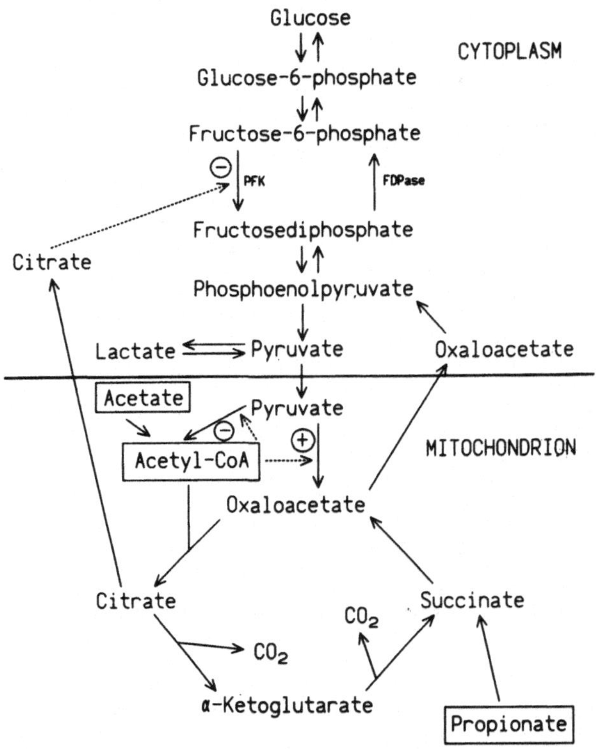

Fig. 29.1. Effects of acetate and propionate on glycolysis and gluconeogenesis. PFK, phosphofructokinase; FDPase, fructosediphosphatase.

& Ball, 1966), by increasing flux through the pentose phosphate pathway (Fig. 29.2).

Effects of propionate

In contrast to fatty acids with an even number of carbon atoms, which are metabolized to acetyl-CoA, propionate and other fatty acids with an odd number of carbon atoms are metabolized to propionyl-CoA, methylmalonyl-CoA and succinyl-CoA, the last of which enters the TCA cycle and is converted to oxaloacetate and thence to glucose (Fig. 29.1). Thus, propionate and other fatty acids with an odd number of carbon atoms are gluconeogenic substrates (Newsholme & Start, 1973). Rectal infusion of 180 mmol (17.5 g) sodium propionate has been shown to increase blood glucose in human subjects (Wolever, Spadafora & Eshuis, 1991; Fig. 29.3).

Propionate decreases glucose production from lactate in isolated hepato-

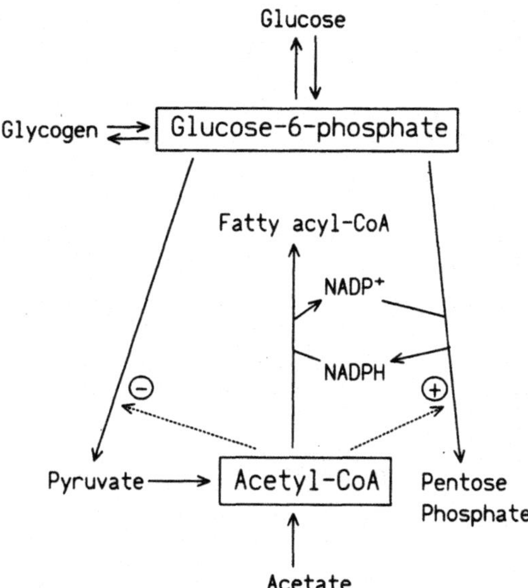

Fig. 29.2. Effect of acetate on intracellular glucose disposal.

cytes (Anderson & Bridges, 1984). It should be noted that under the experimental conditions used, the reduction in the rate of glucose production from lactate induced by propionate was almost equal to the rate of gluconeogenesis from propionate itself (Anderson & Bridges, 1984). Nevertheless, a reduction in hepatic glucose production may be beneficial in established diabetes, since, in the late stages of non-insulin-dependent diabetes, when the fasting level of blood glucose is >140 mg/dl (7.8 mmol/l), hepatic glucose output is directly related to the fasting blood glucose level (DeFronzo, 1988).

Propionate markedly increased glucose utilization by rat hepatocytes *in vitro* which was suggested to be due to a reduction in citrate concentration (Anderson & Bridges, 1984; Fig. 29.1). In the early stages of non-insulin-dependent diabetes (i.e. when the fasting blood-glucose level is <140 mg/dl), fasting hyperglycaemia has been suggested to be due to reduced peripheral glucose clearance (DeFronzo, 1988). Thus, increased glucose utilization would be beneficial in diabetes if it occurred in peripheral tissues. However, since propionate does not appear in peripheral blood under physiological conditions, propionate could only stimulate activity of the glycolytic pathway in the liver. Theoretically, increased hepatic glucose utilization could be deleterious, because it would result in increased VLDL synthesis, increased serum triglyceride levels and an increased risk for coronary heart disease

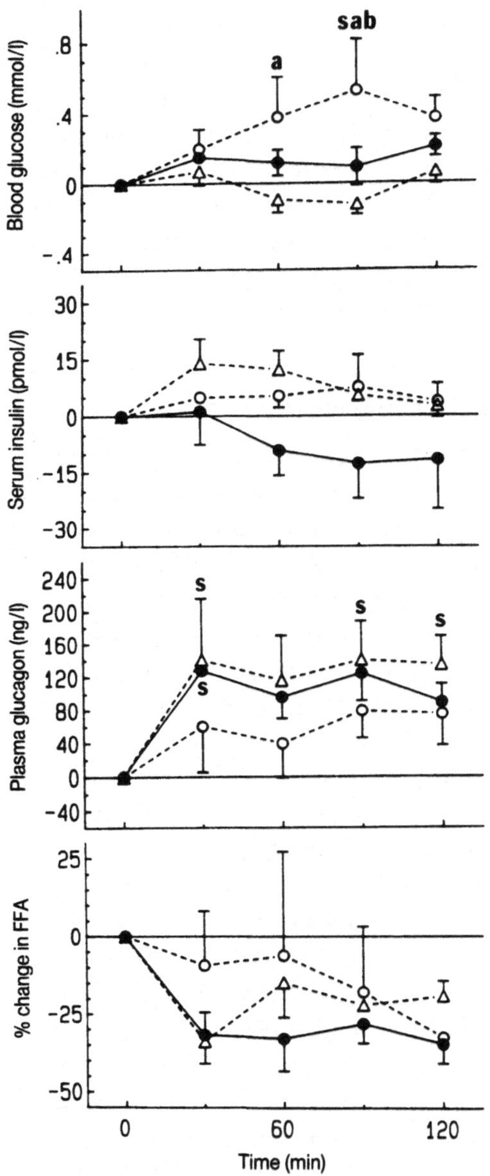

Fig. 29.3. Increments in levels of blood glucose, serum insulin and plasma glucagon, and percentage change in serum levels of free fatty acids (FFA) in six healthy subjects (mean ± SEM) after rectal infusion of 180 mmol sodium acetate (triangles), 180 mmol sodium propionate (open circles) or 180 mmol acetate plus 60 mmol propionate (filled circles) relative to the control infusion of normal saline. Letters above or below points indicate a significant difference ($p < 0.05$) from saline (s), acetate (a) or acetate plus propionate (b). Reproduced from Wolever *et al.* (1991; Copyright, 1991, American Society for Clinical Nutrition).

(West *et al.*, 1983). There is some evidence from two studies that dietary propionate increases serum triglyceride concentrations in healthy subjects (Venter, Vorster & Cummings, 1990; Todesco *et al.*, 1991).

Dietary propionate has been shown to reduce fasting blood glucose levels and maximum serum insulin increments (Venter *et al.*, 1990) which could be consistent with reduced glucose production or enhanced utilization. However, Todesco *et al.* (1991) showed that propionate reduced the rate of digestion of starch by nearly 50% and this may explain some of the effects of oral propionate on blood glucose and insulin levels.

Carbohydrate metabolism in peripheral tissues

In general, acetate has similar effects on glycolysis and gluconeogenesis in peripheral tissues to those in the liver (Newsholme & Start, 1973; Fig. 29.1). Both acetate (Williamson, 1964) and longer-chain fatty acids (Randle, Newsholme & Garland, 1964) have been shown to reduce glucose uptake and oxidation by isolated muscle preparations *in vitro*. However, oral acetate was found to have no effect on oral glucose tolerance (Scheppach *et al.*, 1988*a*) or glucose turnover (Scheppach *et al.*, 1988*b*) in humans. The reason for the lack of effect of acetate on glucose disposal in humans probably relates to the fact that acetate was shown to reduce glucose uptake by rat hearts at a concentration of 10 mM, which is approximately 100 times the concentration normally found in human blood (Cummings *et al.*, 1987) and about 30–50 times greater than the peak achieved after oral acetate administration (Scheppach *et al.*, 1988*a*). In addition, there is evidence that the activity of acetate thiokinase, the enzyme that converts acetate to acetyl-CoA, is much greater in the heart than in peripheral muscles (Ballard, 1972).

Nevertheless, acetate may influence glucose utilization indirectly, since oral (Crouse *et al.*, 1968) and rectal (Wolever *et al.*, 1991) acetate promptly reduce free fatty-acid levels in serum (Fig. 29.3). Physiological increases in free fatty-acid concentrations in the serum have been shown to reduce glucose utilization in humans (Ferrannini *et al.*, 1983; Jenkins *et al.*, 1990). Feeding the fermentable sugar lactulose has been shown to reduce day-long free fatty-acid concentrations in the serum of healthy subjects (Jenkins *et al.*, 1991). Lactulose feeding had no effect on day-long blood concentrations of glucose and insulin in non-diabetics (Jenkins *et al.*, 1991), but has been shown to improve oral glucose tolerance in subjects with non-insulin-dependent diabetes (Genovese, Riccardi & Rivellese, 1992).

Adding acetic acid (2% v/v) to corn starch has been shown to reduce the postprandial blood glucose response in rats, and 60 ml vinegar reduced the serum insulin response to 50 g sucrose in humans (Ebihara & Nakajima, 1988). However, these effects may be due to delayed gastric emptying rather than to a direct effect of acetate on carbohydrate metabolism.

Insulin and glucagon

In ruminant animals (sheep and cows), propionate stimulated pancreatic insulin secretion, and butyrate stimulated both insulin and glucagon (Horino *et al.*, 1967; Brockman, 1982). However, in non-ruminant animals (rats, rabbits and pigs) propionate had no such effect (Horino *et al.*, 1967). The latter finding accords with the fact that rectal infusion of an unphysiologically large bolus of propionate (180 mmol) failed to stimulate insulin in humans, despite raising blood-glucose levels (Wolever *et al.*, 1991; Fig. 29.3). Similarly, feeding the unabsorbed sugar lactulose to healthy subjects had no effect on serum insulin or C-peptide levels throughout the day (Jenkins *et al.*, 1990). However, infusion of SCFA or the fermentable fibre guar gum into the caecum of healthy subjects increased serum glucagon levels in five of six subjects (Stephen *et al.*, 1989). This result was confirmed by rectal infusion studies in which both propionate and acetate resulted in large rises in plasma glucagon levels (Fig. 29.3). Glucagon increases blood glucose levels through increased glucose production (Lins *et al.*, 1983). Further work is required to determine if physiological levels of SCFA influence glucagon secretion in humans.

Acetate metabolism in diabetes

Blood acetate in mammals is derived from endogenous (glucose and fat metabolism) and exogenous (colonic fermentation) sources. In non-diabetic mammals on a normal diet, colonic fermentation is the predominant source of acetate (Ballard, 1972), and blood acetate levels fall after short-term fasting in both rats (Knowles *et al.*, 1974) and humans (Scheppach *et al.*, 1991). However, after longer-term fasting, serum acetate levels rise markedly (Scheppach *et al.*, 1991) and, in this situation, fat oxidation is the major source of acetate production (Seufert, Mewes & Soling, 1984). Serum acetate concentrations are increased in diabetes (Smith, Humphreys & Hockaday, 1986), being directly related to the plasma glucose concentration (Akanji *et al.*, 1989). I am not aware of any evidence suggesting that diabetes is associated with enhanced colonic fermentation, although when diabetic patients were put on mixed high-fibre diets their serum acetate concentration increased (Akanji *et al.*, 1989). Therefore, the high serum acetate level associated with diabetes is most likely to be due to an increased rate of endogenous acetate production or a reduced rate of clearance.

The livers of diabetic animals produce more acetate than do those from control animals, and this has been suggested to be due to impaired oxidation of acetyl-CoA (Seufert *et al.*, 1974). During hyperinsulinaemic, euglycaemic clamps in non-diabetic subjects, serum acetate concentrations fell during the first 90 min, but then rose, suggesting that glucose metabolism is a source of serum acetate in normal subjects (Akanji, Ng & Humphreys, 1988). However, in diabetic subjects, the rise in acetate did not occur. This is consistent with the hypothesis that acetate over-production in diabetes is due to enhanced fat oxidation. In addition, intravenous acetate tolerance tests have shown that diabetic subjects have impaired acetate clearance compared to non-diabetic controls (Akanji & Hockaday, 1990). Taken together, these data suggest that the serum acetate level is high in diabetes because of increased endogenous production and reduced clearance.

Conclusion

Acetate and propionate do not appear to have effects on carbohydrate metabolism which can readily explain the effects of dietary fibre in improving blood glucose control in patients with diabetes (Wolever, 1990). Diabetes is associated with high serum acetate levels, most likely due to increased endogenous acetate production, and reduced acetate clearance. Acetate and propionate have opposite effects on the rates of glycolysis and glucose production. Therefore, the overall effect of colonic fermentation on carbohydrate metabolism may depend upon the relative amounts of acetate and propionate produced, which, in turn, are influenced by many factors, such as the substrate being fermented (Mortensen *et al.*, 1988; McBurney & Thompson, 1988) and the nature of the colonic bacteria (Chen & Wolin, 1977; McCarthy & Salyers, 1988). If propionate is produced in relatively large amounts, its effects on carbohydrate metabolism in the liver may predominate over those of acetate, since propionate has been shown to inhibit hepatic acetate utilization (Smith, 1971).

References

Akanji, A. O. & Hockaday, T. D. R. (1990). Acetate tolerance and the kinetics or acetate utilization in diabetic and nondiabetic subjects. *American Journal of Clinical Nutrition*, **51**, 112–18.

Akanji, A. O., Ng, L. & Humphreys, S. (1988). Plasma acetate levels in response to intravenous fat or glucose/insulin infusions in diabetic and non-diabetic subjects. *Clinica Chimica Acta*, **178**, 85–94.

Akanji, A. O., Peterson, D. B., Humphreys, S. & Hockaday, T. D. R. (1989). Change in plasma acetate levels in diabetic subjects on mixed high fiber diets. *American Journal of Gastroenterology*, **84**, 1365–70.

Anderson, J. W. & Bridges, S. R. (1984). Short-chain fatty acid fermentation products of plant fiber affect glucose metabolism of isolated rat hepatocytes (41958). *Proceedings of the Society for Experimental Biology and Medicine*, **177**, 372–6.

Ballard, F. J. (1972). Supply and utilization of acetate in mammals. *American Journal of Clinical Nutrition*, **25**, 773–9.

Brockman, R. P. (1982). Insulin and glucagon responses in plasma to intraportal infusions of propionate and butyrate in sheep (*Ovis aries*). *Comparative Biochemistry and Physiology*, **73A**, 237–8.

Chen, M. & Wolin, M. J. (1977). Influence of CH_4 production by *Methanobacterium ruminantium* on the fermentation of glucose and lactate by *Selenomonas ruminantium. Applied Environmental Microbiology*, **34**, 756–9.

Consoli, A., Kennedy, F., Miles, J. & Gerich, J. (1987). Determination of Krebs cycle metabolic carbon exchange *in vivo* and its use to estimate the individual contributions of gluconeogenesis and glycogenolysis to overall glucose output in man. *Journal of Clinical Investigation*, **80**, 1303–10.

Crouse, J. R., Gerson, C. D., DeCarli, L. M. & Lieber, C. S. (1968). Role of acetate in the reduction of plasma free fatty acids produced by ethanol in man. *Journal of Lipid Research*, **9**, 509–12.

Cummings, J. H., Pomare, E. W., Branch, W. J., Naylor, C. P. E. & Macfarlane, G. T. (1987). Short chain fatty acids in human large intestine, portal, hepatic and venous blood. *Gut*, **28**, 1221–7.

DeFronzo, R. A. (1988). The triumvirate: beta-cell, muscle, liver: a collusion responsible for NIDDM. *Diabetes*, **37**, 667–87.

Ebihara, K. & Nakajima, A. (1988). Effect of acetic acid and vinegar on blood glucose and insulin responses to orally administered sucrose and starch. *Agricultural Biology and Chemistry*, **52**, 1311–12.

Ferrannini, E., Barrett, E. J., Bevilacqua, S. & DeFronzo, R. A. (1983). Effect of fatty acids on glucose production and utilization in man. *Journal of Clinical Investigation*, **72**, 1737–47.

Flatt, J. P. & Ball, E. G. (1966). Studies on the metabolism of adipose tissue, XIX. An evaluation of the major pathways of glucose catabolism as influenced by acetate in the presence of insulin. *Journal of Biological Chemistry*, **241**, 2862–9.

Garland, P. B. & Randle, P. J. (1964). Regulation of glucose uptake by muscle: 10. Effects of alloxan-diabetes, starvation, hypophysectomy and adrenalectomy, and of fatty acids, ketone bodies and pyruvate, on the glycerol output and concentrations of free fatty acids, long-chain fatty acyl-coenzyme A, glycerol phosphate and citrate-cycle intermediates in rat heart and diaphragm muscles. *Biochemistry Journal*, **93**, 678–87.

Genovese, S., Riccardi, G. & Rivellese, A. A. (1992). Lactulose improves blood glucose response to an oral glucose test in non-insulin dependent diabetic patients. *Diabetes Nutrition and Metabolism*, **5**, 295–7.

Horino, M., Machlin, L. J., Hertelendy, F. & Kipnis, D. M. (1967). Effect of short-chain fatty acids on plasma insulin in ruminant and nonruminant species. *Endocrinology*, **83**, 118–28.

Jenkins, D. J. A., Wolever, T. M. S., Jenkins, A., Brighenti, F., Vuksan, V., Rao, A. V., Cunnane, S. C., Ocana, A. M., Corey, P., Versina, C., Connelly, P., Buckley, G. & Patten, R. (1991). Specific types of colonic fermentation may raise low-density-lipoprotein–cholesterol concentrations. *American Journal of Clinical Nutrition*, **54**, 141–7.

Jenkins, D. J. A., Wolever, T. M. S., Ocana, A. M., Vuksan, V., Cunnane, S. C., Jenkins, M., Wong, G. S., Singer, W., Bloom, S. R., Blendis, L. M. & Josse, R. G. (1990). Metabolic effects of reducing rate of glucose ingestion by single bolus versus continuous sipping. *Diabetes*, **39**, 775–81.

Knowles, S. E., Jarrett, I. G., Filsell, O. H. & Ballard, J. F. (1974). Production and utilization of acetate in mammals. *Biochemistry Journal*, **142**, 401–11.

Lins, P., Wajnot, A., Adamson, U., Vranic, M. & Efendic, S. (1983). Minimal increases in glucagon levels enhance glucose production in man with partial hypoinsulinemia. *Diabetes*, **32**, 633–6.

McBurney, M. I. & Thompson, L. U. (1988). *In vitro* fermentabilities of purified fiber supplements. *Journal of Food Science*, **54**, 347–50.

McCarthy, R. E. & Salyers, A. A. (1988). The effects of dietary fibre utilization on the colonic microflora. In *Role of the Gut Flora in Toxicity and Cancer*, ed. I. Rowland, pp. 295–313. London: Academic Press.

Mortensen, P. B., Holtug, K. & Rasmussen, H. S. (1988). Short-chain fatty acid production from mono- and disaccharides in a fecal incubation system: implications for colonic fermentation of dietary fiber in humans. *Journal of Nutrition*, **118**, 321–5.

Newsholme, E. A. & Start, C. (1973). *Regulation in Metabolism*. London: John Wiley & Sons.

Randle, P. J., Newsholme, E. A. & Garland, P. B. (1964). Regulation of glucose uptake by muscle: 8. Effects of fatty acids, ketone bodies and pyruvate, and of alloxan-diabetes and starvation, on the uptake and metabolic fate of glucose in rat heart and diaphragm muscles. *Biochemistry Journal*, **93**, 652–65.

Roediger, W. E. W. (1980). Role of anaerobic bacteria in the metabolic welfare of the colonic mucosa in man. *Gut*, **21**, 793–8.

Scheppach, W., Cummings, J. H., Branch, W. J. & Schrezenmeir, J. (1988*a*). Effect of gut-derived acetate on oral glucose tolerance in man. *Clinical Science*, **75**, 355–61.

Scheppach, W., Pomare, E. W., Elia, M. & Cummings, J. H. (1991). The contribution of the large intestine to blood acetate in man. *Clinical Science*, **80**, 177–82.

Scheppach, W., Wiggins, H. S., Halliday, D., Self, R., Howard, J., Branch, W. J., Schrezenmeir, J. & Cummings, J. H. (1988*b*). Effect of gut-derived acetate on glucose turnover in man. *Clinical Science*, **75**, 363–70.

Seufert, C. D., Graf, M., Janson, G., Kuhn, A. & Soling, H. D. (1974). Formation of free acetate by perfused livers from normal, starved and diabetic rats. *Biochemical and Biophysical Research Communications*, **57**, 901–9.

Seufert, C. D., Mewes, W. & Soling, H. D. (1984). Effect of long-term starvation on acetate and ketone body metabolism in obese patients. *European Journal of Clinical Investigation*, **14**, 163–70.

Smith, R. F., Humphreys, S. & Hockaday, T. D. R. (1986). The measurement of plasma acetate by a manual or automated technique in diabetic and non-diabetic subjects. *Annals of Clinical Biochemistry*, **23**, 285–91.

Smith, R. M. (1971). Interactions of acetate, propionate and butyrate in sheep liver mitochondria. *Biochemistry Journal*, **124**, 877–81.

Stephen, A. M., Bagby, B., Hoppel, C. & Banwell, J. (1989). Effect of colonic infusion of short chain fatty acids on human glucose and fatty acid metabolism. *FASEB Journal*, **3**, A942.

Todesco, T., Rao, A. N., Bosello, O. & Jenkins, D. J. A. (1991). Propionate lowers blood glucose and alters lipid metabolism in healthy subjects. *American Journal of Clinical Nutrition*, **54**, 860–5.

Underwood, A. J. & Newsholme, E. A. (1967). Control of glycolysis and gluconeogenesis in rat kidney cortex slices. *Biochemistry Journal*, **104**, 300–5.

Venter, C. S., Vorster, H. H. & Cummings, J. H. (1990). Effects of dietary propionate on carbohydrate and lipid metabolism in healthy volunteers. *American Journal of Gastroenterology*, **85**, 549–53.

West, K. M., Ahuja, M. M. S., Bennett, P. H., Czyzyk, A., Mateo-de-Acosta, O., Fuller, J. H., Grab, B., Grabauskas, V., Jarrett, R. J., Kosada, K., Keen, H. Krolewski, A. S., Miki, I., Schliach, V., Teuscher, A., Watkins, P. J. & Stober, J. A. (1983). The role of circulating glucose and triglyceride concentrations and their interactions with other 'risk factors' as determinants of arterial disease in nine diabetic population samples from the WHO multinational study. *Diabetes Care*, **6**, 361–9.

Williamson, J. R. (1964). Effects of insulin and starvation on the metabolism of acetate and pyruvate by the perfused rat heart. *Biochemistry Journal*, **93**, 97–106.

Wolever, T. M. S. (1990). Dietary fiber in the management of diabetes. In *Dietary Fiber: Chemistry, Physiology and Health Effects*, ed. D. Kritchevsky, C. Bonfield & J. W. Anderson, pp. 247–59. New York: Plenum Press.

Wolever, T. M. S., Spadafora, P. & Eshuis, H. (1991). Interaction between colonic acetate and propionate in man. *American Journal of Clinical Nutrition*, **53**, 681–7.

Wolfe, R. R. & Jahoor, F. (1990). Recovery of labeled CO_2 during the infusion of C-1- v. C-2-labeled acetate: implications for tracer studies of substrate oxidation. *American Journal of Clinical Nutrition*, **51**, 248–52.

30

Short-chain fatty acids and hepatic lipid metabolism: experimental studies

D. L. TOPPING AND I. PANT

Introduction

The current interest in the effects of short-chain fatty acids (SCFA) on hepatic lipid metabolism is at two levels, because of their intrinsic capacities to modulate fatty-acid and cholesterol metabolism and also because they may mediate the effects of dietary fibre on plasma lipids. The latter is an important possibility, because one of the major specific health benefits of increased non-starch polysaccharide (NSP; 'fibre') consumption is the lowering of plasma cholesterol levels (Schneeman, 1986). Such reductions have been shown with plant foods high in water-soluble NSP (e.g. oat bran) and isolates of such NSP (e.g. pectin and guar gum) in experimental animals and humans. These NSP preparations are also fermented extensively by the large bowel microflora of omnivores with an increase in the production and absorption of SCFA (Topping, 1991). Therefore, the proposition that NSP preparations may lower plasma cholesterol levels through inhibition of hepatic cholesterol synthesis by one of these SCFA – propionate (Chen, Anderson & Jennings, 1984) – is quite reasonable. Moreover, in rats, diets high in NSP that increase colonic SCFA also lower plasma triacylglycerols (TAG) through reducing hepatic fatty acid synthesis (Mazur *et al.*, 1992). This underscores the potential benefits of SCFA, or of the foods that encourage their production in the hindgut. The effects of SCFA on the metabolism of cholesterol and TAG must be in the context of their production in the hindgut and their portal venous transport, together with their actual metabolism in the hepatocyte.

Hepatic fatty-acid and triacylglycerol metabolism

The liver plays a central role in the regulation of both plasma cholesterol and TAG metabolism. In brief, hepatocytes secrete TAG in very-low-density lipoproteins (VLDL) which also contain apoproteins, cholesterol (free and esterified) and phospholipids (for a review, see Gibbons, 1990). VLDL enter the circulation and are cleared by peripheral tissues through the action of lipoprotein lipase which releases free fatty acids (FFA) and glycerol. These FFA are taken up by the tissue while the non-triacylglycerol components accumulate until they inhibit lipolysis or insufficient TAG remains for enzymic action. The resulting remnant returns to the liver, where it is remodelled into low-density lipoprotein (LDL). The secretion of VLDL is one determinant of LDL concentrations and, therefore, of vascular disease.

Export of VLDL by the liver is driven by the availability of TAG within the hepatocyte which in turn is governed by three main factors – the supply of plasma FFA, fatty acids synthesised *de novo* (lipogenesis) for TAG synthesis and pre-existing TAG within the liver cell. It has been extensively documented *in vitro* that all three contribute to accelerated VLDL secretion, as does the provision of triose phosphates, which promote fatty acid esterification (Mayes & Laker, 1986).

The role of the liver in cholesterol metabolism is equally well understood. In brief, the liver is the site of synthesis of bile acids, which are a major route of loss of cholesterol from the body through faecal excretion (Miettinen, 1981). Normally this loss is relatively small, as there is an extensive enterohepatic circulation. However, it is accelerated by selective agents, such as bile acid sequestrants that bind bile acids in the gut and so limit their reabsorption. The increased loss is made good by a fall in plasma lipoprotein cholesterol concentrations. There is also a rise in hepatic cholesterol synthesis which prevents cholesterol becoming a limiting factor to normal body functions.

SCFA and hepatic metabolism: ruminant studies

The liver is also central to whole-body SCFA metabolism in many animal species. However, interest in the interactions between acetate, propionate and butyrate and hepatic lipid metabolism comes substantially from the field of ruminant nutrition. The important contribution of SCFA to metabolism in ruminant herbivores is axiomatic (and is discussed elsewhere in this volume). The ruminal fermentation of NSP provides most of the metabolizable energy of these species, but it also imposes certain metabolic constraints on them. These limitations include the absence of any significant entry of dietary carbohydrate as monosaccharides into the circulation plus a high degree of dependence on hepatic glucose synthesis (gluconeogenesis) to meet tissue requirements (Ballard, Hanson & Kronfeld, 1969). Propionate plays a key role in this process as, of the major SCFA, it alone can enter the tricarboxylic acid cycle and contribute to the net carbon flux to glucose. In addition, propionate has other important effects, including increased secretion of insulin – a hormone that is a key influence on hepatic lipid metabolism. Ruminant herbivores also have little or no hepatic capacity to synthesize fatty acids *de novo*, very low rates of TAG secretion into the circulation and low concentrations of plasma lipids (Mamo, Snoswell & Topping, 1983).

SCFA in omnivores: factors affecting portal venous concentrations

The appreciation that SCFA may be important in omnivores (as well as herbivores) is also very recent, and there are several good reasons for this neglect. Firstly, under normal conditions, SCFA concentrations in peripheral venous blood of species such as the rat (Illman *et al.*, 1982) and pig (Topping *et al.*, 1985) are very low. This is in marked contrast to the situation in cattle and sheep, where mixed venous SCFA are much higher. Secondly, it was thought that the liver acted only to release SCFA, particularly acetate. Such release occurs during the hepatic metabolism of ethanol and accounts for the very high concentrations of acetate seen chronically in problem drinkers and which decline during ethanol withdrawal (Williamson *et al.*, 1987). The view that the non-ruminant liver was a net source of acetate is supported by the rise in peripheral venous acetate in pigs fed triacetin (Imoto & Namioka, 1978). Triacetin is not a normal dietary component and the true picture emerged from the work of Buckley and Williamson (1977), who showed that acetate was present at quite significant concentrations in rat portal venous plasma and that concentrations were influenced by diet and physiological and hormonal status. Their data indicated that there was a significant release of acetate from the gastrointestinal tract and that, under normal circumstances, the liver was a net remover of acetate. They calculated a set-point concentration of approximately 0.2 μmol/ml, below which release was observed and above which uptake was found. This set-point has been confirmed in perfused rat liver (Snoswell *et al.*, 1982) and also appears to exist in heart (Topping & Trimble, 1985). In perfused liver, acetate uptake rose with increasing concentration up to an inflow concentration of 2 μmol/ml. The acetate taken up appeared to compete with lactate for *de novo* fatty-acid synthesis. This is not surprising, as lactate is a major lipogenic substrate in liver, and acetate has a long history as an index of both fatty acid and cholesterol synthesis in a number of tissues. As the CoA thioester, acetate can also undergo oxidation (via the tricarboxylic acid cycle) and its contribution to *de novo* lipid synthesis and oxidation depends on the supply of acetyl-CoA from other sources.

Clearly, the incorporation of radiolabelled free acetate into lipids does not truly reflect that of total acetyl-CoA and this has been replaced almost completely by ^3H_2O for determination of fatty acid and cholesterol synthesis.

Many *in vivo* studies have shown the presence of propionate and butyrate in addition to acetate in the large-bowel contents and portal venous blood of rats (see e.g. Rémésy & Demigné, 1985). These studies have confirmed that feeding NSP and resistant starch (RS) raises large-bowel and portal venous SCFA concentrations. In all cases, the concentrations in peripheral venous blood remain substantially below those entering the liver circulation. In perfused liver, fractional uptakes of 20–40% have been found for acetate (Snoswell *et al.*, 1982) and propionate (Illman *et al.*, 1988). As we have noted, the greatest increase in SCFA concentrations is with the more fermentable carbohydrates, which also have the greatest potential to reduce cholesterol. Not only do these NSP increase SCFA, but they may modify the profile of the acids present, and it seems likely that they favour an increase in the molar proportions of propionate.

Acetate, propionate and butyrate and hepatic lipid metabolism

The assumption that SCFA mediate the effects of dietary fibre on hepatic lipid metabolism is both simple and convenient. However, it overlooks the fact that all three acids are usually present in the portal vein simultaneously (together with the minor SCFA). Moreover, they may not affect hepatic lipid metabolism in the same way. We have already identified the contribution of acetate to liver lipogenesis and oxidation. The provision of extra acetate through the hepatic metabolism of ethanol is thought to accelerate lipogenesis and so contribute to the raised plasma TAG concentrations seen during excess ethanol consumption (Baraona & Lieber, 1979). Enhanced fatty acid synthesis and raised plasma TAG have also been seen in rats fed oat bran (Roach *et al.*, 1992) – possibly through provision of extra SCFA as lipogenic substrate. However, the effects of dietary NSP on lipogenesis *in vivo* are quite inconsistent, with some studies showing an increase and others a lowering of fatty acid synthesis (Mazur *et al.*, 1992). Most probably the net effect of NSP depends on the total provision of substrate for hepatic lipogenesis, so that if the concentrations of NSP in the diet are increased, it is at the expense of some other component (e.g. starch, sucrose) that can influence synthesis. Small-intestinal carbohydrate digestion and absorption is intrinsically more efficient than that in the large bowel, because of the losses associated with bacterial fermentation (Livesey, 1991). The SCFA produced by bacteria are substrates that may be used by the host and they contain only a fraction (albeit significant) of the total energy contained in fermentable substrates. The remainder, probably some 30%, is used by the bacteria for growth and there are also energy losses due to gas production. This means that, although levels of acetate and other SCFA are raised in animals fed fermentable carbohydrates, the net energy yield is probably 50% or less of the yield that would be obtained from the same carbohydrates if they were absorbed in the small intestine.

In contrast to acetate, very little seems to be known about the impact of butyrate on hepatic lipid metabolism, but much more is documented about the effects of propionate. It is this acid that has been proposed as the main effector of plasma cholesterol reduction by NSP and that is assumed to be pivotal in regulating hepatic lipid metabolism.

Propionate as a mediator of cholesterol reduction by NSP

The proposition that propionate formed by the colonic fermentation of NSP is responsible for cholesterol reduction is very attractive. The concept of cholesterol reduction by dietary propionate is well established and most feeding trials have shown that diets supplemented with propionate reduce plasma levels of cholesterol, with significant reductions in pigs (see e.g. Boila *et al.*, 1981) and rats (see e.g. Illman *et al.*, 1988). In rats, the reduction in plasma cholesterol is of the same order of magnitude as that achieved by feeding water-soluble NSP in oat bran (see e.g. De Shrijver, Fremaut & Verheyen, 1992). However, the support is not unequivocal, as in baboons fed a 'Western-type' of high-fat diet, dietary propionate did not reduce levels of plasma cholesterol relative to controls (Venter *et al.*, 1990). In addition to a direct effect of dietary propionate on plasma cholesterol, feeding fibre preparations (such as oat bran), known to reduce cholesterol concentration, lead to increased propionate concentrations in the large bowel and portal vein of rats (Illman & Topping, 1985). The final piece of supportive evidence is that propionate inhibited hepatic cholesterol synthesis in isolated rat hepatocytes (Chen *et al.*, 1984, Nishina & Freedland, 1990). This decline in synthesis may be due to a reduction in the activity of 3-hydroxy-3-methyl-glutaryl-CoA (HMG-CoA) reductase – an enzyme that is rate-limiting for hepatic cholesterol synthesis.

NSP, plasma cholesterol and hepatic lipid synthesis

If propionate were the mediator of plasma cholesterol reduction, then it would follow that NSP, which lowers cholesterol levels, should always raise the

Table 30.1. *Plasma lipids, portal venous propionate and hepatic lipid synthesis in rats fed oat bran, cellulose or wheat bran. Data from Illman & Topping, 1985 (Experiment 1) and Roach* et al., *1992 (Experiment 2)*

Diet	Plasma concentration (mM)		Portal venous propionate (mM)	Synthesis (μmol/g liver per h)	
	Cholesterol	TAG		Cholesterol	Fatty acids
Experiment 1					
Oat bran	2.13[b]	—	0.29[a]	0.59[a]	4.43[a]
Cellulose	2.50[a]	—	0.08[b]	0.14[b]	2.23[b]
Experiment 2					
Oat bran	2.09[b]	1.60[a]	—	0.13[a]	4.03[a]
Wheat bran	2.46[a]	1.20[b]	—	0.09[b]	2.83[b]

[a,b] In any column, values not sharing a superscript were significantly different for that experiment ($p < 0.05$).
TAG, triacylglycerols.

portal venous propionate concentration and inhibit hepatic cholesterol synthesis. This does not seem to be the case. For example, oat bran lowers the level of plasma cholesterol relative to cellulose and wheat bran (Illman & Topping, 1985; Roach *et al.*, 1992) in rats fed a diet not supplemented with cholesterol and cholic acid. In those animals fed oat bran, propionate concentrations in the caecum and portal venous plasma certainly were increased, but hepatic cholesterol synthesis was higher in the animals fed oatbran than in those fed cellulose or wheat bran (Table 30.1). Two different oat brans were used which may account for the different rates of cholesterol synthesis. Nevertheless, with both, synthesis was increased, consistent with enhanced bile-acid excretion. A similar rise in cholesterogenesis (coupled with increased faecal steroid excretion) has been reported (Turley, Daggy & Dietschy, 1991) in hamsters fed psyllium, which is another water-soluble NSP that lowers plasma cholesterol concentrations. The rat data suggest that although the portal venous propionate level was raised, this was insufficient to block increased cholesterol formation. Examination of studies in which steroid metabolism had been varied by dietary means in experimental animals shows that there is no relationship between large-bowel propionate concentrations and plasma cholesterol levels in pigs (Topping *et al.*, 1993; Marsono *et al.*, 1993). In rats the highest portal venous propionate concentrations that we have found were in rats fed wheat bran aleurone – which also gave high plasma cholesterol concentrations (Cheng *et al.*, 1987).

Table 30.2. *Coprophagy prevention and caecal pools of short-chain fatty acids (SCFA) and plasma levels of cholesterol in rats*

Diet	Coprophagy	Pools (mmol) Propionate	Pools (mmol) Total SCFA	Plasma cholesterol (mM)
Wheat bran	Yes	40[c]	267[b,c]	3.37[a]
	No	23[c]	133[c]	3.45[a]
Oat bran	Yes	161[b]	398[a,b]	2.62[b]
	No	279[a]	556[a]	2.51[d]

[a,b,c] In any column, values not sharing a superscript letter were significantly different ($p < 0.05$).
Modified from Jackson & Topping, 1993.

There are two implicit assumptions in many of these animal studies. The first is that if large-bowel SCFA production is enhanced, then portal venous transport increases solely through a rise in concentration. Such an assumption is true to some degree in the rat, where plasma SCFA concentrations rise following the feeding of fermentable carbohydrates. However, rats are nibbling animals and are caecal fermenters with a complex muscular arrangement for retaining fermentable material in the caecum until fermentation is complete (Graham & Aman, 1982). The rat also practises selective faecal refection, in order to recover vitamins and other nutrients that accumulate as a result of this bacterial activity. Abolition of faecal refection does not alter effects of cereal fibre preparations (specfically as oat and wheat bran) on plasma cholesterol but does modify caecal SCFA and propionate pools (Table 30.2). However, in rats fed fermentable carbohydrate, SCFA transport may also be increased through augmented blood flow (Demigné, Yacoub & Rémésy, 1986), so that the net flow to the liver may be greater than the change in plasma concentration. Blood flow is an important determinant of hepatic O_2 consumption and fatty acid synthesis in its own right (Topping, Trimble & Storer, 1988) and may mediate some of the effects attributed to SCFA. There may also be species differences. For example, the anatomy of the porcine hindgut is much simpler than that of the rat (and is closer to that of humans). In the pig, digesta flow without the reflux seen in rats and relationships between NSP intake and SCFA also seem to be different from those in the rat. For example, we have found that feeding diets high in fermentable carbohydrate increased large-bowel SCFA and digesta but that their distribution along the colon varied considerably with diet (Topping *et al.*, 1993; Marsono *et al.*, 1993). In pigs fed baked (navy) beans, SCFA concentrations in the proximal colon were disproportionately higher than in animals fed oat bran, but in contrast, more SCFA were found in the distal colon in pigs fed brown rice than in pigs fed rice bran. These differences presumably reflect digesta flow. More importantly, we have found in these same studies that portal venous SCFA concentrations correlated only with those in a relatively limited region of the median colon, so that increased fermentation does not automatically mean increased SCFA concentrations in the liver circulation.

The second factor from these animal studies is a challenge to the assumption that altered large-bowel SCFA drive changes in hepatic steroid metabolism. It is well known that dietary fibre can alter metabolism of bile acids and neutral sterols by the colonic microflora. We have found recently that in rats fed various cereal preparations there were large differences in caecal steroid concentrations and hence in faecal excretion (Illman, Storer & Topping, 1993). These differences were also consistent with increased hepatic biliary steroid secretion and with observed differences in plasma cholesterol. Moreover, we found also that there were substantial differences in the molar proportions of caecal SCFA – high propionate and low butyrate – with increased caecal bile acid and neutral steroids. In particular, there was a close correlation between increased coprostanol (the main cholesterol metabolite) and secondary bile acids. These data may be interpreted as showing that the metabolism of steroids by the colonic microflora influenced the proportions of SCFA produced by those bacteria.

Effects of propionate on lipid metabolism *in vivo*

It is a key element in the hypothesis that propionate is the active agent in the reduction in plasma cholesterol and that the acid by itself mimics the effects of dietary fibre on lipid metabolism. This is almost certainly not true. Firstly, propionate fed in the diet is likely to be absorbed with a quite different time-course to that absorbed from the large bowel as a result of fermentation. This is indeed the case in pigs with portal venous cannulae; dietary propionate gave a peak concentration 1–2 h after feeding, followed by a decline (Illman *et al.*, 1988). After 4–6 h, SCFA concentrations rose and these raised levels were sustained for many hours, consistent with the onset and maintenance of large-bowel fibre fermentation. In rats fed propionate-enriched diets, measurement of such a time-course is impractical, but determination of gut and portal venous SCFA in the postabsorptive state showed that propionate concentrations were raised in the portal vein. Propionate was also raised in the stomach, but little appeared in the small

Table 30.3. *Gut and portal venous plasma propionate concentrations and hepatic cholesterogenesis in rats fed propionate*

Diet	Propionate (mM)				Cholesterol synthesis (μmol/g per h)
	Stomach	Duodenum	Ileum	Portal vein	
Control	6.5[b]	1.0	5.2	0.22	0.20
Propionate	26.6[a]	1.2	8.4	0.38	0.21

[a,b] Significantly different ($p < 0.05$).

intestine and liver cholesterol synthesis was unchanged (Table 30.3). In fact, in both rats and pigs, most of the dietary propionate could not be accounted for by portal transport and the question of its fate remains open. Given that propionate appears to be used by the rumen wall, it may be that the rodent and porcine stomach metabolize it also.

Effects of propionate on lipid metabolism *in vitro* – importance of concentration

The concentrations of SCFA found in portal venous plasma of experimental animal models such as the rat and pig are generally in the range 0.5–2.0 μM, depending on diet and hormonal status. In rats fed wheat bran aleurone, concentrations of 2 μM have been recorded with propionate present at 1 μM (Cheng *et al.*, 1987). This appears to be a reasonable maximum and in rats fed other NSP, generally lower concentrations have been found, both by ourselves and others. Measurement of portal venous concentrations in other species is not common, but in pigs we have found broadly similar concentrations to those in rats. It must be emphasized that, although these concentrations may appear to be modest, their contributions to energy are quite considerable – possibly 12% in the pig, which are achieved through the relatively large flow rates of portal venous blood. This is a key issue, as studies *in vitro* (e.g. by Chen *et al.*, 1984) have used propionate at concentrations of >10 mM, which are very high relative to those *in vivo.*

The question of high concentrations is not a trivial issue and there is already a clear example of where the use of unphysiologically high concentrations of a substrate gave quite anomalous results. The substrate was fructose, which is present in the portal vein at <2 μM but has been used in isolated liver studies at >10 mM. At this high concentration, severe liver adenine nucleotide depletion occurred whereas at more physiological conditions, no depletion has been shown (Mayes & Laker, 1986). A concentration dependence is probably true for SCFA. For example, in livers perfused with acetate at concentrations of <5 mM, the acetate was directed towards lipogenesis, but above that, towards fatty acid oxidation (Topping *et al.*, 1984). Effects of propionate also vary with concentration; inhibition of hepatic cholesterol and fatty acid synthesis has been observed at high concentrations in isolated hepatocytes (Chen *et al.*, 1984; Wright, Anderson & Bridges, 1990) and in rat livers perfused with whole blood (Illman *et al.*, 1988), but not at those concentrations more typical of the liver *in vivo* (Illman *et al.*, 1988; Wright *et al.*, 1990). There is a degree of dispute as to the precise concentration at which inhibition occurs, but it appears to be between 1 and 2.5 mM (Wright *et al.*, 1990). There is also some question as to whether propionate inhibits hepatic fatty-acid synthesis *in vivo* at the concentrations found in the portal vein in intact animals. On balance, it appears unlikely that significant inhibition occurs at concentrations below 1 mM.

Conclusions

In considering the effects of SCFA on hepatic lipid metabolism there are, in reality, two questions. The first is: do SCFA affect hepatic lipid metabolism *in vivo*? The unequivocal answer to this question is yes. It is known definitely that acetate at concentrations encountered in the portal vein can contribute to lipid synthesis and to hepatic oxidation. In the instance of butyrate, very little is known and much experimental work needs to be done. The acid that has attracted the greatest attention, propionate, also seems to have generated the greatest confusion. There has been insufficient discrimination between the effects of oral propionate and propionate formed by large-bowel bacterial fermentation. More importantly, studies *in vitro* have been carried out under conditions that do not approximate to the physiological – a criticism that is true of many other experiments with other SCFA. At physiological concentrations and conditions it appears unlikely that propionate is a major inhibitor of hepatic lipid synthesis. However, it is equally true that under these circumstances, hepatic secretion of VLDL and uptake of LDL and HDL have not been studied. In the case of each major SCFA, a clear distinction needs to be made between the acids that enter the liver circulation as a consequence of colonic fermentation and those that enter as a result of oral or other intake.

This leads to the second question: are effects of dietary fibre on plasma cholesterol (and TAG) mediated through effects of SCFA on hepatic lipid metabolism? The answer to that would seem to be (to a significant degree) no. It seems likely that the effects of dietary fibre are confined largely to the gut. Nevertheless, it remains a possibility that SCFA might modify some of those actions by modulating hepatic lipid metabolism and clearly this is a matter that needs addressing.

Acknowledgement

I. Pant is supported by Kellogg (Australia) Ltd.

References

Ballard, F. J., Hanson, R. W. & Kronfeld, D. S. (1969). Gluconeogenesis and lipogenesis in tissues from ruminant and non-ruminant animals. *Federation Proceedings*, **28**, 218–30.

Baraona, E. & Lieber, C. S. (1979). Effects of ethanol on lipid metabolism. *Journal of Lipid Research*, **20**, 289–315.

Boila, R. J., Salomons, M. D., Milligan, L. P. & Aherne, F. X. (1981). The effect of dietary propionic acid on cholesterol synthesis in swine. *Nutrition Reports International*, **23**, 1113–21.

Buckley, B. M. & Williamson, D. H. (1977). Origin of blood acetate in the rat. *Biochemical Journal*, **166**, 539–45.

Chen, W.-J. L., Anderson, J. W. & Jennings, D. (1984). Propionate may mediate the hypocholesterolemic effects of certain soluble plant fibers in cholesterol-fed rats. *Proceedings of the Society for Experimental Biology and Medicine*, **175**, 215–18.

Cheng, B.-Q., Trimble, R. P., Illman, R. J., Stone, B. A. & Topping, D. L. (1987). Comparative effects of dietary wheat bran and its morphological components (aleurone and pericarp-seed coat) on volatile fatty acids in the rat. *British Journal of Nutrition*, **57**, 69–76.

Demigné, C., Yacoub, C. & Rémésy, C. (1986). Effects of absorption of large amounts of volatile fatty acids on rat liver metabolism. *Journal of Nutrition*, **116**, 77–86.

De Shrijver, R. Fremaut, D. & Verheyen, A. (1992). Cholesterol-lowering effects and utilisation of protein, lipid, fiber and energy in rats fed unprocessed and baked oat bran. *Journal of Nutrition*, **122**, 1318–24.

Gibbons, G. F. (1990). Assembly and secretion of hepatic very-low-density lipoproteins. *Biochemical Journal*, **268**, 1–13.

Graham, H. & Aman, P. (1982). The pig as a model in dietary fibre digestion studies. *Scandinavian Journal of Gastroenterology*, **22** (Suppl. 129), 55–61.

Illman, R. J., Storer, G. B. & Topping, D. L. (1993). White wheat flour lowers plasma cholesterol and increases cecal steroids relative to whole wheat flour, wheat bran and wheat pollard in rats. *Journal of Nutrition*, **123**, 1094–100.

Illman, R. J. & Topping, D. L. (1985). Effects of dietary oat bran on faecal steroid excretion, plasma volatile fatty acids and lipid synthesis in the rat. *Nutrition Research*, **5**, 839–46.

Illman, R. J., Topping, D. L., McIntosh, G. H., Trimble, R. P., Storer, G. B., Taylor, M. N. & Cheng, B.-Q. (1988). Hypocholesterolaemic effects of dietary propionate: studies in whole animals and perfused rat liver. *Annals of Nutrition and Metabolism*, **32**, 97–107.

Illman, R. J., Trimble, R. P., Snoswell, A. M. & Topping, D. L. (1982). Daily variations in the concentrations of volatile fatty acids in the splanchnic blood vessels of rats fed diets high in pectin and bran. *Nutrition Reports International*, **26**, 439–46.

Imoto, S. & Namioka, S. (1978). VFA metabolism in the pig. *Journal of Animal Science*, **47**, 479–87.

Jackson, K. A. & Topping, D. L. (1993). Prevention of coprophagy does not alter the hypocholesterolaemic effects of oat bran in the rat. *British Journal of Nutrition*, **70**, 211–19.

Livesey, G. (1991). Energy values of unavailable carbohydrate and diets: an inquiry and analysis. *American Journal of Clinical Nutrition*, **51**, 617–37.

Mamo, J. L. C., Snoswell, A. M. & Topping, D. L. (1983). Plasma triacylglycerol secretion in sheep: paradoxical effects of fasting and alloxan diabetes. *Biochimica et Biophysica Acta*, **753**, 272–5.

Marsono, Y., Illman, R. J., Clarke, J., Trimble, R. P. & Topping, D. L. (1993). Plasma lipids and large bowel volatile fatty acids in pigs fed white rice, brown rice and rice bran. *British Journal of Nutrition*, **70**, 503–13.

Mayes, P. A. & Laker, M. E. (1986). Effects of acute and long-term fructose administration on liver lipid metabolism. *Progress in Biochemistry and Pharmacology*, **21**, 33–58.

Mazur, A., Gueux, E., Felgines, C., Bayle, D., Nasir, F., Demigné, C. & Rémésy, C. (1992). Effects of dietary fermentable fiber on fatty acid synthesis and triglyceride secretion in rats fed fructose-based diet: studies with sugar beet fiber. *Proceedings of the Society for Experimental Biology and Medicine*, **199**, 345–50.

Miettinen, T. A. (1981). Effects of hypolidemic drugs on bile acid metabolism in man. *Advances in Lipid Research*, **18**, 65–97.

Nishina, P. M. & Freedland, R. A. (1990). Effects of propionate on lipid biosynthesis in rat hepatocytes. *Journal of Nutrition*, **120**, 668–73.

Rémésy, C. & Demigné, C. (1985). Stimulation of absorption of volatile fatty acids and minerals in the cecum of rats adapted to a very high fiber diet. *Journal of Nutrition*, **115**, 53–60.

Roach, P. D., Dowling, K., Balasubramaniam, S., Illman, R. J., Kambouris, A., Nestel, P. J. & Topping, D. L. (1992). Fish oil and oat bran in combination effectively lower plasma cholesterol in the rat. *Atherosclerosis*, **96**, 219–26.

Schneeman, B. O. (1986). Dietary fiber: physical and chemical properties, methods of analysis and physiological effects. *Food Technology*, **40**, 104–10.

Snoswell, A. M., Trimble, R. P., Fishlock, R. C., Storer, G. B. & Topping, D. L. (1982). Metabolic effects of acetate in perfused rat liver studies on ketogenesis, glucose output, lactate uptake and lipogenesis. *Biochimica et Biophysica Acta*, **716**, 290–8.

Topping, D. L. (1991). Soluble fiber polysaccharides: effects on plasma cholesterol and large bowel short-chain fatty acids. *Nutrition Reviews*, **49**, 195–203.

Topping, D. L., Illman, R. J., Clarke, J. M., Trimble, R. P., Jackson, K. A. & Marsono, Y. (1993). Dietary fat and fiber alter large bowel and portal venous volatile fatty acids and plasma cholesterol but not biliary steroids in pigs. *Journal of Nutrition*, **123**, 133–43.

Topping, D. L., Illman, R. J., Taylor, M. N. & McIntosh, G. H. (1985). Effects of wheat bran and porridge oats on plasma volatile fatty acids in the hepatic portal vein of the pig. *Annals of Nutrition and Metabolism*, **29**, 325–31.

Topping, D. L., Snoswell, A. M., Storer, G. B., Fishlock, R. C. & Trimble, R. P.

(1984). Dependence on blood acetate concentration of the metabolic effects of ethanol in perfused rat liver. *Biochimica et Biophysica Acta*, **800**, 103–5.

Topping, D. L. & Trimble, R. P. (1985). Effects of insulin on the metabolism of the isolated working rat heart perfused with undiluted rat blood. *Biochimica et Biophysica Acta*, **844**, 113–18.

Topping, D. L., Trimble, R. P. & Storer, G. B. (1988). Effects of flow rate and insulin on triacylglycerol secretion by perfused rat liver. *American Journal of Physiology*, **255**, E306–E313.

Turley, S. D., Daggy, B. P. & Dietschy, J. M. (1991). Cholesterol-lowering action of psyllium mucilloid in the hamster: sites and possible mechanisms of action. *Metabolism*, **40**, 1063–73.

Venter, C. S., Vorster, H. H. & Van der Nest, D. G. (1990). Comparison between physiological effects of konjac-glucomannan and propionate in baboons fed 'western' diets. *Journal of Nutrition*, **120**, 1046–53.

Williamson, P., Pols, R. G., Illman, R. J. & Topping, D. L. (1987). Blood carbonmonoxy-haemoglobin levels are chronically elevated in alcoholics treated for detoxification. *Atherosclerosis*, **67**, 245–50.

Wright, R. S., Anderson, J. W. & Bridges, S. R. (1990). Propionate inhibits hepatocyte lipid synthesis. *Proceedings of the Society for Experimental Biology and Medicine*, **195**, 26–9.

31

Short-chain fatty acids and lipid metabolism: human studies

J. W. ANDERSON

Introduction

Dietary fibre intake can significantly reduce serum cholesterol concentrations in animals (Anderson & Siesel, 1990; Jennings *et al.*, 1988) and humans (Anderson *et al.*, 1984, 1991*a*,*b*). Water-soluble fibres such as psyllium, pectin, guar gum and oat gum have potent hypocholesterolaemic effects. There are two popular hypotheses concerning mechanisms for hypocholesterolaemia: (1) soluble fibres bind bile acids in the intestine, alter lipid and bile-acid absorption and increase faecal loss of bile acids; and (2) soluble fibres are fermented in the colon to short-chain fatty acids (SCFA), which are absorbed into the portal vein and attenuate hepatic cholesterol synthesis (Anderson & Siesel, 1990). The potential role of SCFA in contributing to hypocholesterolaemia in humans is reviewed here.

Our early research (Anderson & Chen, 1979) led to the speculative suggestion that SCFA might contribute to the hypocholesterolaemic effects of dietary fibre. This hypothesis was based on the observations that soluble fibres are fermented in the colon to SCFA, which are absorbed for metabolism in the liver (Cummings, 1981). Furthermore, these SCFA are recognized to have important metabolic effects in animals and in humans (Wright, Anderson & Bridges, 1990). Further mechanistic considerations seemed necessary because the effects of soluble fibres on faecal bile-acid excretion were variable; for example, while both oat bran and beans significantly lowered the level of serum cholesterol in humans, oat bran increased while beans decreased bile-acid excretion (Anderson *et al.*, 1984). Our animal studies that examine this hypothesis are reviewed briefly; the animal work of other investigators is presented in earlier chapters of this volume.

SCFA studies in experimental animals

Preliminary studies using isolated rat hepatocytes indicated that propionate, with three carbon atoms, behaved differently from acetate and butyrate, the major SCFA with even numbers of carbon atoms (Anderson & Bridges, 1981). Whereas propionate tended to inhibit the synthesis of cholesterol and fatty acids, acetate and butyrate had the opposite effect. Propionate also inhibited gluconeogenesis and stimulated glycolysis, whereas acetate and butyrate, acting like long-chain fatty acids and their metabolites, stimulated gluconeogenesis and inhibited glycolysis (Anderson & Bridges, 1984).

The effects of propionate feeding were studied in cholesterol-fed rats. The intake of 0.5% (w/w) sodium propionate for three weeks was accompanied by significantly lower concentrations of serum and liver cholesterol than for control animals given identical diets without propionate. Serum cholesterol was 14% lower ($p < 0.05$) and liver cholesterol was 17% lower ($p < 0.05$) in propionate-fed animals than in controls (Chen, Anderson & Jennings, 1984).

To further assess the physiological significance of propionate, we measured the concentrations of SCFA in the portal vein of rats fed different types of dietary fibre. Oat bran, which significantly decreased concentrations of cholesterol in serum and liver, also significantly increased the excretion of biliary bile acid and cholesterol. Furthermore, oat-bran intake was accompanied by significantly higher portal vein concentrations of acetate, propionate and butyrate than was cellulose intake. Portal vein propionate concentrations, for example, were 92 ± 10 μmol/l (mean $\pm$ SE) in rats fed oat bran and 51 ± 3 μmol/l ($p < 0.005$) in rats fed cellulose. These observations are consistent with those of others (Storer *et al.*, 1983).

The effects of different concentrations of propionate on hepatic cholesterol synthesis were carefully examined using the isolated rat hepatocyte. These studies indicated that propionate levels of 1 mmol/l produced a statistically significant inhibition of cholesterol synthesis from [1-^{14}C]acetate. Propionate also significantly inhibited cholesterol synthesis from ^3H_2O and [2-^{14}C]mevalonate and fatty-acid synthesis from [1-^{14}C]acetate (Wright *et al.*, 1990).

These animal studies support the hypothesis that propionate may mediate some of the cholesterol-lowering effects for serum and liver of rats fed oat bran. Oat-bran feeding increases the loss of faecal bile acids which stimulates synthesis of hepatic cholesterol and bile acids. Propionate may act to attenuate hepatic cholesterol synthesis so that the liver is not able to compensate fully for the sterols being excreted in the stool. While these data lead to hypothesis development for the human, they neither support nor refute the hypothesis that propionate may contribute to the hypocholesterolaemic effects of soluble fibres in humans.

SCFA concentrations in humans

SCFA are major products of anaerobic bacterial metabolism in the human colon. Acetate, propionate and butyrate are the major SCFA produced by bacterial fermentation in the human colon. The relative amounts of these SCFA have been estimated by many investigators (Table 31.1). Measurement of these SCFA in human faeces indicate that the molar ratios of acetate : propionate : butyrate are approximately 60 : 24 : 16 (Table 31.1). Since most of the SCFA are absorbed from the colon, measurements of SCFA in faeces might not accurately reflect SCFA concentrations in the human colon. McBurney *et al.* (1988) used an *in vitro* fermentation system that simulates the human colon to examine relative amounts of different SCFA that might be produced in the human colon. Values obtained with the use of this *in vitro* fermentation system were very similar to values observed for human faeces (Table 31.1).

Different polysaccharides and dietary fibres resulted in production of differing relative amounts of SCFA with *in vitro* fermentation systems. Cummings *et al.* (1987) noted that the molar ratios of acetate ranged from 50 to 83% with different polysaccharides; propionate ranged from 15 to 43% and butyrate ranged from 2 to 29% (Table 31.1). Titgemeyer *et al.* (1991) studied ten different dietary fibres and noted that relative amounts of different SCFA ranged as follows: acetate, 60 to 89%; propionate, 7 to 28%; and butyrate, 3 to 15% (Table 31.1). Starches and sugars tended to generate relatively more butyrate than did dietary fibres (Cummings & Englyst, 1987; Mortensen, Holtug & Rasmussen, 1988; Weaver *et al.*, 1989). Certain dietary fibres resulted in relatively more propionate production (Table 31.1).

Portal vein concentrations of SCFA are the levels presented to the liver for metabolism. Two groups (Dankert, Zijlstra & Wolthers, 1981; Cummings *et al.*, 1987) have examined portal vein SCFA concentrations in humans. Values obtained by Dankert *et al.* (1981) at the time of elective cholecystectomy were lower than values obtained by Cummings *et al.* (1987) from sudden-death victims, probably because the former subjects had been fasting for 12 or more hours while the latter subjects were more likely to be in the postprandial state. Molar ratios of different SCFA in the portal vein were virtually identical (Table 31.1). The colonic epithelium appears to extract butyrate selectively, resulting in lower molar ratios of butyrate in the portal vein than in the colon (Cummings *et al.*, 1987).

Table 31.1. *Concentrations of short-chain fatty acids in humans*

Source	Acetate (μmol/l)	Propionate (μmol/l)	Butyrate (μmol/l)	Acetate (%)	Propionate (%)	Butyrate (%)	Reference
Faeces				60	24	16	Cummings (1981)
Faecal isolate, mixed diet				59	20	21	McBurney *et al.* (1988)
Faecal isolate, purified fibres				60–89	7–28	3–15	Titgemeyer *et al.* (1991)
Faecal isolate, polysaccharides[a]				50–83	15–43	2–29	Cummings & Englyst (1987)
Right colon				57	22	21	Cummings *et al.* (1987)
Portal vein	114	34	9	73	21	6	Dankert *et al.* (1981)
Portal vein	258	88	29	69	23	8	Cummings *et al.* (1987)
Peripheral vein	70	5	4	89	6	5	Cummings *et al.* (1987)
Peripheral vein	61	5	1	91	7	1	Bridges *et al.* (1992)
Peripheral vein	35	2	1	92	5	3	Dankert *et al.* (1981)

[a] Starch, arabinogalactan, xylan and pectin.

Portal vein concentrations of propionate are 20–40-fold higher than peripheral vein values, portal vein butyrate values are about tenfold higher than peripheral vein values and portal vein acetate values are only fourfold higher than peripheral vein values (Table 31.1). This strongly suggests that the liver selectively extracts propionate and butyrate to a greater extent than it does acetate. These observations suggested to us that peripheral venous acetate measurements might be a surrogate measure of SCFA production in the colon. The careful studies of Pomare, Branch & Cummings (1985) are consistent with this suggestion.

Soluble fibre effects on serum acetate in humans

Pomare *et al.* (1985) measured the acute response of serum acetate to the feeding of single doses of non-digestible carbohydrates to healthy subjects. These had avoided foods containing dietary fibre during the day before testing and had a polysaccharide-free evening meal prior to testing the next morning. Oral intake of 20 g of lactulose, a non-digestible disaccharide that is fermented in the colon, was followed by a significant increase in serum acetate level, which peaked at approximately 150 min after administration; serum acetate concentration increased from approximately 50 μmol/l to 181 μmol/l. Intake of 20 g of pectin was followed by an increase in serum acetate level, which peaked at about 6 h and was sustained for 24 h; serum acetate levels increased from fasting levels of approximately 50 μmol/l to 96 μmol/l.

Our group studied changes in serum acetate levels after feeding high-fibre diets for 2–3 weeks. In the first study, hypercholesterolaemic men were admitted to a metabolic research ward for 4 weeks. During the first week they received a low-fibre control diet. They were then randomly assigned to an oat-bran diet or a wheat-bran diet for three weeks. Control and test diets were virtually identical in nutrient content and differed only in the content of oat- or wheat-bran. Fasting and postprandial serum acetate values were measured at the end of one week on the low-fibre diet and after three weeks on oat-bran or wheat-bran diets. For these measurements, blood was drawn at 08.00, 10.00, 12.00, 14.00, 16.00, 19.00 and 22.00 (Anderson *et al.*, 1991*b*; Bridges *et al.*, 1992).

Figure 31.1 summarizes the responses of subjects to oat-bran and wheat-bran diets. Values are given as increments above values at the same time or day on the control diet. Feeding oat-bran diets for three weeks significantly increased fasting serum acetate values. Serum acetate values reached their peak at 16.00 and were 38 μmol/l higher than values at this time on the control diet. Wheat-bran diets also increased serum acetate values, but

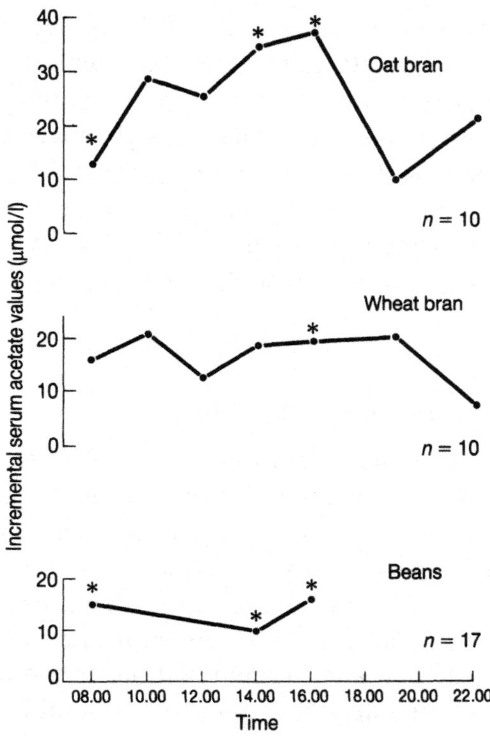

Fig. 31.1. The incremental rise of serum acetate values above values on control diets. All subjects were fed control diets for 2 weeks (beans) or 3 weeks (oat bran and wheat bran). Values shown are the incremental rises computed by subtracting values for control from test diets at each time point. Meals were fed at 08.00, 12.00 and 17.00 and snacks were provided at 10.00, 15.00 and 21.00. Asterisks represent significant differences ($p < 0.05$) from control values.

changes in the fasting state were not statistically significant. The pattern of response to wheat bran differed from that to oat bran in that a distinct peak was not observed. Serum acetate values on wheat-bran diets were sustained at approximately 15 µmol/l higher than control values throughout the day (Bridges *et al.*, 1992).

Recently we assessed the serum acetate response to increased bean intake over a 2-week period. Seventeen hypercholesterolaemic subjects entered the metabolic research ward for the two 2-week study periods with a 4-week washout period between studies. They were randomly assigned to receive a control diet first or a bean diet first. The bean diet provided 114 g (dry weight) of pinto or navy beans. The control diet was essentially identical in nutrient content but contained no bean or oat products (Riddell-Mason, Geil & Anderson, 1993).

Figure 31.1 also summarizes the serum acetate reponses to bean intake over a 2-week period. Values represent the increment above values on the control diet. Bean intake significantly increased serum acetate concentrations in the fasting state (08.00) and at 14.00 and 16.00. Although values were only collected at 14.00 and 16.00, the pattern of response to beans appeared to resemble the response to wheat bran, because no distinct peak was observed.

These studies indicate that diets of oat bran, wheat bran and beans increased fasting serum acetate levels to a similar extent. Macrae *et al.* (1988) reported similar observations for wheat-bran intake in humans. In sharp contrast, oat-bran feeding produced peak serum acetate values almost twice as high as those observed with intake of wheat bran or beans. Increases in acetate concentrations in peripheral blood almost certainly reflect increases in portal vein concentrations of propionate and butyrate. These increases in peripheral blood SCFA concentrations may contribute to the hypocholesterolaemic effects of oat bran.

We also examined the association between changes in serum low-density lipoprotein (LDL)-cholesterol and changes in serum acetate on oat-bran and bean diets. Although these associations were consistent, they were not of statistical significance. For example, with oat-bran diets the five subjects with larger changes in serum LDL-cholesterol ($-19.7 \pm 2.3\%$, mean ± SEM) had larger changes in fasting levels of serum acetate ($+34.4 \pm 24.2$ μmol/l) than the five subjects with smaller changes in serum LDL-cholesterol ($-9.6 \pm 1.4\%$) who had smaller changes in fasting levels of serum acetate (-1.4 ± 6.6 μmol/l). The associations between changes in levels of serum LDL-cholesterol and serum acetate were consistent for each comparison with larger changes in concentrations of serum LDL-cholesterol associated with larger changes in fasting or postprandial values of serum acetate.

With bean intake the associations between serum cholesterol changes and serum acetate changes were less strong and less consistent. However, a consistent relationship was observed between fasting levels of serum LDL-cholesterol and fasting levels of serum acetate. Complete values were available for comparison for 14 subjects. The seven subjects with larger serum LDL-cholesterol changes had larger changes in fasting serum acetate (19.3 ± 3.5 μmol/l) than the seven subjects with smaller cholesterol changes who had smaller fasting serum acetate changes (11.3 ± 1.3 μmol/l).

Strong associations between changes in levels of serum LDL-cholesterol and changes in levels of serum acetate would support the hypothesis that changes in SCFA contribute to the hypocholesterolaemic effects of soluble

Table 31.2. *Metabolic response to the administration of short-chain fatty acids (SCFA) in humans*

SCFA	Administration	Glucose	Free fatty acids	Cholesterol	Triglycerides	Reference
Acetate	Oral		−25%			Crouse *et al.* (1978)
Acetate	IV (CRF)			−8.6%	−6.9%	Port *et al.* (1978)
Acetate	IV (normal)				−32%	Port *et al.* (1978)
Acetate	Oral	Unchanged	Unchanged			Scheppach *et al.* (1988*a*)
Acetate	Oral	Unchanged	Decreased			Scheppach *et al.* (1988*b*)
Acetate	IV	Unchanged	Decreased			Akanji *et al.* (1991)
Acetate	Rectal	Unchanged	Decreased	Increased		Wolever *et al.* (1989)
Acetate + propionate	Rectal	Unchanged	Decreased	Increased	Increased	Wolever *et al.* (1989)
Propionate	Rectal	Increased	Unchanged	Unchanged	Unchanged	Wolever *et al.* (1991)
Acetate + propionate	Rectal	Increased	Decreased	Unchanged	Unchanged	Wolever *et al.* (1991)
Propionate	Oral (7 weeks)	Decreased		Unchanged	Increased	Venter *et al.* (1990)
Propionate	Oral (1 week)	Decreased		Slightly decreased	Slightly increased	Todesco *et al.* (1991)

IV, intravenous; CRF, chronic renal failure.

fibres. Our failure to find strong associations, however, does not negate this hypothesis. Additional studies with larger numbers of subjects are required to assess these relationships further.

Metabolic effects of acetate administration in humans

Because acetate is such an important intermediary metabolite, its effect of glucose and lipid metabolism in humans has been extensively studied. The effects related to glucose and lipid metabolism will be overviewed (Table 31.2) Crouse *et al.* (1978) noted that oral administration of acetate, 143 mg/kg in 30 min (equal to 167 mmol for a 70-kg person), to human subjects was accompanied by a significant decrease in plasma concentrations of free fatty acids of about 25%. Port, Easterling & Barnes (1978) reported that infusion of 180 mequiv. (180 mmol) of sodium acetate over a 30-min period to normal subjects undergoing haemodialysis for chronic renal failure led to a significant reduction in serum cholesterol and triglyceride concentrations. At the completion of the acetate infusion, serum cholesterol values were about 15 mg/dl (8.6%) lower than initial values. Serum triglycerides decreased significantly in both groups, with a fall of 6.9% in dialysis subjects and 32% in control subjects.

Scheppach *et al.* (1988*a*) carefully evaluated the effects of acetate administration on glucose tolerance in healthy human subjects. Subjects took 195 mmol of acetate orally (15 mmol every 15 min for 3 h) and took an oral glucose load (50 g) at 30 min after initiating the acetate. Serum acetate levels rose from baseline values of 66 μmol/l to a plateau of about 800 μmol/l between 180 and 240 min. Changes in levels of plasma glucose, free fatty acid, 3-hydroxybutyrate, insulin, glucagon and gastric inhibitory polypeptide (GIP) were similar to those of administration with control (sodium chloride) and acetate.

To further assess effects of acetate on glucose metabolism in healthy human subjects, Scheppach *et al.* (1988*b*) measured glucose turnover using [U-^{13}C]glucose. Administration of acetate, for a total dose of 135 mmol given orally as 15 mmol every 15 min, did not significantly affect glucose turnover. Although acetate administration produced no observable changes in glucose metabolism, alterations in intermediate metabolism were observed during this study. Consistent with the observations of Crouse *et al.* (1978), acetate administration temporarily halted the rise in free fatty acids but did not affect plasma glycerol levels. These observations suggest that with significantly increased serum acetate levels, acetate is oxidized instead of long-chain fatty acids.

Akanji & Hockaday (1991) examined the effects of acetate administration on glucose tolerance of normal and diabetic subjects. Intravenously infused acetate, at a rate of 2.5 mmol/min for 60 min, did not significantly alter the disappearance rates of intravenously injected glucose for control or diabetic subjects. There was a significant difference in the metabolic clearance rate of acetate between control and diabetic subjects. Acetate infusions significantly decreased plasma concentrations of free fatty acids and glycerol.

Wolever, Spadafora & Eshuis (1991) assessed the effects of rectal infusion of acetate on glucose and lipid metabolism of six healthy subjects. Acetate, 180 mmol, was administered rectally in 800 ml of fluid at a rate of 27 ml/min. A rectal infusion of saline or an oral load of 800 ml of water served as controls. Each subject completed all procedures. Rectal acetate administration increased serum acetate concentration by 300 μmol/l, with peak values occurring at 60 min and incremental values sustained above 250 μmol/l for 2 h. Acetate administration had these effects: concentrations of blood glucose, serum insulin and glucagon were unchanged; serum levels of free fatty acids were significantly decreased; and serum levels of total and LDL-cholesterol were significantly increased by 4–5 mg/dl.

These studies indicate that acetate administration to healthy human volunteers produces significant decreases in serum concentrations of free fatty acids and that glycerol levels may also decrease. In these studies acetate administration did not affect oral glucose tolerance, intravenous glucose tolerance or glucose turnover rates. Acetate administration also did not affect plasma concentrations of hormones such as insulin, glucagon or GIP. Acetate appears to suppress lipolysis and to compete with long-chain fatty acids for oxidation in certain tissues. Acetate administration in humans may promote hepatic cholesterol synthesis.

Metabolic effects of propionate administration in humans

Wolever *et al.* (1989) administered solutions of acetate and propionate by rectal infusion to six healthy subjects to examine their effects on glucose and lipid metabolism. Each subject was given a rectal infusion of 800 ml of fluid at a rate or 27 ml/min for 30 min. The control solution contained saline and the test solutions contained either 90 mmol acetate plus 30 mmol propionate (120-mmol test) or 180 mmol acetate plus 60 mmol propionate (240-mmol test). After the 240-mmol test, serum acetate values increased by 245 mmol/l and remained increased by more than 200 mmol/l 2 h later. Concentrations of blood glucose, serum insulin and serum C-peptide did not change significantly with either test solution. Serum values of free fatty acids decreased significantly with the 240-mmol test. Serum levels of cholesterol and triglycerides increased significantly with the 240-mmol test. These observations suggest that SCFA may be used for hepatic lipid synthesis.

Wolever *et al.* (1991) also compared the effects of acetate alone (180 mmol), propionate alone (180 mmol), and acetate (180 mmol) plus propionate (60 mmol) given by rectal infusion to healthy subjects. The acetate effects are described above. Propionate administration had the following effects: serum propionate values increased by 80 mmol/l, peaked at 60 min and remained increased by more than 60 mmol/l for 2 h; blood glucose values increased significantly by 9 mg/dl; serum insulin and plasma glucagon values did not change; serum levels of free fatty acids did not change; and serum levels of lipids did not change. Acetate plus propionate administration had the following effects: blood glucose levels increased significantly by 2.5 mg/dl; serum levels of free fatty acids decreased significantly; and serum levels of insulin and glucagon as well as serum levels of lipids did not change significantly. The authors concluded that this study was consistent with the hypothesis that propionate resulting from colonic fermentation inhibits the utilization of acetate for cholesterol synthesis.

Venter, Vorster & Cummings (1990) administered 7.5 g of propionate daily in capsule form to healthy subjects for seven weeks. This was a double-blind, placebo-controlled study. Propionate supplementation significantly decreased serum glucose values by 9.5% or 7.2 mg/dl. Propionate use did not affect serum cholesterol levels but significantly increased high-density lipoprotein (HDL)-cholesterol by 11% compared to control changes. Serum triglycerides increased significantly in the propionate group but did not differ significantly from control changes.

Todesco *et al.* (1991) also examined the effects of oral propionate administration on glucose and lipid metabolism of healthy subjects. Six subjects consumed bread containing 9.9 g of propionate per day or white bread without propionate. This was a random-order, crossover study with subjects using each type of bread for one week. Propionate intake was accompanied by significantly lower blood glucose values after a test meal of white bread; the area under the curve was 38% lower ($p < 0.005$). There were no significant differences in serum lipids after one week on propionate bread compared to white bread. However, total cholesterol, LDL-cholesterol and HDL-cholesterol tended to be lower while triglycerides tended to be higher after propionate compared to white bread. The authors concluded that incorporating propionate into bread decreases its digestibility by inhibiting amylase activity. These effects on digestibility would not be seen with propionate produced by fermentation in the colon.

Conclusions

Clinical studies indicate that soluble fibres do not simply act like bile acid by binding resins, since some hypocholesterolaemic fibres increase faecal bile-acid excretion, but others do not (Anderson *et al.*, 1984). Because cholesterol-lowering fibres are fermented to SCFA in the colon, the hypothesis evolved that SCFA might contribute to the hypocholesterolaemic effects of soluble fibres. This hypothesis is still being rigorously examined.

Studies in experimental animals indicate that feeding hypocholesterolaemic fibres (e.g. oat bran) significantly increases portal vein propionate values, while feeding non-cholesterol-lowering fibres (e.g. cellulose) does not. Furthermore, feeding propionate to rats significantly decreases their serum cholesterol concentration. *In vitro* studies indicate that propionate, at physiological concentrations, significantly decreases hepatic cholesterol synthesis. These animal studies support the hypothesis that propionate contributes to the hypocholesterolaemia that accompanies soluble-fibre intake.

Human studies to examine the hypocholesterolaemia effects of propionate will be difficult to perform. Theoretically, administration of a bile-acid binder to mimic the intestinal effects of soluble fibres coupled with short-term (7 days or more) administration of propionate could be done. Whether oral administration of propionate would mimic the colonic source of propionate from fibre is unclear. Administration of lactulose and a bile-acid binder might mimic the effects of a soluble fibre. The goal would be to determine if propionate generation added to the hypocholesterolaemic effects of a small dose of bile-acid-binding resin. Studies to carefully approach this question have not been reported. Oral, intravenous or rectal administration of acetate or propionate do not examine this question fully.

The metabolic effects of acetate and propionate have been carefully studied in humans. Acetate has been administered orally, intravenously and rectally. Propionate has been administered orally and rectally. Mixtures of acetate and propionate have been administered rectally. Most studies were of short duration (a few hours) but two studies examined the longer-term oral administration of propionate. These nine studies are difficult to compare, but some general conclusions can be drawn.

Administration of acetate or propionate does not appear to significantly affect fasting blood glucose values, glucose metabolism or serum levels of important hormones that regulate glucose metabolism. Acetate administration decreases serum concentrations of free fatty acids and appears to decrease lipolysis. Acetate may decrease long-chain fatty-acid oxidation. The effects of acetate or propionate administration on serum cholesterol, LDL-cholesterol, HDL-cholesterol, and triglycerides are unclear.

A wide variety of soluble fibres have cholesterol-lowering effects in animals and humans. The mechanisms responsible for these hypocholesterolaemic effects are unclear; multiple and interacting mechanisms are probably operational. The effects of SCFA on lipid metabolism in humans are yet to be elucidated.

References

Akanji, A. O. & Hockaday, T. D. R. (1991). Acetate tolerance and the kinetics of acetate utilization in diabetic and nondiabetic subjects. *American Journal of Clinical Nutrition*, **4**, 112–18.

Anderson, J. W. & Bridges, S. R. (1981). Plant fiber metabolites alter hepatic glucose and lipid metabolism (abstract). *Diabetes*, **30**, (Suppl. 1) 113A.

Anderson, J. W. & Bridges, S. R. (1984). Short-chain fatty acid fermentation products of plant fiber affect glucose metabolism of isolated rat hepatocytes. *Proceedings of the Society of Experimental Biology and Medicine*, **177**, 372–6.

Anderson, J. W. & Chen, W.-J. L. (1979). Plant fiber. Carbohydrate and lipid metabolism. *American Journal of Clinical Nutrition*, **32**, 346–63.

Anderson, J. W., Floore, T. L., Geil, P. B., O'Neal, D. S. & Balm, T. K. (1991*a*). Hypocholesterolemic effects of different bulk-forming hydrophilic fibers as adjuncts to dietary therapy in mild to moderate hypercholesterolemia. *Archives of Internal Medicine*, **151**, 1597–602.

Anderson, J. W., Gilinsky, N. H., Deakins, D. A., Smith, S. F., O'Neal, D. S., Dillon, D. W. & Oeltgen, P. R. (1991*b*). Lipid responses of hypercholesterolemic men to oat-bran and wheat-bran intake. *American Journal of Clinical Nutrition*, **54**, 678–83.

Anderson, J. W. & Siesel, A. E. (1990). Hypocholesterolemic effects of oat products. In *New Developments in Dietary Fiber, Physiological, Physicochemical, and Analytical Aspects*, ed. I. Furda & C. J. Brine, pp. 17–36. New York: Plenum Press.

Anderson, J. W., Story, L., Sieling, B., Chen, W.-J. L., Petro, M. S. & Story, J. A. (1984). Hypocholesterolemic effects of oat-bran or bean intake for hypercholesterolemic men. *American Journal of Clinical Nutrition*, 40, 1146–55.

Bridges, S. R., Anderson, J. W., Deakins, D. D., Dillon, D. W. & Wood, C. L. (1992). Oat bran increases serum acetate of hypercholesterolemic men. *American Journal of Clinical Nutrition*, **56**, 455–9.

Chen, W.-J. L., Anderson, J. W. & Jennings, D. (1984). Propionate may mediate the hypocholesterolemic effects of certain soluble plant fibers in cholesterol-fed rats. *Proceedings of the Society of Experimental Biology and Medicine*, **175**, 215–18.

Crouse, J. R., Gerson, C. D., DeCarli, L. M. & Lieber, C. S. (1978). Role of acetate in the reduction of plasma free fatty acids produced by ethanol in man. *Journal of Lipid Research*, **9**, 509–12.

Cummings, J. H. (1981). Short chain fatty acids in the human colon. *Gut*, **22**, 763–79.

Cummings, J. H. & Englyst, H. N. (1987). Fermentation in the human large intestine and the available substrates. *Americal Journal of Clinical Nutrition*, **45**, 1243–55.

Cummings, J. H., Pomare, E. W., Branch, W. J., Naylor, C. P. E. & MacFarlane, G. T. (1987). Short chain fatty acids in human large intestine, portal, hepatic and venous blood. *Gut*, **28**, 1221–7.

Dankert, J. Zijlstra, J. B. & Wolthers, B. G. (1981). Volatile fatty acids in human peripheral and portal blood: quantitative determination by vacuum distillation and gas chromatography. *Clinica Chemica Acta*, **110**, 301–7.

Jennings, C. D., Boleyn, K., Bridges, S. R., Wood, P. J. & Anderson, J. W. (1988). A comparison of the lipid-lowering and the intestinal morphologic effects of cholestyramine, chitosan and oat gum in rats. *Proceeding of the Society of Experimental Biology and Medicine*, **189**, 13–20.

Macrae, F. A., Blackley, M., Brouwer, R. & Topping, D. (1988). Measurement of plasma acetate in response to dietary fibre (abstract). *Gastroenterology*, **94**, A276.

McBurney, M. I., Thompson, L. U., Cuff, D. J. & Jenkins, D. J. A. (1988). Comparison of ileal effluents, dietary fibers, and whole foods in predicting the physiologic importance of colonic fermentation. *American Journal of Gastoenterology*, **83**, 536–40.

Mortensen, P. B., Holtug, K. R. & Rasmussen, H. S. (1988). Short-chain fatty acid production from mono- and disaccharides in a fecal incubation system: implications for colonic fermentation of dietary fiber in humans. *Journal of Nutrition*, **118**, 321–5.

Pomare, E. W., Branch, W. J. & Cummings, J. H. (1985). Carbohydrate fermentation in the human colon and its relation to acetate concentrations in venous blood. *Journal of Clinical Investigation*, **75**, 1448–54.

Port, F. K., Easterling, R. E. & Barnes, R. V. (1978). Effect of acetate administration on blood lipids. *American Journal of Clinical Nutrition*, **31**, 1893–6.

Riddell-Mason, S., Geil, P. B. & Anderson, J. W. (1993). Dry bean consumption increases serum acetate in hypercholesterolemic men. *FASEB Journal*, **7**, A740.

Scheppach, W., Cummings, J. H., Branch, W. J. & Schrezenmeir, J. (1988*a*). Effect of gut-derived acetate on oral glucose tolerance in man. *Clinical Science*, **75**, 355–61.

Scheppach, W., Wiggins, H. S., Halliday, D., Self, R., Howard, J., Branch, W. J., Schrezenmeir, J. & Cummings, J. H. (1988*b*). Effect of gut-derived acetate on glucose turnover in man. *Clinical Science*, **75**, 363–70.

Storer, G. B., Trimble, R. P., Illman, R. J., Snoswell, A. M. & Topping, D. L. (1983). Effects of dietary oat bran and diabetes on plasma volatile fatty acids in the rat. *Nutrition Research*, **3**, 519–26.

Titgemeyer, E. G., Bourquin, L. D., Fahey, G. C. Jr. & Garleb, K. A. (1991). Fermentability of various fiber sources by human fecal bacteria *in vitro*. *American Journal of Clinical Nutrition*, **53**, 1418–24.

Todesco, T., Rao, A. V., Bosello, O. & Jenkins, D. J. A. (1991). Propionate lowers blood glucose and alters lipid metabolism in healthy subjects. *American Journal of Clinical Nutrition*, **54**, 860–5.

Venter, C. S., Vorster, H. H. & Cummings, J. H. (1990). Effects of dietary propionate on carbohydrate and lipid metabolism in healthy volunteers. *American Journal of Gastroenterology*, **85**, 549–53.

Weaver, G. A., Krause, J. A., Miller, T. L. & Wolin, M. J. (1989). Constancy of glucose and starch fermentations by two different human faecal microbial communities. *Gut*, **30**, 19–35.

Wolever, T. M. S., Brighenti, F., Royall, D., Jenkins, A. L. & Jenkins, D. J. A. (1989). Effect of rectal infusion of short chain fatty acids in human subjects. *American Journal of Gastroenterology*, **84**, 1027–33.

Wolever, T. M. S., Spadafora, P. & Eshuis, H. (1991). Interaction between colonic acetate and propionate in humans. *American Journal of Clinical Nutrition*, **53**, 681–7.

Wright, R. S., Anderson, J. W. & Bridges, S. R. (1990). Propionate inhibits hepatocyte lipid synthesis. *Proceeding of the Society of Experimental Biology and Medicine*, **195**, 26–9.

32

Colonic short-chain fatty acids in infants and children

C. H. LIFSCHITZ

An infant is born with a sterile colon; as a result, in the first few days of life, the large bowel contains no bacteria to degrade dietary products or endogenous glycoproteins. For that reason, the production and assimilation of short-chain fatty acids (SCFA) are unlikely to occur at significant levels until the infant acquires an anaerobic flora. After birth, however, bacteria rapidly colonize the large bowel, and indirect evidence of carbohydrate fermentation exists at only a few days after delivery. To better understand SCFA formation, most studies have investigated the development of the faecal flora and the various factors that affect its development. Information about the production and utilization of SCFA in infants and children, however, is extremely limited.

The mortality of artificially fed infants during the years preceding the First World War was high. Czerny hypothesized that SCFA, developed by bacterial contamination of cow's milk, might be responsible (Gerstley *et al.*, 1928). Finkelstein, Salge, Moro and others, however, believed that other factors were more relevant. Between 1911 and 1914, Hans Bahrdt and others isolated and measured SCFA from human faeces and observed that the quantities of SCFA were much greater in diarrhoeal stools than in contaminated milk or in the stomach contents.

The early studies of Gerstley (Gerstley *et al.*, 1928) established several important characteristics regarding the influence of diet on faecal SCFA: (1) SCFA and total acid titratability are generally uniform in breast-fed infants; (2) SCFA output is more variable and frequently greater and acetic acid content is higher in the faeces of formula-fed infants than in the faeces of breast-fed infants; and (3) propionic acid is present in measurable amounts only in the stools of infants fed cow's milk. Since the original studies of Moro and Tissier in 1905 (Gerstley *et al.*, 1928), we have known that the faeces of infants fed human milk are more acid and contain a much higher percentage of Gram-positive bacilli, in particular *Lactobacillus bifidus*, than do the faeces

Table 32.1. *Lactate and short-chain fatty acids in fresh faeces of formula-fed and breast-fed infants (mean ± SEM; μmol/g wet weight)*

	Lactate	Acetate	Propionate
Formula-fed	18.5 ± 6.1	98.9 ± 19.4	33.2 ± 3
Breast-fed	22.4 ± 5	44.7 ± 8.1[a]	14.1 ± 4.1[a]

[a] For difference between feeding groups, $p < 0.05$.

of infants fed cow's milk. Barbero *et al.* (1952) identified discernible differences between the faeces of equally well-nourished breast-fed and cow's-milk-fed infants. Breast-fed infants produced a distinctly acid stool with a predominantly Gram-positive flora; cow's-milk-fed infants produced a less acid stool with a mixed bacterial flora. This was corroborated more recently by our own studies (Lifschitz, Wolin & Reeds, 1990).

A recent study has documented that the faeces of breast-fed infants whose diet had been supplemented with formula or cow's milk acquired certain characteristics foreign to the faeces of exclusively breast-fed infants, including a higher pH and the presence of propionate, which is virtually absent in faeces of exclusively breast-fed infants (Ogawa *et al.*, 1992; Table 32.1). These findings contradict a previous study by Bullen, Tearle & Willis (1976), who observed differences in the stool patterns between breast-fed and formula-fed infants, even when breast-fed infants were also fed formula. The development and maintenance of the *L. bifidus* flora in the stool of breast-fed infants has generally been thought to be related to the low protein and high lactose content of human milk. However, our study and that of Ogawa *et al.* indicate that even infants fed modern formulas, in which the lactose and protein content is similar to that of human milk, have differences in the faecal flora. Long & Swenson (1977) found that by the end of the first week of life of term infants (who were delivered vaginally and fed a milk formula), 61% had *Bacteroides fragilis* isolated from the stool. The mode of delivery, gestational age and type of feeding seemed to affect the colonization of the bowel: infants delivered by caesarean section had significantly lower faecal isolates of *B. fragilis* and other anaerobic bacteria at the end of the first week of life than did those delivered vaginally (Fig. 32.1). Significantly fewer anaerobic bacteria were isolated from the stools of preterm infants than from the stools of full-term infants of the same postnatal age. At 48 h after birth, breast-fed and formula-fed infants had similar counts of *B. fragilis*, other anaerobic bacteria, aerobic Gram-negative bacilli, and streptococci, but at 7 days after birth, only

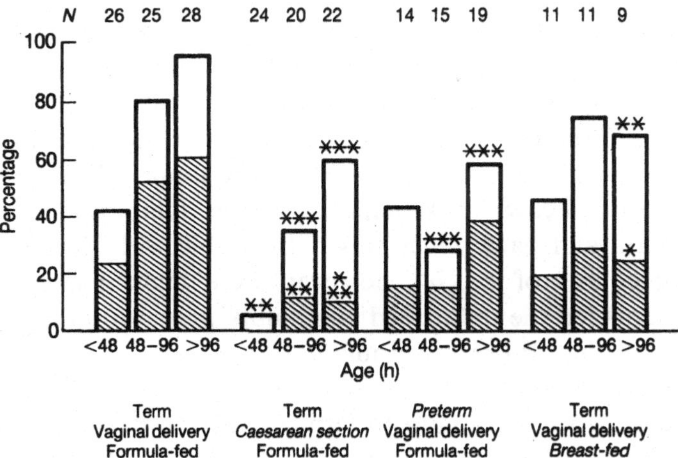

Fig. 32.1. Comparative isolation rates of anaerobic bacteria (white bars) and *Bacteroides fragilis* (hatched bars) from infants' faecal specimens. *N* is the number of specimens cultured. Groups were compared to term infants delivered by the vaginal route who were formula-fed. Significant differences were calculated by the χ^2 technique. * $p < 0.05$; ** $p \leq 0.01$; *** $p < 0.001$. Adapted from Long & Swenson (1977), with permission.

22% of breast-fed infants had *B. fragilis* isolated from the stool compared to 61% of the formula-fed counterparts. The studies of Hall *et al.* (1990) partly supported these findings. The authors studied the faecal flora of 10-day-old infants: 46 were preterm and 52 were full-term. In addition, 37 preterm and 46 full-term infants were studied at 30 days of age, at which time lactobacilli, but not bifidobacteria, were found in high counts in the stool of most of the full-term infants. The mode of delivery, but not the method of feeding, had a significant influence on early colonization. Compared to the number of coliform organisms, the number of lactobacilli was deficient in preterm infants. Previous treatment with antibiotics and having been nursed in an incubator were also significantly associated with a lower rate of early colonization with lactobacilli. These findings indicate that lactobacilli may be an important part of the normal stool flora in early infancy, and that modern methods of neonatal care are associated with delayed or deficient colonization.

Many dietary factors affect the characteristics of the faecal flora. The effects of iron supplementation on the flora were studied by Mevissen-Verhage *et al.* (1985). During the first 12 weeks after the birth of the infants, the authors studied faecal specimens from ten breast-fed infants, six infants fed a cow's-milk preparation supplemented with iron (5 mg/l), and seven infants fed the same product without iron supplement (iron concentration <0.5 mg/l). In breast-fed infants, bifidobacteria were predominant, *Escherichia coli* counts were low, and other bacteria were rarely present. In infants fed the fortified cow's-milk product, *E. coli* counts were high, counts and isolation frequency of bifidobacteria were low, and other bacteria were frequently isolated. In infants fed the unfortified cow's-milk preparation, the isolation frequency of *E. coli*, bifidobacteria and bacteroides was comparable with that found in breast-fed infants; counts of *E. coli*, however, were high. These authors concluded that infants fed the unfortified cow's-milk preparation acquired a faecal flora similar to that of breast-fed infants.

The development of the ability to produce SCFA parallels the development of the faecal flora, as does the ability to ferment carbohydrates and create by-products such as hydrogen gas (H_2). Stevenson *et al.* (1982) collected uniform films of faecal material devoid of solid chunks by inserting the length of a sterile cotton tip applicator into the rectum of preterm infants who did not have clinical evidence of carbohydrate intolerance. The authors also measured changes in the pulmonary elimination of H_2. The end-tidal H_2 excretion correlated with the total count of Enterobacteriaceae in these healthy preterm infants, who were in an apparent steady state of nutrition. In this study, the intestinal colonization of the preterm infants was characterized by a paucity of anaerobes and biotypes of Enterobacteriaceae. The conspicuous absence of anaerobic bacteria and their eventual later appearance in a few infants was very different from the normal pattern of colonization described by Long & Swenson (1977).

To provide information on SCFA in faeces from normal neonates, Rasmussen *et al.* (1988) studied faecal samples collected immediately after birth (meconium) and on the 4th day of life in 13 healthy, full-term neonates. The capacity to produce SCFA was evaluated by a faecal incubation system. Mean ($\pm$SD) concentrations of SCFA were low in meconium (11.2 ± 3.9 mmol/l), equivalent to about 10% of the adult level ($p < 0.01$), but increased significantly during the first 4 days of life to 28.4 ± 20.1 mmol/l ($p < 0.05$). The fermentation pattern (i.e. the relative composition of different acids) differed between adults and neonates, primarily because of a higher proportion of acetate found in the latter. The proportion of acetate : propionate : butyrate : other acids was 89 : 5 : 5 : 1 in 4-day-old neonates and 65 : 18 : 11 : 6 in adults ($p < 0.001$). The establishment of the production of SCFA in the faeces was studied in 30 healthy infants from birth to 24 months of age (Midtvedt & Midtvedt, 1992; Fig. 32.2). Acetic and propionic acids were the principal SCFA produced at 1 and 3 months, followed by butyric, valeric and caproic acids. At 2 years, most of the SCFA had reached adult values. Exposure to foods other than

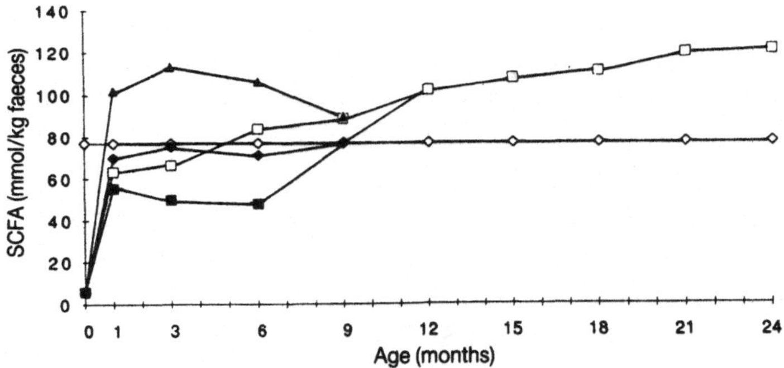

Fig. 32.2. Mean values of the total amount of short-chain fatty acids (SCFA) produced in all children (open squares) and in the three dietary groups separately: group 1, fed human milk exclusively (filled squares); group 2, fed human milk and formula supplement (filled diamonds); and group 3, which received no human milk at the time of the study (filled triangles). Mean values for adults shown for comparison (open diamonds). From Midtvedt & Midtvedt (1992), with permission.

breast milk and to antibiotics seemed to affect the absolute and relative amounts of SCFA only during the first month of life.

Because of the difficulties inherent in the isolation, quantitation and characterization of faecal bacteria, Norin *et al.* (1985) developed a new approach to the study of the colonization of the digestive tract after birth, by examining the development of four microflora-associated characteristics, defined as any anatomical structure or biochemical or physiological function in the macro-organism that had been influenced by the microflora. The following biochemical characteristics were studied in faeces from children at 9–61 months of age: conversion of cholesterol to coprostanol and bilirubin to urobilins, inactivation of trypsin, and degradation of mucin. The results indicated that microbes capable of converting bilirubin to urobilins were established within the second year of life. The mucin-degrading and cholesterol-converting microbes were established in most of the children during the same period. Tryptic activity was absent in meconium, present in faeces from all children up to 21 months of age, and absent in six out of 15 children in the 46–61-month age group. The study indicated that the establishment of microflora-associated characteristics in the digestive tract is a remarkably long process.

We used a similar approach to characterize the carbohydrate fermentation by intestinal flora in formula-fed infants and in breast-fed infants (Lifschitz *et al.*, 1990). We also wished to compare the carbohydrate fermentation process in the two groups to determine whether differences that existed between groups could help explain the observation that breast-fed infants usually have milder forms of acute gastroenteritis. We performed *in vitro* incubations of faecal samples and studied (1) the effect of acid pH on bacterial fermentation and (2) the changes in carbohydrate fermentation in relation to the age of the infant. Faecal samples were incubated, with and without the addition of lactose, at pH 6.8 and at pH 5.5. SCFA and carbohydrates were determined in the incubates. The addition of lactose to the incubate at pH 6.8 resulted in a significant increase in SCFA production and larger amounts of lactose, glucose, and galactose compared with the values observed in 1-h incubates to which no lactose was added. At pH 5.5 SCFA production was significantly lower in both groups compared with those at pH 6.8, and the accumulation of monosaccharides in the incubate of faeces of formula-fed infants increased significantly ($p < 0.05$). In contrast, in stools from breast-fed infants, incubation at pH 5.5 resulted in a greater proportion of saccharides as lactose, i.e. a decrease in the amount of lactose hydrolyzed ($p < 0.01$), accompanied by a non-significant increase in the amount of hexose. The decrease in lactose hydrolysis in breast-fed infants resulted in a lower luminal osmolar load, which may provide a partial explanation for the fact that acute gastroenteritis is milder in this population. We also observed a correlation between age and the sum of faecal SCFA (Fig. 32.3).

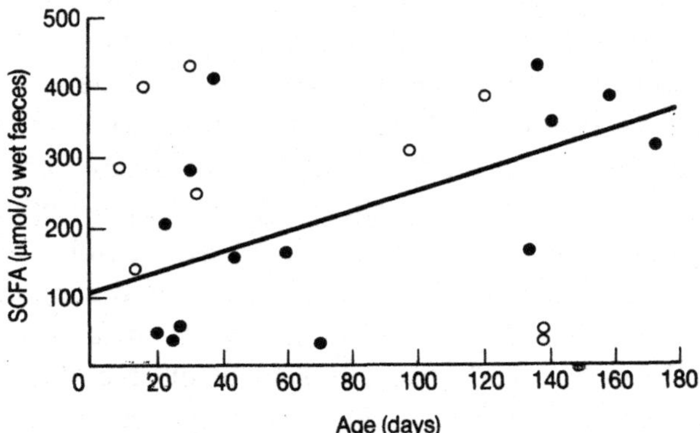

Fig. 32.3. Relationship between the age of infants and the sum of the short-chain fatty acids (SCFA) present in the stool at the end of 1-h incubation with lactose, at pH 6.8. A significant positive correlation ($p = 0.03$) was found for breast-fed infants (filled circles). but not for formula-fed infants (open circles). The regression line was derived from the data from the breast-fed infants. From Lifschitz *et al.* (1990), with permission.

Because it is difficult to perform studies in human infants, and because many aspects of intestinal development and function are similar in the human infant and the pig (Shulman, Henning & Nichols, 1988), many investigators have used the newborn pig as a model to study colonic function. The intestinal flora of the pig, however, is unlikely to be an exact representation of the intestinal flora in the human infant.

Murray *et al.* (1987) studied the profile of SCFA levels in the colonic lumen of pigs over the initial 21 days of life. Newborns produced SCFA in limited amounts as early as the first day of life. Levels were stable between days 5 and 14, and then accumulated abruptly in the lumen. Acetate was predominant early, with propionate and butyrate responsible for late peaks. The production and assimilation of SCFA was nearly complete proximal to the left colon. Age and colon site showed significant interactions for each fatty acid. The combined osmolar contributions of SCFA and electrolytes accounted completely for the luminal osmolarity after the 2nd week of life. Previously there was an 'osmolar gap' suggesting that lactose or its breakdown products were present in the lumen and were being removed by pathways other than the production of SCFA. In another study, the same authors determined the absorption of SCFA and their effects on colonic conservation of water and sodium (Murray *et al.*, 1989). Exclusively suckled, 2–23-day-old pigs were studied. Absorption from a control/electrolyte solution was compared with that from a SCFA solution; SCFA absorption was highest at birth, then declined rapidly over 72 h to a lower and relatively stable level. During the control perfusions, water and sodium absorption increased with age. The addition of SCFA to the perfusate stimulated the uptake of both water and sodium in the first two weeks. After the 14th day, sodium absorption continued to be enhanced by SCFA, but water movement remained unchanged from control levels. Such a result suggests that, although luminal SCFA levels may be limited early in life, the presence of SCFA stimulates the absorption of sodium and water from the colon in newborns.

Argenzio *et al.* (1984) studied the capacity of the colon to absorb water and electrolytes and the production of SCFA by the faecal flora to enhance water absorption and aid in the fermentation of malabsorbed carbohydrate. The authors compared the responses of 3-day-old and 3-week-old pigs infected with transmissible gastroenteritis virus. The older animals did not have diarrhoea, because their capacity to absorb fluids in the large bowel increased by six times over that of the younger animals. Further, carbohydrate that arrived in the colon of the older pigs was completely fermented to SCFA; carbohydrate passed unchanged through the colon of the younger pigs. This study demonstrates that the development of microbial digestion and the ability to absorb SCFA rapidly are the features primarily responsible for the colonic compensation to the viral infection in the older pigs. The diarrhoea frequently observed in infants treated with broad-spectrum antibiotics results from the decrease in bacterial flora and the concomitant decrease in the capacity to ferment dietary carbohydrate as it arrives in the colon. Bhatia, Prihoda & Richardson (1986) evaluated the effects of parenteral antibiotics on carbohydrate tolerance, faecal reducing substances, stool frequency and dietary manipulation in two groups of term neonates: one group received parenteral ampicillin and gentamicin, the other received no antibiotics. Most of the neonates were fed a standard lactose-containing formula and the remainder were breast-fed. Stool frequency, presence of faecal reducing substances and requirement for dietary manipulation were significantly greater in neonates receiving antibiotics than in controls. Infants who manifest symptomatic carbohydrate intolerance while receiving parenteral antibiotics may benefit either from receiving lactose-free formula or from decreasing the intake of carbohydrates that may be incompletely absorbed in the small bowel for the duration of antibiotic therapy.

The relationship between small-bowel carbohydrate malabsorption, colonic fermentation, production of hydrogen gas and SCFA becomes clinically relevant whenever there are large amounts of carbohydrate arriving in the colon, as in diarrhoea. To characterize the process of fermentation, Torres-Pinedo *et al.* (1968) instilled saline and glucose-saline solutions into the distal colons of infants with acute infectious diarrhoea. Samples of the fluid were obtained at hourly intervals. Clear-cut differences in compositional changes were observed with the saline and glucose-saline solutions. The net effects induced by glucose were the generation of organic acids and subsequent formation of poorly absorbable organic acid salts and the osmotic inflow of water. The process led to a net gain of hydrogen ion by the body fluids, a decrease in sodium absorption, an increase in the loss of potassium, and a net increase in the volume of the colonic fluid. These experiments have helped explain the findings observed in the faeces of infants with diarrhoea. When moderate amounts of carbohydrate arrive in the colon and the faecal flora is intact (i.e. not diminished by the previous use of antibiotics), carbohydrate fermentation takes place and is evidenced by the production of H_2, the lack of reducing substances in stools and an increased amount of SCFA, although faecal pH remains above 5.5. If the amount of carbohydrate arriving in the colon increases, fermentation may not be complete and carbohydrate appears in the stool. Alternatively, the amount of SCFA produced is greater than the amount that can be absorbed by the colon, faecal pH falls (particularly when lactic acid is produced) and H_2 production may be impaired, because the luminal pH is lower than the pK of the bacterial enzymes whose activity becomes inhibited (Perman, Modler & Olson, 1981; Lifschitz *et al.*, 1983). The explanation is helpful in the dietary management of infants with diarrhoea. A faecal pH of 5.5 or greater and the absence of glucose (or reducing substances in stools) in the presence of H_2 production indicate that bacteria are almost completely fermenting the carbohydrate to SCFA, which are then absorbed through the intestinal wall. A faecal pH of less than 5.5 and the absence of glucose in stools indicate fermentation but incomplete absorption of the SCFA produced. Finally, a faecal pH of greater than 5.5 and the presence of glucose in stools indicate small-bowel carbohydrate malabsorption and ineffective fermentation: no SCFA are produced and H_2 in breath will be low. It is important to remember that whenever large amounts of carbohydrate arrive in the colon, flux through the glycolytic pathway is increased and bacterial metabolism shifts to the production of lactic acid. The diffusion capacity of lactate through the colonic mucosa may be less than that of acetate. In cases of metabolic acidaemia, seen in premature infants after incomplete disaccharide absorption, serum lactate concentrations are moderately increased, despite the large increase in faecal lactate, and cannot account for the increase in anions observed other than chloride and bicarbonate (Lifschitz *et al.*, 1971).

Premature infants have a certain degree of carbohydrate malabsorption and it has been speculated that carbon arriving in the colon can be scavenged by absorption of the SCFA produced by fermentation. An estimate of carbon scavenging was provided by the study of Kien *et al.* (1992), who, using stable isotopes, determined that the rate of acetate entry to the peripheral circulation was 64 ± 34 μmol/kg per min, which corresponds to $64\% \pm 39$ of the potential two carbon units from dietary lactose.

In the recent past there has been a series of publications about the utilization of SCFA, specifically butyrate, by large-bowel epithelial cells (Roediger, 1980). Based on the information in these publications, several investigators have used SCFA intravenously and in enemas as therapeutic intervention for patients with colitis. Although we are not aware of any such studies in the paediatric population, we have provided indirect evidence that SCFA are important to the welfare of the colon in a case report of an infant who had enterocolitis as a result of Hirschsprung's disease and continued to have a bloody, mucous discharge months after a colostomy (Lifschitz & Bloss, 1985). Biopsies indicated acute and chronic inflammatory changes. A decision was made to restore bowel continuity in this infant, despite the evidence of colitis, which resulted in complete resolution of the symptoms. It is likely that this was a case of 'diversion colitis' in which the large colon, excluded from the flow, does not have a supply of butyrate and the colonic mucosa responds with inflammation. In the forthcoming years, the roles of SCFA in nutrition and colonic health will become better defined, and this information will be useful in developing therapies to treat the paediatric population.

Acknowledgements

This work is a publication of the US Department of Agriculture (USDA)/ Agricultural Research Service (ARS) Children's Nutrition Research Center, Department of Pediatrics, Baylor College of Medicine and Texas Children's Hospital, Houston, TX. This project has been funded in part with federal funds from the USDA/ARS under Cooperative Agreement number 58-6250-1-003. The contents of this publication do not necessarily reflect the views or policies of the USDA, nor does mention of trade names, commercial products, or organizations imply endorsement by the US Government.

References

Argenzio, R. A., Moon, H. W., Kemeny, L. J. & Whipp, S. C. (1984). Colonic compensation in transmissible gastroenteritis of swine. *Gastroenterology*, **86**, 1501–9.

Barbero, G. J., Runge, G., Fischer, D., Crawford, M. N., Torres, F. E. & Gyorgy, P. (1952). Investigations on the bacterial flora, pH, and sugar content in the intestinal tract of infants, *Pediatrics*, **40**, 152–63.

Bhatia, J., Prihoda, A. R. & Richardson, C. J. (1986). Parenteral antibiotics and carbohydrate intolerance in term neonates. *American Journal of Diseases of Children*, **140**, 111–13.

Bullen, C. L., Tearle, P. V. & Willis, A. T. (1976). Bifidobacteria in the intestinal tract of infants: an *in-vivo* study. *Journal of Medical Microbiology*, **9**, 325–33.

Gertsley, J. R., Wang, C. C., Boyden, R. E. & Wood, A. A. (1928). The influence of feeding on certain acids in the feces of infants. I. A comparison of the effects of breast milk and modified cow's milk in the excretion of volatile acids. *American Journal of Diseases of Children*, **35**, 580–9.

Hall, M. A., Cole, C. B., Smith, S. L., Fuller, R. & Rolles, C. J. (1990). Factors influencing the presence of faecal lactobacilli in early infancy. *Archives of Disease in Childhood*, **65**, 185–8.

Kien, C. L., Kepner, J. Grotjohn, K., Ault, K. & McClead, R. E. (1992). Stable isotope model for estimating colonic actate production in premature infants. *Gastroenterology*, **102**, 1458–66.

Lifschitz, C. H. & Bloss, R. (1985). Persistence of colitis in Hirschsprung's disease. *Journal of Pediatric Gastroenterology and Nutrition*, **4**, 291–3.

Lifschitz, C. H., Irving, C. S., Gopalakrishna, G. S., Evans, K. & Nichols, B. L. (1983). Carbohydrate malabsorption in infants with diarrhea studied with the breath hydrogen test. *Journal of Pediatrics*, **102**, 371–5.

Lifschitz, C. H., Wolin, M. J. & Reeds, P. J. (1990). Characterization of carbohydrate fermentation in feces of formula-fed and breast-fed infants. *Pediatric Research*, **27**, 165–9.

Lifshitz, F., Diaz-Bensussen, S., Martinez-Garza, V., Ardo-Bassols, F. & Diaz del Castillo, E. (1971). Influence of disaccharides on the development of systemic acidosis in the premature infant. *Pediatric Research*, **5**, 213–25.

Long, S. S. & Swenson, R. M. (1977). Development of anaerobic fecal flora in healthy newborn infants. *Journal of Pediatrics*, **91**, 298–301.

Mevissen-Verhage, E. A. E., Marcelis, J. H., Harmsen-Van Amerongen, W. C. M., de Vos, N. M. & Verhoef, J. (1985). Effect of iron on neonatal gut flora during the first three months of life. *European Journal of Clinical Microbiology*, **4**, 273–8.

Midtvedt, A.-C. & Midtvedt, T. (1992). Production of short chain fatty acids by the intestinal microflora during the first 2 years of human life. *Journal of Pediatric Gastroenterology and Nutrition*, **15**, 395–403.

Murray, R. D., McClung, H. J., Li, B. U. K. & Ailabouni, A. (1987). Short-chain fatty acid profile in the colon of newborn piglets using fecal water analysis. *Pediatric Research*, **22**, 720–4.

Murray, R. D., McClung, H. J., Li, B. U. K. & Ailabouni, A. (1989). Stimulatory effects of short-chain fatty acids on colonic absorption in newborn piglets *in vivo*. *Journal of Pediatric Gastroeneterology and Nutrition*, **8**, 95–101.

Norin, K. E., Gustafsson, B. E., Lindblad, B. S. & Midtvedt, T. (1985). The establishment of some microflora associated biochemical characteristics in feces from children during the first years of life. *Acta Paediatrica Scandinavica*, **74**, 207–12.

Ogawa, K., Ben, R. A., Pons, S., de Paolo, M. I. L. & Bustos Fernandez, L. (1992). Volatile fatty acids, lactic acid, and pH in the stools of breast-fed and bottle-fed infants. *Journal of Pediatric Gastroenterology and Nutrition*, **15**, 248–52.

Perman, J. A., Modler, S. & Olson, A. C. (1981). Role of pH in production of hydrogen from carbohydrates by colonic bacteria flora. *Journal of Clinical Investigation*, **67**, 643–50.

Rasmussen, H. S., Holtug, K., Ynggard, C. & Mortensen, P. B. (1988). Faecal concentrations and production rates of short chain fatty acids in normal neonates. *Acta Paediatrica Scandinavica*, **77**, 365–8.

Roediger, W. E. W. (1980). Role of anaerobic bacteria in the metabolic welfare of the colonic mucosa in man. *Gut*, **21**, 793–8.

Shulman, R. J., Henning, S. J. & Nichols, B. L. (1988). The miniature pig as an animal model for the study of intestinal enzyme development. *Pediatric Research*, **23**, 311–15.

Stevenson, D. K., Shahin, S. M., Ostrander, C. R., Kerner, J. A., Cohen, R. S., Hopper, A. O. & Yeader, A. S. (1982). Breath hydrogen in preterm infants: correlation with changes in bacterial colonization of the gastrointestinal tract. *Journal of Pediatrics*, **101**, 607–10.

Torres-Pinedo, R., Conde, E., Robillard, G. & Maldonado, M. (1968). Studies on infant diarrhea. III. Changes in composition of saline and glucose-saline solutions instilled into the colon. *Pediatrics*, **42**, 303–11.

33

Short-chain triglycerides in clinical nutrition

S. J. DEMICHELE AND M. D. KARLSTAD

Introduction

A major advance in critical-care medicine has been the aggressive and early administration of a mixed-fuel calorie source for the nutritional support of critically ill patients. Over the past decade there has been rapid evolution of new information that has provided clinicians and the nutritional support team with a more rational but aggressive approach to the intravenous feeding of hospitalized patients. The goal of nutritional support is to provide early administration of an appropriate protein and energy source to sustain the enhanced demands from protein catabolism, to maintain host defences, preserve organ function and avoid malnutrition from severe nutritional depletion, without imposing metabolic demands on the critically ill patient.

It is well accepted that enteral nutrition is a more efficient route for nutritional support than direct intravenous administration of nutrients. Parenteral nutrition is used when complete rest of the gastrointestinal tract is indicated, the gastrointestinal tract is inaccessible, or there is an intolerance or limited capacity for enteral nutrition. However, total parenteral nutrition, when supplied as the sole source of nutrition, has been shown to produce atrophy of the intestinal mucosa, characterized by a decrease in mucosal mass, loss of DNA, decrease in villus height, loss of gut mucosal barrier function and translocation of endotoxin and/or bacteria into the circulatory system (Johnson *et al.*, 1975; Bessey *et al.*, 1984; Alverdy, Aoys & Moss, 1988; Ziegler *et al.*, 1988; Wells, Maddaus & Simmons, 1988). It is thought that the gut may be a portal of entry for bacteria and a cause of bacteraemia in critically ill patients, when no other sources of infection are apparent. It has been estimated that every year in the United States about 500 000 people become bacteraemic and that there are about 70 000 fatalities due to bacteraemia with or without septic shock (Shapiro & Gelfand, 1993). Therefore, one of the goals of parenteral nutrition should be to provide specific nutrients to prevent or limit atrophy of the gastrointestinal tract and maintain the function of the gut mucosal barrier.

This chapter discusses the advantages and disadvantages of currently available intravenous long- and medium-chain triglyceride emulsions and summarizes some of the background and rationale for the use of the short-chain triglycerides, triacetin and tributyrin in nutritional support. Although short-chain triglycerides are not at present available in commercial intravenous lipid emulsions or enteral products for clinical use in patients, the available data in animal models would suggest a potential use of short-chain triglycerides for parenteral as well as enteral alimentation in patients with specific disease conditions.

Intravenous lipid emulsions

Advantages and disadvantages of long-chain triglycerides

Intravenous long-chain triglycerides (LCT) have been widely employed as a calorically dense yet isotonic source of lipid calories that reduces the amount of hypertonic glucose needed and prevents essential fatty-acid deficiency during prolonged use of parenteral nutrition (Goodgame, Lowry & Brennan, 1978; Barr, Dunn & Brennan, 1981). Before the availability of intravenous lipid emulsions, glucose was the only non-protein source of calories. Meeting the caloric requirements of the hospitalized patient with glucose often led to hepatic lipogenesis, with increased carbon dioxide production (Askanazi *et al*., 1980), reduced hepatic protein synthesis, cholestasis and hepatomegaly (Sheldon, Peterson & Sanders, 1978; Lowry & Brennan, 1979; Kaminski, Adams & Jellinek, 1980; Hall *et al*., 1984). The mechanism for these hepatic abnormalities is that of impaired glucose utilization associated with insulin resistance, which accompanies stress.

Intravenous lipid emulsions have also been useful in the patient with impaired pulmonary function. Excess glucose administration can result in the production of large volumes of carbon dioxide by glucose oxidation and lipogenesis. Since the metabolism of fat results in a lower respiratory quotient than that of glucose, the potential benefit of replacing a portion of glucose calories with fat is that it will decrease carbon dioxide production and thereby decrease respiratory complications. However, during the past few years, the extensive use of intravenous lipid emulsions in the clinical setting has resulted in the identification of disadvantages and complications associated with their use. In critically ill patients, hypertriglyceridaemia has been evident as the result of a decrease in the ability to clear exogenous triacylglycerol-rich particles contained in plasma chylomicrons and as a result of the endogenous mobilization of fatty acids exceeding the capacity of fatty-acid oxidation (Nordenstrom *et al.*, 1983). Excessive or prolonged administration of intravenous LCT has been associated with hepatic steatosis (Koga, Ikeda & Inokuchi, 1975), bile-duct proliferation (Salvian & Allardyce, 1980), cholestasis (Allardyce, 1982), splenomegaly (Forbes, 1978) and immune-function derangements such as blockade of the reticuloendothelial system and interference with cellular immunity and bacteriocidal capacity (Koga, Ikeda & Inokuchi, 1975; Jarstrand, Berghem & Lahnborg, 1978; Nordenstrom, Jarstrand & Wiernik, 1979; Wilmore, 1990).

Medium-chain triglycerides

An attractive alternative to LCT lipid emulsons is the use of medium-chain triglycerides for nutritional support. Although these shorter-chain fatty acids would not obviate the need for essential long-chain fatty acids, they might provide useful alternatives to currently available LCT lipid emulsions. Medium-chain triglycerides are attractive, because they would avoid many of the complications outlined above; and they induce ketosis, which may decrease the utilization of glucose by glucose-dependent organs such as the brain. Most of the data available on the effect of medium-chain triglycerides are from enteral feeding studies, which show benefits in a variety of specific metabolic conditions (Bach & Babayan, 1982). However, the intravenous infusion of medium-chain triglyceride emulsions in rhesus monkeys (Rabinowitz *et al.*, 1978), rabbits (Trauner & Adams, 1981) and dogs (Miles *et al.*, 1983) has resulted in encephalopathy, lactic acidosis, and, in some animals, death. As a result, the sole use of medium-chain triglyceride lipid emulsions may have a narrow therapeutic index.

Metabolic role of short-chain triglycerides and fatty acids

Triacetin and tributyrin

The structural formulas of triacetin and tributyrin are shown in Fig. 33.1. Both short-chain triglycerides are chemically synthesized products and are available in pure form. Triacetin (C2:0) and tributyrin (C4:0) are neutral, chemically stable, short-chain triglycerides that are rapidly hydrolyzed by pancreatic (Erlanson & Borgstrom, 1970; Lairon *et al.*, 1980) and gastric lipases (Clark, Brause & Holt, 1969; Gargouri *et al.*, 1986) to glycerol and their respective even-numbered short-chain fatty acids, acetate and butyrate.

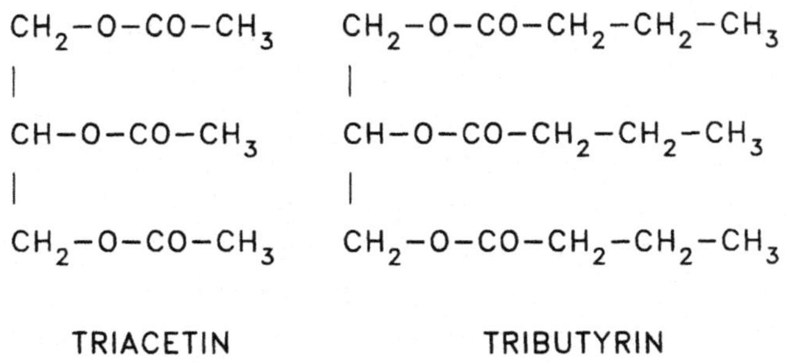

$$
\begin{array}{ll}
CH_2-O-CO-CH_3 & CH_2-O-CO-CH_2-CH_2-CH_3 \\
| & | \\
CH-O-CO-CH_3 & CH-O-CO-CH_2-CH_2-CH_3 \\
| & | \\
CH_2-O-CO-CH_3 & CH_2-O-CO-CH_2-CH_2-CH_3 \\
\\
\text{TRIACETIN} & \text{TRIBUTYRIN}
\end{array}
$$

Fig. 33.1. The structural formulae of triacetin and tributyrin.

Short-chain triglycerides offer additional benefits, as they are easily absorbed in their esterified form or after hydrolysis (Barry, Jackson & Smyth, 1966; Bugaut & Carlier, 1986). Short-chain triglycerides absorbed by intestinal mucosa in the esterified form undergo intracellular hydrolysis in the epithelium (Barry, Jackson & Smyth, 1966; Bugaut & Carlier, 1986). Parenterally administered short-chain triglycerides are readily hydrolyzed to glycerol and free fatty acids in the bloodstream. The solubility of triacetin is 7.1% in water. This makes it versatile and allows it to be added directly to total parenteral or enteral nutritional regimens. Tributyrin is insoluble in water and thus presents the same problems of non-miscibility with aqueous solutions that are encountered with any of the lipid emulsions currently in clinical use.

Metabolic importance of short-chain fatty acids

Considerable evidence has been generated showing the importance of short-chain fatty acids (SCFA) in maintaining the normal physiological function of the mammalian intestinal tract (Demigné & Rémésy, 1985; Roediger, 1990). Briefly, the SCFA acetate, propionate and butyrate are rapidly absorbed by the intestinal mucosa (Cummings *et al.*, 1987), provide an important source of calories (Yang, Manoharan & Mickelsen, 1970), are readily metabolized by intestinal epithelium and liver (Cummings, 1981), stimulate colonic absorption of sodium and water (Roediger & Rae, 1982) and protect against alterations of electrolyte transport induced by bile acids (Roediger, Rigol & Rae, 1984). Most commonly prescribed enteral formulas contain readily digestible polysaccharides, but lack fermentable fibre or resistant starch. Since fermentable fibre and resistant starch are the principal substrates for SCFA production in non-ruminants, atrophy of the distal small bowel and colon have been observed (Janne, Carpentier & Willems, 1977; Ryan *et al.*, 1979; Morin, Ling & Bourassa, 1980).

Trophic effects of short-chain triglycerides and fatty acids

Rombeau and co-workers have provided further supportive evidence that SCFA are essential, by investigating the intracolonic infusions of SCFA in animal models of colonic transection and anastomosis. Rolandelli *et al.* first showed that the inclusion of a fermentable fibre, pectin, in the diet significantly improved the healing of experimental colitis (Rolandelli *et al.*, 1988), colonic anastomosis (Rolandelli *et al.*, 1986*a*) and intestinal adaptation after massive small-bowel resection (Koruda *et al.*, 1986). Since pectin fermentation yields significant amounts of SCFA, the above studies led to the study of the benefits of direct intraluminal infusion of SCFA. Rolandelli *et al.* (1986*b*) demonstrated that the intracolonic infusion of SCFA in rats fed a fibre-free enteral diet enhanced the healing of a colonic anastomosis, as measured by a significant increase in the bursting strength of the anastomosis. In addition, Kripke *et al.* (1989) went on to show that the sole intracolonic infusion of butyrate produced equivalent effects to those of the combined infusion of SCFA in the rat colon. Therefore, intracolonic SCFA replicate the trophic effects of dietary fibre in the absence of bulk.

Provision of either fermentable fibre or starch as substrates for SCFA production may not always be an option. Prescribed bowel rest, alterations in the normal microflora or intestinal loss may be indications for fibre-free elemental diets. These diets, however, have high osmolalities and are not always well tolerated (Kelly, Partick & Hillman, 1983; Flynn, Norton & Fisher, 1987). Therefore, provision of triacetin and tributyrin may be an excellent alternative to SCFA, because they provide a concentrated source of calories and, when hydrolyzed to SCFA, maintain intestinal function and support epithelial repair without increasing the osmolality of enteral formulas as do the free or salt form of SCFA.

Effect of injury on nutritional support

Metabolic response to injury

The clinical characteristic of severe injury, burns, sepsis and other critical illnesses is an integrated metabolic response that is considered to be adaptive and an important and necessary part of the recovery process. The metabolic response, however, may exceed the limits of normal physiological reserves and lead to a rapid deterioration in the nutritional status of the critically ill patient. The metabolic changes are thought to be mediated by elevations in circulating levels of cytokines, eicosanoids, catecholamines, cortisol, glucagon and other mediators of the stress response, resulting in an increase in total-body oxidative metabolism and an increase in metabolic rate (Gelfand *et al.*, 1984; Bessey *et al.*, 1984; Christman, Wheeler & Bernard, 1991). There is a marked degree of muscle wasting that occurs due to an increase in the rate of protein turnover and net catabolism of skeletal muscle protein (Wolfe, 1981; Jahoor & Wolfe, 1987; Shaw & Wolfe, 1987). However, the rate of protein synthesis in skeletal muscle is slightly elevated and responsive to nutritional support (Shaw & Wolfe, 1987).

Early enteral feeding has been shown to lessen the hypermetabolic response and support intestinal mucosal growth in burn injury (Mochizuki *et al.*, 1984). However, conventional parenteral regimens contribute less to the prevention of postburn hypermetabolism and do not provide organ-specific fuels to prevent mucosal atrophy and improve gut function. Attention has focused on SCFA, primarily acetate, propionate and butyrate, as components of nutrition support that are readily utilized. As discussed in several other chapters, the intravenous, intraperitoneal or intracolonic administration of SCFA is used directly by the intestinal mucosa in rats as a source of fuel and has a stimulatory effect on mucosal proliferation (Sakata & Yajima, 1984; Koruda *et al*, 1988; Kripke *et al.*, 1989; Bergman, 1990; Koruda *et al.*, 1990). SCFA have been used clinically with success as a topical agent in treating inflammatory damage to the large-bowel mucosa (Harig *et al.*, 1989). Furthermore, an intravenous infusion of acetate has been shown to have a stimulatory effect on intestinal mucosal proliferation in normal rats (Sakata & Yajima, 1984). This may be due to an improved microcirculation and increased intestinal blood flow, since acetate has been shown to cause vasodilatation in human colonic arteries (Mortensen *et al.*, 1990).

Total parenteral nutrition with triacetin in burn injury

The effect of partial replacement of LCT calories with triacetin in a total parenteral nutrition regimen on protein metabolism and structural parameters of the gastrointestinal tract was studied in hypermetabolic burned rats (Karlstad *et al.*, 1992). Rats were maintained on total parenteral nutrition and received 30% of non-protein calories as triacetin and/or LCT. Parenteral nutrition regimens provided amino acids, dextrose, lipids, electrolytes, vitamins and trace elements. These regimens consisted of lipid compositions of 90% triacetin/10% LCT, 50% triacetin/50% LCT or 100% LCT. The diets were isovolaemic, isocaloric and isonitrogenous and provided 160 kcal/kg per day and 9.6 g amino acids/kg per day for 7 days. LCT was maintained as a component of each parenteral formula to prevent deficiency of essential fatty

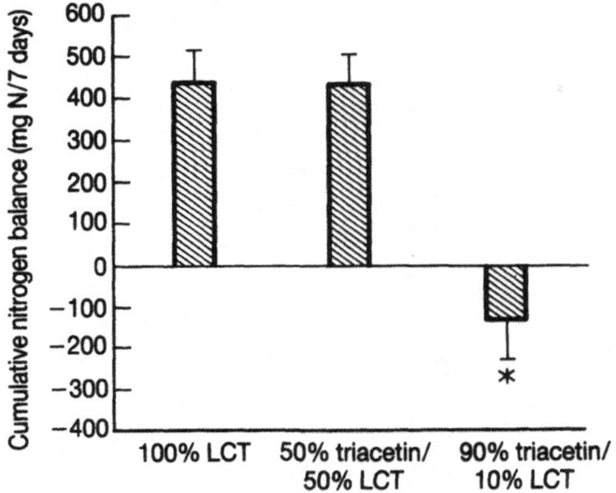

Fig. 33.2. Cumulative nitrogen balance after 7 days of parenteral nutrition in burned rats. Values are mean ± SE. LCT, long-chain triglycerides; asterisk indicates $p \leq 0.05$ compared with 50% triacetin/50% LCT and 100% LCT. Adapted from Karlstad *et al.*, 1992.

acids. The amount of lipid in each diet was calculated on the basis of caloric densities of 6.0 kcal/g for triacetin and 9.0 kcal/g for LCT. Parenteral nutrition with 50% triacetin/50% LCT promoted a positive nitrogen balance, similar to that of 100% LCT (Fig. 33.2), increased the protein content in rectus muscle and liver, resulted in smaller and more numerous mucosal cells in the jejunum and colon, and increased the colonic mucosal weight compared to the effect of other diets in burned rats. However, parenteral nutrition with the highest concentration of triacetin (90% triacetin/10% LCT) resulted in a negative cumulative nitrogen balance (Fig. 33.2) and significantly increased the circulating levels of acetate in burned rats (Fig. 33.3). This elevation of plasma acetate level with the 90% triacetin-supplemented diet indicates that the metabolism of triacetin to acetate exceeded its metabolic fate, because the plasma acetate level was not significantly elevated with 50% and 90% triacetin or 50% triacetin in uninjured controls or burned rats, respectively (Fig. 33.3). The equicaloric provision of triacetin and LCT improved protein utilization and structural parameters of the small and large bowel and reduced the development of intestinal mucosal atrophy associated with conventional parenteral nutrition in burn injury. Therefore, supplementing parenteral regimens with the proper combination of short- and long-chain triglycerides can improve nitrogen utilization following injury and reduce the development of total parenteral nutrition-associated intestinal mucosal atrophy.

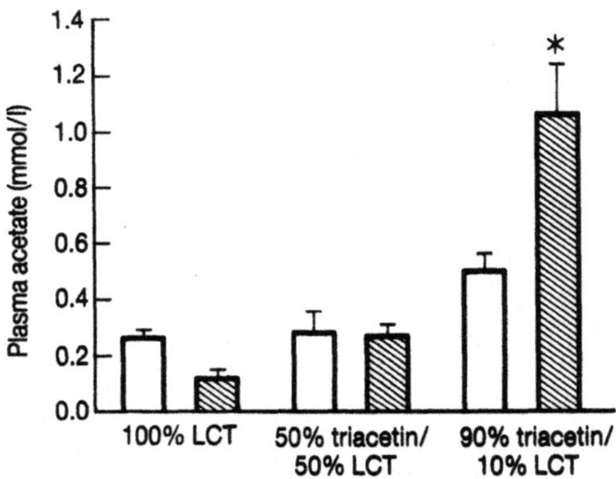

Fig. 33.3. Plasma acetate concentrations after 7 days of parenteral nutrition in control (white bars) and burned rats (hatched bars). LCT, long-chain triglycerides; asterisk indicates $p \leq 0.05$ compared with 50% triacetin/50% LCT and 100% LCT control and burned rats. Values are mean ± SE; n = 5–10. Adapted from Bailey *et al.*, 1992; Karlstad *et al.*, 1992.

Nutrition with short-chain triglycerides after head injury

Metabolic response to head injury

Nutritional support of the neurologically injured patient presents a difficult dilemma for the neurosurgeon and the critical-care physician. During the first 2–3 weeks following a severe head injury, patients are in a hypermetabolic state, consisting of increased resting energy expenditure, excessive protein catabolism and hyperglycaemia (Haider *et al.*, 1975; Clifton *et al.*, 1984; Robertson, Clifton & Grossman, 1984; Young *et al.*, 1985; Robertson, Goodman & Grossman, 1992*b*). The cause of the hypermetabolism is multifactorial and includes elevations in catecholamines, cortisol and cytokines that probably play a rôle in the development of the systemic metabolic abnormalities (Robertson *et al.*, 1992*b*; Goodman *et al.*, 1990.

The increased systemic caloric and protein requirements caused by the neurological injury necessitate early, aggressive nutritional support to minimize complications associated with malnutrition. A reduction in mortality after head injury has been observed with early nutritional support (Rapp *et al.*, 1984). Nutritional support may, however, adversely affect neurological recovery by exacerbating existing hyperglycaemia. Rosner *et al.* (Rosner, Newsome & Becker, 1984) have shown a relationship between severity of injury and the subsequent increase in blood glucose level with poor neurological outcome in an experimental fluid-percussion model of brain trauma. Clinical studies of head-injured patients have demonstrated a direct relationship between hyperglycaemia and a poor neurological outcome with nonketotic hyperglycaemia, hyperosmolar coma being an excellent predictor of poor outcome (Pentelenyi *et al.*, 1979; Auer *et al.*, 1980; Merguerial *et al.*, 1981). The late neurological effects of cerebral ischaemia are consistently worse when the blood glucose level is elevated during periods of cerebral ischaemia or hypoxia, suggesting that the increased cerebral lactic acidosis or other metabolic consequences of glucose metabolism damages nervous tissue.

Short-chain triglycerides as a non-glucose calorie source

Conventional enteral and parenteral nutritional regimens that use carbohydrates as the primary source of non-protein calories commonly cause hyperglycaemia in patients with neurological injuries. In experimental and clinical studies, insulin administration has been used to treat hyperglycaemia following injury to the central nervous system (CNS); however, it is very difficult to consistently maintain fasting blood glucose concentrations in unstable, acutely injured patients who may also be insulin-resistant (Strong, Miller & West, 1985; Robertson & Grossman, 1987; Lemay *et al.*, 1988). Therefore, an alternative strategy to providing carbohydrates is to supplement total parenteral or enteral nutritional formulas with non-glycolytic energy substrates such as short-chain triglycerides. The rationale is that after hydrolysis, short-chain triglycerides are not readily converted to glucose and are metabolized for energy or used for ketone-body production, thus providing the head-injured patient with calories without exacerbating hyperglycaemia. Robertson and coworkers studied the effects of experimental diets, in which the carbohydrate calories were partially replaced with 1,3-butanediol or with triacetin and tributyrin, on ischaemia-induced infarction in rats (Robertson *et al.*, 1992*a*) (Table 33.1). As an alternative substrate, 1,3-butanediol was chosen, because it is converted to β-hydroxybutyrate by the liver and has been shown to be protective during cerebral hypoxia–ischaemia (Lundy *et al.*, 1985; Combs & D'Alecy, 1987). The model of ischaemia-induced infarction in rats was chosen because of the relationship between the temporary occlusion of the middle cerebral artery, and because the size of the cortical infarction is dependent upon the nutritional status of the rat. An infarction of significant size occurs in the fed or glucose-infused rat, whereas a very small infarction occurs in the fasted rat (Nedergaard, 1987; Yip *et al.*, 1991; Robertson *et al.*, 1992). Results from their studies show that plasma glucose concentration was lowest in the fasted rats and higher in the normal rats with the control diet that contained the greatest amount of carbohydrate calories (Fig. 33.4). Diets containing triacetin/tributyrin (diet D) or 1,3-butanediol (diet C) resulted in an intermediate plasma glucose concentration (Fig. 33.4).

Table 33.1. *Contents of the experimental diets, expressed as % calories. Caloric density, 1.5 kcal/ml*

	Diet B (normal control)	Diet C (1,3-butanediol)	Diet D (triacetin/tributyrin)	Diet E (triacetin)	Diet F (tributyrin)	Diet G (high-fat)
Protein	17	17	17	17	17	17
Carbohydrates	51.5	21	21	21	21	21
Long-chain triglycerides[a]	31.5	15	15	15	15	62
Medium-chain triglycerides	0	15	15	15	15	0
Triacetin	0	0	16	32	0	0
Tributyrin	0	0	16	0	32	0
1,3-Butanediol	0	32	0	0	0	0

[a] Given as corn oil.

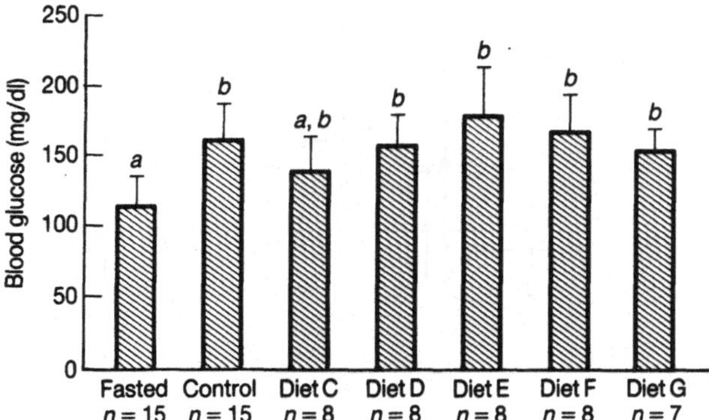

Fig. 33.4. Pre-ischaemia blood glucose concentration in the different dietary treatment groups. *a*, different from control diet ($p < 0.05$); *b*, different from fasted ($p < 0.05$). For definitions of the diets, see Table 33.1. Adapted from Robertson *et al.* (1992*a*).

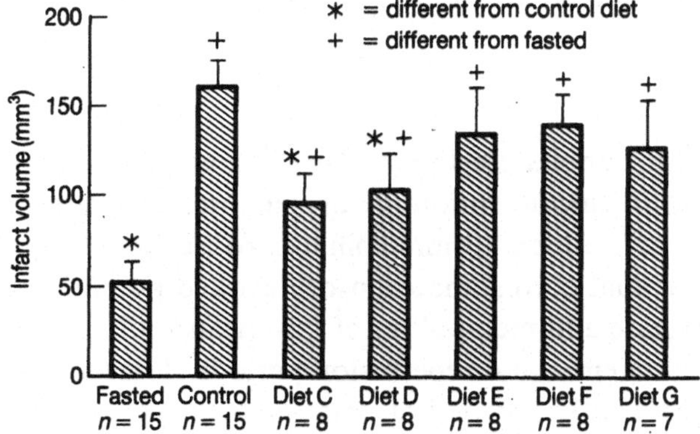

Fig. 33.5. Size of the middle cerebral artery infarct (mean $\pm$ SEM) at 24 h after ischaemia. The groups with the diets containing 1,3-butanediol (Diet C) and triacetin/tributyrin (Diet D) had significantly smaller infarcts than did rats fed the control diet. Adapted from Robertson *et al.* (1992*a*).

Plasma levels of the ketone bodies β-hydroxybutyrate and acetoacetate were highest in fasted rats and with 1,3-butanediol (diet C). Plasma acetate level was elevated only in rats that received triacetin (diet E). Plasma butyrate was not detectable in rats fed tributyrin (diet F). The smallest infarct volume was found in fasted rats and the largest in the normal control (high carbohydrate) group. Of the experimental diets, the smallest infarct volumes occurred in the triacetin/tributyrin (diet D) and 1,3-butanediol (diet C) groups (Fig. 33.5). The volume of the infarct was directly correlated with the pre-ischaemic plasma glucose concentration (Robertson *et al.*, 1992*b*; Fig. 33.6).

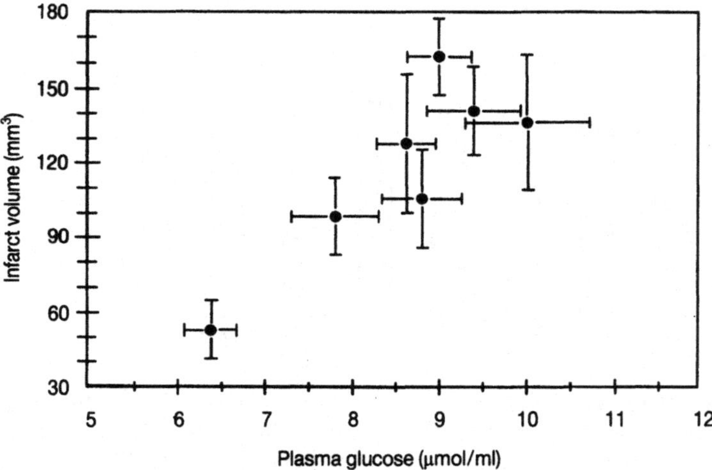

Fig. 33.6. Correlation between the pre-ischaemia plasma glucose concentration and the infarct size. The values are the mean $\pm$ SEM for the seven groups of animals. Reproduced with permission from Robertson *et al.* (1992*b*).

Using a similar model in rabbits, Peek *et al.* (1989) examined the effects of intravenous infusion of isocaloric amounts of glucose, triacetin or 1,3-butanediol on infarct volume after a 10-min spinal-cord ischaemia. Measurements were made of the spinal cord somatosensory evoked potential, as well as the plasma glucose, lactate and metabolites of 1,3-butanediol and triacetin, during the preinfusion, ischaemia and reperfusion periods. Triacetin and 1,3-butanediol infusions significantly elevated plasma levels of acetate while only 1,3-butanediol showed increased levels of β-hydroxybutyrate and acetoacetate. Plasma glucose level was elevated only after glucose infusion, and remained unchanged in the triacetin and 1,3-butanediol groups. Spinal cord electrophysiological recovery after reperfusion was significantly impaired with glucose infusion. Rabbits infused with 1,3-butanediol and triacetin recovered 65% and 64%, respectively, of the amplitude of the pre-ischaemia somatosensory evoked potential, whereas only 19% of the amplitude of the pre-ischaemia somatosensory evoked potential was recovered in glucose-infused rabbits.

These studies suggest that glucose administration during the early period of recovery from severe head injury is a major cause of suppressed ketogenesis and may increase production of lactic acid by the traumatized brain, by limiting the availability of non-glycolytic energy substrates (Robertson *et al.*, 1992*b*). Partial replacement of the non-protein calories from glucose with triacetin and/or tributyrin in total parenteral or enteral nutritional formulas may represent an excellent method for controlling hyperglycaemia while supplying essential energy substrates to intestinal epithelial cells. This would potentially reduce villous atrophy and maintain the barrier to gut bacteria during the prolonged convalescence frequently required after a severe head injury.

Nutritional support in intestinal disease and injury

There has been increasing recognition over the past 30 years of the importance of nutrition in the management of intestinal diseases, particularly inflammatory bowel disease. Current medical treatment is directed toward decreasing the number, frequency and severity of acute exacerbations of inflammatory bowel disease and to prevent secondary complications, but at best, the results are disappointing. Primarily because the aetiology of both Crohn's disease and ulcerative colitis is unknown, no specific treatment for either of these diseases currently exists, and the management of patients with inflammatory disease continues to be symptomatic and supportive. Therefore, adequate nutritional support has become a major component of the management of these patients and has been directed towards correcting malnutrition in adults and growth retardation in children. Moreover, nutritional support is an important aspect that may be initiated to induce a remission of the disease or to treat its complications. Much interest has been generated recently in the use of total parenteral and enteral nutrition as well as in SCFA enemas as adjunctive therapies for the treatment of selected conditions of intestinal dysfunction.

Inflammatory bowel disease

Patients with inflammatory bowel disease (IBD) who are hospitalized for conditions of intestinal dysfunction are commonly prescribed a period of bowel rest that includes the introduction of fibre-free elemental diets and/or total parenteral nutrition. The frequent use of bowel rest with total parenteral nutrition allows the clinician to maintain the nutritional status of a patient with minimal or no stimulation of the gastrointestinal tract (Holm, 1981; O'Morain, Segal & Levi, 1984). Total parenteral nutrition is also frequently employed as primary therapy for patients with severe inflammatory bowel disease who fail to respond to corticosteroids or who are dependent on high-dose steroids for disease control (Sitrin, 1992). Although in some patients bowel rest, achieved through a short course of total parenteral nutrition, has resulted in a decrease in disease activity, there is little physiological evidence to support its use. The confirmed effects of bowel rest, as provided by total parenteral nutrition or fibre-free elemental diets, has been the induction of intestinal atrophy and hypofunction (Levine *et al.*, 1974; Janne *et al.*, 1977; Ryan *et al.*, 1979; Ford *et al.*, 1984). Whether intestinal atrophy is beneficial to the bowel afflicted with acute colitis is open to question. However, patients with active ulcerative colitis generally respond poorly to current regimens of total parenteral nutrition. This may be partially due to the fact that these patients are in need of epithelial regeneration and current regimens of total parenteral nutrition do not provide the primary energy substrates for the small- and large-bowel mucosa. Providing the mucosa with its preferred oxidative fuels intravenously may counteract the lack of luminal nutrients and the atrophy associated with total parenteral nutrition.

Considerable attention has recently been focused on the use of enteral nutrition support as primary or adjunctive therapy for patients with IBD. Selected patients with intestinal dysfunction requiring specialized nutritional support may benefit from supplementation with short-chain triglycerides or fatty acids (Settle, 1988; Rombeau & Kripke, 1990). The stimulatory effects of SCFA on the intestinal mucosa provide a physiological rationale for their inclusion in enteral nutritional regimens in the treatment of selected conditions such as IBD, short-bowel syndrome and colitis.

Intestinal injury and bowel resection

Research by Rombeau and co-workers (Koruda *et al.*, 1988, 1990) has demonstrated that the supplementation of total parenteral nutrition with sodium salts of SCFA retarded the mucosal atrophy associated with total parenteral nutrition in postoperative models of intestinal injury. Additional advantages to providing SCFA in regimens of total parenteral nutrition is that they are water-soluble and provide an alternative source of calories. Although these advantages may be promising, further research must focus on the safety and tolerance of SCFA delivered as the free acid or as a salt.

Recently Kripke *et al.* (1991) showed that a chemically defined diet containing triacetin and tributyrin maintained body weight, nitrogen balance and liver function, and enhanced jejunal and colonic mucosal adaptation in rats with distal small-bowel resection, when compared to short-gut animals receiving a diet without supplemental lipid calories or medium-chain triglycerides. Thus enteral provision of short-chain triglycerides to either the small or large bowel may provide a useful adjunctive therapy in patients with intestinal loss through injury or disease. Clinical complications such as leakage from colonic anastomoses and septic episodes from prolonged use of total parenteral nutrition are associated with a significant increase in postoperative hospital stay and mortality (Fielding *et al.*, 1980). The use of short-chain triglycerides in combination with LCT for essential fatty acids in regimens of total parenteral and enteral nutrition has the potential to decrease the number of incidences of leakage from colonic anastomoses and the rate of intestinal atrophy. Therefore, controlled clinical trials enrolling large numbers of patients are necessary to assess the efficacy of short-chain triglyceride supplementation in decreasing the length of postoperative hospital stay and the incidence of mortality.

Risk/benefits of short-chain triglycerides

Studies by Wretlind (1957) have shown that the LD_{50} of short-chain triglycerides was lowest with triisovalerin (C5:0) when administered intravenously to mice in an emulsified form. The pharmacological dose to produce an LD_{50} increased as the fatty-acid chain length contained fewer than five carbon atoms. Injection of pharmacological doses of triacetin, tripropionin and tributyrin produced a rapid onset of convulsions, respiratory arrest and death. These effects were confirmed by Walker *et al.* (1970) when pharmacological doses of the sodium salts of butyric or octanoic acids were administered intraperitoneally in rats. They proposed that the direct effects of butyrate and octanoate on nerve-cell membrane affected the permeability of ions, thus distrupting normal cerebral function. Samson, Dahl & Dahl (1956) found that the ability to produce CNS effects and narcosis increased as the chain length of the fatty acid decreased. Therefore, further work is needed to assess the risks and benefits of utilizing tripropionin and tributyrin in regimens of total parenteral nutrition. The dose of these two triglycerides required to show metabolic efficacy has yet to be determined, but the possibility of potential side effects may outweigh their benefits.

The data pertaining to the safety and efficacy of triacetin is more encouraging. The fact that triacetin is water-soluble and does not require emulsification like tributyrin to be infused, makes it a very versatile alternative energy source to be incorporated into regimens of parenteral and enteral nutrition. If triacetin is found to be stable in regimens of total parenteral nutrition, it could replace some of the glucose and long-chain triglycerides, making a homogeneous solution for total parenteral nutrition. This would provide a balanced mixture of metabolic fuels and decrease the incidences of side effects from overdelivery of glucose and long-chain triglycerides and reduce the rate of intestinal mucosal atrophy. Triacetin could also be combined with aqueous solutions of dextrose and water for peripheral vein delivery of calories and fluid in hospitalized patients. Because triacetin is less hypertonic than dextrose, there would be a decreased risk of phlebitis and thrombosis, enabling the administration of higher calories by the peripheral venous route. The physiological limits of acid and salt loads as well as the potential toxicity of overdelivering SCFA must also be clearly defined. Preferably, SCFA in their respective triglyceride forms would provide a more concentrated caloric delivery and lower osmolality without the acid and solute loads that are associated with free SCFA.

Potential future use of short-chain triglycerides in nutritional support

At present there is a limited database on the usefulness of short-chain triglycerides in clinical nutrition upon which to draw specific conclusions. Research pertaining to the intravenous infusion of short-chain triglycerides has primarily been performed on triacetin. Results obtained with infusion of triacetin in postabsorptive dogs have shown that it is an efficient caloric source, has rapid intravascular hydrolysis and produces a significant ketonaemia by bypassing the carnitine–acyl transferase system (Bailey *et al.*, 1988; Bailey, Heath & Miles, 1989). Triacetin infused intravenously for up to 120 min at isocaloric or hypercaloric rates (1.5 times resting energy expenditure) in dogs increased the total plasma ketone-body concentration (Bailey, Haymond & Miles, 1991; Fig. 33.7). The ketonaemia was associated with an increase in ketone-body production, presumably due to an increase in acetate conversion to ketone bodies by the liver (Bailey *et al.*, 1991; Fig. 33.8). Triacetin has been shown to have no CNS toxicity and no adverse effects on calcium, magnesium, phosphorus and leucine metabolism when administered

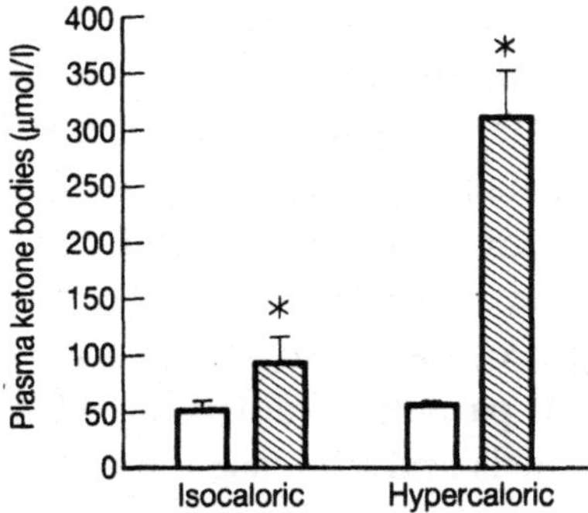

Fig. 33.7. Plasma total ketone-body concentration before (white bars) and 120 min after (hatched bars) the intravenous infusion of isocaloric or hypercaloric triacetin in dogs. Asterisks indicate $p \leq 0.05$. Adapted from Bailey *et al.* (1991).

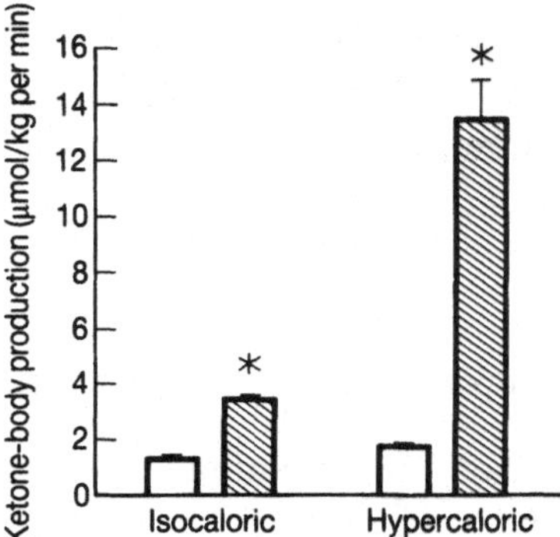

Fig. 33.8. Production rate of ketone bodies before (white bars) and 120 min after (hatched bars) the intravenous infusion of isocaloric or hypercaloric triacetin in dogs. Asterisks indicate $p \leq 0.05$. Adapted from Bailey *et al.* (1991).

intravenously in postabsorptive dogs (Bailey *et al.*, 1988, 1989). Triacetin has also been shown to be metabolically beneficial in hypermetabolic states (Karlstad *et al.*, 1992). We showed that provision of isocaloric amounts of triacetin and long-chain triglycerides compared to long-chain triglycerides alone in a parenteral nutrition regimen improved protein metabolism and reduced intestinal atrophy in burned rats (Karlstad *et al.*, 1992). Triacetin has also been shown to support nitrogen balance in rats when administered as part of a balanced formula for total parenteral nutrition for 7 days (Bailey, Barker & Karlstad, 1992). Although recent studies have not found overt signs of toxicity, further studies with triacetin or other triglycerides of SCFA must be conducted to determine the appropriate dose for optimal efficacy without toxic side-effects. The lack of data pertaining to supplementing regimens of total parenteral nutrition with combinations of tributyrin and tripropionin is due to their potential CNS toxicity and lack of feasibility data pertaining to their stability in sterile intravenous lipid emulsions and their compatibility in regimens of total parenteral nutrition. However, tributyrin has been given as part of an enteral formulation with no apparent difficulties in several studies in animals (Kripke *et al.*, 1991; Robertson *et al.*, 1992*a*).

The use of short-chain triglycerides in enteral nutritional formulas is also encouraging, but the feasibility of incorporating them into specific product matrices must be determined. Assessment of processing concerns such as stability of the triglycerides following sterilization and their effect on product osmolality and organoleptics must be determined. If the challenges outlined above can be met, then further research can be assessed on the effects of incorporating short-chain triglycerides into parenteral and enteral nutrition regimens in a variety of clinical situations, such as trauma, burn injury, sepsis, diabetes and hepatic, renal, cardiac and pulmonary failure.

References

Allardyce, D. B. (1982). Cholestasis caused by lipid emulsions. *Surgery, Gynecology and Obstetrics*, **154**, 641–7.

Alverdy, J. C., Aoys, E. & Moss, G. S. (1988). Total parenteral nutrition promotes bacterial translocation from the gut. *Surgery*, **104**, 185–90.

Askanazi, J., Elwyn, D. H., Silverberg, P. A., Rosenbaum, S. H. & Kinney, J. M. (1980). Respiratory distress secondary to a high carbohydrate load: a case report. *Surgery*, **87**, 596–8.

Auer, L. M., Gell, G., Richling, B., Oberbauer, R., Clarici, G. & Heppner, F. (1980). Predicting lethal outcome after severe head injury. A computer-assisted analysis of neurological symptoms and laboratory values. *Acta Neurochirurgica*, **52**, 225–38.

Bach, A. C. & Babayan, V. K. (1982). Medium-chain triglycerides: an update. *American Journal of Clinical Nutrition*, **36**, 950–62.

Bailey, J., Rodriguez, N., Miles, J. & Haymond, M. W. (1988). Effect of an intravenous short-chain triglyceride infusion on leucine metabolism in dogs (abstract). *FASEB Journal*, **2**, 431A.

Bailey, J. W., Barker, R. L. & Karlstad, M. D. (1992). Total parenteral nutrition with short- and long-chain triglycerides: triacetin improves nitrogen balance in rats. *Journal of Nutrition*, **122**. 1823–9.

Bailey, J. W., Haymond, M. W. & Miles, J. M. (1991). Triacetin: a potential parenteral nutrient. *Journal of Parenteral and Enteral Nutrition*, **15**, 32–6.

Bailey, J. W., Heath, H. III & Miles, J. M. (1989). Calcium, magnesium, and phosphorus metabolism in dogs given intravenous triacetin. *American Journal of Clinical Nutrition*, **49**, 385–8.

Barr, L. H., Dunn, G. D. & Brennan, M. F. (1981). Essential fatty acid deficiency during total parenteral nutrition. *Annals of Surgery*, **193**, 304–11.

Barry, R. J. C., Jackson, M. J. & Smyth, D. H. (1966). Handling of glycerides of acetic acid by rat small intestine *in vitro*. *Journal of Physiology* (*London*), **185**, 667–83.

Bergman, E. N. (1990). Energy contributions of volatile fatty acids from the gastrointestinal tract in various species. *Physiological Reviews*, **70**, 567–90.

Bessey, P. Q., Watters, J. M., Aoki, T. T. & Wilmore, D. W. (1984). Combined hormonal infusion simulates the metabolic response to injury. *Annals of Surgery*, **200**, 264–81.

Bugaut, M. & Carlier, H. (1986). Role of intestinal hydrolases endogenous substrates, and chyloportal partition in fat absorption. In *Fat Absorption*, ed. A. Kuksis, pp. 197–231. Boca Raton, FL: CRC Press.

Christman, J. W., Wheeler, A. P. & Bernard, G. R. (1991). Cytokines and sepsis: what are the therapeutic implications? *Journal of Critical Care*, **6**, 172–82.

Clark, S. B., Brause, B. & Holt, P. R. (1969). Lipolysis and absorption of fat in the rat stomach. *Gastroenterology*, **56**, 214–22.

Clifton, G. L., Robertson, C. S., Grossman, R. G., Hodge, S., Foltz, R. & Garza, C. (1984). The metabolic response to severe head injury. *Journal of Neurosurgery*, **60**, 687–96.

Combs, D. J. & D'Alecy, L. G. (1987). Motor performance in rats exposed to severe forebrain ischemia: effect of fasting and 1,3-butanediol. *Stroke*, **18**, 503–11.

Cummings, J. H. (1981). Short chain fatty acids in the human colon. *Gut*, **22**, 763–79.

Cummings, J. H., Pomare, E. W., Branch, W. J., Naylor, C. P. & Macfarlane, G. T. (1987). Short chain fatty acids in human large intestine, portal, hepatic, and venous blood. *Gut*, **28**, 1221–7.

Demigné, C. & Rémésy, C. (1985). Stimulation of absorption of volatile fatty acids and minerals in the cecum of rats adapted to a very high fiber diet. *Journal of Nutrition*, **115**, 53–60.

Erlanson, C. & Borgstrom, B. (1970). Tributyrin as a substrate for determination of lipase activity of pancreatic juice and small intestinal content. *Scandinavian Journal of Gastroenterology*, **5**, 293–5.

Fielding, L. P., Stewart-Brown, S., Blesovsky, L. & Kearney, G. (1980). Anastomotic integrity after operations for large-bowel cancer: a multicentre study. *British Medical Journal*, **281**, 411–14.

Flynn, K. T., Norton, L. C. & Fisher, R. L. (1987). Enteral tube feeding: indications, practices and outcomes. *Image: The Journal of Nursing Scholarship*, **19**, 16–19.

Forbes, G. B. (1978). Splenic lipidosis after administration of intravenous fat emulsions. *Journal of Clinical Pathology*, **31**, 765–71.

Ford, W. D. A., Boelhouwer, R. U., King, W. W. K., de Vries, J. E., Ross, J. S. & Malt, R. A. (1984). Total parenteral nutrition inhibits intestinal adaptive hyperplasia in young rats: reversal by feeding. *Surgery*, **96**, 527–34.

Gargouri, Y., Pieroni, G., Riviere, C., Sauniere, J. F., Lowe, P. A., Sarda, L. & Verger, R. (1986). Kinetic assay of human gastric lipase on short- and long-chain triacylglycerol emulsions. *Gastroenterology*, **91**, 919–25.

Gelfand, R. A., Matthews, D. E., Bier, D. M. & Sherwin, R. S. (1984). Role of counterregulatory hormones in the catabolic response to stress. *Journal of Clinical Investigation*, **74**, 2238–48.

Goodgame, J. T., Lowry, S. F. & Brennan, M. F. (1978). Essential fatty acid deficiency in total parenteral nutrition: time course of development and suggestions for therapy. *Surgery*, **84**, 271–7.

Goodman, J. C., Robertson, C. S., Grossman, R. G. & Narayan, R. K. (1990). Elevation of tumor necrosis factor in head injury. *Journal of Neuroimmunology*, **30**, 213–17.

Haider, W., Lackner, F., Schlick, W., Benzer, H., Gerstenbrand, F., Irsigler, K., Korn, A., Krystof, G. & Mayrhofer, O. (1975). Metabolic changes in the course of severe acute brain damage. *European Journal of Intensive Care Medicine*, **1**, 19–26.

Hall, R. I., Grant, J. P., Ross, L. H., Coleman, R. A., Bozovic, M. G. & Quarfordt, S. H. (1984). Pathogenesis of hepatic steatosis in the parenterally fed rat. *Journal of Clinical Investigation*, **74**, 1658–68.

Harig, J. M., Soergel, K. H., Komorowski, R. A. & Wood, C. M. (1989). Treatment of diversion colitis with short-chain-fatty acid irrigation. *New England Journal of Medicine*, **320**, 23–8.

Holm, I. (1981). Benefits of total parenteral nutrition in the treatment of Crohn's disease ulcerative colitis. *Acta Chirurgica Scandinavica*, **147**, 271–6.

Jahoor, F. & Wolfe, R. R. (1987). Regulation of protein catabolism. *Kidney International*, **22** (Suppl.), S81–S93.

Janne, P., Carpentier, Y. & Willems, G. (1977). Colonic mucosal atrophy induced by a liquid elemental diet in rats. *American Journal of Digestive Diseases*, **22**, 808–12.

Jarstrand, C., Berghem, L. & Lahnborg, G. (1978). Human granulocyte and reticuloendothelial system function during intralipid infusion. *Journal of Parenteral and Enteral Nutrition*, **2**, 663–70.

Johnson, L. R., Copeland, E. M., Dudrick, S. J., Lichtenberger, L. M. & Castro, G. A. (1975). Structural and hormonal alterations in the gastrointestinal tract of parenterally fed rats. *Gastroenterology*, **68**, 1177–83.

Kaminski, D. L., Adams, A. & Jellinek, M. (1980). The effect of hyperalimentation on hepatic lipid content and lipogenic enzyme activity in rats and man. *Surgery*, **88**, 93–100.

Karlstad, M. D., Killeffer, J. A., Bailey, J. W. & DeMichele, S. J. (1992). Parenteral nutrition with short- and long-chain triglycerides: triacetin reduces atrophy of small and large bowel mucosa and improves protein metabolism in burned rats. *American Journal of Clinical Nutrition*, **55**, 1005–11.

Kelly, T. W., Partick, M. R. & Hillman, K. M. (1983). Study of diarrhea in critically-ill patients. *Critical Care Medicine*, **11**, 7–9.

Koga, Y., Ikeda, K. & Inokuchi, K. (1975). Effect of complete parenteral nutrition using fat emulsion on liver. *Annals of Surgery*, **181**, 186–90.

Koruda, M. J., Rolandelli, R. H., Bliss, D. Z., Hastings, J., Rombeau, J. L. & Settle, R. G. (1990). Parenteral nutrition supplemented with short-chain fatty acids: effect on the small-bowel mucosa in normal rats. *American Journal of Clinical Nutrition*, **51**, 685–9.

Koruda, M. J., Rolandelli, R. H., Settle, R. G., Saul, S. H. & Rombeau, J. L. (1986). The effect of a pectin-supplemented elemental diet on intestinal adaptation to massive small bowel resection. *Journal of Parenteral and Enteral Nutrition*, **10**, 343–50.

Koruda, M. J. Rolandelli, R. H., Settle, R. G., Zimmaro, D. M. & Rombeau, J. L. (1988). Effect of parenteral nutrition supplemented with short-chain fatty acids on adaptation to massive small bowel resection. *Gastroenterology*, **95**, 715–20.

Kripke, S. A., De Paula, J. A., Berman, J. M., Fox, A. D., Rombeau, J. L. & Settle, R. G. (1991). Experimental short-bowel syndrome: effect of an elemental diet supplemented with short-chain triglycerides. *American Journal of Clinical Nutrition*, **53**, 954–62.

Kripke, S. A., Fox, A. D., Berman, J. M., Settle, R. G. & Rombeau, J. L. (1989). Stimulation of intestinal mucosal growth with intracolonic infusion of short-chain fatty acids. *Journal of Parenteral and Enteral Nutrition*, **13**, 109–16.

Lairon, D., Nalbone, G., Lafont, H., Leonardi, J. Vigne, J. L., Chabert, C., Hauton, J. C. & Verger, R. (1980). Effect of bile lipids on the absorption and activity of pancreatic lipase on triacylglycerol emulsions. *Biochemica et Biophysica Acta*, **618**, 119–28.

Lemay, D. R., Gehua, L., Zelenock, G. B. & D'Alecy, L. G. (1988). Insulin administration protects neurologic function in cerebral ischemia in rats. *Stroke*, **19**, 1411–19.

Levine, G. M., Deren, J. J., Steiger, E. & Zinno, R. (1974). Role of oral intake in maintenance of gut mass and disaccharidase activity. *Gastroenterology*, **67**, 975–82.

Lowry, S. F. & Brennan, M. F. (1979). Abnormal liver function during parenteral nutrition: relation to infusion excess. *Journal of Surgical Research*, **26**, 300–7.

Lundy, E. F., Dykstra, J., Luyckx, B., Zelenock, G. B. & D'Alecy, L. G. (1985). Reduction of neurological deficit by 1,3-butanediol induced ketosis in Levine rats. *Stroke*, **165**, 855–60.

Merguerial, P. A., Perel, A., Wald, U., Feinsold, M. & Cotev, S. (1981). Persistent nonketotic hyperglycemia as a grave prognostic sign in head-injured patients. *Critical Care Medicine*, **9**, 838–40.

Miles, J., Cattalini, M., Wold, L., Gerich, K. & Haymond, M. (1983). Toxicity of intravenous medium chain triglyceride emulsion in dogs. *Clinical Research*, **31**, 243A.

Mochizuki, H., Trocki, O., Dominioni, L., Brackett, K. A., Joffe, S. N. & Alexander, J. W. (1984). Mechanism of prevention of postburn hypermetabolism and catabolism by early enteral feeding. *Annals of Surgery*, **200**, 297–310.

Morin, C. L., Ling, V. & Bourassa, D. (1980). Small intestinal and colonic changes induced by a chemically defined diet. *Digestive Diseases and Sciences*, **25**, 123–8.

Mortensen, F. V., Nielsen, H., Mulvany, M. J. & Hessov, I. (1990). Short chain fatty acids dilate isolated human colonic resistance arteries. *Gut*, **31**, 1391–4.

Nedergaard, M. (1987). Transient focal ischemia in hyperglycemic rats is associated with increased cerebral infarction. *Brain Research*, **408**, 79–85.

Nordenstrom, J., Carpentier, Y. A., Askanazi, J., Robin, A. P., Elwyn, D. H., Hensle, T. W. & Kinney, J. M. (1983). Free fatty acid mobilization and oxidation during total parenteral nutrition in trauma and infection. *Annals of Surgery*, **198**, 725–35.

Nordenstrom, J., Jarstrand, C. & Wiernik, A. (1979). Decreased chemotactic and random migration of leukocytes during intralipid infusion. *American Journal of Clinical Nutrition*, **32**, 2416–22.

O'Morain, C., Segal, A. W. & Levi, A. J. (1984). Elemental diet as primary treatment of acute Crohn's disease: a controlled trial. *British Medical Journal*, **288**, 1859–62.

Peek, K. E., Robertson, C. S., Priessman, A. & Goodman, J. C. (1989). Ketone precursors as nutritional substrates may improve neurological outcome following ischemia (abstract). *Journal of Neurotrauma*, **6**, 204–5.

Pentelenyi, T., Kammerer, L., Peter, F., Fekete, M., Koranyi, L., Stutzel, M., Veress, G. & Bezzegh, A. (1979). Prognostic significance of the changes in the carbohydrate metabolism in severe head injury. *Acta Neurochirurgica*, **28**, 103–7.

Rabinowitz, J. L., Staeffen, J., Aumonier, P., Blanquet, P., Vincent, J. D., Daviaud, R., Ballan, P., Ferrer, J., Terme, R., Series, C. & Myerson, R. M. (1978). The effects of intravenous sodium octanoate on the rhesus monkey. *American Journal of Gastroenterology*, **69**, 187–90.

Rapp, R. P., Young, B., Twyman, D., Bivins, B. A., Haack, D., Tibbs, P. A. & Bean, J. R. (1984). The favorable effect of early parenteral feeding on survival in head-injured patients. *Journal of Neurosurgery*, **58**, 906–12.

Robertson, C., Goodman, J. C., Grossman, R. G., Claypool, M. & White, A. (1992*a*). Dietary nonprotein calories and cerebral infarction size in rats. *Stroke*, **23**, 564–8.

Robertson, C. S., Clifton, G. L. & Grossman, R. G. (1984). Oxygen utilization and cardiovascular function after severe head injury, *Neurosurgery*, **15**, 307–14.

Robertson, C. S., Goodman, J. C. & Grossman, R. G. (1992*b*). Blood flow and metabolic therapy in CNS injury. *Journal of Neutrotrauma*, **9**, S579–S594.

Robertson, C. S. & Grossman, R. G. (1987). Protection against spinal cord ischemia with insulin-induced hypoglycemia. *Journal of Neurosurgery*, **67**, 739–44.

Roediger, W. E. W. (1990). The starved colon-diminished mucosal nutrition, diminished absorption, and colitis. *Diseases of the Colon and Rectum*, **33**, 858–62.

Roediger, W. E. W. & Rae, D. A. (1982). Trophic effect of short chain fatty acids on mucosal handling of ions by the defunctioned colon. *British Journal of Surgery*, **69**, 23–5.

Roediger, W. E. W., Rigol, G. & Rae, D. (1984). Sodium absorption with bacterial fatty acids and bile salts in the proximal and distal colon as a guide to colon resection. *Diseases of the Colon and Rectum*, **27**, 1–5.

Rolandelli, R. H., Koruda, M. J., Settle, R. G. & Rombeau, J. L. (1986*a*). The effect of enteral feedings supplemented with pectin on the healing of colonic anastomoses in the rat. *Surgery*, **99**, 703–7.

Rolandelli, R. H., Koruda, M. J., Settle, R. G. & Rombeau, J. L. (1986*b*). Effects of intraluminal infusion of short-chain fatty acids on the healing of colonic anastomosis in the rat. *Surgery*, **100**, 198–204.

Rolandelli, R. H., Saul, S. H., Settle, R. G., Jacobs, D. O., Trerotola, S. O. & Rombeau, J. L. (1988). Comparison of parenteral nutrition and enteral feeding with pectin in experimental colitis in the rat. *American Journal of Clinical Nutrition*, **47**, 715–21.

Rombeau, J. L. & Kripke, S. A. (1990). Metabolic and intestinal effects of short-chain fatty acids. *Journal of Parenteral and Enteral Nutrition*, **14**, 181S–185S.

Rosner, M. J., Newsome, H. H. & Becker, D. P. (1984). Mechanical brain injury: the sympathoadrenal response. *Journal of Neurosurgery*, **61**, 76–86.

Ryan, G. P., Dudrick, S. J., Copeland, E. M. & Johnson, L. R. (1979). Effects of various diets on colonic growth in rats. *Gastroenterology*, **77**, 658–63.

Sakata, T. & Yajima, T. (1984). Influence of short chain fatty acids on the epithelial cell division of digestive tract. *Quarterly Journal of Experimental Physiology*, **69**, 639–48.

Salvian, A. J. & Allardyce, D. B. (1980). Impaired bilirubin secretion during total parenteral nutrition. *Journal of Surgical Research*, **28**, 547–55.

Samson, F. E., Dahl, N. & Dahl, D. R. (1956). A study on the narcotic action of the short chain fatty acids. *Journal of Clinical Investigation*, **35**, 1291–8.

Settle, R. G. (1988). Short chain fatty acids and their potential role in nutritional support. *Journal of Parenteral and Enteral Nutrition*, **12**, 104S–107S.

Shapiro, L. & Gelfand, J. A. (1993). Cytokines and sepsis: pathophysiology and therapy. *New Horizons*, **1**, 13–22.

Shaw, J. H. F. & Wolfe, R. R. (1987). Energy and protein metabolism in sepsis and trauma. *Australian and New Zealand Journal of Surgery*, **57**, 41–7.

Sheldon, G. F., Peterson, S. R. & Sanders, R. (1978). Hepatic dysfunction during hyperalimentation. *Archives of Surgery*, **113**, 504–8.

Sitrin, M. D. (1992). Nutrition support in inflammatory bowel disease. *Nutrition in Clinical Practice*, **7**, 53–60.

Strong, A. J., Miller, S. A. & West, I. C. (1985). Protection of respiration of a crude mitochondrial preparation in cerebral ischaemia by control of blood glucose. *Journal of Neurology, Neurosurgery and Psychiatry*, **48**, 450–4.

Trauner, D. A. & Adams, H. (1981). Intracranial pressure elevations during octanoate infusion in rabbits: an experimental model of Reye's syndrome. *Pediatric Research*, **15**, 1097–9.

Walker, C. O., McCandless, D. W., McGarry, J. D. & Schenker, S. (1970). Cerebral energy metabolism in short-chain fatty acid-induced coma. *Journal of Laboratory and Clinical Medicine*, **76**, 569–83.

Wells, C. L., Maddaus, M. A. & Simmons, R. L. (1988). Proposed mechanisms for the translocation of intestinal bacteria. *Reviews of Infectious Diseases*, **10**, 958–79.

Wilmore, D. W. (1990). Pathophysiology of the hypermetabolic response to burn injury. *Journal of Trauma*, **30**, S4–S6.

Wolfe, R. R. (1981). Review: acute versus chronic response to burn injury. *Circulatory Shock*, **8**, 105–15.

Wretlind, A. (1957). The toxicity of low-molecular triglycerides. *Acta Physiologica Scandinavica*, **40**, 338–43.

Yang, M. G., Manoharan, K. & Mickelsen, O. (1970). Nutritional contribution of volatile fatty acids from the cecum of rats. *Journal of Nutrition*, **100**, 545–50.

Yip, P. K., He, Y. Y., Hsu, C. Y., Garg, N., Marangos, P. & Hogan, E. L. (1991). Effect of plasma glucose on infarct size in focal cerebral ischemia–reperfusion. *Neurology*, **41**, 899–905.

Young, B., Ott, L., Norton, J., Tibbs, P., Rapp. R., McClain, C. & Dempsey, R. R. (1985). Metabolic and nutritional sequelae in non-steroid treated head injury patients. *Neurosurgery*, **17**, 784–90.

Ziegler, T. R., Smith, R. J., O'Dwyer, S. T., Demling, R. H. & Wilmore. D. W. (1988). Increased intestinal permeability associated with infection in burn patients. *Archives of Surgery*, **123**, 1313–19.

Index

A–PV (arterio–porto venous) concentration difference, SCFA absorption 437–8
AAD *see* Antibiotic-associated diarrhoea (AAD)
Acetate
administration (humans)
glucose tolerance 518
metabolic effects 517–18
rectal 518
arterial *in vitro* and *in vivo* resistance experiments 392–9
blood acetate 50, 447
colonic production 454
colorectal cancer 379–80
fibre effects, humans, bran feeding experiments 513–17
infants, breast-fed v. formula-fed 526
liver metabolism 171–7
enzymes 172–4
metabolic effects 176–8
substrates and hormones, influence 174–6
measurement by enzymatic methods 35–55
activation with acetyl-CoA 35–6
cyclic assay 44
interfering substances 50–2
metabolic pathways 36
sample preparation and storage 47–9
type-1, using acetyl-CoA 35–42
formation of acetyl-CoA 35–7
maleate dehydrogenase 37–41
sulphanilimide 41–2
type-2, acetate–acetyl phosphate cycling, hexose phosphotransferase 43–5
type-2, using acetyl phosphate 42–5
acetate kinase and hydroxylamine 42–3
type-3, measuring ADP 45–7
summary and discussion 49–53
metabolism
activation
in diabetes 175
mitochondrial 172–3
in starvation 175
activation to acetyl-CoA 484
antilipolytic effect 452
carbohydrate metabolism effects 485–8
concentrations and proportions in gut contents, healthy v. adenoma/carcinoma 380
endogenous v. exogenous production in human colon 453–4
heat released 460
insulin secretion in sheep 224–9
synergism with glucagon 229
isotope dilution studies 453–4
lipogenesis 175–6
metabolizable energy in ruminants 246–51
oxidative acetogenesis 107, 107–17
reductive acetogenesis
bacteriology 109–12
competition between acetogenesis and other hydrogenotrophic activities 112–13
quantitative aspect of acetogenesis 113–15
respiratory quotient (RQ) 458–9
uptake by muscles 185
pharmacological use 428
radiolabelling studies 453–4
rumen
formation in 62
variation with diet 67–8
tissue extracts 48
peripheral venous circulation (human) 50, 447
transport in ruminant forestomach 133–47
turnover 454
decrease with age 454
utilization
liver 450
other human tissues 447–50
see also Acetic acid
Acetate kinase 36, 47
and hydroxylamine, acetate measurement by enzymatic methods 42–3
Acetate thiokinase 484, 488
in heart tissue 488
Acetic acid
absorbance change due to, formula 38–9
ATP production from direct oxidation 456
heat released in metabolism 460
metabolism in animals, oxidation efficiency 457
pK_a values, in various mixtures 23
resonance 23–4
respiratory quotient (RQ) 458–9
Acetogenesis
hydrogen sink 443
reductive/oxidative 107–17

Acetogenic bacteria 109–12
  enumeration 109
  inhibition of methanogenesis 110
  main characteristics 108, 109–11
  radiolabelling 111–12
  various species 111
  various substrates 110
Acetomaculum ruminis, characteristics 108
Acetonaemia, lactating ruminants 253–4
Acetonema longum, requirements 108
Acetyl adenilic acid 49
Acetyl-CoA
  activation of acetate 35–6
  CoA–acetate recycling 453–4
  mitochondrial 447
Acetyl-CoA synthetase 36
  activation of SCFA 341
  inhibition 175–6
  liver 172
  mitochondrial 173
Acetyl-CoA transferase 37
Acetylcarnitine 47
  acylcarnitine transferase 181
Acid–base regulation, SCFA in human colon 457–61
Acidaminobacter hydrogenoformans, in humans 99
Acidaminococcus fermentans, in humans 98
Acidification
  and colorectal cancer 443
  in cytoplasm, by SCFA 366–8
  and methanogenesis 443
Acidity of carboxylic acids 18–26
Acidosis, ruminants, gastrointestinal motility 191–7
Actin (cytoskeletal) network
  activation 367–9
  pertussis blocking 368
Actinomycin, cancer cells, *n*-butyrate effects 277
Acyl-CoA, activation of *n*-butyric acid 463
Acyl-CoA dehydrogenase, genetic defects 346
Acylcarnitine transferase, bypass 552
Acylcarnitine transferase, inhibition, sheep liver 181
ADP, measurement 45–6
Albumin, bound *n*-butyrate 447
Alcohol
  conversion to SCFA, efficiency 432–3
  liver metabolism, and acetate 428
Alcoholism, acetate concentrations 497
Alkaline phosphatase
  n-butyrate effects 278
  colon cancer 321
Alkanes, molecular weights, and boiling points 29
Amino acids
  colonic
    amino acid bacteria 98
    fermentation producing SCFA 97–101
  Stickland reactions 97, 99
Aminopeptidase, colon cancer 321–2
Ammoniagenesis, SCFA in human colon 459
Ammonium ion, interactions with SCFA in reticulorumen 143
Amphibians, SCFA concentrations in hindgut 74
Amylase, rumen protozoa 62
Amylomaize, in rats 182–3
Anaerobic fermentation
  BCFA production 461
  hydrogen sinks 439–41
  triglyceride production, toxicity 461
Anaerovibrio lipolytica, properties 60
Animal models
  colitis 347
  neonatal model of colonic function 531–2
  SCFA studies 510–11
  see also Ruminants; specific animals
Anion transport inhibitor DIDS 394, 397
Antibiotic-associated diarrhoea (AAD) 373–8, 462
  infants 532
Antibiotic-induced colitis 413–14
Antibiotics
  as feed additives, rumen dysfunction 68–9
  SCFA effects 373–8
Antipodes, defined 17
APC gene 328
Apical and basolateral membranes, absorption of SCFA 162–3
Appetite control in ruminants 257–73
  and pancreatic hormones 264–8
Aquatic herbivores, SCFA concentrations in hindgut 75, 76
Arabinogalactans 432
  energy as acetate, propionate and *n*-butyrate 442
Arterial *in vitro* and *in vivo* resistance experiments 392–9
Arterio–porto venous (A–PV) concentration difference, SCFA absorption 437–8
  see also Portal venous concentrations of SCFA
ATP production
  formation in rumen 63
  from SCFA, stoichiometry 454–7
  from various substrates 456
Atropine, intestinal secretory response 212
Auerbach's plexus 210
Autonomic nervous system *see* Enteric nervous system (ENS)
Avoparcin, feed additives 69

Bacteria of rumen *see* Acetogenic bacteria; Rumen bacteria
Bacterial infections 361–72
  bacteraemia, incidence, USA 537
  gut barrier 466
Bacterial metabolism
  human colon, faecal protein excretion 435–6
  rat hindgut, trophic effect of SCFA 298–9
Bacterial overgrowth, pouchitis 417
Bacterial production of SCFA 428–30, 432, 435–6
Bacterial translocation and sepsis, SCFA administration 466
Bacteroides fragilis
  infants 526–7
  SCFA released during growth 362–4, 366
Bacteroides ovatus
  in humans 94, 96
Basal metabolic rate, energy contribution of SCFA 149

BCFA (branched-chain fatty acids)
colon 100–1, 171
liver 171
production in anaerobic fermentation 461
Benzoic acid, pK_a values, in various mixtures 23
Bicarbonate ion
and absorption of SCFA in colon 157–8, 445–6
and interactions with SCFA in reticulorumen 139
Bicarbonate-induced shift to ureagenesis 459
Bifidobacterium breve, in humans 94, 95
Biotin, propionate metabolism 178
Birds, SCFA concentrations in hindgut 75–6
Bloat 68
Blood, *n*-butyrate 447
Blood circulation *see* Intestinal blood circulation
Blood–brain barrier, penetration by triglycerides 461
Boiling points 289
Bowel rest, SCFA administration 463, 550
Bran feeding
cholesterol-lowering effects 510–11
energy as acetate, propionate and *n*-butyrate 442
hypercholesterolaemic subjects 513–17
large-bowel neoplasia 313
SCFA rise in non-ruminants 498–502
Branched-chain fatty acids *see* BCFA
Bread, incorporation of propionate 519
Breath hydrogen *see* Hydrogen breath test
Bromoethane sulphonic acid, methogenesis inhibition 112–13
Brush border membrane hydrolases 321
Bulk, kaolin v. fermentable fibre 408
Burn injury *see* Injury, nutritional support
n-Butyrate
amylase secretion enhanced 224–5
arterial *in vitro* and *in vivo* resistance experiments 392–9
cell morphology and ultrastructure effects 277–80
colon tumorigenesis 310–11, 320–3, 378–82
neoplastic cells, paradoxical effects 326, 327–8
colonic epithelium, normal and paradoxical 323–8
concentrations and proportions in gut contents, healthy v. adenoma/carcinoma 380
gene expression and regulation, effects 276–80, 282
genetic effects 330–2
human blood 447
liver metabolism 182
rats, gluconeogenesis 184–5
metabolism
atrophic effects 312
β-oxidation pathway 338
colonocytes, sulphide effects 343
regulation 341–3
cell proliferation effects 275–6
colonic effects 211–13
benefits 378
colonocytes
animal models 339–40
human biopsy 339–40
formation in rumen 63
heat released in metabolism 460
histone deacetylase effects 379–81
inhibition of acetate metabolism in liver 174
insulin secretory response 225, 296
metabolizable energy in ruminants 246–51
pivalyloxymethyl 282
poly(ethylene glycol) 282
rectal irrigation in colitis treatment 353–60
therapeutic use 282
n-Butyric acid
activation by acyl-CoA 463
ATP production from direct oxidation 456
heat released in metabolism 460
Butyrivibrio fibrisolvens, properties 60, 61, 62
Butyryl-CoA, oxidation 446–7

C_2, C_3, C_4 carboxylic acids *see* Acetate; *n*-Butyrate; Propionate
c-*fos*, *n*-butyrate effects 280
c-*myc*
n-butyrate effects 279
genetic rearrangements 329
c-*ras*
and cell cycle 330–2
c-*ras* mutation, colorectal cancer 328–9
Caecal motility, SCFA effects, rat, dog 199–200
Caecectomy 415
Caecum fermenters, v. colon fermenters, size 121
Calcium, cellular messenger in SCFA-induced responses 226–8
Calorimetry, classic studies in humans 458
Cancer cells
n-butyrate effects 277
n-butyrate therapy 282
tumorigenesis 310–11, 320–3, 326–8, 378–82
see also Colorectal cancer
Caprylic acid (caproate)
colonic effects 211–13
see also Octanoate
Carbohydrate
non-digestible *see* Lactulose
polymerized, list and structures 88
replacement by SCFA 182–3
resistance to absorption in small bowel 376–7
substrates fermented in human colon 431
unavailable
defined 428–9
distribution of energy 429–30
energy release 429
intake and fermentability 434–5
see also Starch, resistant
Carbohydrate intolerance, antibiotic-associated diarrhoea (AAD) 532
Carbohydrate metabolism 483–93
colonic 90–7, 404, 408
conversion to SCFA, efficiency 432–3
diabetes 489–90
fermentation in colon 90–7, 182–3, 404, 408
bacterial breakdown of polymers 88
control 93–7
major pathways 92

Carbohydrate metabolism (*cont.*)
  insulin and glucagon 489
  liver 483–8
    acetate effects 484–5
    propionate effects 485–8
  malabsorption syndromes 367–8, 381
  peripheral tissues 488–9
  propionate effects 179–81
  substrate
    ruminants
      cereal processing 245
      effect on molar proportions of SCFA 244
  see also named carbohydrates
2,7-*bis*carboxyethyl-5(6)-carboxyfluorescein, leukocyte marker 366
Carboxylic acids
  acidity 18–26
    acid dissociation 20
    electron-donating inductive effects 25–6
    electron-withdrawing inductive effects 25
    hydrogen bonding 27–8
    inductive and electrostatic effects 24
    resonance effect 19–24
  boiling points 289
  defined 15
  dimerization constant and distribution constant 32
  hydrogen bonding 26–33
    and acidity 27–8
    dimerization constant 28–33
    and solubility in water 28
  molecular weights, and boiling points 29
  pK_a values 19, 20, 21
    various di- and tri-carboxylic acids 20
    in various solvents 22
  terminology 15–16
Carnityl–acyl transferase system 181
  bypass 552
Cattle
  acetogenic bacteria 111
  glucagon, role in appetite control 267
  see also Ruminants
CCPR *see* Crypt cell production rate (CCPR)
Cell morphology and ultrastructure, *n*-butyrate effects 277–80
Cell proliferation
  n-butyrate effects 275–6
  differentiation 325–7
  G-1 phase, differentiation 322
  ruminant/non-ruminant digestive tract 289–305
  see also Colonic epithelial cells
Cellodextrins, digestion by rumen bacteria 61
Cellulases
  rumen fungi 61
  rumen protozoa 61
Cellulolysis, rumen bacteria 61–2
Cellulose, energy as acetate, propionate and *n*-butyrate 442
Cereals
  amylomaize, in rats 182–3
  incorporation of propionate into bread 519
  processing
    effect on molar proportions of SCFA 244–5
    ruminants, effect on molar proportions of SCFA 245
  see also Bran feeding
Chemistry of SCFA 15–34
  geometrical isomers 15–17
  notation 18
  optical isomers 17–18
Children *see* Infants and children
Chloride
  interactions with SCFA in reticulorumen 140–2
  propionate-induced secretion in colon 210–13
  role in absorption of SCFA, colon 162
3-Chloropropionate, cross-inhibition of propionate effects 217
Cholecystokinin, release by SCFA 224
Cholesterol, plasma
  acetate inhibition 176
  fibre and hepatic lipid synthesis 499–502
  propionate inhibition 499–500
Cholesterol reduction
  human studies 511–23
  hypercholesterolaemic subjects 513–17
  hypotheses 509
  propionate mediation 499
Chromatin
  proteins, phosphorylation 280
  structure and expression, *n*-butyrate effects 281
Chromatography methods 243–4
Clinical nutrition, short-chain triglycerides (SCT) 537–54
Clostridium bifermentans, in humans 96
Clostridium butyricum, in humans 93
Clostridium difficile
  antibiotic-associated diarrhoea 373–8
  colitis 413, 415
Clostridium formicoaceticum 107
Clostridium mayombei 109
Clostridium perfringens, in humans 94, 96
Clostridium sporogenes, in humans 96
Clostridium thermoaceticum 107
  acetogenesis 112
Colitis
  animal models 347
  antibiotic-induced 413–14
  Crohn's colitis 345
    SCFA administration 464
  defined 343
  distal, management 356–9
  diversion colitis 343, 345, 413
    Hirschsprung's disease colostomy 533
    management 353–6
    SCFA administration 463–4
  management 353–60
  pouchitis 356, 417
    management 356
  pseudomembranous 413
  see also Ulcerative colitis
Collagen index, hydroxyproline 410
Colon
  absorption of SCFA 149–70
    apical and basolateral membranes 162–3

bicarbonate ion 157–8, 445–6
n-butyrate effects 211–13
n-caproate effects 211–13
chain length and lipid solubility 153–5
chloride, role 162
colonic starvation 377
concentration, dependence 150–1
intracellular pH 156–7
luminal nutrition 403–4
model, apical and basolateral membranes 162–3
motility effects 199–204
paracellular pathway 155
pH dependence 151–2
potassium transport 162
proton antiport systems in applied membrane 156
sodium transport 160–1
study methods 150
unequal intramural fluxes 159–60
arterial *in vitro* and *in vivo* resistance experiments 392–9
atrophy 463
'bowel rest', SCFA administration 419–20, 463, 537, 549–50
distal, structural requirement for stimulation of secretory response 215–17
epithelium *see* Colonic epithelial cells
flow dynamics of digesta 122–8
infants
acute infectious diarrhoea, carbohydrate fermentation 532–4
neonatal model of colonic function 531–2
metabolism, *see also* Energy source, SCFA in human colon
microbiology 87–105
potential-difference response 214–15
production of SCFA
amino acid fermentation 97–101
breakdown of polymers 90, 102
carbohydrate fermentation 90–7
fermentation rates
horse, pig, wombat 128–9
human implications 129–30
fermentation substrates 89–90
quantitation of SCFA 101–3
SCFA concentration, range 395
propionate-induced secretion of chloride 210–13
structure and motility of human colon 121–2
tumorigenesis 310–11, 320–3, 326–8, 378–82
animal models 307–18
APC gene 328
n-butyrate effects 319–35, 378–82
major effects 319–20
DCC gene 328
human therapy implications 313–14
multistep process 328–9
role of *n*-butyrate 310
SCFA protective mechanisms 311–13
secretion of urokinase 328
n-valerate effects 211–13
wall tension, Laplace law 410
see also Hindgut
Colon fermenters
v. caecum fermenters, size 121
principal characteristics 129
Colonic diversion
post-colostomy 412–15
see also Diversion colitis
Colonic epithelial cells
barrier function 337
cell adhesion 324–5
colon tumorigenesis 309
differentiation as key factor in cell behaviour 322
differentiation markers 321–2
faecal desiccation 324
growth indicators 402
gut mucosal barrier 466, 537–8
luminal nutrition, defined 403
metabolism 337–41
β-oxidation pathway 338
n-butyrate metabolism, atrophic effects 312
n-butyrate utilization 533–4
energy supply 323, 377, 444–6
fasting and starvation 343
HMG-CoA β-oxidation pathway 338
lumen trophic factor 291
normal and paradoxical effects of *n*-butyrate 323–8
regulation of β-oxidation of *n*-butyrate 341–3
SCFA effects *in vivo* 289–305
non-ruminants 296–302
ruminants 290–6
sodium absorption 377
ulcerative colitis 344–6
mitotic index 292
proliferation and differentiation 325–7
rectal irrigation in colitis treatment 353–60
SCFA effects 289–305
SCFA utilization 533–4
Colonic starvation 377
Colonic surgery 401–25
Colonocytes *see* Colonic epithelial cells
Colorectal cancer
and acidification 443
adenoma, hypomethylation, histones 329
biomarker for susceptibility 466
cell cycle, and proto-oncogenes 330–2
colon tumorigenesis 310–11, 320–3, 326–8, 378–82
concentrations and proportions of SCFA in gut contents, healthy v. adenoma/carcinoma 380
differentiation, steps 328–9
epidemiology 378
and fibre 378
genetic alterations 328–9
pH effects 382–3
SCFA administration 466–7
wheat-bran study 313
Coprophagy (faecal refection), and SCFA studies 501
Coronary artery disease 451

Coupled non-ionic diffusion 11
Cow *see* Cattle; Ruminants
Crohn's colitis 345
  SCFA administration 464
Crotonate, cross-inhibition of propionate effects 217
Crypt cell production rate (CCPR) 297–8
Cycloheximide, cancer cells, *n*-butyrate effects 277
Cytoplasmic acidification, by SCFA 366–8
Cytosine, hypermethylation 280
Cytoskeletal network, activation 367–9
Cytosolic activation, ATP production from direct oxidation 456

DCC gene 328
Dehydroxycholate, intestinal secretory response 212
Diabetes mellitus
  acetate effects on carbohydrate metabolism 489–90
  acetate utilization 185
  lactulose, oral glucose tolerance in non-insulin-dependent diabetes 488
  thermogenesis 451–2
Dialysis, metabolism of acetate 428
Dialysis capsules 8–10
Diaminopeptidylpeptidase, colon cancer 321–2
Diarrhoea
  antibiotic-associated (AAD) 373–8, 462
  infants with acute infectious diarrhoea, carbohydrate fermentation 532–4
  post-operative, sodium absorption and SCFA 312
  prevention strategies 463
  SCFA administration 462–3
DIDS anion transport inhibitor 394, 397
Dietary fibre *see* Fibre
Dietary sources of SCFA 428–33
Digestive systems, historical notes
    human gut 5–10
    in vivo faecal dialysis 8–10
    non-ruminant studies 3–5
    ruminant studies 2–3
Digestive tract, hind *see* Colon; Hindgut
Dimerization 28–33
Dimerization constant 28–33
  and distribution constant, carboxylic acids 32
Diploplastron affine, properties 62
Dipole interactions *see* Hydrogen bonding
Dipole moment, defined 24
Distribution constant, and dimerization constant, carboxylic acids 32
Diversion colitis
  fasting/starvation 343, 345
  following surgery 413
  Hirschsprung's disease colostomy 533
  management 353–6
  SCFA administration 463–4
DNA hyperacetylation, colon tumorigenesis 310–11
DNA methylation, *n*-butyrate effects 280, 330
Dog
  colonic effects of SCFA 199–200
  gastric and small-intestinal responses to SCFA 198–9
  SCFA concentrations in hindgut 77–9
Dugong, SCFA concentrations in hindgut 75
Dumping syndrome, peptide tyrosine (PYY) 300–1, 313

Electrostatic effects of acids and ions 24–6
Embden–Meyerhof–Parnas pathway 64
Enamel, salivary composition and SCFA 239
Enema
  n-butyrate, ulcerative colitis 467
  retrograde administration of SCFA 420–1
Energy
  bacterial, efficiency of conversion 436
  total metabolizable (ME) 434–5
Energy source, SCFA 10–11
  ratio (acetate:propionate:*n*-butyrate) 436
Energy source, SCFA in human colon 10–11, 427–81
  acid–base regulation 457–61
  ammoniagenesis 459
  contribution to energy requirements 434–9
    based on arterio–venous exchanges 437–8
    faecal protein excretion 435–7
    intake of unavailable carbohydrates 434–5
    supply limiting metabolism 438
  endogenous v. exogenous acetate production 453–4
  heat production 458–9, 460
  interorgan transport and systemic metabolism 446–53
  intestinal surgery 403–4
  percentage of energy intake 435
  proportion of requirement met by SCFA 435–6
  sources in diet 428–33
    other unavailable carbohydrates 430–3
    unavailable starch 428–9
  stoichiometry of ATP production from SCFA 454–7
  stoichiometry of fermentation 439–44
    n-butyrate as major hydrogen sink 441–3
    hydrogen sinks during anaerobic fermentation 439–41
    inferences 443–4
  unavailable carbohydrates, distribution of energy 428–30
  uptake from colon 444–6
  ureagenesis 459
Energy source, SCFA, in ruminants 243–56
  metabolizable energy 246–51
  see also Liver, SCFA metabolism
ENS *see* Enteric nervous system (ENS)
Enteral feeding, fibre-free, effects 463, 538–9
Enteric nervous system (ENS) 209–10
  neuroblocking agents, effects on intestinal secretory response 212
  secretory response to reflex 213–14
  stimulation by SCFA 405–7
  vagal receptors 196–7

Enteroglucagon
location of secretory cells 408
monitoring of SCFA 408
trophic effects of SCFA 300–1
see also Glucagon
Enterotrophic effects of SCFA *see* Trophic effects of SCFA
Enterotrophic GI hormones
stimulation by SCFA 278–9, 407–9
see also Enteroglucagon; Gastrin; Intestinal peptide YY
Epithelial cells *see* Colonic epithelial cells
Escherichia coli
n-butyrate oxidation 343
infants 528
SCFA inhibiting phagocytic cell function 363–4
Ethanol
conversion to SCFA, efficiency 432–3
liver metabolism, and acetate 428
Eubacterium limosum
n-butyric acid production 111
requirements 108, 109
Eubacterium ruminantium, properties 62

FAD dehydrogenase, 'suicide inactivation' by propionyl CoA 181
Faecal dialysis *in vivo*
historical notes 8–10
ionic composition 8
Faecal protein excretion, human colon, measure of bacterial metabolism 435–6
Faecal SCFA 373–89
and colonic cancer 378–82
pH effects 382–3
infants 512, 526–31
ratios 511, 512
reflection 501
Familial adenomatous polyposis
risk of carcinoma 415
SCFA investigations 313–14
steps 328–9
wheat-bran study 313
Fermentation, stoichiometry 439–44
Fibre
cholesterol-lowering action 495, 499–504
and colorectal cancer 378
feed for ruminants
v. concentrates 243, 254–5, 295
hay and grass 238–9
fermentability
propionate effects 180–1
and tumorigenesis 307–8
hepatic lipid synthesis, plasma cholesterol and 499–502
intake, European countries 430–1
lipid-lowering effect 183–4
low-fibre diets 404
protective role in colon tumorigenesis 307–8, 378
SCFA rise in non-ruminants 498–502
and total food intake 452
wheat-bran study, large-bowel neoplasia 313
see also Arabinogalactans; Bran feeding; Cellulose; Guar gum; Pectin; Polysaccharides; Xylan
Fibre-containing diets
LDL-cholesterol studies 515–17
serum acetate 513–17
Fibre-free enteral feeding, diarrhoea 463
Fibrobacter succinogenes, properties 60, 61
Fish, SCFA concentrations in hindgut 75
Flow dynamics of digesta 122–8
application of chemical reactor theory 123–5
Forestomach *see* Reticulorumen
Fructose isomers 431–2
Fumaric acid, pK_a values, effect of hydrogen bonding 27
Fungi of rumen 61
Fusobacterium nucleatum, in humans 97, 98

G-proteins 330
Galactose, of milk 431–2
Gastric responses to SCFA 198–9
Gastrin, trophicity to GI segments 407–8
Gastrointestinal motility
motor effects of SCFA
modulation 191–7
physiological implications 202–4
ruminants/non-ruminants 191–207
sensory mechanisms for SCFA 209–21
Gene expression, *n*-butyrate effects 276–80
Gene promotion and regulation, *n*-butyrate effects 282
Geometrical isomers 15–17
Globin gene, *n*-butyrate effects 276
Glucagon
carbohydrate metabolism 489
and oral acetate 450
role in appetite control
ruminants 267–8
sheep 267
secretory response in sheep
n-butyrate infusion 225
cell proliferation 294–5
see also Enteroglucagon
Gluconeogenesis
effects of acetate and propionate 485
enzymes, activity 175
human, and ethanol 184
propionate as substrate 179
3-C substrates (propionate, lactate, alanine) 179
ruminants 496
propionate metabolism 184–5
Glucose
ATP production from direct oxidation 456
glycolysis and gluconeogenesis, tricarboxylic acid cycle 485
metabolism, acetate effects 517–18
replacement by SCFA, metabolic consequences in the liver 182–4
Glucose deficiency, lactating ruminants 253–4
Glucose intolerance 451

Glucose tolerance, administration of acetate, diabetic v. normal (humans) 518
Glutamine
  ileal pouch 464–5
  small bowel nutrition 401
Glycerols of SCFA
  ATP production from direct oxidation 456
  enteral nutrition 428
Glycine, pK_a values, in various mixtures 23
Grains *see* Cereals
Grass feeding 238–9
Guar gum
  conversion to SCFA, efficiency 432–3
  glucagon levels 489
  gum arabic, energy as acetate, propionate and *n*-butyrate 442
Guinea pig
  energy contribution of SCFA to BMR 149
  propionate, colonic effects 213
  SCFA absorption from hindgut 149–65
    unidirectional fluxes 154
Gut contents, SCFA concentrations and proportions 380
Gut epithelial cells *see* Colonic epithelial cells
Gut mucosal barrier, bacterial infections 466, 537–8

Haemoglobin, *n*-butyrate effects 276
Hartmann's procedure, *in vivo* effects of SCFA in patients 392
Hay and grass 238–9
  see also Fibre
Head injury *see* Injury, nutritional support
Heart tissue, acetate thiokinase 488
Heat production, SCFA in human colon 458–9, 460
Hepatic lipid synthesis, fibre, plasma cholesterol and 499–502
Hepatic metabolism of SCFA
  non-ruminant studies 497–8
  ruminant studies 496–7
Hepatic steatosis, LCT i.v. 539
Hexamethonium, intestinal secretory response 212
Hexokinase, contaminant of acetate 47
Hexose phosphotransferase–acetyl phosphate, acetate measurement by enzymatic methods 43–5
Hindgut
  caecum fermenters v. colon fermenters, size 121
  endogenous SCFA utilization 81
  epithelial cells, SCFA effects *in vivo* 296–302
  horse 125
  microbiological aspects 87–105
  SCFA concentrations
    as indicators of microbial fermentation 80–1
    various species 73–80
  SCFA sensation, physiological significance 219
  see also Colon; Colonic
Hirschsprung's disease, inflammation following colostomy reversed by bowel continuity restoration 533
Histone deacetylase, *n*-butyrate effects 379–81
Histones
  hyperacetylation
    n-butyrate effects 280
    colon tumorigenesis 310–11
  hypomethylation, colonic adenoma 329
  phosphorylation 280
Historical notes
  colonic epithelial cells 337–40
  non-ruminant studies 3–5
  ruminant studies 2–3
  SCFA as energy source 10–11
HMG-CoA β-oxidation pathway, colonocytes 338
HMG-CoA reductase, activity, and MCFA 183
Holotrichs, rumen protozoa 60–1
Hormone receptors, *n*-butyrate effects 278
Hormones
  n-butyrate effects 278, 279
  pituitary glycoprotein hormones, *n*-butyrate effects 278
  vitamin D_3, *n*-butyrate modulation of effects 281
Horse
  colonic SCFA production 128–9
  energy contribution of SCFA to BMR 149
  hindgut 125
  SCFA absorption from hindgut, unidirectional fluxes 154
  SCFA concentrations in hindgut 79
Human gastric and small-intestinal responses to SCFA 199
Human large bowel *see* Colon
Human salivary flow, SCFA effects 239
Hydrogen bonding
  carboxylic acids 26–33
    and acidity 27–8
Hydrogen breath test, malabsorption syndromes 373, 381
Hydrogen sinks, during anaerobic fermentation 439–41
Hydroxylamine, and acetate kinase, acetate measurement by enzymatic methods 42–3
Hydroxyproline, collagen index 410
Hyrax, energy contribution of SCFA to BMR 149

Ileal brake 203
Ileal pouch
  glutamine 464–5
  ileo-anal pouchitis 356, 417, 464–5
  post-total proctocolectomy 415–18
Infants and children 525–35
  carbohydrate fermentation 530
  development of bacterial flora 525–31
  faeces
    breast-fed v. formula-fed 526
    faecal flora 526–31
  historical notes on SCFA 525–6
  lactose in feeds, and antibiotic-associated diarrhoea (AAD) 532
Inflammatory bowel disease
  peptide tyrosine (PYY) 300–1, 313
  TPN and bowel rest 419–20, 463, 537, 549–50
Inflammatory reaction 361–5
Injury, nutritional support 541–54
  metabolic response 541–2, 544–5

SCT as non-glucose calorie source 545–9
TPN with triacetin 542–4
Insects, SCFA concentrations in hindgut 74–5
Instillation of SCFA, rectal 353–60, 392, 398–9
Insulin
carbohydrate metabolism 489
lactating ruminants 253–4
mitotic index effects 294
resistance 451
role in appetite control 264–7
rumen, and SCFA as trophic factor 294
secretion in sheep 225–9
secretory response, *n*-butyrate infusion 225
stimulus–secretion coupling model 228
Insulin–pancreatic–acinar axis 223–31
Interferons, *n*-butyrate effects 281–2
Interorgan transport, and systemic metabolism 446–53
Intestinal blood circulation 391–400
arterial *in vitro* relaxation experiments 392
in vivo effects of SCFA in Hartmann's procedure patients 392
stimulation, rationale for use of SCFA in intestinal surgery 404–5
Intestinal and colonic surgery 401–25
colonic anastomosis, SCFA administration 410–12, 465–6
postcolostomy colonic diversion 412–15
rationale for use of SCFA 402–3, 402–9, 550–1
enterotrophic GI hormones 407–9
luminal contact and provision of energy 403–4
pancreatobiliary secretions 405
stimulation of autonomic nervous system 405–7
stimulation of intestinal blood flow 404–5
resection, TPN with SCFA supplementation 550–1
risks/benefits of use of SCT 551–2
Intestinal disease and injury *see* Injury, nutritional support
Intestinal peptide YY (PYY)
location of secretory cells 408–9
trophic effects of SCFA 300–1, 313, 408–9
Intestinal secretory response 198–9
adaptation 214–15
neuroblocking agents, effects 212
see also Enteric nervous system (ENS)
Intestine, motility *see* Gastrointestinal motility
Inulin 431
Ionic strength, defined 19
Ionogram, *in vivo* faecal dialysis 9
Ionophores, feed additives 69
IP3, calcium channel opening 228
Isomers of SCFA 15–18
cis and *trans*, defined 17
notation 18
Isotope dilution, SCFA production measurement 126–8
IUPAC nomenclature of SCFA 15–16

Jejunal morphometrics, rat, SCFA effects 405–7

K^+/H^+ antiport 445
Kangaroo, forestomach, SCFA production 125–8
Kaolin, v. fermentable fibre, bulk, study 408
Ketogenesis
acetate utilization by liver 450
from *n*-butyrate, colon 338
SCT infusion 552
Ketosis, lactating ruminants 253–4
Kidney dialysis, metabolism of acetate 428
Krebs cycle 485
acetate utilization 185
Kwashiorkor 343

Lachnospira multiparus, properties 60
Lactate
absorption 444
and acetate uptake 497–8
infants, breast-fed v. formula-fed 526
interference with gastrointestinal motility 193–6
interference with liver metabolism of SCFA 176–7
metabolism by rumen organisms 65
Lactation, ruminants 253–4
Lactic acidosis
human 461
rumen dysfunction 68
Lactobacillus bifidus, breast-fed infants 525–8
Lactose
infant feeding
and antibiotic-associated diarrhoea (AAD) 532
carbohydrate fermentation effects 530
Lactulose
acidification of stool 443
availability to absorption 432, 513
effects on serum acetate levels 513
effects on serum triglyceride levels 484
energy as acetate, propionate and *n*-butyrate 442
hydrogen breath test 373
and oral glucose tolerance in non-insulin-dependent diabetes mellitus 488
Laplace law 392
tension of bowel wall 410
Large bowel (intestine) *see* Colon; Hindgut; named species
Large-bowel epithelium *see* Colonic epithelial cells
Large-bowel neoplasia *see* Colorectal cancer
Lasalocid, feed additive 69
LCT *see* Long-chain triglycerides
LDL-cholesterol studies 515–17
Leukocytes
inhibition, mechanisms 365–9
phagocytic killing capacity, SCFA effects 363
superoxide production, SCFA effects 367
Lidocaine, intestinal secretory response 212
Lipid emulsion, intravenous 538–9
Lipid metabolism
human studies 511–23
lipogenesis
abnormal, ruminants 251–3

Lipid metabolism (*cont.*)
acetate as substrate
enzymes, activity 175
inhibition 176
glucose v. alcohol as substrate 451
propionate effects 502–4
propionate effects *in vitro* 502–4
Liposomes, *n*-butyrate encapsulation 379–81
Liver
carbohydrate metabolism 179–81, 483–8
disease states
hepatic coma 448
hepatic steatosis, LCT intravenous 539
lipid synthesis, fibre, plasma cholesterol 499–502
metabolism of ethanol to acetate 428
steroid metabolism, and large-bowel SCFA 502
Liver, SCFA metabolism 171–90, 467, 495–8
acetate 171–7
adaptation to high fermentable carbohydrate diet 175
comparative aspects 184–5
lactate interference 176–7
and lipid metabolism 498–502
non-ruminants 497–8
propionate 177–81
effects on carbohydrate metabolism 179–81, 483–8
ruminants 496–7
SCFA extraction 447
and triacylglycerols 495–6
see also named SCFA and organisms
Long-chain triglycerides, as intravenous lipid emulsion in nutrition 538–9
Low-density lipoproteins (LDL)
LDL-cholesterol, fibre-containing diets 515–17
and VLDL secretion by hepatocytes 495–6
Lumen trophic factor 291–302

Magnesium ion, interactions with SCFA in reticulorumen 142
Malabsorption syndromes
carbohydrate 376–7, 381
infants 533–4
hydrogen breath test 373, 381
peptide tyrosine (PYY) 300–1, 313
Malate dehydrogenase, measurement of acetyl-CoA 37–41
Maleic acid, pK_a values, effect of hydrogen bonding 27
Maltitol 433
Manatee, SCFA concentrations in hindgut 75
Mannitol 433
Marsupial GI tract
kangaroo 125
wallaby 126
MCT *see* Medium-chain triglycerides
ME (metabolizable energy) 246–51, 434–5
Medium-chain triglycerides, as alternative to LCT 539
Megasphaera elsdenii, properties 60, 63, 65
Metabolizable energy, energy sources 246–51, 434–5
Metallothionein, *n*-butyrate effects 278
Methanobrevibacter ruminantium, properties 60
Methanogenesis
and acidification 443
inhibition by bromoethane sulphonic acid 112–13
stoichiometry 439–41
Methylmalonic aciduria 178
Methylmalonyl-CoA 485
Mitochondrial oxidation
activation, ATP production 456
defects, SCFA and 342, 346
TCA cycle 485
Mitotic index
epithelial cells 292
insulin effects 294
Monensin, feed additive 69
Monoacetacetin, monobutyrin, heat released in metabolism 460
Mucosal and submucosal plexus 210
Mucosal barrier 537–8
Myenteric (Auerbach's) plexus 210

N-*ras*, *n*-butyrate effects 280
Na^+/H^+ antiport 162, 445, 462
Neosugar 432
Neuroblocking agents, effects on intestinal secretory response 212
Neurological injury *see* Injury, nutritional support
Nomenclature of SCFA
IUPAC 15–16
polarized light 17–18
S/R system 18
Non-starch polysaccharides (NSP) *see* Fibre
Nutrition, clinical, short-chain triglycerides (SCT) 537–54

Octanoate
increase of calcium in pancreatic cells 226
inhibition of acetate metabolism in liver 174
inhibition of *n*-butyrate metabolism in liver, rat 463
Oleate, inhibition of acetate metabolism in liver 174
Oligosaccharides
heats of combustion 433
raffinose 432
Oncogenes, *n*-butyrate effects 279–80, 330–2
Ophryoscolecidae, rumen protozoa 60–1
Ophryoscolex caudatus, properties 62
Optical isomers 17–18
enantiomers, defined 17
Ornithine decarboxylase, colonic mucosa 402
Osmoreceptors, rumen 264
Oxalate, conversion to SCFA 432

p53 gene, cancer and adenoma 329
Pancreatic hormones, ruminants, appetite control 264–8
Pancreatic secretion, effect of SCFA
exocrine/endocrine 223–31
cellular mechanisms 226–8

clinical implications 228–9
structural requirements for SCFA 225–6
Pancreatobiliary secretions, use of SCFA in intestinal surgery 405
Parenteral feeding *see* Total parenteral nutrition infusion
Pectin
anticolitis effects 463
antidiarrhoea effects 463
conversion to SCFA
as acetate, propionate and *n*-butyrate 442
efficiency 432–3
nutritional effects 409–10
Pentose phosphate pathway, acetate effects 484
Peptide tyrosine *see* Intestinal peptide YY (PYY)
Peptostreptococcus anaerobius, in humans 96
Peptostreptococcus productus, requirements 108, 109
Peripheral vein, SCFA ratios, humans 512
Peroxisomes, acetogenesis 173
Pertussis toxin, blocking actin polymerization 368
pH
and colon carcinogenesis 378–82
gastric and small-intestinal responses to SCFA 199
pH dependence, absorption of SCFA 151–2
pH-partition hypothesis 151–2
Phagocytic cell function 361–72
Phosphofructokinase, glycolytic flux 484
Phospholipids, SCFA solubility 33
Phosphotransacetylase 36
Phycomycetes, rumen fungi 61
Pig
colonic SCFA production 128–9
absorption 149–65
unidirectional fluxes 154
acetogenic bacteria 111–12
concentrations 79
energy contribution of SCFA to BMR 149
propionate effects on lipid metabolism 502–4
gut, gross morphology 120
insulin
and adiposity 267
and satiety control 266
neonatal, model of colonic function 531–2
Pituitary glycoprotein hormones, *n*-butyrate effects 278
pK_a values, defined 19
Plasminogen activation inhibitor-1 (PAI-1) 319
Plug-flow reactor theory 123–5
PMNs *see* Leukocytes
Polarized light, optical isomers, *dextro* and *laevo* 17–18
Polyplastron multivesiculatum, properties 62
Polysaccharides
cell-wall 432–3
heats of combustion 433
non-starch (NSP) *see* Fibre
polydextrose, conversion to SCFA, efficiency 432–3
substrates fermented in human colon 431
see also Fibre; named polysaccharides
Porphyromonas asaccharolytica, in humans 98
Portal venous concentrations of SCFA
arterio–porto venous (A–PV) concentration difference 437–8
and hepatic lipid metabolism 498–9
human studies 511–13
non-ruminants 497–8
SCFA ratios 512
Post-colostomy colonic diversion 412–15
Potassium ion, and absorption of SCFA, colon 162
Pouchitis 356, 417
SCFA administration 464–5
see also Colitis
Poultry, SCFA absorption from hindgut 149–65
Prevotella ruminicola, properties 60, 61, 62
Primates, SCFA concentrations in hindgut 80
Propionate
administration (humans)
chronic 519
metabolic effects 518–19
oral, incorporation into bread 519
analogues 216–17
arterial *in vitro* and *in vivo* resistance experiments 392–9
human blood 447
liver metabolism 177–81
effects on carbohydrate metabolism 179–81
and lipid metabolism 181
metabolism
antiketogenic effects 181
carbohydrate metabolism effects 485–8
colorectal cancer 379
concentrations and proportions in gut contents, healthy v. adenoma/carcinoma 380
cross-inhibition by crotonate 217
effects on lipid metabolism 502–4
formation in rumen 62–3
from crossfeeding 65
heat released in metabolism 460
inhibition of acetate metabolism in liver 174
inhibition of starch digestion 431
intestinal secretory response 212–14
lipid metabolism effects, *in vitro* 502–4
metabolizable energy in ruminants 246–51
pathway in liver 178
rats, gluconeogenesis 184–5
ruminants, gluconeogenesis 184–5
Propionate-induced secretion of chloride, colon 210–13
Propionic acid
ATP production from direct oxidation 456
heat released in metabolism 460
infants, breast-fed v. formula-fed 526
Propionyl-CoA 485
Propionyl-CoA synthetase, conversion to methylmalonyl-CoA synthetase and succinyl-CoA 177–8
Protein, colon, fermentation producing SCFA 97–101
Proto-oncogenes *see* Oncogenes

Proton antiport systems in applied membrane, SCFA in colon 162, 445, 462
Protozoa of rumen 60–1
Pseudomembranous colitis 413
Pseudomonas aeruginosa 417
Pyruvate carboxylase, propionate metabolism, effects 179
Pyruvate–ferredoxin oxidoreductase 62
PYY *see* Intestinal peptide YY (PYY)

Rabbit and other lagomorphs
  energy contribution of SCFA to BMR 149
  PYY, interaction with ENS 408
  SCFA concentrations in hindgut 77, 78
Raffinose oligosaccharides 432
Rat
  acetogenic bacteria 111
  caecal motility, SCFA effects 199–200
  cholesterol-fed 510
  colon
    effects of SCFA 199–200
    SCFA absorption 149–65
      unidirectional fluxes 154
    structural requirement for stimulation of secretory response 215–17
  coprophagy (faecal refection) and SCFA studies 501
  fibre, fermentation, propionate effects 180–1
  gastric and small-intestinal responses to SCFA 198–9
  gut, gross morphology 120
  jejunal morphometrics, SCFA effects 405–7
  liver, *n*-butyrate metabolism 184–5
  SCFA as lumen trophic factor 296–302
  starch diet, glucose replacement by SCFA 182–3
Rectal, *see also* Colorectal
Rectal instillation of SCFA 392, 398–9
  in colitis treatment 353–60
Reptiles, SCFA concentrations in hindgut 74, 75
Respiratory quotients (RQ) 458–9
Reticulorumen (and rumen)
  biochemistry 61–5
  diet
    acetate, variation with diet 67–8
    effects of SCFA infusions on food intake, rumen fluid 261–4
    food intake, effects on blood SCFA 258
    and saliva secretion 237–9
  dysfunction
    antimicrobials, feed additives 68–9
    bloat 68
    lactic acidosis 68
  epithelial cells, SCFA effects *in vivo* 290–6
  functions 57–8, 133–4
  microbiology 57–71
    metabolic pathways 58
  motility
    other gut segment SCFA effects 192–3
    ruminal SCFA effects 192
    SCFA properties that inhibit 193–7
      mechanisms 196–7
  osmolality of rumen fluid 262–4
  transport of SCFA 133–47
    capacity for absorbing SCFA 134–6
    influence of:
      diet 135, 136
      pH 137, 138
      SCFA chain length and metabolism 137–9
      SCFA concentration 137
    interactions with:
      ammonium ion 143
      bicarbonate 139
      chloride 140–2
      magnesium 142–3
      sodium 140
    mechanisms 137–43
    methods 134
    summary and conclusions 143–4
  see also Rumen; Ruminants
Retinoic acid, *n*-butyrate, modulation of effects 281
Ricinoleate, intestinal secretory response 212
Rodents, SCFA concentrations in hindgut 77, 78
Roughage *see* Fibre
Rumen bacteria
  microbial physiology
    carbohydrate fermentation, major pathways and species 92
    cellulolysis 61–2
    cross-feeding and hydrogen transfer 65–6, 67
    dietary effects 67–8
    protein metabolism 64
    regulatory mechanisms 66–7
    SCFA production from pyruvate 62–4
  principal genera 59–60
  properties 60
  substrates and products 60
Rumen fungi, cellulases 61
Rumen protozoa, cellulases 61
Ruminants
  appetite control
    feeding behaviour 257–73
    glucagon 267–8
    insulin 264–7
  digestive tract
    historical studies 2–3
    see also Reticulorumen
  energy sources, SCFA utilization 243–56
    absorption of SCFA 245
    caecal effects of SCFA 199–200
    carbohydrate substrate, effect on molar proportions of SCFA 244–5
  fat synthesis, abnormal 251–3
  food intake 257–73
    concentrates v. roughage 243, 254–5
    effects on blood SCFA 258
    effects on rumen SCFA 259
    effects of SCFA infusions on food intake
      blood 259–61
      rumen fluid 261–4
    hay and grass 238–9
  forestomach *see* Reticulorumen
  hepatic metabolism 496–7
  lactation 253–4
  pancreatic hormones, appetite control 264–8

saliva, composition and SCFA 233–9
SCFA
as lumen trophic factor 290–6
stimulation of insulin secretion 225, 452
see also named examples of ruminants
Ruminobacter amylophilus, properties 60, 62
Ruminococcus albus, properties 60, 61
Ruminococcus flavefaciens, properties 60, 61

S/R system 18
Salinomysin, feed additive 69
Salivary flow
humans 239
non-ruminants 233
ruminants 233–9
SCFA in mouth 235–7
SCFA in reticulorumen 237–8
Salting effects 31
Satiety
control in ruminants 257–73
glucagon control in humans 267
SCFA
absorption, role of chloride 162
acidic forms v. salt forms 459
administration, practical aspects 420–1
antimicrobials
effects 373–8
as feed additives 68–9
ATP production, stoichiometry 454–7
bacterial infections, effects 361–72
chemistry 15–34
chain length, and lipid solubility 153–5
colon 73–85
colon concentration, human 395
colonocyte metabolism, pathway 342
defined 1–2
energy *see* Energy source, SCFA in human colon
energy ratio (acetate:propionate:*n*-butyrate) 436
enterotrophic effects, possible mechanisms 403
gastrointestinal motility
motor effects 191–207
sensory mechanisms 209–21
gut contents, concentrations and proportions 380
hepatic metabolism 171–90
extrahepatic metabolism 185
non-ruminant studies 497–8
ruminant studies 496–7
hindgut 73–85
in human diet 239
as lumen trophic factor
rat 296–302
ruminants 290–6
mucosal metabolism 171
pancreatic secretion effects 223–31
phagocytic cell function effects 361–72
pharmacological use 428
production, isotope dilution 126–8
ratios, humans, portal vein 512
rectal instillation 353–60, 392, 398–9
rectal irrigation in colitis treatment 353–60
relaxant effects in colonic arteries 392–9
respiratory quotients (RQ) 458–9
rumen 57–71
acetate, variation with diet 67–8
SCFA stimuli, effect on GI function 210–13
SCFA-sensitive receptors, non-ruminants 201–2
sensation in hindgut, physiological significance 219
substrates 460
useful in metabolic studies 460
supplementation of TPN 550–4
potential future use 552–4
risks/benefits of SCT 551–2
supply, limiting metabolism 438–9
transport in ruminant forestomach 133–47
trophic effects 291–302, 313, 398, 402–9, 541
CCPR 297–8
use
acidic forms v. salt forms 459
in colonic surgery 401–25
Western diet
percentage of energy intake 435
total metabolizable energy (ME) 434
see also Acetate; *n*-Butyrate; Propionate
SCFA receptor
characterization 218–19
rat colon, structural requirement for stimulation of secretory response 215–17
SCT *see* Short-chain triglycerides (SCT)
Secretin, release by SCFA 224
Selenomonas ruminantium, properties 60, 62, 63, 65, 66, 69
Sensory mechanisms for SCFA 209–21
adaptation 214–15
cross-adaptation and self-adaptation 214
chemosensation in GI tract 209–10
effect on GI function 210–13
structural requirement for stimulation of secretory response 215–17
Sheep
acetogenic bacteria 111
caecal motility, SCFA effects 199–200
glucagon, role in appetite control 267
insulin secretion 225
reticuloruminal motility and SCFA infusion 194–5
SCFA absorption from hindgut, unidirectional fluxes 154
see also Ruminants
Short-bowel syndrome 418
SCFA administration 465, 550
Short-chain triglycerides (SCT) 460, 537–54
heat released in metabolism 460
infusion, ketogenesis 552
metabolism 460, 539–40
non-ruminant studies 497
potential future use 552–4
risks/benefits 551–2
trophic effects 541
Sickle cell anaemia, *n*-butyrate therapy 277, 282
Silage 238–9
Small intestine *see* Intestinal
Smooth muscle of GI tract, effect of SCFA on contractility 202

Sodium
  absorption by colonic epithelial cells 377
    post-operative diarrhoea 312
  interactions with SCFA in reticulorumen 140
  transport, interactions with SCFA 160–1
Sodium hydrogen sulphide, effects on β-oxidation pathway 343
Sodium mercaptoacetate 343, 347
Sodium sulphite 343
Sodium/hydrogen antiport 162, 445, 462
Solvent extraction 31
Sorbitol 433
Sporomusa termitida, characteristics 108, 111, 113
Starch
  breakdown in rumen 62
  energy as acetate, propionate and *n*-butyrate 442
  malabsorption syndromes 381
  resistance to absorption in small bowel 182–3, 376–7
  resistant
    defined 430
    feeding experiments 182–3
    SCFA rise in non-ruminants 498
  unavailable, distribution of energy 428–30, 434–5
Starch diet, rat, glucose replacement by SCFA 182–3
Stickland reactions
  amino acids 97, 99
  electron donors 99
Stoichiometry
  ATP production 454–7
  fermentation 439–44
Streptococcus bovis, properties 60, 62, 68
Succinate
  leukocyte inhibition 366
  production 461
  protonation 365
Succinomonas amylolytica, properties 62
Succinyl-CoA 485
Sugar alcohols, conversion to SCFA, efficiency 432–3
Sulphanilamide, measurement of acetyl-CoA 41–2
Sulphate reduction 443
  and methanogenesis 439–41
Sulphide, effects on colonocytes, β-oxidation pathway 343, 347
Surgery *see* Intestinal and colonic surgery; *specific procedures*
Sympathetic nervous system *see* Enteric nervous system (ENS)

TCA cycle 485
Teeth, enamel, salivary composition and SCFA 239
Teleosts, SCFA concentrations in hindgut 75
Termites, acetogenic bacteria 111–14
Tetrodotoxin, intestinal secretory response 212
β-Thalassaemia, *n*-butyrate therapy 277, 282
Thermogenesis, acetate, normal and diabetic subjects 451–2
Total parenteral nutrition (TPN) infusion
  administration of SCFA 418–21
  and blood–brain barrier 461
  effects on mucosa 537
  LCT as intravenous lipid emulsion in nutrition 538–9
  MCT as alternative 539
  with SCFA supplementation 550–1
    potential future use of SCT 552–4
    risks/benefits of SCT 551–2
  TPN-induced bowel rest 419–20, 463, 537, 549–50
  see also Triacetin; Tributyrin
TPN *see* Total parenteral nutrition (TPN) infusion
Transport of SCFA, reticulorumen 133–47
Triacetin
  advantages over tributyrin 551–2
  structure 540
Triacetin, Tributyrin, Tripropionin, *see also* Short-chain triglycerides
Triacylglycerols (TAG), metabolism, and hepatic fatty-acid metabolism 495–6
Tributyrin
  disadvantages 551–2
  structure 540
Tricarboxylic acid (TCA) cycle 485
Triglycerides
  blood–brain barrier 461
  production in anaerobic fermentation 461
  serum levels, lactulose effects 484
  short-chain, medium-chain, long-chain *see these headings*
Tripropionin, side effects 553
Trophic effects of SCFA 291–302, 313, 398, 402–9
  direct intraluminal infusion 541
  mechanisms
    possible mechanisms (flow chart) 403
    rat 296–302
  ruminants 290–6
Trypticase, breakdown products, rumen 64
Tyrosine aminotransferase, *n*-butyrate effects 182

Ulcerative colitis
  acyl-CoA dehydrogenase, genetic defects 346
  n-butyrate enemas 467
  distal, management 356–9, 550
  hypothesis 343
    mitochondrial oxidation defects 346
  metabolism of colonic epithelial cells 344–6, 549–50
    quiescent v. acute ulcerative colitis 342
  SCFA administration 463–4
  see also Colonic epithelial cells
Ungulates, SCFA concentrations in hindgut 79
Uptake of SCFA, from colon 444–6
Ureagenesis
  SCFA effects compared 180
  SCFA in human colon 459
Urokinase, secretion, colon cancer cells 328
Ussing chamber 158

Vagal receptors
  reticulum and rumen 196–7
  see also Enteric nervous system

n-Valerate
colonic effects 211–13
colorectal cancer 379
Vascular supply *see* Intestinal blood circulation
Veillonella parvula, properties 60, 65, 69
Very low-density lipoproteins (VLDL), secretion by hepatocytes 495–6
Vitamin (hormone) D_3, *n*-butyrate, modulation of effects 281
VLDL *see* Very low-density lipoproteins (VLDL)

Wallaby, stomach, SCFA production 126–8
Weaning, physiological change in ruminants 290–2
Wombat, colonic SCFA production 129

Xylan
breakdown in rumen 62, 88
energy as acetate, propionate and *n*-butyrate 442

Printed in the United States
By Bookmasters